DIAGNOS
PROCEDU
IN HEARING,
SPEECH, AND
LANGUAGE

Edited by **Sadanand Singh, Ph.D.**, Professor; and **Joan Lynch, Ed.D**, Associate Professor and Associate Director; both at Speech and Hearing Institute, University of Texas Health Science Center at Houston

Written by clinicians primarily for clinicians, this is the only book that combines diagnostic procedures in hearing, language, and speech. It is a comprehensive text in diagnostics in these fields and presents a complete state of the art review entailing a concise synthesis of classical and recent literature and diagnostic trends.

The book contains 14 chapters divided into four main sections. The first is an overview presenting the art and science of diagnostic testing. The second section consists of five chapters on different aspects of audiologic testing. The third section covers the evaluation of linguistic disorders in children and adults with special attention to the identification of the normal bilingual individual. The final section covers evaluation of speech, voice, and fluency disorders. Each of the distinguished authors draws upon extensive clinical insight and personal experience in diagnostics to present a protocol for testing individuals with hearing, language, or speech problems. Their presentations highlight matters of current concern, such as bilingualism and recent legislative guidelines for examiners.

The volume provides insights for speech pathologists and audiologists, who often function as a diagnostic team. For audiologists it clarifies the evaluation of language and speech problems, while speech pathologists will find it helps their understanding of diagnosing audiologic disorders.

Diagnostic Procedures in Hearing, Language, and Speech is recommended as the primary text for undergraduate and graduate students in diagnostic courses and as a key reference source for practicing clinicians, audiologists, speech pathologists, and educational diagnosticians in public schools. It is also particularly valuable for advanced students in special education and clinical psychology specializing in evaluation of persons with hearing and language/learning impairments.

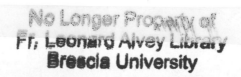

Diagnostic Procedures in Hearing, Language, and Speech

Diagnostic Procedures in Hearing, Language, and Speech

Edited by
Sadanand Singh, Ph.D.
Professor
Speech and Hearing Institute
University of Texas
Health Science Center at Houston
and
Joan Lynch, Ed.D.
Associate Professor and Associate Director
Speech and Hearing Institute
University of Texas
Health Science Center at Houston

University Park Press
Baltimore

UNIVERSITY PARK PRESS
International Publishers in Science and Medicine
233 East Redwood Street
Baltimore, Maryland 21202

Copyright © 1978 by University Park Press

Typeset by Action Comp. Co., Inc.
Manufactured in the United States of America by
The Maple Press Company

Library of Congress Cataloging in Publication Data
Main entry under title:
Diagnostic procedures in hearing, language, and speech.
Bibliography: p.
Includes index.
1. Speech, Disorders of—Diagnosis. 2. Hearing
disorders—Diagnosis. I. Singh, Sadanand. II. Lynch,
Joan. [DNLM: 1. Hearing disorders—Diagnosis.
2. Language disorders—Diagnosis. 3. Speech disorders
—Diagnosis. WV270.3 D536]
RC423.D48   616.8′55′075   78-1280
ISBN 0-8391-1217-3

Contents

ART AND SCIENCE OF DIAGNOSIS

HEARING

LANGUAGE

62182

SPEECH

Contributors

John Bernthal, Ph.D.
Associate Professor and
Coordinator of Speech Pathology
Oklahoma State University
Stillwater, Oklahoma 74074

Denzil N. Brooks, M. Fc.
Physicist in Charge
Manchester Audiology Clinic
Manchester, M3 3HD
England

Marina K. Burt, Ph.D.
President
Bloomsbury West, Inc. and
Executive Director
Bloomsbury West Lau Center
545 Sansome Street
San Francisco, California 94111

J. C. Cooper, Jr., Ph.D.
Associate Professor
University of Texas
Health Science Center at San Antonio
San Antonio, Texas 78284

Jeffrey L. Danhauer, Ph.D.
Assistant Professor
Communications Sciences Laboratory
Bowling Green State University
Bowling Green, Ohio 43403

Heidi C. Dulay, Ph.D.
Vice President
Bloomsbury West, Inc. and
Director
Bloomsbury West Lau Center
545 Sansome Street
San Francisco, California 94111

Donna Russell Fox, Ph.D.
Professor
Department of Audiology and Speech
  Pathology
University of Houston;
Private Practice, Kelsey-Seybold
  Clinic
Houston, Texas 77004

Harvey Halpern, Ph.D.
Professor
Department of Communication Arts
  and Sciences
Queens College
City University of New York
Flushing, New York 11367

Eduardo Hernández-Chávez, Ph.D.
Vice President
Bloomsbury West, Inc. and
Language Analyst
Bloomsbury West Lau Center
545 Sansome Street
San Francisco, California 94111

Stephen B. Hood, Ph.D.
Professor
Programs in Communication
  Disorders;
Coordinator of Clinic Services
School of Speech Communication
Bowling Green State University
Bowling Green, Ohio 43403

James Jerger, Ph.D.
Professor and Head
Division of Audiology and Speech
  Pathology
Department of Otorhinolarnygology
  and Communicative Sciences
Baylor College of Medicine
Houston, Texas 77030

Joan Lynch, Ed.D.
Associate Professor and Associate
  Director
Speech and Hearing Institute
University of Texas
Health Science Center at Houston
Houston, Texas 77030

Lorraine I. Michel, Ph.D.
Assistant Professor
Department of Speech;
Director, Speech and Hearing Clinic
The University of Kansas
Lawrence, Kansas 66045

Donald M. Morehead, Ph.D.
50 Mallorca Way
San Francisco, California 94123

Kevin P. Murphy, Ph.D.
Deputy Director
Audiology Unit
Royal Berkshire Hospital
London Road
Reading, Berks. RG1 5 AN
England

Norma S. Rees, Ph.D.
Dean of Graduate Studies
Graduate School
City University of New York
New York, New York 10036

Jon K. Shallop, Ph.D.
Professor
School of Hearing and Speech
  Sciences
Ohio University
Athens, Ohio 45701

Sadanand Singh, Ph.D.
Professor
Speech and Hearing Institute
University of Texas
Health Science Center at Houston
Houston, Texas 77030

Henry Tobin, Ph.D.
Associate Professor
Department of Audiology and Speech
Gallaudet College
Washington, D.C. 20052

Frederick F. Weiner, Ph.D.
Associate Professor
Department of Speech Pathology and
  Audiology
The Pennsylvania State University
University Park, Pennsylvania 16802

Foreword

In 1976 the American Speech and Hearing Association celebrated its fiftieth anniversary—fifty years of teaching, research, and clinical services in the field of human communication and its disorders. During the first quarter of this growth period, professors of speech pathology and audiology laid the groundwork for the future of the profession. Many of these pioneers published texts that provided what was then a comprehensive presentation of the state of knowledge in all areas of speech pathology or audiology. In the years that followed, these were the texts that supplied the impetus for specialization in the many facets of hearing, language, and speech disorders. Today we are well aware that knowledge of the total field has grown beyond the grasp of one person. A review of the literature over the past quarter of a century enables us to recognize the increasing complexity of our profession and the inevitable trend toward smaller compartments of knowledge and research. The results of this necessary trend have provided us with experts in a variety of subfields in the area of human communication.

This text, *Diagnostic Procedures in Hearing, Language, and Speech,* is an example of the trend from the global view of human communication and its disorders to the component parts of this highly specialized field. The book focuses entirely upon measurement in the discipline of communication disorders including the three facets of hearing, language, and speech. The editors, Professors Singh and Lynch, have combined his adroitness in the field of research with her expertise in clinical application of research data to develop a format for this text. They have selected contributors, each of whom is an expert in his/her area of interest. The contributors, in addition to their presentation of facts and suggested techniques for diagnostic procedures, have demonstrated sensitivity to the value of historical data, theoretical constructs, and the morass of what is not known in their specialized disciplines.

The underlying attributes of this book include three prime areas: consideration of the total child or adult in the diagnostic process, validity and reliability in the selection and use of diagnostic tools, and ethical practices. In a differential diagnosis of hearing, language, and speech disorders, the diagnostician not only must know the scope and sequence of behaviors and how to obtain baseline data, but must be concerned also with the total person. This implies the differentiation between language disorders and language differences in bilingual speakers, the family crises that may result from the diagnostic report, and consumer costs, to name but a few of these basic principles covered by several of the authors.

The second attribute is related to discussions in the text that emphasize the need for the development, selection, and use of diagnostic tools based on theory, research, and follow-up studies. The authors leave no room for bandwagon and cookbook approaches to diagnostic procedures. Attribute three is concerned with ethical practice and the necessity for qualified diagnosticians.

The contributors to this text have written in the mode of the behavioral scientist dealing with research and keen observations of behaviors in the evaluation process. Collectively they have provided a comprehensive, practical yet critical presentation of the state of knowledge in the diagnosis of children and adults who present hearing, language, and speech disorders. This text will appeal to a large professional audience.

Tina E. Bangs, Ph.D.
Professor and Director
Speech and Hearing Institute
The University of Texas
Health Science Center at Houston

Preface

The art and science of diagnosis in the professions of hearing, language, and speech have now reached a state of maturation that requires an overall accounting. Current theories of diagnosis, and the practice emerging therefrom, have been enriched by a cross-disciplinary approach drawing heavily from areas such as life sciences, psychology, and linguistics. Nonetheless, even while gaining insight from these allied fields, the art and science of diagnosis have continuously maintained independence and uniqueness.

Our major undertaking has been to assemble under one cover the highlights of diagnostic procedures in the sister disciplines of hearing, language, and speech—procedures applicable both to children and to adults. The diversity of diagnostic procedures now extant, and the myriad claims by proponents of alternative (and sometimes conflicting) theories, impelled us to set forth as a guideline for each author the inclusion of historical perspective and theoretical discussion in addition to presentation of diagnostic procedures.

This book contains fourteen chapters arranged in four sections. The first section, consisting of one chapter, is devoted to diagnostic theories in hearing, language, and speech. The next three sections—hearing, language, and speech—are preceded by introductory overviews written by specialists from the fields. Five chapters pertain to audiologic diagnosis; four chapters to language, of which one presents normal language development among bilingual children and three deal with the diagnosis of linguistically handicapped persons; and four chapters to the assessment of speech disorders. In all, this material encompasses a comprehensive overview of areas most relevant to the needs of a practicing hearing, language, and speech clinician. The authors are practicing diagnosticians, teachers of diagnosis, and research scientists specializing in diagnostic work. Each has taken a theoretical stand in his/her discipline; each has made a significant impact on the state of the diagnostic art today.

This text is primarily intended for practicing clinicians and students of diagnosis, in hearing, language, and speech. It will provide both theoretical background and a firm basis for diagnostic practice to the clinician with some surface knowledge in these fields. Students in hearing, language, and speech pathology will gain insight into current diagnostic procedure presented in a unified manner. In addition, students in special education and clinical psychology will gain an understanding of the contribution of these areas to differential diagnosis. Even experienced audiologists and speech pathologists will no doubt find in this volume much that will deepen their understanding of their discipline.

The editors wish to express appreciation to Mary Lilly for her assistance in the preparation of this manuscript.

This volume is dedicated to those diagnosticians who know this material and more, and who daily apply their knowledge to serve the communicatively handicapped. Their willingness to share their clinical insights with their students and colleagues is reflected in this volume.

Diagnostic Procedures in Hearing, Language, and Speech

ART AND SCIENCE
OF DIAGNOSIS

Art and Science of Diagnosis in Hearing, Language, and Speech

Norma S. Rees

CONTENTS

As a profession, audiologists and speech pathologists are still defining their identity. This dilemma is reflected in the nine fundamental questions Professor Rees poses concerning diagnosis in hearing, language, and speech. Although they seem philosophical, these are the questions that every competent diagnostician must resolve before proceeding with the practical business of evaluation. Students of diagnostics, in particular, will find that their choice of one of Professor Rees' alternative responses to each of these questions will guide them in choosing specific evaluation protocols that will contribute to the type of diagnostic service they deem appropriate to their professional competence and role. This chapter has relevance for all subsequent chapters. It is not possible to provide high quality diagnostic service until the diagnostician has defined the nature and proper objective of diagnosis. —Eds.

Let us begin with a definition. Dictionaries agree that "diagnosis" derives, via the Latin form, from the Greek διαγιγμώσκω, meaning to discern or distinguish. Current dictionary definitions refer to determining the cause or nature of a disorder, the types of disorder mentioned ranging from medical problems through economic upheavals to malfunctioning of the family car.

Diagnosis, therefore, wherever it applies, seems to pertain to specifying the disorder, although the degree of specification is not given in any dictionary definition. What are the definitional implications for disorders of hearing, language, and speech? A search for answers will turn up a number of controversies and unresolved questions, and may reveal some unexamined assumptions. To a very real degree the issues underlying these unresolved questions are the issues fundamental to the evolving structure of the discipline itself. This overview of the subject of diagnostic procedures in hearing, language, and speech is organized around such questions and the differing answers that have been offered.

WHAT IS THE PROPER BUSINESS OF DIAGNOSIS IN HEARING AND SPEECH?

Alternative A 1: Diagnosis in hearing, language, and speech focuses on the use of language in communication. Any diagnostic activity that does not contribute to an understanding of the individual's functioning with regard to the use of language in communication is either tangential or unrelated to the object under consideration.

Alternative A 2: Speech pathologists and audiologists have special technical skills that may be applied to acquiring information about a patient's physiologic, biologic, cognitive, or emotional functioning that will contribute to medical, dental, psychologic, or educational diagnosis. They may perform their professional roles partly or wholly in these directions.

The unifying core of all work in hearing, language, and speech is the focus on the use of language in communication. The potential users of services by specialists in hearing, language, or speech are those children or adults with possible or actual disorders of communication. Although these disorders take a wide variety of forms and levels of severity, their common theme is that the persons so characterized perform less than adequately in terms of their own and their community's expectations for participation in interpersonal communication via the spoken language. It seems then, that to the degree that the speech-language pathologist or audiologist engages in diagnostic activity that does not directly contribute to an apprecia-on of the subject's disorder of communication, he is performing tasks that are peripheral to his primary goal.

Agreement on this point need not imply that speech-language pathologists and audiologists never do, or never should, engage in these activities, here termed peripheral or tangential. It does, however, imply that when they are so engaged, they are using their skills for purposes other than those directly related to the nature of the dis-cipline. Speech-language pathologists and audiologists are involved in such activities to varying degrees, usually without embarrassment. For example, in reviewing the components of the battery of audio-logic tests, Rosenberg (1972) makes several suggestions about mea-surement of function that have little or nothing to do with com-munication; Emerick and Hatten (1974) recommend that the speech pathologist perform at least gross assessment of motor abilities during the clinical examination. When the speech-language pathologist mea-sures and describes tongue-thrust movements in the absence of any articulation disorder or assesses the young child's level of motor func-tioning; when the audiologist performs electronystagmography to contribute to the site-of-lesion decision or studies backward masking phenomena to add to the body of hearing science knowledge; these data may or may not be useful to the final outcome of diagnosis, but nonetheless can hardly be viewed as direct investigation of the subject's functioning with regard to the use of language in communi-cation.

Whatever tangential concern may engage his attention, Tillman and Olsen (1973) observed that the clinician in hearing, language, and speech ultimately focuses on communication. These authors, commenting on the value of speech audiometry, state that pure tone audiometry is of questionable validity when used for the purpose of estimating handicap. "Since hearing is the primary communicational sense, a valid estimate of the practical consequences of hearing loss should utilize speech as the test stimulus. The desire to obtain this more valid measure led to the development of speech audiometry as a tool to supplement pure-tone techniques" (Tillman and Olsen, 1973, p. 37).

These comments lead directly to the interesting question of what purpose or purposes may properly be assigned to diagnosis. It fol-lows from the foregoing discussion that the purpose of diagnosis in hearing, language, and speech is to initiate the process that results in improved communication. The improvement, moreover, must be measured in terms of the subject's performance in language production and comprehension as a participant in dialogue or discourse. The goal is little more than an ideal, inasmuch as our available tools of measurement give relatively little information about these matters. This view of the proper business of diagnosis in hearing, language, and speech is not universally shared, some audiologists being notable dissenters. It is the point of view of this writer that when professionals in hearing, language, and speech provide data (however complex) from which a member of another profession reaches a diagnosis, they are serving essentially in the capacity of technicians; when they produce data that contribute to basic knowledge about human communication, they are functioning as speech and hearing scientists. All of these are options, and should be so recognized; but it is important not to confuse such activities with diagnosis in these areas.

IS THE OBJECTIVE OF DIAGNOSIS IN HEARING, LANGUAGE, AND SPEECH CLASSIFICATORY OR DESCRIPTIVE?

Alternative B 1: Diagnostic procedures have the fundamental purpose of allowing the patient or his disorder to be assigned to a recognized category of pathology. True diagnosis is differential diagnosis in which the presenting symptoms are identified in etiologic terms and possible disorders are ruled out until the correct classification is made.

Alternative B 2: Diagnostic procedures have the fundamental purpose of describing the disorder in all its relevant dimensions. The purposes of the description are to determine areas of weakness or deficit so that they may be 1) remediated, or 2) measured again at a later time to determine progress and the results of remediation, if any.

As many others have pointed out, alternative B1 is the one most closely associated with the medical model. Classifying the disorder under investigation according to its category of pathology is likely to be useful when specific treatments are associated with specific etiologic classifications. Johnston and Harris (1968) point out that such an approach to speech and language disorders is limited, if not actually misleading. In the case of a child with defective language, they state that "labeling a language disorder in terms of etiology, when no treatment for the causative factors involved is available, contributes relatively little to planning treatment procedures" (p. 41). The history of the development of diagnostic approaches to speech and language disorders shows, however, that differential diagnosis has occupied an important place. Even in the most recent edition of Charles Van Riper's *Speech Correction* (1963), he offers procedures for both describing the disorder, such as articulation inventories, and for determining the (probable?) cause of the disorder, such as tests of "phonetic discrimination." In Van Riper's list of recommended diagnostic procedures both descriptive and etiology-directed approaches appear together generally without further ado.

Although the speech and language area has moved away recently from diagnostic approaches aimed primarily at labeling and classifying the disorder, the same movement has not characterized audiology. A recent quote from one of Jerger's (1973) influential works illustrates his point of view:

> In a sense, all audiometry is diagnostic since it contributes, in some sense, to the ultimate location of the auditory disorder. The relationship between air-conduction and bone-conduction thresholds, for example, is one of the principal bases for differentiating conductive from sensorineural hearing loss. (p. 75)

For Jerger, then, diagnosis is a matter of determining the site of lesion. In contrast, Schultz (1972) laments the labeling emphasis in audiology. Although he admits the usefulness of etiologic labels for the purposes of record-keeping and even for research, he points out that in the management of the hearing-impaired subject the label has little or no practical value. He states,

> ...there is little relationship between formalized audiologic assessment and audiologic therapy, so that the individual clinician is more or less successful depending upon the additional observations he makes and the individual insights with which he interprets his observations. In other words, audiologic evaluation is a highly complex process and very little of the observational material necessary to these clinical decisions arises from the formalized results of audiologic assessments. (p. 69)

Although Schultz' cogent comments may help to explain the well known separation between "diagnostic audiology" and "rehabilitative audiology," in all fairness it is necessary to point out that the apparently different state of affairs in speech-language pathology may be more illusory than real, a point that is explored in the discussion of alternatives D1 and D2.

Alternative B2 has a somewhat virtuous ring. It is clear that the descriptive goal of diagnosis is more compatible with educational models than with the medical model. The controversy about which alternative is the right one for speech-language pathologists and audiologists is essentially the question of whether the profession has a primarily medical or primarily educational orientation. The developing interest during the 1960s in behavior modification approaches to speech and language disorders may be credited with much of the shift toward description rather than labeling. For example, Brookshire (1967) clearly outlined the "experimental analyst's" interest in measuring the subject's baseline behavior in order to have a frame of reference against which to measure the effects of treatment. Johnston and Harris (1968) stress the role of descriptive data in diagnosis of childhood language disorders:

> Direct and systematic observation of the child's verbal behavior does furnish pertinent diagnostic information that is immediately useful, serving to provide an objective evaluation of the child's actual speech repertoire and the antecedent and consequent events relevant to his use of language. Such data provide a record of the speech sounds, words, phrases, and sentences that the subject uses before treatment and supply the basis for planning treatment procedures that start with the language the child already has. Observation also establishes the extent to which the child is able to attend and respond to cues and directions from the therapist, and the extent to which the subject's language is under the control of experimental stimuli. (p. 41)

Despite their different orientation toward the nature of language and learning, the psycholinguists in the Chomskian tradition also stressed the need for collection of language samples from which observations about the child's mastery of the language could be made. As a result of these movements, approaches to diagnosis in language disorders moved away from the medical model by the 1960s, although these changes had relatively little effect on fundamental issues in audiologic diagnosis.

WHAT IS THE NATURE OF DIAGNOSTIC
DATA IN HEARING, LANGUAGE, AND SPEECH?

Alternative C 1: The basic data in diagnostic procedures in hearing language, and speech are behavioral in nature.

Alternative C 2: For at least some diagnostic purposes, physiologic data are more desirable than behavioral data.

It follows from the earlier discussion that different diagnostic procedures may produce different types of data. Probably most diagnostic procedures in hearing, language, and speech are based on the collection and analysis of behavioral data. Perkins (1971) calls these data "psychologic" in contrast to biologic or physiologic data, and points out that "although physiologic processes underlying speaking behavior and acoustic characteristics of speech sounds produced can also be measured directly, they should not be confused with the speaking behavior with which they are correlated" (p. 24). Perkins (1971) makes it clear that however the clinician collects, organizes, and interprets the data, and whatever he infers from the data, the data are essentially behavioral in nature.

For much of audiologic diagnosis the same point applies. For example, Clarke and Bilger (1973) show that in ordinary practice the audiologist makes inferences about the auditory system by specifying "a relation between an acoustic input to the auditory system and an output, usually behavioral, from a motor subsystem of the organism" (p. 439). Although it is true that in audiometry the input is usually specified with far greater precision than in speech and language testing, the output data are nonetheless behavioral, an observation over which audiologists have agonized in their search for "objective" procedures that bypass behavioral variables.

Physiologic procedures were developed to overcome the audiologist's dependence on the subject's voluntary responses to acoustic stimuli. These procedures, which have been based on measurement of changes in the organism's electrical properties, or heart rate, use physiologic data rather than the usual behavioral data. According to Goldstein (1973), the physiologic procedures have their major value in determining presence and severity of peripheral hearing impairment in subjects who cannot be counted upon to give reliable behavioral responses. If that is so, the audiologic procedures based on physiologic data provide the information that may be useful for both medical and educational purposes. In contrast, if physiologic data are regarded as essential to something like site-of-lesion decisions, they would play a role in the "labeling" approach to diagnosis and have relatively little to contribute to an understanding of the subject's function with regard to ordinary communication.

WHAT TYPES OF BEHAVIORAL DATA
SHOULD BE COLLECTED IN DIAGNOSTIC PROCEDURES?

Alternative D 1: The behavioral approach requires the diagnostician to analyze the subject's behavior in terms of a set of discrete abilities, which together comprise the function in question.

Alternative D 2: The behavioral approach requires that the function in question be examined synergistically and in a realistic context.

Given that at least some of the data the diagnostician in speech and hearing collects are behavioral in nature, further questions arise about the nature of the behavioral data worth gathering. This is where models of the communicative process come in, and significantly affect the types of data that the diagnostician collects. The type of model of the communicative process that has been most characteristic of the field of speech and hearing is one that attempts to separate communication into its component units in a sort of building-block fashion. Probably most familiar is the model described by Irwin, Moore, and Rampp (1972), wherein the communicative process is viewed as composed of three types of activities: decoding, central processing, and encoding, and supported by the basic processes of "acuity, discrimination, association, motor patterns, and discrete movements" (page 241). This model is related to the possible diagnostic labels so that the input disorders of acuity, discrimination, and symbolic association were correlated with deafness, agnosia, and receptive aphasia, whereas the output disorders were dysarthria, apraxia, and expressive aphasia.

This kind of model allows the diagnostician to investigate specific areas individually. Numerous familiar tests have been based on such an approach. Part of the presumed usefulness of test batteries based on this kind of model is that it presupposes "simple" abilities, like hearing acuity, to be prerequisite for more "complex" abilities, like auditory comprehension. To pursue this example, however, although hearing acuity may be necessary for auditory comprehension, it is not sufficient. The building-block type of model tends to overlook that adding together all the components does not produce the total behavior in question. Possibly this weakness in the reductionist-type model accounts for the observation by Irwin, Moore, and Rampp (1972) that the traditional model of the communication, applied to diagnosis in speech and hearing, neither described linguistic functioning nor served the purpose of prediction.

Schultz (1972) also calls attention to the possibility that information about the hearing-impaired individual's ability to process the speech he hears may be viewed as some combination of an undetermined number of specific abilities: for example, temporal resolution of 30 msec or better, or a dynamic range of amplitude (from barely detected to too painful) of greater than 20 dB. The examiner can then appraise each of these abilities, weigh each of the component results, and combine them to obtain a speech-intelligence estimate (page 72). The difficulties involved in determining all the requisite specific abilities, finding ways to measure them accurately in human subjects, figuring out the correct differential weighting, and combining them meaningfully seem, however, insurmountable given the present state of the art. The notion that specific abilities can be assessed in a hierarchical fashion from simplest to most complex, with the corollary assumption that each step on the abilities scale is prerequisite for the next step, has become popular, especially in the assessment of auditory processing disorders. The notion that a hierarchy of auditory processing abilities can account for the listener's operations in the comprehension of spoken language was questioned by Rees (1973, 1977) and Sanders (1977).

The model on which the Illinois Test of Psycholinguistic Abilities (ITPA) is based is similar to the one described by Irwin, Moore, and Rampp (1972) and criticized by Rees (1973) in that it assumes a set of specific abilities that together comprise the language function. The ITPA approach (1968) and similar systems have been enormously influential in diagnostic and remedial work in speech, language, and learning disorders although, as noted earlier, it is not unlike some recent approaches to assessment in audiology. Bloom and Lahey (1978) take exception to the specific abilities orientation, pointing out the unspoken assumption underlying this approach that "first, there are certain cognitive abilities that are required for language and second, that these abilities can be identified, measured, and remediated." On the subject of auditory processing, Bloom and Lahey state,

> There seems little question that learning and using language involves the processing of sequences of auditory information. It is easy to assume that deficiency in the reproduction of sequences of auditory stimuli reflects the cause of a language disorder—or that such a deficiency interferes with learning language....It is not clear how many unrelated words one must be able to repeat in order to learn language—perhaps only one or two, or perhaps none. The correlation between memory span for sequential auditory information and language development in children may be related to some third factor influencing both, and improvement in one skill may not influence the other.

In contrast to the "discrete abilities" approach to diagnosis are approaches that seek to examine the function in question in a holistic manner and in appropriate context. In audiologic diagnosis, an example might be assessing the subject's ability to comprehend spoken language against a background of competing noise. In diagnosis for language disorder, analyzing naturalistic language samples also falls into this category. In articulation disorders of various etiologies, assessment of the speaker's intelligibility would serve as an example of the holistic approach, as contrasted with the evaluation of discrete phonemes in their varying phonetic contexts. Far more examples of the "fragmentized, discrete abilities" approach may be found in diagnosis in speech, language, and hearing, however, in part reflecting the recent emphasis on the production of quantifiable data for the purposes of ready "accountability."

WHEN THE DIAGNOSTICIAN IN SPEECH AND HEARING COLLECTS BEHAVIORAL DATA, HOW MAY THEY BEST BE USED?

Alternative E1: The most practical uses of behavioral diagnostic data are to identify areas of deficit so that these areas may be remediated directly.

Alternative E2: Behavioral diagnostic data are primarily useful to provide a measure of the severity of the problem, identify the goals of remediation, and provide a basis for measuring change or progress.

The foregoing discussion has shown that, irrespective of numerous issues, the bulk of data collected in speech and hearing diagnosis are of a behavioral type. Data collection, however, is not the final objective, and behavioral data may be used in different ways according to the clinician's point of view. The pivotal question here is how the data that result from diagnostic procedures relate to the remedial program that may follow.

According to one point of view, (alternative E1), the relationship is direct and intimate. In this case the results of assessment procedures are supposed to determine not only the goals but the process of remediation. The familiar concept of diagnosis-and-prescription is an example of this approach. It essentially seeks to identify specific areas of weakness in the subject's functioning or achievement so that the remedial program may be designed to focus on these areas only.

This approach to the relationship between diagnosis and remediation is highly consistent with the "specific abilities" notion discussed earlier. If a major area of functioning like language can be viewed as composed of a set of discrete abilities, then it should be possible to assess these abilities individually, determine which show the greatest deficit, and concentrate on those in the remedial program. An illustration of this theory is the popular emphasis on "auditory sequencing" as a specific skill component of linguistic functioning. The procedure is to assess the subject's ability on an auditory sequencing test or subtest, and if the results show a weakness in this skill as compared to test norms, attacking the problem by training the child in auditory sequencing using the same types of materials found in the test or subtest. A post-test of the same type is typically used to measure the results of remediation. This approach, sometimes characterized as teaching-to-the-test, lends itself neatly to accountability systems. Teaching programs based on the ITPA (Kirk et al. 1968) are examples, as is the *Interactive Language Development Teaching* system for training grammatical structure (Lee, Koenigsknecht, and Mulhern, 1975).

Gray and Ryan's (1973) approach to language training express a similar point of view about what to do with behavioral assessment data, although with an interesting twist. Their carefully organized, step-by-step remedial procedure based on operant conditioning principles was developed first, and the assessment procedure followed as a means for identifying the step in the program at which to begin the subject's training. The result is a reversal of the teaching-to-the-test approach, but the presumed relationship between the behavioral diagnostic data and the remedial program is no less direct. These examples are but a few of many formal and informal systems for testing and teaching children and adults with communication disorders that rest on the assumption of an isomorphic relationship between results of assessment procedures and the content of therapy procedures.

In contrast is the approach that whatever the value of collecting behavioral data during diagnostic sessions, the data do not necessarily determine the structure of the remedial program. According to this point of view, diagnostic data allow the clinician to assess the severity of the communication disorder and to determine the objectives of a remediation program for the subject in question. The behavioral data collected during diagnostic sessions also provide a handy baseline for measuring change over time. The results of assessment do not, in this case, translate directly into a design for remediation. In this appoach it is possible that the remedial program may attack the problem directly, as in the foregoing examples, but it is also possible that the remedial approaches may be largely indirect. An extreme example of the indirect approach might be the clinician who uses play therapy techniques with a child manifesting an articulatory disorder, at no time instructing the child about how to produce the sounds of speech. Alternative E2 is therefore characterized by greater flexibility in the use of behavioral diagnostic data, whereas alternative E1 generally leads to the development of a single set of training procedures presumably applicable to all subjects who score the same on the tests.

DOES DIAGNOSIS IN HEARING, LANGUAGE, AND SPEECH HAVE A UNIFORM SET OF UNDERLYING PRINCIPLES?

Alternative F1: Yes. The answers to the issues of purpose apply equally to diagnosis in speech and language and to diagnosis in audiology.

Alternative F2: No. Speech and language pathology, on the one hand, and audiology, on the other hand, are characterized by differing principles determining the purpose of diagnostic activities.

In dealing with this question, and its alternative answers, it is important to distinguish between current reality and desirable ideals. In fact, speech and language pathologists have tended to think differently from audiologists about the principles that underlie diagnosis. The medical model has been better received by audiologists, as the references cited from Rosenberg (1972) and Jerger (1973) reveal, whereas what Emerick and Hatten (1974) term the learning or education model, emphasizing the "nature of the behavioral disability," as already noted, has strongly influenced diagnostic concepts in speech and language pathology. The fact that speech and language pathologists have assumed the responsibility for remediation more typically than have audiologists may help to account for this division in diagnostic approaches. It is interesting to note that few writers on the subject of diagnosis in speech and hearing have attempted to take on both. A notable exception is Schultz (1972), who opts for a single set of principles. Schultz also offers some caustic comments about the "depersonalization" that characterizes some of the approaches to evaluation in hearing handicaps, as well as the audiologist's abrogation of the responsibility for rehabilitation. He argues that "the development of audiology in recent years has been primarily and almost completely from an acute-disease orientation rather than a more appropriate chronic disease orientation. The climate in which the audiologist functions can be characterized by a philosophy of immediate treatment, expressed sometimes through surgery, sometimes through hearing-aid fitting with little follow-up of associated therapy" (p. 75).

Schultz' proposed solution to these ills includes adopting a set of goals for audiologic assessment that relate to the subject's capacity and potential for communication, suggesting that the principles currently characteristic of much of speech and language pathology ought to apply to audiology also. That professionals in speech and hearing are impressed by a similar need may be inferred from recent trends in some training programs to produce a group called "hearing clinicians" who will take on the role of assessment and remediation for the hearing impaired with specific regard to the use of language in communication. Indeed, it is on the subject of the principles that apply to diagnosis that the disunity between speech pathology and audiology originates. This writer, like Schultz (1972), concludes that a common set of principles would not only make better sense but would also be in the greater interest of the clinical population served by professionals in speech and hearing.

IS DIAGNOSIS A DISCRETE ENTITY, OR IS IT PART OF SOME OTHER ONGOING PROCESS?

Alternative G1: Diagnosis is a segment of overall management that can be conceptually and operationally separated from segments pertaining to remediation.

Alternative G2: Diagnosis is an ongoing process inseparable from remediation.

The traditional, although by no means only, approach in the management of communication disorders has been to separate diagnosis, temporally as well as conceptually, from ongoing remediation. The basic textbooks in speech pathology and audiology train the embryonic professional to complete the steps of diagnosis/evaluation/

assessment before designing and initiating therapy. Bangs (1968), for example, describes in intensive detail the tools and techniques of assessment in language and learning disorders that will result in reports to parents, physicians, and teachers, the latter person being responsible for "structuring her training program." Shelton, Hahn, and Morris (1968) explain that speech diagnosis in cleft palate covers the status of the speech disorder, its etiology, its prognosis, and "development of a plan for the remediation of the problems involved." Again, the medical model seems to have greatly influenced these traditional approaches. Standardized tests, in particular, are designed for use before or after training or remediation, but ordinarily not as integral components in remediation. In audiology especially, the diagnostic session has been viewed as a separate entity with remediation not only beginning after the evaluation is completed but typically carried on by different personnel.

A number of writers have expressed a different point of view about the diagnostic evaluation. For Berry (1969), diagnostic teaching is the focus: "We think we can learn more about the child's language disorder by observing him when he is actively involved in language learning than by his answers to questions or nonverbal performance in a formal test situation." Emerick and Hatten (1974), although generally treating diagnosis as a phase preliminary to treatment, also state that the conduct of the diagnostic session has an important impact on therapy and, furthermore, that therapy itself often provides diagnostic information. In the management of subjects with voice disorders, Boone (1971) stresses an integral relationship:

> Evaluation and therapy are highly overlapping: What is found at the evaluation and "fed back" to the patient may be highly therapeutic; similarly, the constant probing for the right combination of factors to produce the "best" voice is an evaluative part of every therapy session. (p. 72)

Again, a strong statement is made by Schultz (1972), who bluntly recognizes that greater prestige seems to be attached to the diagnostician than to the rehabilitator, especially in audiology. For Schultz, the goal of evaluation in speech and hearing is to provide data from which clinical decisions may be "made with confidence," and inasmuch as clinical decisions are made continually during the ongoing rehabilitation process, the evaluative data can hardly be viewed as having been fully collected at some prior time.

Another way of stating the issue is that one viewpoint has it that the clinician/diagnostician can determine a subject's problem, and perhaps also what needs to be done about it and how, by administering the right battery of standardized tests in the right order. Contributions to the literature on assessment that offer extensive summaries of existing standardized tests seem to underscore this approach (Carrow, 1972; Irwin, Moore, and Rampp, 1972). Emerick and Hatten (1974) put it succinctly:

> Almost every training program in speech pathology conducts an active out-patient diagnostic clinic in which patients are seen for short periods of time and a "diagnostic evaluation" is conducted, complete with parent interview, test administration, and concluding interview. We contend that such practices contribute to the "ninety-minute wonder" syndrome to which many young clinicians succumb in their early years of practice.

Although this approach is easy to tear down when applied to speech-language pathology, it is almost unchallenged in the case of diagnosis in audiology.

The contrasting viewpoint is that the results of standardized tests are unilluminating or, at best, incomplete, and that test results need to be replaced or supplemented by naturalistic, longitudinal data including observations on how the subject learns in exploratory teaching sessions. The language sample dear to some psycholinguistically oriented language clinicians seems to fit here, although there is by no means complete agreement on how best to collect and analyze the sample (Longhurst and Schrandt, 1973). It is noteworthy that both the standardized test and naturalistic behavior sample approaches share an underlying assumption; namely, that from a sample of a subject's behavior, standardized or not, it is possible to reach a generalized conclusion about the area of functioning under consideration.

It seems reasonable to conclude that the combined influence of the traditional diagnostic model and the development of standardized tests leads to the notion that diagnosis in speech and hearing is a primary, discrete, and prestigious stage in the management of persons with communication disorders; whereas the growing emphasis on the goal of improved communication through language and the use of longitudinal samples of communication behavior in naturalistic settings is more compatible with the view of diagnosis as inseparable from the ongoing process of remediation.

IS ASSESSMENT OF THE FACTORS
THAT WILL AFFECT THE OUTCOME OF
REMEDIATION A LEGITIMATE PART OF DIAGNOSIS?

Alternative H1: Yes. Evaluation of the psychodynamic and other prognostic factors that may influence the course of remediation is essential to adequate diagnostic evaluations.

Alternative H2: No. Although factors of motivation, the subject's perception of his problem, and style of interpersonal functioning are of significance to the clinician, they are not considered part of the diagnostic evaluation pe se.

If one accepts Schultz' (1972) dictum that the goal of diagnostic evaluation is to structure the clinical process, the diagnostician will inevitably be interested in learning anything about the subject that will help determine how best to improve his level of communicative functioning. Boone (1971) and Emerick and Hatten (1974) likewise stress the importance of determining which factors of the individual's perceptions, adjustments, and motivations will affect the course and outcome of therapy. On the other hand, if one views the assessment component as limited to the collection of relevant baseline behavioral data, as Brookshire (1967) and Johnston and Harris (1968) do, gathering information about perceptions and motivations will seem irrelevant or at best peripheral to the real business of evaluation. Audiologic diagnosis, as typically conducted in the current period, similarly omits investigation of the subjects' motivations or interpersonal relationships, with the notable exception of assessment of psychogenic hearing disorders. It may be reasonable to say that the more diagnosis is viewed as a separable component from remediation, the less the diagnostician may be concerned with the psychodynamic factors that will influence the success of the remedial program. In contrast, clinicians who view diagnosis as an integral part of ongoing remediation are more likely to pay serious attention to evaluating interpersonal factors at every step of the way.

HOW IS SCREENING RELATED TO
DIAGNOSIS IN HEARING, LANGUAGE, AND SPEECH?

Alternative I1: Screening is essentially a much shortened version of diagnosis for clinicians who don't have the time to collect data that are primarily useful for research purposes anyhow.

Alternative I2: Screening is the use of any procedure that identifies subjects needing further attention to their functioning in speech, language, and hearing.

Standardized tests sometimes allow the clinician to use a limited number of items for the purpose of screening. The Templin-Darley Tests of Articulation (Templin and Darley, 1970) include instructions for using certain items only for screening purposes, and this checklist approach has become traditional in screening for articulation disorders with large groups of school children. The distinction between screening and diagnostic evaluation in the case of articulation disorders, therefore, seems to be primarily a matter of the depth at which the evaluation is conducted. Although Emerick and Hatten (1974) state that screening data are insufficient for planning treatment for articulation disorders, it is likely that in some settings clinicians faced with large case loads never conduct in-depth diagnostic evaluations for children with articulation disorders. The generally accepted purpose of screening, however, is merely to identify subjects probably in need of closer examination with regard to the function in question. Screening in this sense seems to have reached its peak of efficiency in the case of identification audiometry.

In standard clinical practice children and adults who have failed screening tests of hearing do not enter remedial programs directly, but are referred for diagnostic evaluation. The distinction between the handling of articulatory disorders and hearing disorders probably derives from the different goals of the clinicians involved. The speech and language pathologist in a school setting, for example, aims to get large numbers of children into remedial programs, improve their performance in a measurable way, and dismiss them from therapy. The audiologist in a hospital setting, on the other hand, may be responsible for diagnostic evaluations only, with the goals of producing diagnostic information for the use of other practitioners altogether. It is unsurprising that one of these clinicians views diagnosis as often unnecessary while the other views diagnosis as his primary function. These are extreme examples, but they present the noteworthy contrasts of opinion regarding the relationship between screening and diagnosis.

It is also questionable that the techniques of identification audiometry have relevant analogues in other areas of communication disorders. Once again the state of the art may be inadequate to the objectives. In diagnosis for language disorders, for example, no fully satisfactory screening instrument has yet been designed, and clinicians frequently resort to referrals from teachers, physicians, and parents in place of direct identification (Siegel and Broen, 1976). In the case of stuttering and voice disorders, screening typically consists of a subjective indication on the part of the clinician that dysfluency or dysphonia has been noted. However, referrals and subjective impression seem to be considerably effective in identifying communication handicaps, and will no doubt continue to be used until more rigorous procedures are developed.

CONCLUSION

The purpose of this chapter is to provide an overview of the issues characterizing diagnostic procedures in hearing, language, and speech. To gain a broad perspective, the review identified a number of underlying questions to which contrasting, if not mutually exclusive, answers have been offered both implicitly and explicitly. A major point that emerges from the review is that the preferred answer to any of the unresolved questions depends on who is being asked. For example, on the issue of whether the purposes of diagnostic data are primarily descriptive or classifying, speech-language pathologists tend to react quite differently from audiologists. A similar division may be found on the question of whether diagnosis is conceptually separable from remediation. On the issue of whether diagnostic data are largely about performance or a set of discrete abilities to be trained directly during remediation, the clinician with behaviorist orientation is inclined to respond differently from the clinician with psychodynamic training. On the matter of screening, the school clinician's point of view may be quite different from that of the clinician in a hospital setting.

It seems that the combined factors of 1) the setting in which the specialist in communication disorders works and 2) whether the specialization is speech-language pathology or audiology are likely to predict the answers to the questions posed. An inescapable conclusion is that the profession lacks a set of unified principles underlying current approaches to diagnosis. If a move in the direction of unity would be desirable, as it is in the opinion of this writer, the starting point should be on the very first issue raised above: namely, that diagnosis in hearing, language, and speech must take as its primary and proper subject the use of language in communication, considering the human subject as both speaker and listener.

REFERENCES

Bangs, T. E. 1968. Language and Learning Disorders of the Pre-Academic Child. Appleton-Century-Crofts, New York.

Berry, M. F. 1969. Language Disorders of Children. p. 193. Appleton-Century-Crofts, New York.

Bloom, L., and Lahey, M. 1978. Language Development and Language Disorders. John Wiley & Sons, New York.

Boone, D. 1971. The Voice and Voice Therapy. p. 241. Prentice-Hall Inc., Englewood Cliffs, N.J.

Brookshire, R. H. 1967. Speech pathology and the experimental analysis of behavior. J. Speech Hear. Disord. 32:215–227.

Carrow, E. 1972. Assessment of speech and language in children. In: J. E. McLean, D. Yoder, and R. Schiefelbusch (eds.), Language Intervention with the Retarded, pp. 52–88. University Park Press, Baltimore.

Clarke, F. R. and Bilger, R. C. 1973. The theory of signal detectability and the measurement of hearing. In: J. Jerger (ed.), Modern Developments in Audiology, pp. 437–467. Academic Press, New York.

Cox, B. P. and Lloyd, L. L. 1976. Audiologic considerations. In: L. L. Lloyd (ed.), Communication Assessment and Intervention Strategies, pp. 123–193. University Park Press, Baltimore.

Emerick, L. L. and Hatten, J. T. 1974. Diagnosis and Evaluation in Speech Pathology. Prentice-Hall Inc., Englewood Cliffs, N.J.

Goldstein, R. 1973. Electroencephalic audiometry. In: J. Jerger (ed.), Modern Developments in Audiology, pp. 407–435. 2nd Ed. Academic Press, New York.

Gray, B. B., and Ryan, B. 1973. A Language Program for the Non Language Child. Illinois Research Press, Champaign.

Irwin, J. V., Moore, J. M., and Rampp, D. L. 1972. Nonmedical diagnosis and evaluation. In: J. V. Irwin and M. Marge (eds.), Principles of Childhood Language Disabilities. p. 241. Appleton-Century-Crofts, New York.

Jerger, J. 1973. Diagnostic audiometry. In: J. Jerger (ed.), Modern Developments in Audiology, pp. 75–115. Academic Press, New York.

Johnston, M. K., and Harris, F. R. 1968. Observations and recording of verbal behavior in remedial speech work. In: H. N. Sloane and B. C. MacAulay (eds.), Operant Procedures in Remedial Speech and Language Training. p. 41. Houghton Mifflin Company, Boston.

Kirk, S. A., McCarthy, J. J., and Kirk, W. D. 1968. The Illinois Test of Psycholinguistic Abilities (revised). University of Illinois Press, Urbana.

Lee, L. L., Koenigsknecht, R. R., and Mulhern, S. T. 1975. Interactive Language Development Teaching. Northwestern University Press, Evanston, Ill.

Longhurst, T. M., and Schrandt, T. A. M. 1973. Linguistic analysis of children's speech: A comparison of four procedures. J. Speech Hear. Disord. 38: 240–249.

O'Neill, J. J. 1975. Measurement of hearing by tests of speech and language. In: S. Singh (ed.), Measurement Procedures in Speech, Hearing, and Language, pp. 219–252. University Park Press, Baltimore.

Perkins, W. H. 1971. Speech Pathology. p. 24. The C. V. Mosby Company, St. Louis.

Perkins, W. H. and R. F. Curlee. 1969. Causality in speech pathology. J. Speech Hear. Disord. 34:231–238.

Rees, N. S. 1973. Auditory processing factors in language disorders. The view from Procruster's bed. J. Speech Hear. Disord. 38:304–315.

Rees, N. S., and Shulman, M. I don't understand what you mean by comprehension. Journal of Speech and Hearing Disorders. In press.

Rosenberg, P. E. 1972. The test battery approach. In: J. Katz (ed.), Handbook of Clinical Audiology, pp. 271–279. The Williams & Wilkins Company, Baltimore.

Sanders, D. 1977. Auditory Perception of Speech: An Introduction to Principles and Problems. Prentice-Hall, Englewood Cliffs, N.J.

Schultz, M. C. 1972. An Analysis of Clinical Behavior in Speech and Hearing. p. 72, 75. Prentice-Hall Inc., Englewood Cliffs, N.J.

Shelton, R. L., Hahn, E., and Morris, H. L. 1968. Diagnosis and Therapy. In: C. C. Spriesterbach and D. Sherman (eds.), cleft Palate and Communication. Academic Press, New York.

Siegel, G. M., and Broen, P. A. 1976. Language assessment. In: L. L. Lloyd (ed.), Communication Assessment and Intervention Strategies, pp. 73–122. University Park Press, Baltimore.

Templin, M., and Darley, F. 1970. The Templin-Darley Tests of Articulation. 2nd Ed. University of Iowa Bureau of Educational Research and Service, Iowa City.

Tillman, T. W., and Olsen, W. O. 1973. Speech audiometry. In: J. Jerger (ed.), Modern Developments in Audiology, pp. 37–74. 2nd Ed. Academic Press, New York.

Van Riper, C. 1973. Speech Correction. Prentice-Hall Inc., Englewood Cliffs, N.J.

HEARING

Introduction

James Jerger

The diagnostic evaluation of hearing disorders has evolved, over the past two decades, from the simple application of a limited number of hearing tests into a sophisticated examination in which testing strategy plays an even more important role than test administration.

Twenty years ago, the audiologist's repertoire was limited to conventional pure tone audiometry by air and bone, rudimentary speech audiometry in the form of a spondee threshold and a phonetically balanced (PB) score at a single suprathreshold level, and an assortment of functional tests, of which only the Stenger test survives. Specialized diagnostic tools were limited to the Alternate Bilateral Loudness Balance Test (ABLB) and a scattering of techniques purporting to measure difference limina for intensity change. Békésy's automatic audiometer had been invented, but its clinical applications had not yet been exploited.

The testing of children was almost exclusively by behavioral techniques graduated according to their suitablility at various ages. Play audiometry was in its formative stage and we saw the development of several techniques more renowned for their technologic complexity than their efficacy in pediatric evaluation.

Virtually the only electrophysiologic test was the psychogalvanic skin response (PGSR), a technique whose anticipated promise for children never quite materialized.

Screening was by pure tones set at a level just audible in the school cafeteria, and follow-up was by thresholds in the teacher's lounge. This technique seldom missed a child with acoustic trauma but usually failed to identify mild middle ear disorders, the most prevalent source of hearing loss in childhood.

Hearing aid performance was measured by the ubiquitous PB list. One proceeded from the assumption that somewhere a "best aid" for the patient existed. Finding it was just a matter of perseverance in testing a sufficient number of different brands until one PB score burst gloriously upward from the commonality of it brethren.

Three technologic developments have had profound impact on the modern evaluation of hearing disorders. One was the development of the electroacoustic impedance audiometer; the second was the development and low cost commercial availability of the averaging computer; and the third was the development of new materials to broaden the scope of speech audiometry.

The impedance audiometer has changed our basic approach to a wide variety of measurement problems, from pediatric screening to the measurement of hearing aid performance. In routine audiometric assessment the impedence audiometer is undoubtedly the most important tool at our disposal. It enjoys this status for two reasons: first, it is the most sensitive indicator of middle ear disorder, short of microscopic examination of structure; second, it makes possible the measurement of the acoustic reflex which, in knowledgable hands, is probably the most versatile test of hearing disorder that exists.

The relations among acoustic reflex thresholds for contralateral and ipsilateral stimulation are uniquely different in middle ear, cochlear, VIIIth nerve, brain stem, and temporal lobe disorders, a versatility unmatched by any other test at our disposal.

The averaging computer was responsible for a good deal of fruitless effort during the slow wave or "V" potential phase of evoked response audiometry (ERA). Several thousand man hours were lost in search of the elusive "objective audiogram." But the great hope that slow wave potentials in the 100–300 msec latency range would provide independent thresholds at any audiometric frequency in difficult-to-test children has yet to be realized. The lability of the slow wave potential, and its dependence on state variables, especially stages of sleep, seem to be its principal problems.

But those who impatiently abandoned ERA did so prematurely. The recognition and exploitation of early (2–10 msec) evoked responses from brain stem structures has given audiologists an invaluable new tool. For difficult-to-test children, the principal virtue of the brain stem evoked response (BSER) is its virtual independence of state variables. Indeed it is so resistant to such factors that some neurologists consider its absence to mean brain death.

A second important feature of the BSER is the stability and repeatability of its latency. The exquisite precision of the latency measure makes possible an array of diagnostic distinctions quite independent of other audiometric measures. Because of their dependence on synchronized neural activity from the basal turn of the cochlea, BSER responses will probably never yield satisfactory estimates of auditory sensitivity at discrete frequencies. They will not give an "objective audiogram." What they will give, however, is an extremely dependable and accurate gross estimate of overall sensitivity in the 1,000–4,000 Hz region that is entirely independent of behavioral data. The value of this becomes apparent in the testing of multiply involved children.

In spite of the profound implications that both impedance and BSER audiometry have had for audiologic practice, the new development with broadest long range implications for our field lies in the area of speech audiometry. For too many years this area could count among its resources 36 spondee words and no more than 12–16 monosyllabic word lists, materials notorious for their sensitivity to high frequency loss and to virtually nothing else.

As long as people believed that disorders of speech perception began and ended with how well you could hear 3,000 Hz, these materials were well suited to the task. In the early 1950s, however, several investigators, notably an Italian team under Professor Bocca, began a series of investigations of central auditory disorders. This work, coupled with concurrent Canadian studies of dichotic stimulation, have added vast new dimensions to the scope of speech audiometry. The clinical exploitation of these important findings required the development of new speech testing materials, especially techniques employing sentences rather than single words. This development, in process for more than 10 years in several laboratories, has already yielded a number of promising sets of test materials. As these materials come to enjoy more widespread application among clinicians, the breadth and depth of audiometric evaluation may exceed anything we can currently imagine.

These three new technologic developments—impedance, BSER, and new speech materials—have given us much more than just a series of new auditory tests. They have altered our fundamental approach to diagnostic strategy. Twenty years ago there was little need for diagnostic strategy. The adult test battery was pretty much the same for everyone unless a functional problem was suspected. The judicious use of impedance audiometry, however, leads to a strategy in which tedious, time-consuming, and variably accurate bone-conduction threshold measurements need be carried out only after the presence of middle ear disorder has been defined by the impedance battery. At an even more sophisticated level, the combination of impedance data and air conduction thresholds determines whether a peripheral or central battery of tests is more appropriate.

One of the most important new concepts in pediatric evaluation is the cross-check principle, a stragety made possible by the advent of two methods for estimating sensitivity loss independent of behavioral audiometry: 1) the SPAR index based on relations among acoustic reflex thresholds for pure tones and white noise; and 2) the BSER sensitivity estimate. Behavioral responses to sound certainly constitute the ultimate test of hearing, and the clinician has a number of techniques at his disposal for observing responses. Yet it must be said that, so long as we had to rely on behavioral responses alone, all of us made mistakes with children. When the child does not want to play the audiologist's games, it is often not clear who is being tested.

The cross-check principle says that you never believe behavioral results alone. You always insist that they be confirmed by cross-check against an independent estimate of hearing sensitivity. In fact, with children you never believe the result of any single procedure, no matter how valid you think it might have been. Behavioral testing is cross-checked by SPAR. If middle ear disorder precludes SPAR, then BSER is the cross-check. For children who cannot be validly tested behaviorally, the combination of SPAR and BSER is usually a sufficient cross-check. The application of this cross-check strategy, based on SPAR and BSER, will certainly permit us to do much better, and more honest, pediatric evaluation.

In the chapters that follow each author has tried to give us something of the flavor of the excitement that these new developments have brought to specific areas of diagnostic evaluation.

Identification of Hearing Loss in Young Children: Prenatal to Age Six

Kevin P. Murphy and Jon K. Shallop

CONTENTS

The responsibility of the audiologist testing young children extends beyond the test suite to concerns about the child's linguistic and social development. Dr. Murphy and Professor Shallop distinguish "detection," which merely identifies the child, from "diagnosis," which represents the beginning of the management procedures for the infant or child. They note that the entire family is threatened by the discovery of a child's hearing loss. Criteria for identifying infants at high risk for hearing loss are given. The procedures for neonatal screening include behavioral response observation and automated instrumentation (Simmons and Russ, 1974; Bennett, 1975a,b). Throughout the chapter the need for follow-up audiometric testing is stressed. Normal hearing in the first few months of life does not preclude future problems. At any one time almost one-third of young hearing aid users may be affected with middle ear problems. The testing procedures suggested for use with very young children are described in considerable detail, supplemented by a series of excellent figures in which Dr. Murphy and Professor Shallop illustrate exact positioning of the child within the audiometric suite and the maturational sequence of expected head movements as the child's ability to localize sound matures through four different stages. The special problems of very young hearing aid users are discussed, including the need to instruct those responsible for the child in the care and use of the hearing aid.   —Eds.

Audiology is concerned with the management of all patients who suffer from sufficient hearing loss to affect their psychologic, educational, or career potentials. It should also be clear that with children much of our work is related to the development of speech and language pathologies that affect potential learning and factors of attention, which can preclude normal intellectual and vocal skills. In addition, we should be concerned with the domestic stresses and the consequential developments that can accompany hearing loss.

HISTORICAL PERSPECTIVES
AND CURRENT STATUS OF QUALITY SERVICE

Historically, hearing loss has often been described from the points of view of effect as well as cause. Such view points remain as major concerns today and we may benefit from some past views regarding the effects of hearing loss. One such example is a quotation taken from William Buchan's book entitled *Domestic Medicine*, which was first published in 1769. He indicated that hearing "...may be injured by wounds, ulcers, or anything that hurts its fabric" (p. 500). He cited additional causes and indicated the serious nature of profound congenital deafness: "When this is the case, it admits of no cure; and the unhappy person not only continues deaf, but generally likewise dumb, for life" (p. 501). Although this statement that the deaf cannot speak is typical of past and sometimes current opinions, he offers an interesting historical comment regarding the work of a teacher, Thomas Braidwood. Buchan states:

> Though those who have the misfortune to be born deaf are generally suffered to continue dumb, and consequently are in a great measure lost to society, yet nothing is more certain than that such persons may be taught, not only to read and write, but also to speak, and to understand what others say to them. Teaching the dumb to speak will appear paradoxical to those who do not consider that the formation of sounds

is merely mechanical, and may be taught without the assistance of the ear. This is not only capable of demonstration, but is actually, reduced to practice by the ingenious Mr. Thomas Braidwood of Edinburgh. This gentleman has, by mere force of genius and application, brought the teaching of dumb persons to such a degree of perfection, that his scholars are actually more forward in their education than those of the same age who enjoy all their faculties. They not only read and write with the utmost readiness, but likewise speak, and are capable of holding conversation with any person in the light. What this a pity any of the human species should remain in the state of idiotism who are capable of being rendered as useful and intelligent as others! We mention this not only from humanity to those who have the misfortune to be born deaf, but also in justice to Mr. Braidwood, whose success has far exceeded all former attempts this way; and indeed it exceeds imagination itself so far, that no person who has not seen and examined his pupils can believe what they are capable of. As this gentleman, however willing, is only able to teach a few, and as the far greater part of those who are born deaf cannot afford to attend him, it would be an act of great humanity as well as of public utility, to erect an academy for their behoof. (p. 501)

Buchan's words have relevance to our concerns in this chapter, i.e., the importance of early and accurate detection of hearing loss. It is hoped this will lead to an accurate diagnosis in order to establish the following objectives:

1. Rapid general remediation of the total family situation
2. Improved social roles of the child
3. Improved linguistic abilities of the child
4. Realistic educational plans for the child
5. Realistic career objectives for the child

To establish the above objectives requires the concern and cooperation of many persons and agencies. In the United Kingdom, for example, the government has statutory responsibilities for the health and well being of its citizens. Organized efforts are made to detect and diagnose health problems (including hearing loss) of children as early as possible and certainly within the 1st year of life. When children with hearing loss are identified, it becomes the responsibility of the local school authority and the National Health Service (in the United Kingdom) to plan for the education and continue the diagnosis and management of that child. It is difficult to state the quality of such services objectively; however, it can be stated that, at present, more than 98% of all severely hearing-impaired children in the United Kingdom are identified before the age of 1 year.

There are other nations with similar systems of health and educational care for their younger citizens. However, in the United States, we do not yet see a comprehensive national plan to detect and manage hearing-impaired children at the earliest possible age. Excellent efforts are made in many sectors of the United States, but a comprehensive plan remains for the future. Thus, the quality of service is variable. Preschool hearing-impaired children do not have equal access to an early education in all parts of the United States, and such is the case in many parts of the world.

It is our contention that a plan for early detection and diagnosis of hearing loss is essential to the five objectives stated above. Such a plan improves the prognosis of a better life for the child and his family.

DETECTION AND DIAGNOSIS

Butterworth's Medical Dictionary defines diagnosis as follows:

> The art of applying scientific methods to the elucidation of the problems of a sick person. This implies the collection and critical evaluation of all the evidence obtainable from every possible source and by the use of any method necessary. From the facts so obtained, combined with a knowledge of basic principles, a concept is formed of the aetiology, pathological lesions, and disordered functions which constitute the patient's disease. This may enable the disease to be placed in a certain recognized category, but of far greater importance it provides a sure basis for the treatment and prognosis of the individual patient.

Although a knowledge of etiology has its place, the identification of pathologies and disorders of function are at least equally important. The primary purpose of such activity, as Butterworth emphasizes, is to provide a sure basis for the treatment and prognosis of the individual patient.

At this point we shall make a distinction between diagnosis and detection or identification. Some persons, by nature of their responsibilities, are more concerned with the detection of children with hearing impairment. Detection of hearing loss does not resolve etiology of the hearing loss or the child's subsequent educational prognosis. Detection is accomplished by various means, including high risk registration, neonatal nursery screening, and follow-up of children previously suspected of having hearing loss. The primary concern in the detection of hearing loss is to examine incidence and prevalence in specific populations and to initiate diagnosis. Diagnosis is fundamentally concerned with the consequences of hearing loss.

Diagnosis follows, but is distinct from detection and, as we just said, their purposes are fundamentally different. Diagnosis is primarily concerned with the child and family, and most important, their futures. We should begin with the idea of concern for children who have individual assets and deficiencies. Our task should be to help the parents and child deal with the problems of hearing loss. The child is a person entitled to the same rights, privileges, and responsibilities as all other human beings. For the parents, however, the hearing-impaired child may represent a blow to their aspirations and pride. The entire family is somewhat threatened and their lives are certainly altered as a result of hearing loss.

Very often, the parents are the first to recognize the existence of a problem. It is often the parents who insist that they have detected a hearing loss in their child, although professional opinion may be contrary. As a result, parents are without adequate support for their problems and concerns.

Diagnosis can be a bewilderment for the parents and the child, or it can become the point at which their questions are answered and habilitation truly begins. Diagnosis can be shrouded with the mystique of technical jargon and "tests," or it can be a time when factual information about a child is set forth in understandable language to the parents. At this point, parents need support and reassurances.

In clinicial practice we meet large numbers of parents whose somewhat naive hopes may be summarized as follows.

1.   Their child does or does not have a hearing loss.
2.   If he does have a hearing impairment, that it can be cured.
3.   If it cannot be cured, that it is not serious.
4.   If it is serious, that by some means, especially amplification and special education and training, it can be ameliorated.
5.   That their child will be no different from other children except for wearing a hearing aid.
6.   That their child will not be like other unfavorable hearing-impaired children the parents may have known or their child will be more like a "normal" child is most respects.

Each of these points must be discussed honestly with the parents. They must not be misled concerning the facts, abilities, or prognosis for their child. We must remember that the primary purpose of the diagnosis is to effect a cure and that this will be paramount in the minds of the parents. When a hearing loss is confirmed and a cure cannot be effected per se, the parents may deny that their child has a hearing loss. Denial is followed by rationalization, sorrow, and ultimate acceptance. The need for professional support should be evident to the clinician.

The diagnosis, then, is the formulation of all available factual information concerning the child and his parents. Etiology must be determined, if possible, to aid in all treatment and training procedures, as well as for the well being of the parents and as a basis for genetic counseling, where relevant. Subsequently, the prognosis, insofar as it can be ascertained, must be clearly and simply stated and a plan of management should be initiated or continued in cooperation with other professional persons and agencies. During all of this, the parents will seek someone to advocate various aspects of the management procedures for their child. This may very well be the audiologist.

Some words of caution: 1) The diagnosis of hearing loss in children is often not accomplished in a short period of time. Various aspects may be completed quickly, but the true diagnosis is a continuing process that requires renewed validations. The clinician should make this clear to the parents and other professionals from the beginning. However, the need for a prolonged diagnostic period should not become an excuse for misdiagnosis, or for the clinician's inability to deal with the situation. 2) The cases of deafness often result in other complicating conditions. When the additional symptoms are severe, differential diagnosis may be relatively easy. Where, however, secondary pathologies are of relatively minor nature they may be easily missed. 3) Other severe and easily identified disabilities may be complicated by relatively minor degrees of hearing impairment. It is wise to exclude the phenomenon of hearing loss in every case of a serious sensory or intellectual deficit. 4) It is not uncommon for certain types of congenital hearing loss to manifest themselves in the 2nd or 3rd year of life. Where there are genetic factors (e.g., familial deafness) or rubella embryopathies, regular follow-up studies should be made until at least the age of 4 years. 5) The hearing-impaired child is at least as vulnerable to conductive deafness as is the infant with normal hearing. Between 20 and 30% of children between ages 1 and 7 years (Brooks, 1975) and between 10 and 15% of the remaining school age population are affected by middle ear disorders at any one time of the year. In other words, at any one period of time almost one-third of young hearing-aid wearers may be affected by middle ear problems. This phenomenon raises serious problems of supervision and management and should be foremost in the mind of the educational and pediatric branches of audiology.

PRENATAL AND NEONATAL TESTING

Prenatal Testing

There is little doubt that the unborn infant can respond to sound. By the 20th week, the human cochlea is mature (Elliot and Elliot, 1964). Responses of the fetus can and have been measured primarily by assessment of fetal movement and fetal heart rate change (Sontag and Wallace, 1935; Murphy and Smyth, 1962; Bench, 1968). The "noise" level reaching the fetal ear has been estimated to be 72 dB (Bench, 1968).

The clinical measurement of prenatal hearing does not seem to be routinely applicable. Its use is limited presently for research purposes. The techniques of amniocentesis (transabdominal perforation of the uterus to test amniotic fluid) and genetic mapping may provide more useful information for the diagnosis of prenatal deafness.

Neonatal Testing

The evaluation of the neonate's hearing has been somewhat of a controversy in recent years. The primary controversies have concerned methodologies for screening of potential hearing problems of the newborn. The two major procedures are a high risk registry and auditory stimulus screening.

The high risk registry seeks to identify infants with potential hearing loss by studying prenatal history and the postnatal physical condition. The eight high risk factors recommended by the 1971 Conference on Newborn Hearing Screening include:

1. All infants with a family history of childhood deafness in some member of the immediate family, i.e., father, mother, or sibling.
2. All infants whose mothers have had rubella documented or strongly suspected during any period of pregnancy.
3. All infants with a family history of congenital malformations of the external ear, cleft lip, or palate.

4. All infants with a family history of deafness in other relatives, with onset in childhood.
5. All infants found to have a structural abnormality of the external ear, cleft lip, or palate, including bifid uvula.
6. All infants having bilirubin values of 20 mg/1,000 ml or more, who also had exchange transfusions, are at high risk for bilirubin encephalopathy.
7. All infants under 1,500 g of body weight.
8. All infants with abnormal otoscopic findings.

Infants who are identified as "at risk" should receive regular follow-up pediatric, otologic, and audiologic evaluations. These assessments should enable confirmation of the hearing capabilities of the infant within the first few months of life.

Neonatal auditory screening has been accomplished by two primary procedures, behavioral response observation and instrumented response recordings. In each instance, specific stimuli are presented to the neonate and the responses are observed and recorded. Guidelines for a neonatal screening program have been available for the past decade (Downs and Sterritt, 1967).

Automated instrumentation for recording the responses of newborn infants has been reported by Simmons and Russ (1974), and Bennett (1975b). These techniques seem promising because they potentially remove the problems associated with observer bias inherent in any observational procedure (Bench, Hoffman, and Wilson, 1974).

Hearing assessment of a child during the first few weeks of life should be conducted only by persons experienced with this population. Behavioral responses can be observed during the first hours of life, but they are difficult to observe and quantify. However, the urgency for early detection is more important than early diagnosis. The confirmation of a diagnosis can perhaps wait a few months without causing undue harm to the infant while providing emotional protection for the parents. Therefore, the assessment of infants and young children is stressed in the next section of this chapter.

Perhaps more important is the need to observe caution in ensuring satisfactory follow-up procedures. The fact that a child has been classified in the first months of life as normal hearing should never preclude the possibility of repeated testing either at parental request or, where feasible, as routine follow-up.

INFANTS AND YOUNG CHILDREN

Presenting Problem

The initial concern that an infant or child has a hearing loss is typically suggested by a parent, usually the mother, or a relative or friend of the family. Suspicion of a hearing loss is discussed within the family until enough doubt exists for the parents to seek professional advice. Most likely the parents will seek the advice of their family physician or a pediatrician or, in the United Kingdom, of the community health services. Where available, an audiologist or otologist is the next most likely to be consulted. Thus, the presenting problem is often simply a fear on the part of parents that their child may have a hearing loss or, in the United Kingdom, the identification by a local authority infant welfare clinic that auditory responses are not satisfactory.

Ideally the child with a congenital hearing impairment will be identified during the first 12 months of life, but unfortunately, such is not always the case. Even if these children are identified early, the subsequent steps of diagnosis and management may not be as successful as they should be especially in those cases where there are multiple pathologies, as stated previously.

Children with adventitious hearing losses are detected primarily by behavioral changes observed by the parents, teachers, etc. The audiologist should be alerted by descriptions of inattentiveness, hyperdistractibility, snoring, mouth-breathing, poor appetite, apparent solitariness, lethargy, slow development of communication skills, persistence of early infantile vocalizations up to the 10th month of life or deterioration of quality and quantity of vocalizations subsequently, dullness in school, difficulties of discrimination of speech, etc. The subsequent diagnosis and treatments are also obtained most often through some aspect of a health delivery system as previously described. It should be clear that most adventitious hearing-impairment is mild and commonly associated with middle ear disorders; it is most widely distributed among minority and lower income groups. Hence, to get such children to the relevant clinical services may well involve considerable community support and education. In the United Kingdom the use of a mobile test clinic proved a very helpful service to one of the present writers.

Behavioral and Observational Audiometry

General guidelines In all assessments of auditory function, the clinician should be sure that what he is evaluating is the auditory state and that all other sensory stimulation is rigorously excluded. For example, when evaluating young children, the clinician should be aware of possible visual and olfactory stimulation. Set up a situation that is as free as possible from these stimuli and also make sure that the position in which you place the child is one most children will tolerate. For young infants, simply place them on their back and reduce the room illumination. For older children, a high chair or another type of child's chair would be appropriate. Make the situation comfortable and pleasant for the child.

When the child is settled and comfortable, have the parent put the child in and out of the chair, etc., in a playful manner. If it seems that the parents are needed to calm the child, they should not be touching the child or be a source of visual stimulation. However, if necessary, the child could sit on a parent's lap. The clinician must then watch that the parent does not cue the child either deliberately or inadvertently by leaning and turning. Also be aware that reflective surfaces can cause problems. An observation window or any other glazed surface might well lead the child to detect you and become so absorbed in his own reflection that he ignores the auditory stimuli.

When one is using various sound field auditory signals, the position of the child in the chair must be very carefully determined and marked. The sound pressure levels must be accurately determined with large speakers at close range, especially when working with very young children. An inch may make 10–15 dB of difference. If 10 or 15 dB is significant, then a way must be found to present the stimuli in such a way that this difference can be overcome. In view of this, it is better not to have the speakers too close. If the speakers are more than 2 feet away, then movements are not going to affect the sound pressure level at the ear as much as if the child moves within 1 foot from the speakers. In the latter case, there is going to be much more variation in the sound pressures.

In Figure 1, we illustrate some suggested arrangements for placing a child in a sound field. Each speaker is 2 feet from the child's ear at 30° above or below midline. We also employ the use of front versus back placement of the speakers because younger children seem to localize better in the horizontal plane than the vertical plane illustrated in Figure 1 (Conway and Shallop, 1975). Each speaker is also equipped with a lighted finger puppet for visual reinforcement.

When using behavioral audiometry and, therefore, when the child is expected to give behavioral cues, make certain that the be-

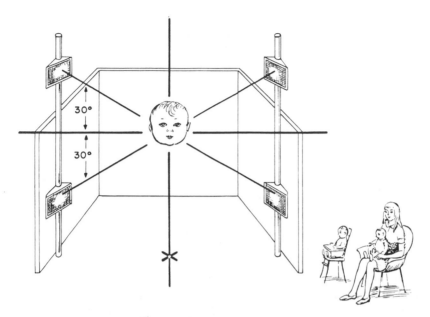

Figure 1. Suggested arrangements for placing a child in a sound field.

havioral cues are within the child's repertoire. One should read the case history carefully and make predictions as to what the child ought to be able to do and also check visual stimulation to verify that the child can make adequate head movements. Never take for granted that the child will be able to respond with an audiomotor pattern or any behavioral task until the motor functioning and basic task performances have been satisfactorily assessed.

When using criteria based on the sound pressure of the stimuli and their spectral characteristics, make certain that these parameters are carefully measured. Examine every stimulus as closely as possible and check it regularly. Everything that you use, if it is going to be diagnostically valid, must be checked regularly. If responses are elicited by many kinds of interesting "toys" that are known to have certain acoustic properties, then these are not necessarily tests. Rather, it has been determined that the child can turn his head to these stimuli and, thereby, the parent may be relieved to observe the child responding to the sound. To obtain a threshold evaluation, pure tones or preferably warble tones must be presented at descending sound pressure levels. Play audiometry should be perfectly feasible for a 2½-3 year old child in a sound field. Many 2½-3 year olds can also cope with headphones. However, it must be remembered that modern headphones can distort the meatal cavity. It may be necessary to use some other device that is not going to be as tight or to verify the ear canal sound pressures with a probe microphone.

Sound localization   The sound localization abilities can be a very useful technique to determine auditory responses. Any responses obtained with this technique do not necessary imply "hearing" for the purposes of language acquisition and learning. As with so many aspects of human behavior, sound localization is a developmental ability.

The maturation of sound localization in children is illustrated in Figure 2 by the type of responses that will be observed. The earliest type of response will be a combination of eye movement and head movement. The head movement will be contingent upon the motoric capabilities of the child, regardless of age. Initial head movements are mostly horizontal, even though the sound source may be placed below the child, as indicated by the *star* in Figure 2. Eventually sound localization responses mature to a direct diagonal pattern. These four patterns will now be described as stages of maturation.

Stage 1   This stage will be observed in the infant from the 14th–20th week of life. As illustrated in Figure 3, this stage consists of a primary horizontal head movement in the general direction of the sound, regardless of its exact position. The clinician should anticipate

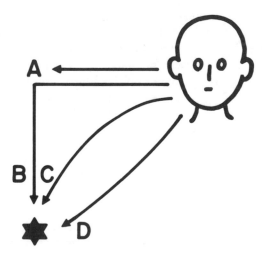

Figure 2.   Maturation of head movement in localizing sound. Types of head movement: *A*, horizontal; *B*, horizontal and vertical; *C*, arc; *D*, diagonal.

that these responses will not be abrupt, but rather it will take the infant a few seconds to respond. Infants will show this response provided they are comfortable, dry, and not hungry. For very young children, i.e., until they are mature enough to control head movements in the seated position, this response should be initiated with the child lying supine.

Stage 2 As illustrated in Figure 4, about 22 weeks of age, infants begin to exhibit a combination of horizontal and vertical head movements while searching for sound stimuli placed below the ear. Again, a response delay should be expected, although it will be less than the delay in stage 1. The clinician is also advised to carefully observe eyelid movements, eye movements, breathing, general body movement cessations, and vocalization—imitations of the sound stimuli.

Stage 3 The arcing stage is illustrated in Figure 5. It is characterized by a moderately quick arced movement toward the sound source. This response pattern is to be expected of a child by about the 26th week.

Stage 4 When children reach 8-9 months of age, they should begin to localize sounds directly on a diagonal to the source, as shown in Figure 6. Generally, the older the child, the quicker and more accurate this response will be. In most cases such responses will occur after stimuli in the 45-55 dB sound pressure level (SPL) range. Increased intensities below threshold of startle tend to speed up response patterns or, in a number of cases, produce apparent matura-

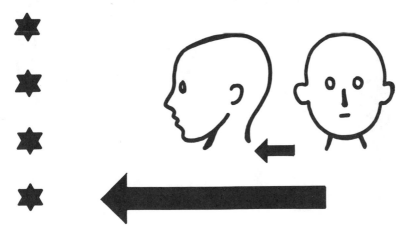

Figure 3.   Stage 1. Pure horizontal movement in general direction of sound source.

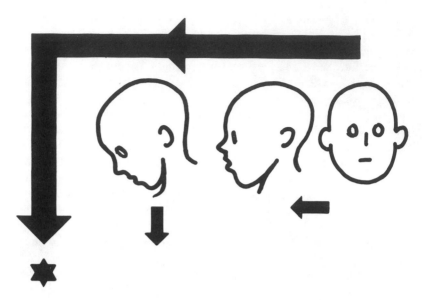

Figure 4. Stage 2. At 22 weeks, horizontal and vertical movement commences in localizing sound below the ear.

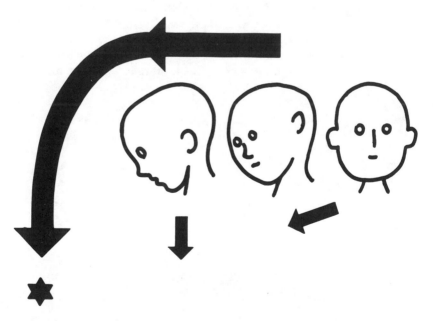

Figure 5. Stage 3. At 26 weeks, arc movement commences in localizing sound below the ear.

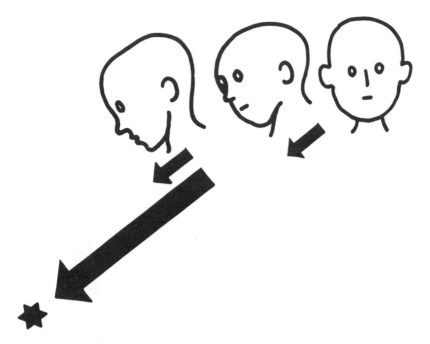

Figure 6.   Stage 4. At 32 weeks, diagonal movement commences in localizing sound below the ear.

tion e.g., a 6-month-old child should respond to a 50-dB SPL stimulus at stage 2, but would usually respond at stage 3 if the intensity of the original stimulus were increased to 70 dB SPL.

Some additional comments regarding the sound localization abilities of children may be helpful to the clinician. From our experience, about 60% of the children who have no apparent hearing loss will localize dominantly to the right side. Subsequently, this activity also develops toward the left side. In other words, if stimuli are presented to the child's right he will turn right. When presented left there may be no orienting response. In the case of monaural deafness the child responds to the unaffected side regardless of the source of the auditory stimuli. To summarize, in the age range 5–7 months:

1. response to right only, for stimuli presented right, indicates normal maturation patterns;
2. response to right but not to left for ipsilateral stimuli is also normal at that age (after 10 months persistent monaural responsivity is not normal);

3. response to right or left for contralateral stimuli should raise suspicions of either monaural malfunction or of aversive behavior should the phenomenon occur in the case of both ears.

Another point of interest relates to the results of sound localization obtained from the situation illustrated in Figure 1. In this situation, downward localization develops before the corresponding upward movement. When using this technique, the clinician is advised to use some type of visual or tangible reinforcement; an illuminated toy or dry cereal may be appropriate. In many instances, assurance such as, "That's good," will also be helpful.

Visual reinforcement is an essential element of the assessment of sound localization abilities of infants. Wilson (1978) reports that localization responses are more prevalent when the visual reinforcement is complex (animated toy). Progressively, the prevalence of responses lessens with simple visual reinforcement, social reinforcement, and no reinforcement, respectively.

The sound pressure levels and specific sound stimuli used in sound localization procedures should be appropriately selected. For example, the clinician might employ warble tones at two frequencies and two sound levels as presented in Table 1. Such a paradigm enables the clinician to predict, generally, the specific audiometric results that may be obtained in the future. For example, the child with a high frequency sensorineural loss may respond to all stimuli except the 4,000 Hz signal at 30 dB hearing threshold level (HTL), whereas the child with a low frequency conductive hearing loss may fail to respond only at 30 dB for 500 Hz.

Again, it must be emphasized that sound localization is an ability to do just that, localize sounds. It does not imply any present or eventual intellectual or linguistic competence on the part of the child. It does, however, provide a relevant paradigm for evaluating young

Table 1. Paradigm that can be used for evaluating hearing loss in young children

	30 dB	70 dB
500 Hz	Evaluate response	Evaluate response
4,000 Hz	Evaluate response	Evaluate response

children. Additional methods and procedures are detailed by Northern and Downs (1974), Eisenberg (1976), and Wilson (1978).

Visual Reinforcement Audiometry (VRA)   VRA is an extension and modification of Conditioned Orientation Reflex Audiometry (COR), as described by Suzuki and Ogiba (1961). COR is a sound field technique and is essentially the same as sound localization, which was described in the previous section. VRA is a similar technique, except that definite sound localization is not required of the child and earphones or bone conduction transducers can be used in addition to a sound field environment (Reddell and Calvert, 1967; Liden and Kankkunen, 1969; Matkin and Thomas, 1974). The essential difference between VRA and sound localization techniques is that in VRA thresholds are the objective. In sound localization procedures, although responses are related to known stimulus intensities, developmental patterns of response are the primary objective.

VRA should be conducted in a sound-treated audiometric booth and employ sound field earphone or bone-conducted signal presentations (warble tones or speech). The child is observed carefully to be "ready" and a signal is presented. If any type of alerting response occurs that is time-locked with the stimulus, visual reinforcement is presented. The visual reinforcement is typically a lighted or animated toy. As previously mentioned, complex reinforcers seem to produce more responses (Wilson, 1978). The reinforcement schedule is usually recommended to be 100%. VRA can produce responses at sound levels that are 10-15 dB less than the levels observed in behavioral observation audiometry (BOA), COR, and sound-localization techniques in general. However, it must be pointed out that' VRA minimal response levels decrease with the aging of the children. This point is illustrated in Figure 7, which is from the paper of Matkin and Thomas (1974). Their results are in good agreement with the results described by Wilson (1978), which are based on several years of study at the Child Development and Mental Retardation Center in Seattle, Washington.

Tangible Reinforcer Operant Conditioning Audiometry (TROCA)   TROCA is an audiometric procedure in which threshold measures are also the objective. Reinforcements are tangible, such as small toys, candy, dry cereal, etc. The reinforcements are presented to the child when a button-pushing response by the child is satisfactorily time-locked to the stimulus presentation. This technique has been successful with children as young as 7 months of age, although such procedures on these normal hearing infants were rather time con-

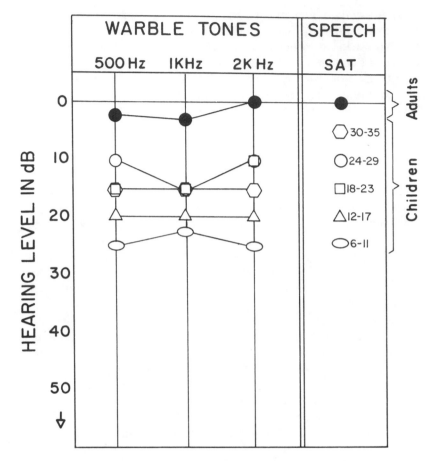

Figure 7. Minimal response levels obtained with VRA, 6–35 months (*N* = 100). (From Matkin and Thomas, 1974, reprinted by permission.)

suming compared to VRA procedures (Wilson, 1978). TROCA is also a valuable procedure to be employed with the mentally retarded (Fulton and Lloyd, 1975; Niswander, Ruth, and Speilberg, 1976).

Play audiometry   Between 2 and 3 years of age, children can usually be conditioned to respond to audiometry in a play situation. Typically, the child is given an opportunity (or is enticed) to wear audiometric earphones or by incorporating them in a baseball helmet or other attractive headgear (Miller, 1967). This can often be accomplished for reluctant children by having the parent and others also wear earphones. The responses to pure tone presentations should then be based on a simple task that is appropriate and pleasant for the child. Some examples include stacking blocks, dropping small objects in a container, assembling simple puzzles, peg boards, backlighted peg boards, etc. Audiologists should develop a variety of techniques and be prepared to use and quickly change techniques for any child.

The goal of any audiometric procedure is a reliable and valid record of auditory behavior. With children, the reliability and validity of audiograms are often very dependent upon the skills of the audiologist and the specific play technique employed. Where mimimal losses are suspected, careful control of the acoustic and visual environment is essential.

Speech Audiometry

Speech stimuli should be used as soon as possible because pure tone, narrow band, or warble tone audiometry may not produce the desired results with children. Moreover, these nonspeech stimuli do not give us any guide to the child's eventual ability to cope with vocal structures. In fact, nonspeech stimuli may not get past the right cerebral hemisphere; so the evaluation of the association pathways between the left and the right hemispheres may be neglected. To determine a speech reception threshold, we often use conversation with a very young child, e.g., "Where's your nose?" "What's your name?" etc. This could provide a behavioral test that covers the maximum range of phonemic elements without going into a lengthy standardized test. It is good information when a child can point out parts of his body, or colors, or respond to a question, e.g., "Where's Mummy?", and the child turns around and gives a big grin to Mummy. Then if you say, "Where's Daddy?", you're lucky if he says, "Gone, gone work," or something similar. The use of pictures of selected spondaic words is also helpful. Responses to the above stimuli are especially meaningful at a 30-dB HTL presentation level. Speech discrimination can be evaluated with children by using selected single syllable words appropriate for the child's age level. Examples of such a task are the Word Intelligibility by Picture Identification (WIPI), which enables the child to select a response from four or five pictured words, or the Reed Pictures Series, produced in the United Kingdom by the Royal National Institute for the Deaf.

Middle Ear Assessments

The assessment of middle ear function is a most helpful technique to use with infants and children. The feasibility and applicability of such measurements with children has been reported by many authors (Keith, 1973; Brooks, 1968; Jerger, Jerger, Mauldin, and Segal, 1974; Shallop, 1975; Bennett, 1975a). Middle ear function assessment should be routine for all infants and children with suspected hearing loss. The audiologist, otologist, and pediatrician will be the persons most likely to interpret and act upon results of such assessments.

Middle ear function assessment should include at least a tympanogram of each ear and, if possible and indicated, studies of the acoustic reflexes and Eustachian tube function. The assessment of middle ear function is not an audiometric procedure per se; rather, it is a procedure by which the status of the middle ear is determined by an electroacoustical approach. Additional applications and requirements of middle ear measurements have enabled its valuable use in the prediction of hearing loss in children, as proposed by Neimeyer and Sesterhenn (1974) and Jerger, Burney, Mauldin, and Crump (1974). This procedure has also been applied to the evaluation of Eustachian tube functioning by Bluestone, Berry, and Andrus (1974).

Electrical Response Audiometry (ERA)

In the past, ERA has had various definitions. As the term is used here, it simply refers to the procedures to measure the various evoked electrical potentials that are time-locked responses to auditory stimuli. These procedures include electrocochleography, brain stem evoked response audiometry (BSER), and cortical evoked response audiometry (CERA). It has become evident in the past few years that various levels of the auditory system can be assessed by the measurement of these various electrical potentials. Additional refinement and standardization of each procedure is presently in continued development.

ERA should not be viewed as the only assessement procedure; rather, it should complement behavioral assessments, particularly in cases of differential diagnosis or multipathology. Behavioral and ERA measures provide the diagnostician with comparative results and they provide the clinician with specific assessments to aid in prognosis. Some recent references are suggested regarding ERA procedures for further reading: electrocochleography (Ruben et al., 1976); BSER (Hecox and Galambos, 1974); and CERA (Barnet et al., 1975).

Criteria for Choice of Tests

In evaluating the hearing of infants and children, we must not take excessive amounts of time to perform many "tests." Many such tests may have relevance, but the question is, is it essential to traumatize a child in order to obtain results, or even to place him under an anesthetic simply to complete the battery? How relevant is it for the younger child that we complete a battery of tests in a short time span? Could we not give one test today, another test in 2 weeks, and another test in another 2 weeks, so that over a period of time each aspect needing evaluation is completed? Each test should be relevant to the condition presented. A benefit of this technique is that developmental changes could be observed.

The criteria for test selections should be based on the nature of the presenting problem and the sequential unfolding of the diagnostic impressions of the audiologist. If a history of middle ear problems is evident, then middle ear function should be one of the primary evaluations. If a history of congenital deafness is evident, then the selection of tests should be relevant to establishment of a clear diagnosis in this regard.

Case History and Developmental Assessment

While taking the case history, there should be continual observation of the child. The history taking should establish a bond between the doctor and the parent relating the history. If this is done sympathetically and quietly, the child will be in a more relaxed state. Observe the child and maybe, if different people are making noises, it can be seen whether or not the child responds. History taking also gives the child time to adapt to this new environment. If he begins to struggle to get down, let him down, and observe his voluntary behavior. It is often useful to place the parent and child alone in a room and to observe them remotely. Such information is very relevant indeed. If the child is put directly in a test situation and someone else who has not been observing behavior takes the history, very valuable information may be lost to the audiologist. Some audiologists may feel that taking a case history is something a clerk can do satisfactorily or that, in some ways, it is not important. Whoever takes the history should do the testing. It may be done under observation or supervision, but this person should be the one who maintains the rapport established during history taking.

During the history taking, observe carefully and ask all relevant questions: how long has he had this cold? How long has he had this inflamed eye? Does he always rub this ear? Is he teething now? He has this little red spot up there, hasn't he? I see he has a little birth mark, does he have any more? Where are they? How big are they? Is he walking yet? Has he always walked like this? All of these things are essential in a preliminary developmental assessment.

Developmental assessment should come before the testing and include the study of the child's ability to move around, his locomotive skills, and his general alertness. Look especially for his distractions and his ability to focus attention on anything placed before him. Observe how he approaches objects and try to make some kind of rough estimation about his ability to focus attention, and his alertness. A detailed developmental assessment may not be necessary, depending upon the reason the child has come for evaluation. If someone thinks he is deaf and, in fact, it is found that he has severe negative pressure, then there is not much point in doing a complete developmental assessment until the negative pressure has been dealt with. If the child then persists in being disinterested in sound, then obviously the investigations of the child must be intensified. Developmental assessments can best be performed by a multidisciplinary team including, where applicable, psychologic, educational, social, medical, occupational, speech-language, and audiologic evaluations.

REPORTING RESULTS AND RECOMMENDATIONS

Formulation of Diagnosis

In forming the diagnosis, emphasis should be placed on what has been discussed above. Diagnosis will probably not be a one-time procedure; it may be prolonged. It involves a team approach that is not simply the audiologist or the speech pathologist. Again, we stress the need for a distinction between the detection and the diagnosis of hearing loss. Detection merely identifies the child, whereas a diagnosis represents the beginning of the management procedures for the infant or child. All results and recommendations should be subsequently communicated to the parents and other professionals who are and will become a part of the child's future management.

Hearing Aid Evaluation

If the provision of a hearing aid is indicated, a hearing aid evaluation should be performed by an audiologist. Amplification benefit must be validated; in particular, one has to be assured that there will not be a deterioration of etiologic factors of a sensorineural nature or of conductive factors ranging from very simple things like impacted wax all the way to complex middle ear disorders. Perhaps it should be said that the rubella-deafened child and the cleft palate child are particularly prone to modification of middle ear function.

Hearing aid evaluation is a continuing process. The evaluation must be well planned from the very beginning. In other words, the auditory training aspect should precede the prescription of the hearing aid. A trial use of the hearing aid should also precede the prescription of the aid or aids. The aid should only be provided after trial and the child should not be traumatized. While wearing the hearing aid, the child should be observed for evidence of increased voice production and improved responses to sound. If it is a very young infant, increased vocalizations or improved responses to parents' voices should be apparent, and later on, discrimination should also improve.

The notion of hearing aid evaluation without carefully evaluating the ear mold is somewhat naive. Why should we remove the aid from its mold for testing? Ideally, hearing aid response characteristics and distortions should be measured from the ear canal of the hearing aid user. Such a technique may become more feasible in the future. It is not only the ear mold shape and quality of fit that are so terribly important but, in particular, the length of the meatal peg. Another point to be stressed is that the profoundly deaf child may be in receipt of two or three different qualities of signal. In school, he may have a group auditory trainer, an FM system, or a loop system. These may be in addition to, or instead of, the hearing aid. This needs to be taken into account when a hearing aid is provided for the child. In reality, the hearing aid may be worn only in the evening or during vacation time. On the other hand is the partially hearing child who is placed in an environment where there is a lot of ambient noise. We have to ask ourselves how helpful the aid is for speech discrimination in ambient noise. If the ambient noise is complicated by reverberation, then an additional problem exists. The term "hearing aid evaluation" may be a misnomer in some cases because although we do prior tests including responses to speech stimuli, we usually do not measure benefits of the hearing aid in noise or in reverberant conditions. Both of these conditions can and should be simulated in a hearing aid evaluation.

Whatever amplification procedures are recommended for a child, the audiologist is obliged to coordinate this important aspect of the child's habilitation. The reasons for amplification, as well as care and use of the hearing aid, should be effectively communicated to the parents. This can often be accomplished more effectively through the provider of the hearing aid, but the audiologist should provide effective follow-up. Complete details of the amplification recommendations should also be provided to the hearing aid dealer, the pediatrician, the otologist, and especially the child's teachers. Aside from the parents, teachers will have the most contact with the child and they should be thoroughly prepared to deal with the child and his hearing aid.

Parent Counseling

Parent counseling should begin before the child comes for diagnosis. Counseling, in many ways, has led the child to the first screening program, and counseling may have persuaded the parents to bring the child in for extended diagnosis. Counseling should be part of the extended diagnosis. Parents need to provide intensive support to a hearing-impaired child. If the parrents cannot give this kind of support, either for reasons of intelligence, occupation, or preparedness to work with the child, it may be best for the child to be educated in a residential school.

Ideally, the hearing-impaired child should benefit from living at home with his family. The family needs to be assisted so that they can provide the best possible emotional and communicative environment for the child. In a residential program, it would be helpful if a parent could accompany the child to school for the first few months and actually take on the role of a teaching assistant. This would enable the child and parents to adapt better to the entire situation, if it is necessary for the child to be placed in a residential program. It may also assure the school that overall educational objectives are carried out.

Preschool Training

Preschool training of the child should begin in the home as soon as the child has been detected, preliminary diagnosis has been completed, and the hearing aid has been fitted. There are various preschool programs that might be used as guides. In the United States such programs might include the John Tracy Clinic Correspondence Program when planned programming is not available locally through schools or some other agency. In England, the local school authority is responsible for this program and provides for preschool home instruction. There is movement in this direction in the United States, but unfortunately many hearing-impaired children are not presently receiving adequate preschool education. This fact is a particular burden for the parents and a detriment to the child.

Follow-up

Medical follow-up should be a routine part of the diagnostic process. A typical situation might be a rubella-deafened child who automatically is referred to an ophthalmologist and a pediatrician for investigation. If retinitis pigmentosa has been detected, then there should be automatic follow-up over an extended period, because there is considerable likelihood of visual deterioration. Unfortunately, there is nothing easier than to label a child as psychologically ill because he is hyperactive, hyperdistractible, or his language is delayed. However, careful follow-up of a child will help identify misdiagnosis and provide continual support to the child and family.

Once a child has been evaluated, the whole program is in continuing supervision and management. Audiologic follow-up should be routine for all hearing-impaired children. After a diagnosis has been validated and an educational program has been initiated, the parents should be encouraged to bring their child in at least annually. They should also be instructed to be alert for changes in auditory responsiveness that may be the result of hearing deterioration, middle ear dysfunction, or a malfunction of the hearing aid. Emphasis should be placed on awareness that conditions can deteriorate, and a child who was gaining 40–50 dB from his hearing aid is likely to lose that or most of it with a conductive overlay. A conductive overlay can easily exceed 30 dB. This, in addition to an already severe loss with the possibility of sound distortion, may cause many children to discontinue using their hearing aids. In the past, it has sometimes been a policy to prescribe a more powerful aid in such cases. This is inappropriate because if the child subsequently recovers from his conductive loss, he will then find that the aid is too powerful.

As stated at the beginning of this chapter, audiology is concerned with the management of all persons who suffer from sufficient hearing loss to affect their pyschologic educational, or career potential. The audiologist is obliged to provide follow-up for hearing-impaired children. Successful educational and habilitation programming are very dependent upon a continued accurate hearing assessment.

REFERENCES

Barnet, A. B., Ohlrich, E. S., Weiss, I. P., and Shanks, B. 1975. Auditory evoked potentials during sleep in normal children from ten days to three years of age. Electroenceph. Clin. Neurophysiol. 39:29–41.

Bench, J. 1968. Sound transmission to the human fetus through the maternal abdominal wall. J. Genet. Psychol. 113:85–87.

Bench, J., Hoffman, E., and Wilson, I. 1974. A comparison of live and videorecorded viewing of infant behavior under sound stimulation. I. Neonates. Dev. Psychobiol.

Bench, R. J., and Murphy, K. P. 1970a. The Papoisek cradle: a device for measuring babies' head movement responses to auditory stimulation. J. Laryngol. Otol. 84:521–523.

Bench, J., and Murphy, K. P. 1970b. Auditory rehabilitation with special reference to children. In: R. Hinchcliffe and D. F. N. Harrison, (eds.), Scientific Foundation of Otolaryngology. William Heinemann Ltd., London.

Bennett, M. J. 1975a. Acoustic impedance bridge measurements with the neonate. Br. J. Audiol. 9:117–124.

Bennett, M. J. 1975b. The auditory response cradle: a device for objective assessment of auditory state in the neonate. Symp. Zool. Soc. Lond. 197: 291–305.

Bluestone, C. D., Berry, Q. C. and Andrus, W. S. 1974. Mechanics of the eustacian tube as it influences susceptibility to and persistence of middle ear effusions in children. Ann. Otol. Rhinol. Laryngol. 83(II):1–8.

Brooks, D. N. 1968. An objective method for detecting fluid in the middle ear. Int. Audiol. 8:280–286.

Buchan, W. 1774. Domestic Medicine. pp. 500–502. W. Strahan and T. Cadell. London.

Conference on Newborn Hearing Screening. 1971. A. G. Bell Association for the Deaf. pp. 11–12.

Conway, S. M., and Shallop, J. K. 1975. Sound localization abilities of infants using the Murphy Chair. Presented at the Convention of the American Speech and Hearing Association. November 21–24, Washington, D.C.

Downs, M. P., and Sterritt, G. M. 1967. A guide to newborn and infant hearing screening programs. Arch. Otolaryngol. 85:15–22.

Eisenberg, R. 1976. Auditory Competence in Early Life, the roots of communicative behavior. University Park Press, Baltimore.

Elliott, G. B., and Elliott, K. A. 1964. Some pathological rediological and clinical implications of the precocious development of the human ear. Laryngoscope. 74:1160–1171.

Fulton, R., and Lloyd, L. (eds.), 1975. Auditory Assessment of the Difficult-to-Test. The Williams & Wilkins Company, Baltimore.

Jerger, J., Burney, P., Mauldin, L., and Crump, B. 1974. Predicting Hearing Loss from the Acoustic Reflex. J. Speech Hear. Dis. 39:11–22.

Jerger, S., Jerger, J., Mauldin, L., and Segal, P. 1974. Studies in impedance audiometry II. Children less than 6 years old. Arch. Otolaryngol. 99:1–9.

Keith, R. W. 1973. Impedance audiometry with neonates. Arch. Otolaryngol. 97:465–467.

Hecox, K., and Galambos, R. 1974. Brain stem auditory evoked responses in human infants and adults. Arch. Otolaryngol. 99:30–33.

Lidén, G., and Kankkunen, A. 1969. Visual reinforcement audiometry. Arch. Otolaryngol. 89:87–94.

Matkin, N. D., and Thomas, J. 1974. A longitudinal study of visual reinforcement audiometry. Presented at the Convention of the American Speech and Hearing Association, November, Las Vegas.

Miller, J. 1967. Personal communication and demonstration to K. P. Murphy at Kansas University Medical Center.

Murphy, K. P. 1962a. Ascertainment of hearing in children. Panorama, 3.

Murphy, K. P. 1962b. Development of hearing in babies. Child and Family, 1.

Murphy, K. P. 1973. Deaf children with assitional difficulties. In: E. Kampp (ed.), Evaluation of Hearing Handicapped Children. Fifth Danavox Symposium, Ebeltoft, Denmark.

Murphy, K. P., and Smyth, C. M. 1962. Responses of Fetus to Auditory Stimulation. Lancet 1:972–973.

Neimeyer, W., and Sesterhenn, G. 1974. Calculating the hearing threshold from the stapedius reflex for different sound stimuli. Audiology 13:421–427.

Niswander, P. S., Ruth, R., and Speilberg, S. E. 1976. Testing the Hearing of Children. Nisonger Center, Columbus.

Northern, J. L., and Downs, M. P. 1974. Hearing in Children. The Williams & Wilkins Company, Baltimore.

Reddell, R. C., and Calvert D. R. 1967. Conditioned audiovisual response audiometry. Voice. 16:52–57.

Ruben, R. J., Elberling, C., and Salomon, G. 1976. Electrocochleagraphy. University Park Press, Baltimore.

Shallop, J. K. 1975. The measurement of middle ear function. In: S. Singh (ed.), Measurement Procedures in Speech, Hearing and Language, pp. 279–321. University Park Press, Baltimore.

Simmons, F. B., and Russ, F. N. 1974. Automated newborn hearing screening, the Crib-o-gram. Arch. Otolaryngol. 100:1–7.

Sontag, L. W., and Wallace, R. F. 1935. The movement response of the human fetus to sound stimuli. Child Dev. 6:253–258.

Suzuki, T., and Ogiba, Y. 1961. Conditioned orientation reflex audiometry. Arch. Otolaryngol. 74:192–198.

Swannie, E. M. 1966. Impedance Audiometry in Clinical practice. Proc. R. Soc. Med. 59 (10):971–974.

Wilson, W. 1978. Sensory assessment: auditory. In: F. D. Minifie and L. L. Lloyd (eds.), Communicative and Cognitive Abilities—Early Behavioral Assessment. University Park Press, Baltimore.

Disordered Functions Approach to Audiologic Diagnosis

Henry Tobin

CONTENTS

This chapter is among the first to take a disordered functions approach to standard audiologic diagnostic practice. This approach presumes that the responsibility of the audiologist rests largely in the area of audiologic habilitation. Professor Tobin differentiates between the disordered systems approach to audiologic diagnosis, in which the audiologist is providing an essential service for the physician, and the disordered functions approach in which the audiologist holds the primary responsibility for case management. The emphasis throughout this chapter is on audiologic habilitation and the diagnostic information necessary to meet this responsibility.

The chapter establishes the principles for approaching audiologic diagnosis from the disordered functions point of view. Many of the procedures available in the test battery commonly used by the audiologist can still be used, but with certain modification of technique, leading to a different final goal. The shortcomings of some of the standardly used tests are discussed, including the problem of relating the audiometric data currently generated for real life communication functioning. The purpose behind the disordered functions approach is to determine signal processing capabilities of the hearing-impaired individual and his potential for signal processing and communication in general. The results of the assessment are intended to be used for the planning and implementation of audiologic habilitation. Regardless of whether the reader agrees with Professor Tobin's premise, this chapter represents a unique contribution to the literature by discussing the role of the audiologist as the professional charged with the comprehensive audiologic habilitation of the hearing-impaired individual.   —Eds.

AN OVERVIEW

Introduction to Audiologic Diagnosis

The role of the audiologist   Through the years that the human develops, evolves, and ultimately declines, his interaction with the also changing environment and a changing social milieu presents him with conditions that require constant adaptation, habituation, and other forms of learning governed by fresh situations and new rules. As it is said, "The only thing that is constant in life is that there is nothing constant." Our task in this chapter on diagnosis in audiology (the 6th year through adulthood) is to specify the role of the audiologist in this life process.

In this chapter the audiologist will be seen as a professional primarily engaged in providing a unique educational service based on his knowledge of the science of hearing. The diagnostic responsibilities associated with this service at times will be supportive of medical as well as psychologic evaluation. However, the primary diagnostic role of the audiologist will relate to the speech perceptual-communicative needs of individuals with hearing impairment, and the unique expertise, training, and insight audiologists can bring to such problems. Audiologic habilitation is the raison d'être of audiologic diagnosis.

The objectives   Audiologic habilitation is a term intended to signify a comprehensive service meeting the needs of hearing-impaired people from birth through advanced age, those whose hearing loss is congenital as well as those whose hearing loss is acquired, those who were prelingual when hearing was impaired as well as those who were postlingual when hearing was impaired. Audiologic habilitation is intended for those with residual hearing as well as for those without residual hearing, those with temporary hearing losses, changing hearing losses, permanent hearing losses, and even individuals with a need for a hearing loss. It encompasses individuals with central as well as peripheral auditory problems.

Audiologic habilitation is concerned with helping the hearing-impaired individual improve his speech perceptual-communicative adequacy. It has as its major objectives:

1. Helping the hearing-impaired individual evolve the rules of language, i.e., the rules as they pertain to the phonologic, morphologic, syntactic, and semantic levels of language as well as the idiomatic structure of the language,
2. Meeting the language-communicative needs and desires of the hearing-impaired individual, and
3. Helping the hearing-impaired individual speech perceive and speech produce language in its natural form.

The stages of audiologic habilitation   Four fundamental stages can be defined for carrying out audiologic habilitation. Audiologic diagnosis is inherent in all four stages, i.e., assessment, planning, implementation, and re-evaluation. The description of these stages follows.

1. Assessment of the hearing-impaired individual's communicative status, which includes determination of:
   a. his knowledge and current use of the rules and idioms of the language
   b. his ability to meet his current communicative needs
   c. his auditory signal processing and ability to perceive and produce speech
   d. his listening strategy
   e. his criterion or willingness to receive and respond to messages
   f. his ability to use amplification or other aids and the appropriateness-efficiency of such amplification or other aids,
   g. his psychosocial and physical problems and related needs
   h. his speech perceptual-communicative problems related to learning disabilities and central difficulties in perceptual, integrative, associative, and retrieval processing that some hearing-impaired individuals may exhibit
   i. his listening-speaking function when he is required to communicate in noisy environments, distracting situations, and over various distances
2. Formulation of remedial plans to meet the evident needs of the hearing-impaired individual as shown by the assessment including

means of improving communication and resolving associated educational, social, and vocational problems
3. Implementation of remediation, which includes carrying out the therapy or teaching plans according to the desires, needs, and interests of the hearing-impaired individual
4. Continuing evaluation of remediation and reassessment to determine changing needs of the hearing-impaired individual.

The above represents the basis for diagnosis in audiology and is the framework for the subsequent approach to audiologic evaluation and techniques that follows. A comparison of our taxonomy for assessment with that provided by the American Speech and Hearing Association Committee on Rehabilitative Audiology (1974) finds ours to be without direct reference to testing for site of lesion. Determination of site of lesion can be inferred under item 1c in the outline.

Historical Perspectives and Directions

Man undoubtedly has been aware of the functional consequences of hearing loss since quite early in his existence. Today he generally still assesses his own problem if it is severe enough. He can tell his physician or audiologist that he is not hearing well and he can define the conditions under which he has the greatest difficulty. He even may be aware of the general site of lesion. He is not so much concerned about what the problem is as what we can do about it. To do something about it we require information of two types: the site of lesion, and the rules and strategies of communication that he is currently employing to cope with his hearing problem. It was not until the first century that we began to see writings concerned with the site of lesion. It was centuries later before any aspect of communicative adequacy was investigated. In the early 1800s Itard, director of the Institute for the Deaf in Paris, demonstrated the application of hearing tests for the study of progress being made through auditory training (Feldmann, 1970).

The disordered functions approach to diagnosis   Today both the otologist and audiologist are concerned about hearing management. They approach their respective roles differently. The physician is concerned about the medical implications of the site of lesion and what can be done about it medically. The audiologist is concerned about the functional implications of the site of lesion and the consequences it presents for audiologic habilitation. We can differentiate between a disordered systems approach to diagnosis, generally associated with the role of the physician, and that of a disordered functions approach often associated with the role of the audiologist. These approaches are depicted in the following analogy.

The human and his journey through life can be likened to that of a spacecraft plummeting onward, changing direction and mode of operation to fit changing circumstances and goals. Accompanying this "spacecraft" might be two crewmen. One who can fix things when they go wrong, although there are always limits as to what can be done to correct maladies in flight, and the other who can teach the individual how best to operate according to new rules when an uncorrectable flight malady has occurred. If we limit ourselves to communication difficulties associated with an auditory problem, we see that once the physician has done all that can be done to correct the physical malady of the ear, it is then that the audiologist assumes case management and tries to help the individual devise techniques for steering the communication spacecraft.

The search for the site of lesion   In recent history we can view diagnosis in audiology as progressing through three overlapping and continuing phases: the 1950s saw us searching for the site of lesion; the 1960s was devoted to predicting the course of hearing impairment; and the 1970s, to trying to determine signal processing and its effects on the rules of language. Each of these three areas continues to serve as a focal point for research in audiology. Because of the time and effort devoted to it, it is not surprising that we have made our greatest gains in our search for the site of lesion.

Compared to the 1950s we are now quite sophisticated in our attempts to establish site of lesion. There are still shortcomings. We still lack precision in the identification of the location of central auditory lesions, and we still can be fooled by various combinations of peripheral or central lesions. We still lack norms for many of our central tests. We have not agreed upon the tools to use or the structure of these central measures (Keith, 1977). In central testing we emphasize the use of the speech signal and tend to disregard the use of nonspeech signals that may be just as effective or more effective, particularly in the presence of confounding peripheral problems.

We are in greater agreement in evaluation of the periphery, but there is the tendency to use traditional tools that may be irrelevant, unproductive, or even invalid for our diagnostic goals. Bone conduction measurement still remains a troublesome procedure, but may be supplanted to a great extent by impedance audiometry (Feldman, 1975). We continue to use pure tones as the bastion of audiology.

Some even infer site of lesion based on the audiogram. The reception of pure tones is certainly not species-specific to the human. Continued overdependence on pure tones to the neglect of speech signals undoubtedly has had a retarding effect on the field of audiology (Bilger, 1973).

We can employ behavioral audiometry as well as so-called objective audiometry for evaluating the periphery. In general we are not in need of objective audiometry, except for impedance audiometry, for establishing presence of hearing loss or site of lesion for the people in the 6th year through adulthood category. These procedures are expensive, time consuming, and often unreliable (Mendel and Harker, 1974; Russ and Simmons, 1974). This notwithstanding, brain stem evoked response audiometry (Reneau and Hnatiow, 1975) and electrocochleography (Ruben, Elberling, and Salomon, 1976) have proved useful in special situations. Impedance audiometry (Jerger, 1975; Feldman and Wilber, 1976) is indispensible at this time and is probably the most important step forward in the last 20 years in our search for the site of lesion.

Predicting the course of hearing impairment   Among the earliest questions asked by our hearing-impaired clients is "Will it get worse?" Some of the response can only be provided medically, but some answers can be obtained through audiometric data. The answers and the methodology used to derive them are not representations of absolutes. Serial hearing measurement (Macrae, 1968; Jacobson, Downs, and Fletcher, 1969; Downs, 1976) still represents the best way to establish trends. It can tell us about changing threshold caused by overstimulation by a hearing aid, the effects of noise exposure, the improvement over time or following otosurgery of a hearing impairment with a conductive basis, and progressive losses caused by presbycusis, systemic problems, late onset hereditary losses, and losses of unknown origin. The relative speed at which the hearing seems to be changing can be inferred, permitting the impact for social adequacy to be estimated and the development of strategies for audiologic habilitation to be initiated.

The most notable effort to predict the course of hearing impairment is the work devoted to establishing damage risk levels (Ward, 1963; Kryter, 1973). We now have tables for damage risk that relate type and level of noise to the exposure times that are tolerable. Damage risk tables represent the best current guidelines for those exposed to noise, although they are still limited as predictors of individual differences.

Serial tympanograms are now being used to follow the course of middle ear problems. For individuals with chronic middle ear difficulties, frequent routine screening by impedance audiometry is used in an attempt to spot the problem in its early stages (Feldman, 1975).

Speech audiometric tests also have been used to follow improvement or degradation of speech perceptual performance (Bergstrom and Thompson, 1976). This has been the least systematic and the least successful approach to predicting the course of hearing loss, but it is appealing because of the face validity that speech provides in relation to social adequacy. Thus far we have no good method for relating any of our audiometric data to real life functioning.

Signal processing and effects on the rules of language   Schubert has pointed out that there is "...an astonishing dearth of terms about audition—terms that reliably describe what people hear. Almost all the terms people do use to describe what they hear are specific to the source of the sound" (Merzenich, Schindler, and Sooy, 1974, p. 151). In other words, we know very little about the processing of signals, particularly speech signals. Audiology, unlike psychology, has never gone through the introspective phase of investigation (Graham and Ratoosh, 1962). The hearing-impaired individual does not seem to know how to describe his auditory experiences, and we need to develop language that will permit this form of introspection.

Only in the last few years have we begun to re-evaluate speech audiometry. Most of the materials traditionally used in speech audiometry were not designed for the evaluation of hearing-impaired people. They were designed for the evaluation of telephony and other types of communication systems (Bilger, 1973). They tell us little or nothing about how the individual is using the auditory rules of language, i.e., the prosodic and phonemic structure of the language, or what his potential might be for the processing of speech. Clinically, we have begun to study speech processing for phonemic error patterns or confusions that occur when individuals are asked to respond to speech materials that can be confused. The basis for this work was well established through experimental studies done in the 1950s (Peterson and Barney, 1952; Miller and Nicely, 1955).

We continue to lag in the application of basic research findings, but we are moving in the right direction and momentum may be increasing. We are beginning to see the clinical application of such psychoacoustic standbys as masking level difference (Goldstein and Stephens, 1975; Olsen, Noffsinger, and Carhart, 1976; Bocca and

Antonelli, 1976), temporal processing (Sheeley and Bilger, 1964; Wright, 1968; Gengel and Watson, 1971), critical bands (Scharf, 1970; Flottorp, Djupesland and Winther, 1971; Jerger, Burney, Mouldin and Crump, 1974; Niemeyer and Sesterhenn, 1974), directional hearing (Link and Lehnhardt, 1966; Tonning, 1975; Bosastra and Russolo, 1976) and binaural hearing (Moncur and Dirks, 1967; Carhart and Tillman, 1970) for the study of signal processing capabilities.

There are many things we have yet to do to meet the diagnostic needs of our hearing-impaired clients. We tend to want to do the things we did and use the tools we know just because that is how we have been doing it. We need to overcome this form of inertia and employ an armamentarium of tests and measures based on the needs of our client and the relevance and usefulness of our tools.

APPROACHING AUDIOLOGIC DIAGNOSIS

Principles of Audiologic Evaluation

The role of the psychophysicist   It has been said that the primary role of the psychophysicist is the defining of his signal. Without a clear and precise understanding of the parameters of the signal he is using, the audiologist can say little about the response that he obtains. In his role as a psychophysicist the audiologist manipulates the four attributes of sound, i.e., frequency, intensity, time and spectrum, and the figure-to-ground relationship referred to as the signal-to-noise ratio. We need to remind ourselves that every auditory event, including speech, can be defined according to these physical attributes. Imprecision in signal definition often leads to equivocal diagnosis or worse yet, misinformation.

Signal definition is not a simple matter. Many audiologists think they are avoiding this responsibility by the purchase of commercially packaged audiometers whose characteristics are supposed to be within the limits specified by the American National Standards Institute (1969). Aesthetic packaging does not guarantee the performance characteristics of the instrument nor is it a substitute for understanding its limitations in terms of signal parameters and paradigms that might be needed for presentation (Melnick, 1973). The days of the audiologist as the rugged individualist devoted to understanding his equipment and making conscious decisions about his signal seem to have been forgotten. We need to retrieve this by reminding our-

selves of our role as psychophysicist and psychoacoustician. Sources
that may be of use to the reader are Hirsh (1952); Rosner (1962);
Harris (1969); Ventry, Chaiklin and Dixon (1971); Harris (1974);
Marks (1974); and Green (1976).

Psychophysics is the study of the responses of organisms to various
stimulating configurations. It should be kept in mind that we really
are not dealing with a stimulus-response situation. It is more appropriate to say we are dealing with a signal-to-response paradigm.
As audiologists we are limited to the presentation of signals that (it
is hoped) are perceived as stimuli and elicit some particular responses.
In classic terms the psychophysical experiment can be represented
by the following formula: $R = f(S)$, i.e., the response is a function
of the stimulus. With that portion of the new psychophysics, known
as the theory of signal detection (TDS), we now recognize the complexities of the stimulus. What is a necessary and sufficient stimulus
for one person may not be enough for another person, regardless of
his sensitivity. Stimulus implies all the factors that are operating and
converging on a listener at a given moment. Because of this we are
limited in our ability to define the stimulus. We can only define that
which we can completely control, the signal. (The terms "stimulus"
and "signal" as used here are at variance with the typical way they
are used in the audiologic literature. TSD does not differentiate between the use of these terms in the manner shown. It is the author's
intention to show that these terms can be used to depict the physical
event, the signal, and the psychophysical event, the stimulus. Webster's Third New International Dictionary, the unabridged version,
does not clearly delineate between these two terms. The term "stimulus"
is, however, associated with physiologic change, whereas the term
"signal" is not given this direct association. The term stimulus is
being used in this chapter in a manner similar to that employed by
Gibson (1966): "A stimulus may specify its source, but it is clearly
not the same thing as its source" (p. 28).

Signal specification must include the spectrum of the wave form,
duration, level, rise-decay rate, signal-to-noise ratio, and distortion.
In addition, if the signal is not automatically controlled, the vagaries
of the audiologist using the signal-generating device must be known
and appreciated. Such things as the duty cycle, which includes the
on-time of the signal and the intersignal interval, the rhythm pattern,
and the pacing of the listening trials will all have an effect on the
observer. The instructions, the tedium of the task, and the personal
interaction and rapport with the examiner are important variables.

All of the abovementioned factors have a cumulative effect on the observer, his response strategy, response criterion, and ultimate response.

TSD and listener response criterion   Our knowledge of TSD forces us to re-evaluate the response phase of our paradigm. Response is not an all-or-none phenomenon. It is graded and is confounded by the listener's response criterion. Although the methodology of TSD is rarely used for clinical purposes, (it is too time consuming), we need to be aware of the theoretical implications. Classical psychophysics did not devote much attention to the observer's response. As audiologists, even if we are not directly measuring it, we need to be thinking about the criterion the individual has adopted for a particular response. This criterion may shift because of changing conditions of the signal, fatigue, attitude, or just the reverie that the observer may be going through at that moment.

Pure tone audiometry, although overused and limited because of the form of the signal, can serve as a model for the application of the spirit if not the total methodology of TSD. The least complicated psychophysical response paradigm is the single interval or yes-no decision. Many researchers prefer the forced choice multiple interval experiment in which the signal can appear in any one of two or more intervals. The forced choice procedure tends to reduce the influence of criterion. As currently practiced, pure tone audiometry does not allow for single interval or multiple interval observations. Response is limited to some kind of indication when a signal has occurred, but no conscious indication when it has not occurred. TSD assumes two signal conditions: signal-plus-noise or noise alone. Noise exists in every listening situation. The noise may be from external ambient sources, or from internal physiologic noise. It may be generated intentionally through the signaling device, or unintentionally as some form of distortion. Regardless of the source, noise always exists and needs to be included as an alternative in the response paradigm.

TSD and audiometry   The search for "threshold" represents a vigilance task requiring a high degree of attention. In general, we probably can make do with the typical methods of collecting threshold data. However, if we need a technique that aids in maintaining attention, differentiates between noise and signal-plus-noise conditions, and in addition permits us to use each potential presentation for the evaluation of signal processing and response criterion of the observer, then single interval or multiple interval responses may be worth pursuing. This approach might be needed when tinnitus is present,

when the observer is unfamiliar with auditory signals because of congenital deafness, or when there are special problems such as central
hearing loss, exaggerated hearing loss, or retardation. Although best
done automatically (Levitt and Bock, 1967; Mahaffey, 1975), it would
not be difficult to manually indicate to the observer when the signal
interval was going to appear. The observer would be required to provide a yes-no response or an indication in which interval the signal
appeared. Because the chance score for these type responses is 50%,
we should establish at least a 75% criterion for acceptable performance.

An element of TSD to be added to the Carhart-Jerger (1959)
recommendation for the use of the Hughson-Westlake modification
of the method of limits procedure might involve nothing more than
the addition of an observation interval. The scenario for such a revision follows. We should start, if possible, with a signal preview at
whatever level is clearly perceivable to the listener. The simplest
method for doing this is to ask the observer when the signal is at a
comfortable level. The next step is to quickly bring the signal down
to the listener's inaudible level. The quick search for this level should
establish the "ballpark" area of threshold. The ascending approach
toward threshold can now begin in 5-dB steps. Once a response has
occurred, the traditional adaptive technique of dropping 10 dB and
coming back up in 5-dB steps should be followed. The use of 5-dB
steps for pure tone measurement is clinically within the range of
appropriate precision. The yes-no approach permits us to observe
the influence of criterial factors, and is the easiest to administer manually (Dember, 1964). This form of response should be required for
each observation interval. The examiner shows the time domain of
the signal in a manner similar to that used in studio broadcast cueing.
He raises his hand and forefinger alerting the observer to the im-
pending presentation of the signal. The observation interval is indicated by pointing the forefinger at the listener. The hand is brought
back to the starting position indicative of signal termination and the
beginning of the response interval. Dropping of the hand ends that
trial. If we use a 1-sec alerting interval, a 1-sec observation interval,
and a 3-sec response interval, we have a total of 5-sec per trial, which
is clinically quite acceptable. This could be somewhat longer or shorter
depending upon the speed of response or reaction time of the observer. The trials can be individually paced to meet the special needs
of the elderly, the child, the uncertain observer, and others. The
instructions to the listener should include the explanation that the

signal will be presented most of the time; some of the time the signal will be too weak for them to hear it, and occasionally there will not be a signal presented. When they think they hear the signal, they should indicate "yes"; if not, "no."

If signal-plus-noise is presented and the individual indicates that he hears it, we credit him with a "hit." If signal-plus-noise is presented but he apparently does not hear it, this is called a "miss." If noise alone is presented and he indicates he does not hear the signal, he is credited with a "correct rejection." If, however, the observer says "yes" when noise alone is presented, we consider this to be a "false alarm," and an indication of some kind of criterial problem that will need attention.

In 1948 Pollack reported two paralleling threshold curves, one for tonality and the other for audibility. Variability of response for both types of thresholds was apparently the same. The appreciation of tonality required a greater energy level than audibility. In traditional measurement it is unclear which threshold the observer is indicating, an additional source of variability. In TSD the threshold task is really a difference limen rather than a search for the elusive absolute threshold. In the yes-no and multiple interval approaches the issue of tonality threshold versus audibility threshold is removed. The signal-plus-noise is always being compared to the apparent noise alone category. Clinically this is important for inexperienced listeners (the deaf), some individuals with central problems, as well as others who do not have a complete appreciation of tonality (individuals with cochlear implants seem to fit this category).

Threshold The modification of the traditional procedure that has been described for the clinical application of an aspect of TSD by no means provides us with a complete statistic of threshold. "Threshold," in clinical practice, has never really been the energy level that has elicited a response from the observer 50% of the signal presentation time. A more realistic operational definition for clinical threshold might be the lowest energy level that generally elicited a correct response from the observer during that particular evaluation session. Over the years the pure tone audiogram came to represent the inferred physiologic status of that individual's hearing mechanism compared to the inferred status of the hearing mechanisms of a large group of otologically and, it is hoped, otherwise healthy young adults who had had minimal life exposure to noise (Corso, 1958; Egan and Clarke, 1966). "Threshold" never was what it was thought to be, and we need to be reminded of this. There are no perfect answers in clinical measurement, only approximations. The reader may refer to Campbell, to Taylor and Creelman, and to Levitt for examples of more precise application of TSD to audiometry (Campbell, 1965; Taylor and Creelman, 1967; Campbell and Moulin, 1968; Levitt, 1971). The application of TSD to the clinical realm, even in an incomplete form, is long overdue (Clarke and Bilger, 1973).

Tests and measures   Psychophysics interests itself in things that are measurable, i.e., $R = f(S)$. In this measurement task we have no preconceived notion about the response we will obtain. If we specify or measure all the attributes of the signal, we can supposedly define the response according to the signal parameters. Audiologic evaluation is not just concerned with measures; it also uses tests. In a test the signal becomes a function of the expected response, i.e., $S = f(R)$. For example, if the signal were $1 + 1$, the expected response would be 2. A test usually provides a percent correct score, and an indication that something is right or wrong. We get no right or wrong answers in psychophysical measurement, only a posteriori relationships.

Most of speech audiometry, as generally practiced today, is in the form of tests (Hirsh, Davis, Silverman, Reynolds, Eldert and Benson, 1952; Tillman and Olsen, 1973). Tests are a priori in nature and depend on our insight and value judgments for appropriateness. For example, if we wanted to evaluate how well a particular telephone receiver worked compared to several other handset receivers, we could administer some kind of speech test to a large group of normal listeners, such as a list of monosyllabic relatively familiar words in the form of an identification task (Egan, 1948; Hirsh et al., 1952). Several lists of these words might be used for each receiver. In addition, we might select another speech test of similarly selected words for comparison of tests. From the number of subjects to whom the tests were administered, the number of versions of the two tests per subject per receiver as well as across receivers, and the repetition of these different tests for each receiver over a few days we could derive a reasonably strong statistic of some measure of central tendency that would permit us to state, within a specific degree of confidence, which telephone receiver was best. Because of the large number of forms of the two similar tests administered as well as the number of times these tests were repeated for each telephone receiver, we can evaluate the similarity of the different versions of the two tests as well as the tests' reliability or repeatability, i.e., whether the tests give us essentially the same distribution of values for the data across the several days that the tests were used. Knowing that the supposedly parallel or equivalent forms of each test are in fact similar and that the tests are reliable, we now have some evidence supportive of the internal, construct, and criterion forms of validity. Internal validity can be inferred if the several versions of each test produce similar responses that are highly correlated. Construct validity can be inferred if the two different tests produced essentially similar responses. In order to meet the criterion for criterion validity we have to accept some amount of circular reasoning. Criterion validity is said to exist if the test devised is able to predict the success or level of performance established as the criterion for success. College entrance exams are an example of this. Because only those who meet the criterion are accepted, we cannot know if others who did not meet the criterion could have achieved success. Our criterion in the case of the telephone receivers was to systematically differentiate their potential effectiveness as part of a communication system. Our tests permitted us to do that, but we still do not really know if the receiver we have selected as being the best is in fact best under all conditions relating to speech signal processing. Criterion validity only taps a portion of behavior and cannot be generalized to all behavior. In other words, face validity, also referred to as content validity, may still be in question. The assumption has been made that the processing of relatively familiar monosyllabic words can in fact represent speech processing in general. (The reader may notice the similarity between the testing just described and that which is often used in hearing aid evaluations for differentiating among wearable amplifiers.) Face validity, or content validity, a deceptively simple concept, is really the most crucial for establishing a truthful and meaningful test. The other forms of validity will not stand if the basic assumptions are false, regardless of the consistency or reliability of the tests that are used (Thorndike and Hagen, 1967).

Audiologic tests, as a general class, are more difficult and troublesome to use than measures. The clinical assumptions made on the basis of tests need to be put in perspective. Tests do not permit us to make specific or general assumptions about the signal-processing abilities of individuals. Tests are of little help in establishing the individual's auditory language ensemble, i.e., the prosodic and phonemic rules actually employed by the individual. The prosodic and phonemic rules described by linguists (Jacobson, Fant and Halle, 1952; Chomsky and Halle, 1968) are represented differently for hearing-impaired individuals. Tests generally are based on the assumption that everyone uses auditory language rules according to the way normal hearing individuals use them. Phonetically balanced word lists are an example of this premise. The premise may only be true for an individual who has had normal hearing at least through the adolescent years and has been in the language mainstream of society. Even for this individual it may not be true. Hearing impairment has changed the rules of language and listening. Auditorially things cannot be the same as they were.

A complaint that is often heard about tests when we try to apply them clinically is that they are insensitive. That is, people get either too high or too low scores on a given test. When we try to use the percent correct values to differentiate among conditions, as for the evaluation of telephone receivers, we are trying to use the test as if it were a measure. Because we cannot really define the signal, we cannot make a measure. It is often assumed that if we are to use tests for purposes of differentiating conditions, it would be desirable that the scores obtained fall somewhere within the mid range. This is thought to permit us to see change in direction when we change conditions. The tests should be difficult enough so that they provide clinical sensitivity. However, a 76% score for an individual may be no more useful than a 96% score, if all that has been done is shift the location of the variance without also providing the possibility of a change in variance related to the observation variables. It must also be remembered that these tests still do not necessarily tell anything about real life functioning (Carhart, 1965).

There are other approaches to speech audiometry that seem to be clinically useful. In the last several years closed-response sets of rhyming words requiring a discrimination task have come into increased clinical use (Fairbanks, 1958; House, Williams, Hecker, and Kryter, 1965; Black, 1968; Kreul, Nixon, Bell, Kryter, Land, and Schubert, 1968; Owens and Schubert, 1968; Pederson and Studebaker, 1972; Wang and Bilger, 1973; Jones and Studebaker, 1974; Sher and Owens, 1974). Several versions of rhyming single syllable word lists, generally referred to as the Modified Rhyme Test (MRT), are available. None of these lists taps the complete phonemic ensemble, nor do they examine the phonemes in the most clinically useful way. As with other speech materials, their original purpose was the evaluation of communication systems. However, the arrangement of the foils in each set permits us to derive confusion matrices for the phonemic oppositions. The phonemic error patterns that can be derived from the confusion matrix, although incomplete, represent a measure of speech signal processing capabilities. The rhyming signals in a closed-response format, although complex and confounded by the very nature of speech, can be defined with more precision than the traditionally used open set materials.

Most MRT lists use a closed-response set of six opposing words for each trial, thus providing a 16% chance score for each word as well as an overall 16% score for the speech audiometric measure. The MRT has been used with profoundly hearing-impaired individuals in three communication modes; look-alone, listen-alone, and the combination of look-and-listen. Knowledge of the chance score permits us to measure the relative contribution of audition to speech processing for these observers. With the MRT there is no a priori assumption of how the observer will process the speech signal, nor should we have a preconceived notion of how he should; after all, perception is still in the private domain of the listener. Paraphrasing an observation made by Arthur House (Levitt and Nye, 1971, p. 75): light cannot convince the blind; sound may not convince the deaf.

It would be nice to have a speech audiometric measure specifically designed for hearing-impaired people that would yield clinically useful data. The essential criteria for such a tool should be as follows. We should be able to derive multifaceted information about the speech signal processing of the observer. This should include both his current abilities and his potential. The procedure should be easy to administer, of reasonable length, and sufficiently challenging so that interest can be maintained. It should be structured so that tedium is avoided. The material should be in the form of a closed-response set of not more than 7 ± 2 items, which is well within the channel capacity for most individuals for speech-related materials (Miller, 1956; Corliss, 1971; Liberman, Mattingly, and Turvey, 1972). We would then also have the advantage of a known chance score. The foils in any set should deviate from each other in a systematic way and only by the number of variables that can be displayed in a confusion matrix. The error patterns derived from the confusion matrix should elucidate something about the phonetic processing that the individual is able to use. The materials should be such that anyone 6 years of age or older should be able to manage. The materials should be general enough to be applied across all subcultures and dialects within a language area such as encompassed by English. They will need to be easy enough so that even foreign born individuals with a limited knowledge of the phonemic rules of English or deaf individuals with limited oral language experience could be quickly trained to perform the task. The materials should be such that they have little or no meaning, so that the observer is forced to analyze differences based on phonetic structure rather than on a phonemic or other linguistic basis. The presentation should be recorded so as to avoid problems of reliability introduced by live voice. This also will permit more complete definition of the signal. The response could be in the form of a pencil-and-paper response with the individual circling the item in the set that he thinks is appropriate, or better yet, the response could be automated. For some individuals with physical handicaps we may need to use communication boards or other special arrangements. The material should lend itself for use under different and difficult listening conditions, producing clearly different percent correct scores and phonetic error distributions. Male and female talkers as well as children's voices should also be used with these materials. The Articulation Gain Function (Miller, Heise, and Lichten, 1951) for this material should exhibit an essentially linear rise as the signal-to-noise ratio approaches more favorable listening conditions. The material should be able to be used at different intensity levels so that a Performance-Intensity Function (PI) (which can be clinically useful) can be displayed for the observer (Speaks, 1967; Jerger and Jerger, 1971). The material should be organized in such a way as to permit criterion measures to be made on it. This should be particularly helpful during the course of training when individuals are trying to determine their maximum processing capabilities for these types of materials.

Nonsense syllable materials (Fletcher and Steinberg, 1929) seem the most likely candidates to meet the criteria we have set forth. The nonsense syllable measure developed by Resnick (Resnick, Dubno, Hoffnung and Levitt, 1975; Resnick, Dubno, Hawie, Hoffnung, Freeman, and Slosberg, 1976) seems to have considerable merit for clinical application. It follows a presentation format in which there are many trials of each signal item. The signals are presented in random order, and they are represented an equal number of times. The closed-response format of the nonsense syllable procedure is a true discrimination task. The multiple uses and measurement features of the nonsense syllable procedure are appealing. As it is applied clinically we will have the opportunity to evaluate its usefulness.

Objectivity   Among the issues that are raised regarding tests and measures is the quesion of "objectivity." We are told that in order to be good, a test or measure should be "objective." It also is inferred that the only audiologic tests or measures that are objective are those designed to elicit an electrophysiologic response.

There are four criteria that must be met for objectivity. There is no audiometric procedure that meets all of these criteria. To be completely objective the procedure must require no overt purposeful response from the observer, the observer must not be able to cause intentional or unintentional artefacts of measurement that can go undetected, the procedure should be automated so that it is not under the control of the examiner who can introduce a considerable number of variables, and finally the results should be so explicit as to require no interpretation on the part of the examiner. Obviously there will never be a completely objective procedure in any area of measurement. In audiology we have degrees of objectivity, none of which is any guarantee of validity.

Table 1 displays the relative objectivity for seven audiologic procedures. The pluses and minuses are not indications of goodness or badness, only a relationship to objectivity. Those procedures that show both plus and minus for the interpretation of response indicate the existence of elements of subjectivity as well as objectivity. The objective procedure is generally considered a reliable procedure. Our experience with evoked response audiometry indicates that reliability is not always attainable (Goldstein, 1973). Usually the more standardized the procedure, the more reliable it is, and the more objective it is. Standardization requires that the method of signal presentation, the response form, and the scoring be precisely fixed so that the same procedure can be used at different times with the same individual and different individuals, the same examiner and different examiners, at the same place and at different places. If the traditional approach to speech audiometry routinely included (as it should) recorded signal presentation, then all seven procedures in Table 1 could be considered as standardized methods, regardless of how closely they approach the ideal of objectivity (Hirsh, 1952; Chronbach and Meehl, 1955). This description of objectivity and standardization differs from others (Goldstein, 1973) in that response form and response artefacts are considered an integral part of the procedure.

Variability of response   All measurements attempt to classify things and put them in their proper order. With the human, we need to consider at what point in his experience his data are most representative of his true behavior. Logically, asymptotic behavior should be sought. However, we know performance is statistical and practice effects exist. Depending upon the degree of accuracy or appropriate precision we seek, it may require a few hundred trials to achieve asymptotic performance related to simple tasks. More complex tasks

Table 1. Relative objectivity for selected audiologic procedures

Criteria for Objectivity		Audiologic procedures						
		Conventional pure tone audiometry	TSD-modified pure tone audiometry	Conventional speech audiometry (PB lists)	Nonsense syllable speech audiometry	Békésy audiometry	Evoked response audiometry	Impedance audiometry
Presentation form	Examiner controlled	−	−	−	+	+	+	+
	Automated							
Response form	Overt—voluntary	−	−	−	−	−	+	+
	Covert—involuntary							
Response artefacts	Not always detectable	−	+	−	+	+	−	−
	Usually detectable							
Interpretation of response	Examiner decision	−	− +	−	+	− +	− +	− +
	Without examiner decision							

may require several sessions, and very complex tasks may continue to show observer improvement over several thousand trials. Also, the reliability of the response cannot be used to determine whether the observer was performing near his maximum level of capability (Robinson and Watson, 1972). This is because of motivational or criterial factors. We will have to establish pragmatic considerations. "A difference, to be a difference, has got to make a difference" (Van Riper, personal communication).

As clinicians, it is our responsiblity to decide what is acceptable and what is unacceptable in performance. There is, in fact, acceptable variability as well as unacceptable variability. We are more willing to accept criterial forms of variability from someone inexperienced in listening than from someone whom we believe has some particular need to obfuscate. We can accept the variability shown by those who have fluctuating middle ear problems or someone with Meniere's Syndrome, and, with some experience, we learn to understand the variability shown by someone with a central auditory problem.

Some of the variability in our clients' performance arises from our unwillingness to spend the time necessary for conditioning, motivating, and training these individuals. Among the sources of help that we have ignored is the payoff condition of TSD (Green and Swets, 1966). Payoff can be in the form of a reward or punishment, depending upon whether the individual is assuming too strict a response criterion and needs encouragement, or too lax a criterion and needs to be discouraged from precipitous response or too many guesses. Until the willingness to respond or criterion level can be estimated, it is generally best to permit the observer to establish his own operational level. If that level seems to need change, we can then attempt to modify it. For the school-age child, actual rewards can be used and a game made of responding. For the adult this can also be done, but usually a tangible reward is unnecessary. The challenge of playing the game may be enough, particularly as they are provided feedback about their performance. The initial phase of any type of listening task may require feedback information. If automation is unavailable, this can be done by the examiner simply nodding or shaking his head. For the individual with criterial problems it may be necessary to review his relative success rate with him after the initial training phase.

Response bias   The assumption should not be made that only those individuals with nonorganic aspects to their hearing problems demonstrate criterial problems. Anyone who is unfamiliar with the rules involved in the processing of a signal can have this problem. This includes the congenitally deaf individual as well as the postlingual, adventiously hearing-impaired individual who is confounded by a change in listening rules and who does not know how to fit what he remembers into what he hears now. Part of the consequences of hearing loss for all people, including the receivers as well as the senders of messages, is the criterial problems that arise. Criterial problems are not trivial matters, and they need to be studied by the audiologist if he intends to effect positive change in his observer.

There are times when it would be helpful to know the relative contribution of criterion to the response. This process can be formalized. TSD permits us to isolate the effects of response bias. In TSD the response bias or criterion level is referred to as the beta level (β). Thus a threshold of detectability (d') in TSD would be said to be β-extracted, i.e., the contribution of response bias has been removed from the overall performance. The data obtained from an observer on some listening task can be plotted in the form of what Swets (1973) calls the relative operating characteristic (ROC). " The ROC is a curve whose overall location corresponds to a particular degree of discrimination, while the position of any point along the curve represents a particular degree of bias in the report" (Swets, 1973, p. 991). For details of this analysis the reader is referred to Green and Swets (1966) and Swets (1973). There are two types of ROC curves that can be generated. Type I ROC involves a signal-to-response contingency, and is the approach typically used in experimental audiology. The type II ROC is derived by a response-to-response contingency (Pollack, 1959). The type II approach has been generally less acceptable in experimental audiology because it is not as clearly definable mathematically as the signal-to-response contingency. It involves asking the observer not only to give a response to a signal but also to rate his confidence in his response. The four-celled matrix for a response-to-response contingency is shown in Figure 1. A hit is credited to the observer when he correctly identifies the signal and rates his confidence in his response as positive. A miss occurs when he gives the right response to the signal but fails to believe he is right. A false alarm occurs when he is incorrect but believes his identification was correct. A correct rejection is a failure to identify the signal correctly and at the same time realizing his response was inappropriate. Each cell in the matrix shows the simple computation necessary to derive the percent value for that response condition.

Despite experimental limitations, the type II ROC can be clini-

Response to the Signal

	% Responses Correct	% Responses Incorrect
+	# plus/# correct HIT	# plus/# incorrect FALSE ALARM
−	# minus/# correct MISS	# minus/# incorrect CORRECT REJECTION

Confidence Rating of Responses

100%   100%

Figure 1.   Response-to-response contingency matrix. Derivation of the four-celled response-to-response contingency matrix. (Consult TSD sources for calculating d' and β.)

cally useful. For example, whenever we attempt to derive a PI function, as with open-set monosyllabic words, we are faced with the possibility of significant changes in β as the speech intensity is raised to high levels. Observer intimidation may become a criterial factor at these high levels. Egan, Greenberg, and Schulman (1961) noted that hit rates could drop under certain conditions while sensitivity remained essentially the same. This occurs when the false alarm rate also drops. This is attributed to criterial changes and is associated with a rise in the correct rejection rate. It is possible that percent correct scores obtained with monosyllabic words can show this same effect for some individuals. We need to investigate the possible association of response bias to rollover demonstrated by PI-PB functions. It is not clear what this association will be, but individual criterial differences can be expected.

Order effect is a well known form of response bias. This usually is controlled by counterbalancing test materials and the ear to which the materials are presented. However, a response-to-response contingency task also may have to be administered if we are to separate critierion from sensitivity or acuity. If the signals we are presenting are considered unpleasant, too difficult to follow, or boring, the observer may consciously or unconsciously withdraw from the listening task. Assuming that the right ear was tested first and then the left ear, we might find significant differences that turn out to be criteria related. The left ear might show poorer response than the right ear. In this case it could be that the individual knew what to expect and was having difficulty accepting the task. For another individual it might have worked in just the opposite fashion. Knowing what to expect, because of previous experience on the other ear, he now performs better. As audiologists we need to be alert to the response changes we may provoke in our observers either through our manner, the testing ambience, the ordering of tasks, or the unpleasantness of the signals we generate.

Type I and type II errors   Audiologic diagnosis is akin to hypothesis testing in statistics. TSD in fact derives from the statistical theory of probability. Audiologic diagnosis is decision making and this involves hypothesis testing. Two major hypotheses confront us in our form of diagnosis: something is or something is not. In relation to these two hypotheses we can and do make two types of errors. The type I error (α) is made when we reject the significance of a finding or condition, i.e., there really was a problem and we failed to recognize it. We established our level of acceptance of significance at such a stringent criterion point that we failed to appreciate information that could help in the diagnosis. This includes subtle responses that we tend to overlook, as well as clear responses that we ignore because we are unfamiliar with the tools, or fail to understand their meaning. Because of the crudeness of our procedure, we may be afraid to believe what it can tell us. Audiologists also have been known to act as if data did not exist when applicability or recommendations for audiologic habilitation based on the audiologic diagnosis were not yet apparent. The type II error (β) is made when we attribute significance to a finding, when in fact the true condition is either not what we thought it was, erroneous, or trivial in nature. This β is directly related to the β we use in TSD. To a very great extent the TSD β is controlled by the false alarm rate. The type II error is essentially describing a false alarm situation. As audiologists we need to minimize type I errors and be willing to make type II errors. Clinically, it is better to err toward the side of too many positive findings than to fail to meet a client's needs. With the use of a battery of procedures and repeated measures we can usually correct our type II errors. The type I errors are often lost clinically and are not corrected. The reader wishing to pursue the theoretical basis for the testing of statistical hypotheses may find the discussion by Winer (1962) helpful.

Averaged data   In addition to other concerns about measurement, we need to proceed cautiously when trying to associate individual performance with averaged data. The example of the limits of interpretation for damage risk tables has already been mentioned. In a study on the perception of dichotically presented vowels Weiss and House found their results supporting "the idea that, when a group of listeners is assembled essentially at random, the individuals **may differ considerably in ear preference, making it difficult to generalize about population ear preferences when responses are averaged** for a number of listeners" (1973, p. 55). With averaged data it is possible for only a few listeners to skew the results. The complexity and alternatives for response also need to be considered. For dichotic listening, Weiss and House identify six different response patterns available to the observer, any one or combination of which an observer may tend to use: "(1) no response; (2) one correct identification; (3) one incorrect identification; (4) two correct identifications; (5) two responses, consisting of one correct identification and one incorrect identification; and (6) two incorrect identifications" (1973, p. 55).

Tests are dependent upon normative data for interpretation. It is difficult to talk about deviation if there is no norm for a comparitor. Acceptance of normative data cannot be made without interpretation of how the data were collected, the range of subjects, the effects of individual differences on the norms, the comparability of testing conditions (both the facilities currently being used and those under which the normative data were collected), the congruence of testing materials (the same or similar and how similar; and if recorded, is it a first-, second-, or third-generation recording). Normative data generally represent a range of supposedly acceptable responses. In **many cases we will have to use the individual as his own control and reject the hypothesis of responses within normal limits.** This may occur when the two ears of an individual seem to be considerably different, although both are still within the so-called normal range.

Under those circumstances, and maybe under all circumstances, we need to ask, "Normal for whom?" Properly controlled normative data can help in the interpretation of responses, but they are no substitute for understanding the task and the individual's idiosyncratic behavior.

Examiner bias It is known that preconceived notions about an observer can affect the test as well as measurement results. The examiner's response criterion, although generally not as difficult to control as the listener's response criterion, can have a distorting influence on audiologic diagnosis. Before even seeing the client, we have often begun to form ideas about the nature of the problem, its severity, how difficult the observer will be to test, and so forth. This is not altogether negative; however, we must be careful not to involve ourselves in some kind of clinical self-fulfilling prophecy. Our expectations may cause the audiologic problem to seem better or worse than it really is. Our bias could lead to misdiagnosis. It may cause us to overlook more significant problems, or problems which, because of our bias, we consider trivial. What may seem to be a trivial problem to the audiologist may be the critical problem for the client. It is often assumed that a high frequency hearing loss or a unilateral hearing loss will not have a major impact on an individual's life. However, it may be just that problem, coupled with the individual's life style and communication demands, that needs our attention. Our expectations may cause us to ignore or consider irrelevant certain findings that may be important in the overall audiologic diagnostic picture.

Among the criteria that can influence evaluation are age, socioeconomic status, sex, race, otologic diagnosis, and empathy with the client. The cuteness of the child, the attractiveness of the individual, or unwillingness to be objective are other factors that can lead to errors of leniency or severity. We want to bend over backwards to give the benefit of the doubt to someone we find likable. Rynes (1969), in a study of examiner bias in auditory data collection, found both an additive and a subtractive effect for the factors of age and otologic diagnosis. If an elderly person was supposed to have a sensorineural loss, he was found to perform at a lower level than the elderly person with a supposed conductive loss, even though the actual performance was the same. The subjects, both experienced and inexperienced audiologists, were asked to evaluate recorded speech recognition responses to CID W-22 words spoken by difficult-to-understand subjects whose voices would not reveal their ages.

When subjects were informed of age and otologic diagnostic factors, subsequent scores were assigned that reflected preconceived notions about performance. The experienced audiologist tended not to be as greatly influenced by age as the inexperienced audiologist. Both, however, showed an expectancy bias favoring the conductive loss. The chief means of controlling examiner bias is awareness. In addition, procedures that require the least interpretation should be employed.

The anamnesis and the examiner as a good listener   Throughout this discussion of the principles of audiologic evaluation, measurement techniques and associated problems have been stressed. A major portion of the assessment that assists in differential diagnosis is the anamnesis, which includes all the information and background concerning the client that may help to analyze his difficulty. The anamnesis is a reminiscence of previous and current communication experiences, felt needs, as well as a general case history.

The anamnesis provides the opportunity for the audiologist and the client to establish rapport, explore matters that relate to disordered systems and disordered functions in audition, and express general concerns related to perceived needs. The anamnesis should be considered as the beginning of audiologic habilitation. The audiologist is not only exploring relevant aspects of the auditory problem and providing information about audition and signal processing, but he is also providing the understanding, acceptance, and other forms of counseling necessary during this highly vulnerable time for the client. Positive regard and commitment to the helping relationship must be apparent to the client. We must be particularly cautious not to impose our own value system upon the client, his life style, or situation. We owe the client unconditional acceptance. The reader may find the discussions by Rogers (1951, 1961) helpful.

The anamnesis is often used for the development of a hypothesis relating to the client's problems and needs. It is this hypothesis, based on the anamnesis, the rapport, interpersonal attitude, and clinical intuition and experience, that affects the selection of first approximation clinical procedures. If we control for examiner bias, the hypothesis testing approach can be helpful toward establishing a differential diagnosis. The uncritical approach that uses a routine battery of tests, regardless of the client, can be deceiving. The initial procedures should be thought of as screening for purposes of testing the hypothesis. If the individual fails some aspect of the screening battery, this should lead toward other procedures that may define more clearly the nature of the problem.

We are all familiar with the assertion in audiology that no one test or measure gives all the information needed for diagnosis. A battery of tests and measures is needed. Signal processing, particularly speech processing, is a complex perceptual task. We need to observe behavior associated with varying kinds of signal presentations. In addition to this we need to add the human ingredient. The examiner should be a good listener and observer. It is the catamnesis, or follow-up to the anamnesis, that will cause us to confirm or reject the initial hypothesis. The catamnesis should be thought of as an ongoing process that occurs during the active assessment phase, immediately following it, and at more remote times when we try to determine whether our last hypothesis and course of action was appropriate. Time often has a way of providing answers that are not obvious during the initial phases of assessment. The catamnesis should also be thought of as the process of active listening during and between formal evaluations. Although introspective terminology is limited, we can still learn a lot by asking our observers what they heard and then giving them the time to explain their experiences as fully as possible. It is often something that is said or the manner of response that suggests the need for hypothesis modification and the selection of other evaluative tools.

Diagnosis for Audiologic Habilitation

The communication process For an individual with a communication problem of an auditory nature, it seems that rehabilitation is possible only if the disordered system, the ear, can be fixed, i.e., made to operate essentially as before. As audiologists we really do not rehabilitate; we habilitate. Rehabilitation implies the return of a system to a prior desirable state. Habilitation implies coming to terms with the disordered system and making the best possible accommodation to the situational demands for functioning. This is true whether the functional difficulty was of a congenital and prelingual origin or occurred after the auditory rules of language were established.

The individual with the postlingual adventitious loss faces new rules for signal processing of the auditory language. The signal still is encoded in the same way, but the stimulation is different. If the hearing loss continues to change over time, the rules for decoding the language continue to change, often without the individual being aware of it. For the individual with congenital loss the rules evolved in an idiosyncratic fashion, but even here the rules may not be invariant. Every time the individual must change his amplification system, his hearing aid, he may find that several months go by before he adjusts to the new unit. The adjustment process involves the relearning of the auditory rules of language.

An example of shifting rules, one that can continually fluctuate for some individuals with severe losses, is the /i/ sound. The average first formant for adult males is about 270 Hz, and the second formant is around 2,290 Hz. This may present little, if any, problem for individuals with hearing in this second resonant frequency range. However, if confronted with an adult female voice, the rules may shift sometimes or always, depending upon whether the observer has hearing at 2,790 Hz, the second formant for a woman. The 500-Hz difference may be a difference that makes the difference. The shifting fundamental frequency during inflectional excursions will also cause some shifting of the formant structure bringing the second formant of /i/ in and out of focus for some individuals. Clearly, the child's voice and formant structure will present similar problems for many hearing-impaired individuals. If the child is himself hearing-impaired, he may not be able to appreciate the rule for /i/ even for his own production of the sound. It may be years before he will have an opportunity to appropriately monitor his own production of the formant rule for /i/. By that time he may have internalized a rule for /i/ other than the one typically used by normal hearing individuals. The shifting or modification of rules for the phonemes is a universal problem for all but the conductively hearing-impaired individual.

The communication process is complicated for the hearing-impaired individual and the person trying to talk to him. Figures 2, 3, and 4 are an attempt to show the communication process that goes on between the audiologist and listener with the auditory problem. The communication process is displayed in flow chart fashion using the block diagram model of Shannon (Shannon and Weaver, 1949). The model is depicted in three parts. Figure 2 shows the variables and criterion for communication associated with the role of the audiologist and the role of the hearing-impaired listener. Figure 3 shows the many things that can go wrong at each stage in the communication process. Figure 4 depicts the clinician-client interchange of information. Factors and questions that relate to audiologic diagnosis pervade the three-part model.

The first part of the model (Figure 2) lists several forms in which a signal can be transmitted. Typically, a message is transmitted as a multidimensional display. The audiologist needs to be aware of the coincident and paralleling signals that are conveying information. Signal processing may involve several of the factors listed under "Transmitter." The signals that we transmit can be analyzed so that we know the several variables that can effect response. The signals must be delimited so that we can determine specific signal processing ability.

It is hoped that the signal is received as a stimulus. The receiver is quite complicated. We are dealing with an auditory system that anatomically includes an external ear, middle ear, inner ear, auditory nerve, central auditory pathways, an auditory cortex, and association areas. In addition, this system has the following characteristics. It is a distance receptor responding to frequency, intensity, time, and spectral parameters of acoustic signals. It receives afferent as well as efferent stimulation. It is binaural and expected to extract signal from noise as well as to localize sound sources. It is tonotopic, i.e., neural auditory structure is organized in a systematic frequency arrangement. It responds to very quiet as well as very loud sounds. It is expected to process rapidly changing auditory events that, once produced, apparently cannot be retrieved or naturally scanned again. It is thought to show a species-specific bias for speech, although it is also called upon to process environmental sounds, machine produced sounds, and music. We often require it to interact with an amplifying system that affects signal perception because of its frequency response, gain, maximum power output, and distortion characteristics. We expect it to have the capability of a short term as well as a long term holding mechanism so that we can put together segments to form words, words to form sentences, and so that we can retrieve previous speech experiences. As complicated as the auditory system and the signals that it must process are, we also have other modalities (particularly vision and the haptic senses) that often must interact with this system for signal perception. All of this is confounded by the observer's age, experience with audition, speech and language, strategies, and criteria for signal processing. The response capabilities of the auditory system also can be viewed based on the kinds of learning that can take place. The principle types of learning that we are aware of are adaptation, habituation, conditioning and trial and error learning. Our view of the response capabilities of the auditory system is attributable largely to our current limits in tapping this system, rather than the complete characteristics that it may possess.

The second part of the model (Figure 3) lists the factors that interfere with the communication associated with the audiologist

SOURCE → TRANSMITTER → Signal in Channel → RECEIVER → DESTINATION

Audiologist Encodes Message for Purpose of:

1. Communication with client:
   a. to develop rapport
   b. to convey information
   c. to take case history
2. Identification of auditory disorders
3. Assessment of auditory status and communication efficiency
4. Synthesizing a therapy plan which meets the evident communication needs and desires of the client
5. Implementing audiologic habilitation including:
   a. selection of appropriate prosthetic devices
   b. counseling and guidance
   c. training methods for learning rules of language
   d. applied techniques for improvement of social adequacy and quality of life
6. Reassessment and modification of audiologic habilitation management
7. Seeking answers to research questions

Message Form Transmitted Via:

1. Speech mechanism:
   a. providing language information
      (1) phonologic
         (a) prosodic
         (b) phonemic
      (2) morphologic
      (3) syntactic
      (4) idiomatic
      (5) semantic
   b. providing paralanguage information
      (1) affective
      (2) stylistic
      and characterized by:
      (1) Pitch
      (2) Loudness
      (3) Duration
      (4) Tempo
      (5) Rhythm
      (6) Stress
      (7) Inflection
   c. providing non-language information
   d. producing speech and non-speech acoustic signals live-voice or recorded
   e. producing speech and non-speech speechreading signals live or recorded
2. Visual Clues:
   a. gesture
   b. body kinesics
   c. proxemic distance
3. Tactile-kinesthetic clues:
   a. touch
   b. tactile-kinesthetic analog of acoustic signal
   c. electro-tactile analog of acoustic signal
4. Situational-contextual clues

Message Form Received Via:

1. Auditory system which:
   a. anatomically includes:
      (1) external ear
      (2) middle ear
      (3) inner ear
      (4) auditory nerve
      (5) central auditory pathways
      (6) cortex
      and
   b. has the following characteristics:
      (1) it is a distance receptor responding to frequency, intensity, time and spectrum parameters of acoustic signals
      (2) it receives afferent-efferent stimulation
      (3) it is binaural
      (4) it is tono-topic
      (5) it responds to very quiet as well as very loud sounds
      (6) it is species-specific for speech and often must interact with
   c. an amplifying system which affects signal perception due to its:
      (1) frequency response
      (2) gain
      (3) maximum power output
      (4) distortion characteristics
2. Other modalities which include:
   a. visual sense
   b. tactile-kinesthetic sense

Listener with Auditory Problem Decodes Message for Purposes of:

1. Communication with audiologist:
   a. to determine extent, nature and resolution of his problem
   b. to gain information
2. Improving communication abilities:
   a. by learning how to extract information from limited acoustic clues
   b. by learning to effectively utilize the rules of language
   c. by improving ability to perceive speech and produce speech for better communication with hearing individuals
   d. by learning to listen effectively through amplification
   e. by improving ability to use visual and tactile-kinesthetic clues
   f. by improving ability to use situational-contextual clues
   g. by improving ability to communicate via manual communication
3. Promoting psychological well-being, social adequacy and the quality of life

5. Manual communication:
   a. sign language
   b. fingerspelling and signed English
   c. cued speech
   d. other
6. Visual materials:
   a. written language
   b. actual objects
   c. representational materials
7. Acoustic signals not produced by speech mechanism:
   a. music
   b. non-musical sounds
   c. creature produced sounds
   d. other environmental sounds
8. Special teaching devices
9. Non-speech language systems

Figure 2. Audiologic habilitation: a flow chart of the communication process.

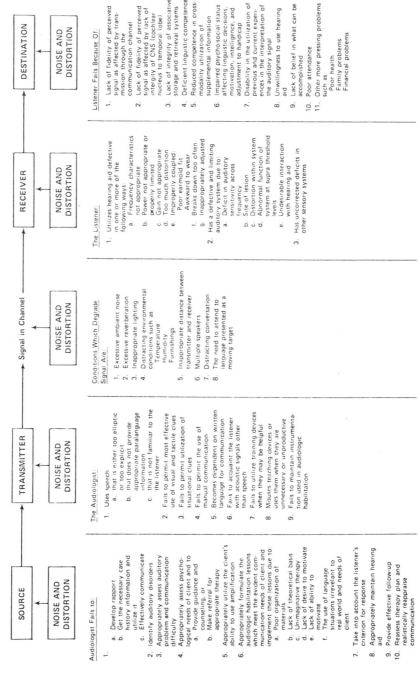

Figure 3.   Audiologic habilitation: factors leading to a decrement in listener performance.

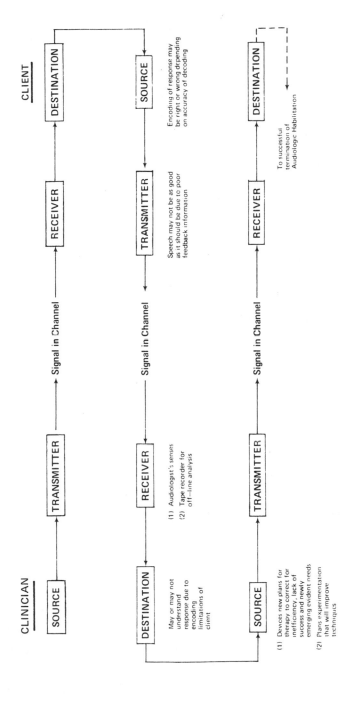

Figure 4. Audiologic habilitation: the speech production-speech perception inter-change. The model can be used to represent both short term as well as long term goals. The simultaneous interchange of information between the clinician and client is recog-nized but not depicted in this model.

and his client. It can be used as a checklist in a disordered functions approach to audiologic diagnosis. Conditions that degrade the signal are listed under *Signal in Channel*. We need to know how these conditions degrade communication for a hearing-impaired individual.

The third part of the model is a reminder of the reciprocal process of communication. The audiologist is not only concerned about the messages he is sending; he also is just as concerned about the messages he is receiving. Figure 4 should be read by the following the *arrows*.

The performance evaluation   The complete realm of audiologic habilitation, i.e., assessment, planning, and training, can be categorized under 10 headings. These are:

1. Intensity
2. Time
3. Frequency
4. Spectrum
5. Signal-to-noise relationships
6. Listener-speaker strategy
7. Listener response criterion
8. Contrast
9. Opposition
10. Redundancy

These 10 categories can subsume all of what we now consider, and probably all that in the future will be considered, within the realm of audiologic habilitation.

In our role as psychophysicists we are concerned about defining our signal, i.e., the four attributes of sound and the signal-to-noise ratio. As audiologists concerned with audiologic habilitation we need to know how our hearing-impaired observer processes the parameters of sound under different listening conditions. The signal we are particularly interested in is speech. We can categorize the auditory rules of language according to some distinctive feature system or we can view the features according to their acoustic production. For simplicity we can use the four attributes of sound to depict the auditory rules of language. Thus intensive rules of language can be categorized as stress and accent. Timing rules relate to durational and rhythmic patterns of speech and to the syllable. Both intensity and time rules of speech are produced and controlled by the lungs and associated musculature. Frequency is produced by the laryngeal system, and we derive intonational and voicing rules of language from it. Paralanguage information of vocal pitch for identification of age and sex of the speaker is also derived from frequency. Time and intensity also play a role in affective and stylistic aspects of paralanguage, as does frequency. The length of the vocal tract, the width of the vocal tract, and the place of major constriction as determined by the placement of the tongue determine the spectral production. Spectrum can be used to describe the elements of speech that are referred to as phonemes. Time, intensity, and frequency completely describe the prosodic features and rules of speech; spectrum, the phonemic rules.

Signal-to-noise relationships can refer to signal processing with various kinds of noises. The presentation may be in sound-field, or diotic or dichotic if under earphones. If two ears are involved and the phase relationships of the signal and noise are manipulated, then binaural unmasking becomes a consideration. Room acoustics and reverberation are factors in signal processing particularly if a hearing aid is involved. These factors, and amplification systems, are included under the category of signal-to-noise relationships.

Listener-speaker strategy includes all those things that a hearing-impaired individual does to communicate. A hearing impairment has consequences for speech production as well as speech perception. We need to examine both aspects of communication behavior. The three major categories of learning, i.e., adaptation, habituation, and conditioning, modify our approach to communication. We are generally unaware of the strategies that we adopt for communication under varying kinds of conditions. The assessment should explore this aspect of communication to determine if inappropriate strategies are being used.

Listener response criterion influences response in real life as well as in contrived assessment conditions. The importance and relationships of this factor to the assessment have been indicated earlier in this chapter. The assessment should explore the modification of criterion behavior that may improve real life functioning. We will need to determine if the listener is in a speech-receiving mode or in an analytic type mode. (House, Stevens, Sandel, and Arnold, 1962).

If our goal is to determine or modify rules of language, there are only two ways materials can be presented, i.e., by contrasting or opposing them. The simplest contrasting task is the same-different task. In the contrasting task the materials that are to be contrasted are presented in close proximity so that the observer can make some judgment about the relative similarities and differences and the attributes of the signals. In the opposition task the observer draws upon his auditory memory of things that logically might be opposed when he is presented with one item from this possible set. The MRT lists are examples of opposition tasks. The observer hears one word and must select out of a closed response set of six words the one to which it comes closest, based on how he thinks it was encoded and which mental model or engram provides him with the best match.

Finally, the assessment will need to determine which methods for restoring redundancy will be best for a particular hearing-impaired observer. Hearing problems reduce the redundancy of the message. We can, through visual and tactile means, restore some of this redundancy. Look-and-listen as well as comparable look-alone and listen-alone tasks will have to be used to suggest the relative contribution that speechreading might make.

Audiologic assessment should be a predictor of communication adequacy. It is not enough to know what the individual is doing now; it is what he may be capable of doing that is important. Diagnosis is here defined as the investigation or analysis of the cause or nature of a condition, situation, or problem and it is intended to lead to action. The disordered functions approach to diagnosis should lead to an indication of etiology and an audiologic habilitation plan based on the functional cause of the problem and the evident needs of the hearing-impaired individual.

The performance evaluation includes both those procedures that have gained some acceptance through experimentation and clinical trial, and those procedures that have had limited application. In addition we are faced with many gaps in the disordered functions armamentarium. Figure 5 displays in cuboidal fashion a language-related evaluation and training protocol. It is adapted from a two-dimensional display by Erber (1977). The model in fact has many more than a dozen dimensions. Those speech-related stimuli that we display certainly are not exhaustive for speech. The display does not show our concern for other auditory experiences. The listing under *Transmitter* in Figure 2 is more complete. The criterion to be used for choosing materials, particularly as they exhibit semantic content, is not at all clear. Many choices are available, and they may be equally appropriate. We certainly want the materials to be within the experiential background of the observer. The materials could be displayed in an auditorily explicit fashion, i.e., clearly produced although not assuming pedantic characteristics, or they could be produced in some elliptic manner ranging from normal uncareful production to highly slurred and distorted production. The materials

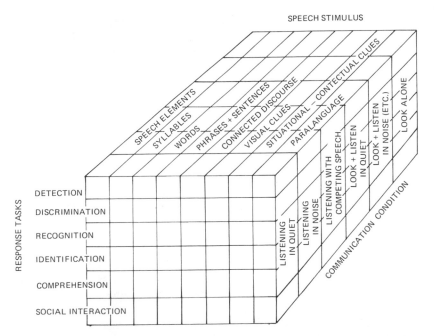

Figure 5.   An Evaluation and Therapy Matrix. All communication tasks and situations can be displayed by this cuboidal matrix. Evaluation and therapy may include open as well as closed set materials. The materials may be presented in an explicit manner or in an elliptic manner. Listener Response Criterion and Listener-Speaker Strategy exists in all communication situations and needs to be considered for each cell. (The matrix is adapted from a two-dimensional display by Erber (1977)).

can be in either an open or closed set. The communication conditions in this model also are not all inclusive. We can and should use different types of noise or competing messages at different levels of presentation. We also may wish to explore tactile-kinesthetic inputs, cued speech, or signing in a simultaneous communication form. The response tasks we have included are: 1) detection—a sensitivity measure that involves an indication of presence or absence of some signal; 2) discrimination—considered an acuity measure requiring the observer to differentiate between or among stimuli; 3) recognition—which requires a report indicating the message, and is achieved by providing a set of signals that are matched to a target signal; 4) identification—the same as the recognition task but the alternatives are unspecified; 5) comprehension—requires some indication of understanding of the message; 6) social interaction—requires performance in a communication interchange. For discussion of tasks 1-4 the reader may wish to consult Dember (1964, pp. 16–26). Other response tasks also could be required. Rosenblith and Vidale (1962) consider reaction time data as among the most sensitive indicants of sensory-information processing. In addition to all of these considerations each cell within the cuboidal matrix requires evaluation of listener response criterion and listener-speaker strategies. Clearly it is not possible to do all of these things with every client or any client. We should let the needs of the client determine the range of signal processing procedures that will be used. For many of the cells within this model, tests and measures do not yet exist.

THE REPORTING OF RESULTS AND RECOMMENDATIONS

The Need to Effect Change

The individual The purpose of audiologic assessment is to effect some positive change in the individual. It is of little help to him if all that can be said at the end of the evaluation is what he already knew before he came in, i.e., "You have a hearing problem." The evaluation process itself should have been a learning experience for the listener. Assessment is not just the precursor for habilitation, it can be the start of habilitation. Each evaluative procedure provides another opportunity for systematic listening and discussion of the perceptual experience. By the compeltion of the evaluation phase the client as well as the audiologist should have a better understanding of signal processing abilities and potential.

Each individual has a different reason for wanting audiologic assessment. Some individuals want to understand their problem better so they seek information. Others want confirmation of their problem and reassurance that what they are doing is what they should do. In many cases they want to continue to do nothing, and some want to believe that nothing can be done anyway. Others are seeking a sympathetic person who understands their problem, although they really do not expect help. A formal treatment program is not necessary for everyone nor is it acceptable to many who might benefit from it. If the assessment phase has been designed to educate the observer, then it should be natural to structure the discussion of results so that in essence it is a continuation of a short term hearing orientation program. The assessment and discussion of results should form a hearing orientation program that covers the following areas: 1) the educational, social, vocational, and interpersonal consequences of hearing difficulty; 2) signal processing, particularly speech processing, limitations, and likely potential; 3) the basics of the anatomy and physiology of hearing and fundamentals of acoustics; 4) the potential benefit of a hearing aid with some opportunity for informal trial; 5) the listener's response criterion; 6) listener-speaker strategies that can be employed to improve communication functioning; 7) special devices (for telephone, television, and other situations) that can assist a hearing-impaired individual; 8) environmental restructuring for better communication; and 9) methods to improve interpersonal relations through open and frank discussion of the individual's hearing impairment, education of those with whom he must communicate, and an appropriate degree of assertiveness.

If the assessment and follow-up discussion includes this orientation program, then very few individuals will not have gained something from audiologic evaluation regardless of their initial motivation. The orientation program can be as long or as short as it seems appropriate. Portions of it can be presented via captioned video tape. Aside from that portion of the orientation program that is integrated into the assessment, no one should be required to participate. Audiologists will find few unreceptive individuals in the 6th year through adulthood category. Materials, of course, will have to be modified so that all individuals can gain maximum benefit from an orientation program. There is sometimes the tendency to exclude the young school-age child from discussions about his hearing problem. He, above all, has to cope with it and deserves as much information as he can use to improve his communication situation. The hearing-impaired individual has a right to know and we are obliged to help him understand as much as possible about the auditory problem. It is important that we leave our client with a clear sense of direction and a feeling of closure. The individual needs to know what our recommendations are and how he can implement them or how we intend to implement them. If audiologic habilitation is needed, the details need to be arranged. Similarly, if further medical management or consultation is called for, this needs to be arranged.

Others and the environment   The hearing-impaired individual is rarely an island unto himself. He generally has family, friends and colleagues with whom he must interact. These individuals may also need to understand the consequences of hearing impairment. Except in the case of the child, how and what information will be conveyed to the family and others will be largely determined by the hearing-impaired individual himself. In the case of the child the parents or guardians generally determine who will receive information. The teacher, principal, school nurse, speech or hearing clinician, psychologist or guidance counselor may need to be apprised of the nature of the hearing problem. The physician, preferably an otologist or other appropriate specialist, may need to be informed in the case of both the child and the adult.

If the problem falls within the realm of audiologic habilitation, the audiologist will maintain case management and try to serve as an advocate for the hearing-impaired individual. If the problem is essentially medical or if extensive counseling seems necessary, case management should be transferred to the appropriate service. As the hearing-impaired individual's advocate, the audiologist is expected to represent the needs of his client to educational programs, health and welfare agencies, and occasionally to employers. He should know the laws that may assist his client. Matters that the audiologist appropriately can discuss on behalf of his client and at the request of his client must pertain to audiologic habilitation. In his role as advocate the audiologist is trying to improve the communication situation for his hearing-impaired client. In discussion or exchange of information with other service professionals the audiologist will need to have the permission of the client for matters that are of a confidential nature.

Audiologic intervention on behalf of our client may involve studying his home, school, social, or work environment to determine sources of communication problems. Recommendations should then be made on how these problems can be corrected, or how the hearing-impaired individual can modify his own attempts to improve the situation. Structural changes generally are costly and unrealistic as a recommendation. Induction loops, ear protectors, accoustical treatment of rooms including carpeting and drapes, and special seating and lighting arrangements generally are appropriate as recommendations.

Whenever there is a hearing impairment and the issue is largely a matter of a disordered function (a speech receptive or speech productive problem), audiologic management and intervention are appropriate. There is no one more qualified for determining educational placement, establishing needs, and developing and carrying out programs for the hearing-impaired school-age child than the audiologist. Similarly the audiologist is the most qualified individual for meeting the audiologic habilitative needs of the complete range of adult hearing-impaired individuals.

The Report

Freedom of information It is generally assumed today that a client can have access to evaluative data and reports that pertain to him. It is good policy to share the report with the client. He may want his own copy, including graphic representations of his hearing, i.e., audiogram, tympanogram, confusion matrix, and other summary tables. It is this report and associated data that the client can carry back home with him for further study, reflection, and reminder of his signal-processing abilities, consequence of the hearing problem and the recommendation for effecting change. The findings of the audiologist may not always agree with the beliefs and feelings of the client. This is all the more reason to share the documental information so that the client can confront the audiologist with his own views of the analysis. The report becomes part of the learning process and offers opportunities for counseling that may be necessary.

If the report essentially focuses on signal processing capabilities of the client and recommendations for audiologic habilitation, then it is desirable that all parties concerned, including the client, receive the same document. Less misunderstanding is created if everyone involved receives the same report. This is important for parents who may need to discuss their child's problem with several professionals.

The professional jargon that is often employed by audiologists is useful if one is talking to another audiologist, but is usually unacceptable in a report. If it is necessary to use technical terms, then they should also be clearly explained. The report should be as long as necessary to tell the complete story. Some amount of redundancy is usually helpful. The story that is told should be such that the reader will want to refer back to it many times as a guide to directions to be taken on behalf of the client. The format or report writing style need not always be the same. Although clinics and clinicians usually adopt some uniform report style, this is only helpful if neatness of files counts. Individualizing of the report can improve its readability and permits the telling of the client's story as it needs to be told.

The follow-up Audiologic habilitation is the "raison d'etre" of audiologic assessment. The writing of the report does not complete our responsibility to the client. One of the most important traits of an audiologist is tenacity. One must be willing and prepared to work through problems. If the recommendations that were made are unrealistic, cannot be carried out, or are wrong, then the audiologist must be prepared to change his views and make the appropriate modifications. Having accepted the hearing-impaired individual as a client, it is the audiologist's responsibility to try to effect change. Audiologic management is not relinquished until the hearing-impaired person has established control of his situation.

The follow-up is intended to determine if recommendations have been implemented and the desirable changes are taking place. The follow-up should be considered a test for the validity of the audiologic diagnosis and recommendations. Periodically the client or we may wish to re-evaluate the situation. This relationship with the client may cover several years. Changes in the need of the client can and should be expected. Changes in our own way of viewing audiologic habilitation problems and treating them should also be expected. This is all part of the growth and change process that takes place for both the audiologist and the hearing-impaired individual.

REFERENCES

American National Standards Institute. 1969. Specifications for audiometers. S36.

Bergstrom, L., and Thompson, P. 1976. Ototoxicity. In: J. L. Northern (ed)., Hearing Disorders, pp. 136–152. Little, Brown and Company, Boston.

Bilger, R. 1973. Research frontiers in audiology. In: J. Jerger (ed.), Modern Developments in Audiology, pp. 469–501. Academic Press, New York.

Black, J. W. 1968. Responses to multiple-choice intelligibility tests. J. Speech Hear. Res. 11:453–466.

Bocca, E., and Antonelli, A. R. 1976. Masking level difference: Another tool for the evaluation of peripheral and cortical defects. Audiology 15: 480–487.

Bosastra, A., and Russolo, M. 1976. Directional hearing, temporal order and auditory pattern in peripheral and brain stem lesions. Audiology 15: 141–151.

Campbell, R. A. 1965. Thresholds and (or?) signal detection theory. J. Speech Hear. Res. 8:97–98.

Campbell, R. A., and Moulin, L. K. 1968. Signal detection audiometry: An exploratory study. J. Speech Hear. Res. 11:402–410.

Carhart, R. 1965. Problems in the measurement of speech discrimination. Arch. Otolaryngol. 82:253–260.

Carhart, R., and Jerger, J. 1959. Preferred method for clinical determination of pure-tone thresholds. J. Speech Hear. Dis. 24:330–345.

Carhart, R., and Tillman, T. W. 1970. Interaction of competing speech signals with hearing losses. Arch. Otolaryngol. 91:273–279.

Chomsky, N., and Halle, M. 1968. The Sound Pattern of English. Harper and Row, New York.

Chronbach, L. J., and Meehl, P. E. 1955. Construct validity in psychological tests. Psychol. Bull. 52:281–302.

Clarke, F. R., and Bilger, R. 1973. The theory of signal detectability and the measurement of hearing. In: J. Jerger, Modern Developments in Audiology, pp. 437–467. Academic Press, New York.

Committee on Rehabilitative Audiology, American Speech and Hearing Association. 1974. The audiologist: Responsibilities of the auditorily handicapped. Asha. 16:68–70.

Corliss, E. L. R. 1971. Estimates of the inherent channel capacity of the ear. J. Acoust. Soc. Am. 50:671–677.

Corso, J. F. 1958. Proposed laboratory standard of normal hearing. J. Acoust. Soc. Am. 30:14–23.

Dember, W. N. 1964. Psychology of Perception. Holt, Rinehart & Winston, New York.

Downs, M. P. 1976. The handicap of deafness. In: J. L. Northern, Hearing Disorders, pp. 195–206. Little, Brown and Company, Boston.

Egan, J. P. 1948. Articulation testing methods. Laryngoscopy. 58:955–991.

Egan, J. P., and Clarke, F. R. 1966. Psychophysics and signal detection. In: J. B. Sidowsky (ed.), Experimental Methods and Instrumentation in Psychology. McGraw-Hill Book Company, New York.

Egan, J. P., Greenberg, G. Z., and Schulman, A. I. 1961. Operating characteristics, signal detectability, and the method of free response. J. Acoust. Soc. Am. 33:993–1007.

Erber, N. P. 1977. Developing materials for lipreading evaluation and instruction. Volta Rev. 79:35–42.

Fairbanks, G. 1958. Tests of phonemic discrimination: The rhyme test. J. Acoust. Soc. Am. 30:596–601.

Feldman, A. S. 1975. Acoustic impedance-admittance measurements. In: L. Bradford (ed.), Physiological Measures of the Audiovestibular Ear System, pp. 87–145. Academic Press, New York.

Feldman, A. S., and Wilber, L. A. 1976. Acoustic Impedance and Admittance: The Measurement of Middle Ear Function. The Williams & Wilkins Company, Baltimore.

Feldmann, H. 1970. A History of Audiology. Translations of the Beltone Institute for Hearing Research, Chicago.

Fletcher, H., and Steinberg, J. C. 1929. Articulation testing materials. Bell Systems Tech. J. 8:806.

Flottorp, G., Djupesland, G., and Winther, F. 1971. The acoustic stapedius reflex in relation to critical bandwidth. J. Acoust. Soc. Am. 49:457–461.

Gengel, R., and Watson, C. 1971. Temporal Integration: 1) Clinical implications of a laboratory study, 2) Additional data from hearing impaired subjects. J. Speech Hear. Dis. 36:213–224.

Gibson, J. J. 1966. The Senses Considered as Perceptual Systems. Houghton Mifflin Company, New York.

Goldstein, R. 1973. Electroencephalic audiometry. In: J. Jerger (ed.), Modern Developments in Audiology. Academic Press, New York.

Goldstein, D. P., and Stephens, S. D. 1975. Masking level difference: A measure of auditory processing capability. Audiology 14:354–367.

Graham, C. H., and Ratoosh, P. 1962. Notes on some interrelations of sensory psychology, perception and behavior. In: S. Koch, Psychology: A Study of a Science, pp. 485–487. McGraw-Hill Book Company, New York.

Green, D. M. 1976. Introduction to Hearing. Lawrence Erlbaum Assoc. Hillsdale, New York.

Green, D. M., and Swets, J. A. 1966. Signal Detection Theory and Psychophysics, John Wiley & Sons, Inc., New York.

Harris, J. D. 1969. Forty Germinal Papers in Human Hearing. J. Auditory Res.

Harris, J. D. 1974. Psychoacoustics. The Bobbs-Merrill Co., Inc., New York.

Hirsh, I. J. 1952. The Measurement of Hearing. McGraw-Hill Book Company, New York.

Hirsh, I. J., Davis, H., Silverman, S. R., Reynolds, E. G., Eldert, E., and Benson, R. W. 1952. Development of materials for speech audiometry. J. Speech Hear. Dis. 17:321–337.

House, A. S., Stevens, K. H., Sandel, T. T., and Arnold, J. B. 1962. On the learning of speech-like vocabularies. J. Verb. Learn. Verb. Behav. 1:133–143.

House, A. S., Williams, G. E., Hecker, M. H. L., and Kryter, K. D. 1965. Articulation testing methods: Consonantal differentiation with a closed-response set. J. Acoust. Soc. Am. 37:158–166.

Jacobson, E. J., Downs, M. P., and Fletcher, J. L. 1969. Clinical findings in high-frequency thresholds during known ototoxic drug usage. J. Audiol. Res. 9:379–385.

Jacobson, R., Fant, C. G. M., and Halle, M. 1952. Preliminaries to Speech Analysis: The Distinctive Features and their Correlates. The MIT Press, Cambridge, Massachusetts.

Jerger, J. 1975. Handbook of Clinical Impedance Audiometry. American Electromedics Corporation, Dobbs Ferry, New York.

Jerger, J., Burney, P., Mouldin, L., and Crump, B. 1974. Predicting hearing loss from the acoustic reflex. J. Speech Hear. Dis. 39:11–22.

Jerger, J., and Jerger, S. 1971. Diagnostic significance of PB word functions. Arch. Otolaryngol. 93:573–580.

Jones, K. O., and Studebaker, G. A. 1974. Performance of severely hearing impaired children on a closed-response auditory speech discrimination test. J. Speech Hear. Res. 17:531–540.

Keith, R. 1977. Central Auditory Dysfunction. Grune & Stratton, Inc., New York.

Kreul, E. J., Nixon, J. C., Bell, D. W., Kryter, K. D., Land, J. S., and Schubert, E. D. 1968. A proposed clinical test of speech discrimination. J. Speech Hear. Res. 11:536–552.

Kryter, K. D. 1973. Impairment to hearing from exposure to noise. J. Acoust. Soc. Am. 53:1211–1234.

Levitt, H. 1971. Transformed up-down methods in psychoacoustics. J. Acoust. Soc. Am. 49:467–477.

Levitt, H., and Bock, D. 1967. A sequential programmer for psychophysical testing. J. Acoust. Soc. Am. 42:911–913.

Levitt, H., and Nye, P. W. (eds.). 1971. Sensory Training Aids for the Hearing Impaired. National Academy of Engineering, Washington, D.C.

Liberman, A., Mattingly, I. G., and Turvey, M. T. 1972. Language codes and memory codes. In: A. W. Melton and E. Martin (eds.), Coding Processes in Human Memory. V. H. Winston & Sons, Inc., Washington, D.C.

Link, R. and Lehnhardt, E. 1966. The examination of directional hearing, a simple clinical method. International Audiol. 5:67–70.

Macrae, J. H. 1968. Recovery from TTS in children with sensori-neural deafness. J. Acoust. Soc. Am. 43:1451.

Mahaffey, R. B. 1975. The measurement of hearing by computer. In: S. Singh (ed.), Measurement Procedures in Speech, Hearing and Language. University Park Press, Baltimore.

Marks, L. E. 1974. Sensory Processes: The New Psychophysics. Academic Press, New York.

Melnick, W. 1973. Psychoacoustic instrumentation. In: J. Jerger (ed.), Modern Developments in Audiology, pp. 253–300. Academic Press, New York.

Mendel, M. I., and Harker, L. A. 1974. Comment on "Five years of experience with electric response audiometry." J. Speech Hear. Res. 18:221–222.

Merzenich, M. M., Schindler, R. A., and Sooy, F. A. (eds.). 1974. Proceedings of the First International Conference on Electrical Stimulation of the Acoustic Nerve as a Treatment for Profound Sensorineural Deafness in Man. Velo Bind, Inc., San Francisco.

Miller, G. A. 1956. The magical number seven, plus or minus two: Some limits on our capacity for processing information. Psychol. Rev. 63:81–97.

Miller, G. A., Heise, G. A., and Lichten, W. 1951. The intelligibility of speech as a function of the context of test materials. J. Exp. Psychol. 41: 329–335.

Miller, G. A. and Nicely, P. E. 1955. An analysis of perceptual confusions among English consonants. J. Acoust. Soc. Am. 27:338–352.

Moncur, J. P., and Dirks, D. D. 1967. Binaural and monaural speech intelligibility in reverberation. J. Speech Hear. Res. 10:186–195.

Niemeyer, W., and Sesterhenn, G. 1974. Calculating the hearing threshold for the stapedius reflex threshold for different sound stimuli. Audiology. 13:421.

Olsen, W. O., Noffsinger, D., and Carhart, R. 1976. Masking level differences encountered in clinical populations. Audiol. 15:287–301.

Owens, E. and Schubert, E. D. 1968. The development of consonant items for speech discrimination testing. J. Speech Hear. Res. 11:656–667.

Pederson, O. T., and Studebaker, G. A. 1972. A new minimal contrasts closed-response-set speech test. J. Audiol. Res. 12:187–195.

Peterson, G. E., and Barney, H. L. 1952. Control methods used in a study of the vowels. J. Acoust. Soc. Am. 24:175–184.

Pollack, I., 1948. The atonal interval. J. Acoust. Soc. Am. 20:146–149.

Pollack, I. 1959. On indices of signal and response discriminability. J. Acoust. Soc. Am. 31:1031.

Reneau, J. P., and Hnatiow, G. Z. 1975. Evoked Response Audiometry. University Park Press, Baltimore.

Resnick, S. B., Dubno, J. R., Hawie, D. G., Hoffnung S., Freeman, L., and Slosberg, R. M. 1976. Phoneme Identification on a closed response nonsense syllable test. Presented at 52nd Annual Convention of the American Speech and Hearing Association.

Resnick, S. B., Dubno, J. R., Huffnung, S., and Levitt, H. 1975. Phoneme Errors on a Nonsense Syllable Test. Presented at the 90th Meeting of the Acoustical Society of America.

Robinson, D. E., and Watson, C. S. 1972. Psychophysical methods in modern psychoacoustics. In: J. V. Tobias (ed.), Foundations of Modern Auditory Theory, Vol. II. Academic Press, New York.

Rogers, C. R. 1951. Client-Centered Therapy. Houghton Mifflin Company, Boston.

Rogers, C. R. 1961. On Becoming a Person. Houghton Mifflin Company, Boston.

Rosenblith, W. A., and Vidale, E. B. 1962. A quantitative view of neuro-electric events in relation to sensory communication. In: S. Koch (ed.), Psychology: A Study of a Science. McGraw-Hill Book Company, New York.

Rosner, B. S. 1962. Psychophysics and neurophysiology. In: S. Koch (ed.), Psychology: A Study of a Science, pp. 280–333. McGraw-Hill Book Company, New York.

Ruben, R., Elberling, C., and Salomon, G. 1976. Electrocochlegraphy. University Park Press, Baltimore.

Russ, F. M., and Simmons, F. B. 1974. Reply to Mendel's and Harker's comments on "Five years of experience with electric response audiometry." J. Speech Hear. Res. 18:222–223.

Rynes, E. J. 1969. The Effect of Examiner Expectancy in Auditory Data Collection. Doctoral Dissertation, Case Western Reserve University, Cleveland.

Scharf, B. 1970. Critical bands. In: J. V. Tobias (ed.), Foundations of Modern Auditory Theory, Vol. I, pp. 157–202. Academic Press, New York.

Shannon, C. E., and Weaver, W. 1949. The Mathematical Theory of Communication. University of Illinois Press, Urbana.

Sheeley, E., and Bilger, R. 1964. Temporal integration as a function of frequency. J. Acoust. Soc. Am. 36:1850–1857.

Sher, A. E., and Owens, E. 1974. Consonant confusions associated with hearing loss above 2000 Hz. J. Speech Hear. Res. 17:669–681.

Speaks, C. 1967. Performance-intensity characteristics of selected verbal materials. J. Speech Hear. Res. 10:344–347.

Swets, J. A. 1973. The relative operating characteristics in psychology. Science. 182:990–1000.

Taylor, M. M., and Creelman, C. D. 1967. PEST: Efficient estimates on probability functions. J. Acoust. Soc. Am. 41:782–787.

Thorndike, R. L., and Hagen, E. 1967. Measurement and Evaluation in Psychology and Education. John Wiley & Sons, Inc., New York.

Tillman, T. W., and Olsen, W. O. 1973. Speech audiometry. In: J. Jerger (ed.), Modern Developments in Audiology. Academic Press, New York.

Tonning, F. M. 1975. Auditory localization and its clinical applications. Audiology 14:368–380.

Van Riper, C. Personal communication.

Ventry, I. M., Chaiklin, J. B., and Dixon, R. F. (eds.). 1971. Hearing Measurement. Appleton-Century-Crofts, New York.

Wang, M. D., and Bilger, R. 1973. Consonant confusions in noise: A study of perceptual features. J. Acoust. Soc. Am. 54:1248–1266.

Ward, W. D. 1963. Auditory Fatigue and masking. In: J. Jerger (ed.), Modern Developments in Audiology, pp. 240–286. Academic Press, New York.

Weiss, M. S., and House, A. S. 1973. Perception of dichotically presented vowels. J. Acoust. Soc. Am. 53:51–58.

Winer, B. J. 1962. Statistical Principles in Experimental Design. McGraw-Hill Book Company, New York.

Wright, H. H. 1968. Clinical measurement of temporal auditory summation. J. Speech Hear. Res. 11:109–127.

Evaluation of "Hard to Test" Children and Adults

Denzil N. Brooks

CONTENTS

History shows that yesterday's "hard-to-test" individual has become the routine subject of today, and no doubt many of today's hard-to-test patients will be routine evaluations tomorrow. Dr. Brooks' chapter is rich in practical case studies of the special problems presented by such patients as those with cerebral palsy and functional hearing loss. The problems presented by the mentally retarded, emotionally disturbed, blind, geriatric, and other special patients are also illustrated. Guidelines are presented to assist the audiologist in deciding which tests have the greatest potential for providing accurate evaluations of hearing thresholds in these populations. Suggestions, such as those described by St. James-Roberts (1976), Coles and Priede (1971), Ames et al. (1970), Kronholm (1968), Harper (1971), and Groen (1963) are given for ways in which the standard test procedure may be modified to obtain optimum responses from these different types of patients. Finally, Dr. Brooks describes the four most common diagnostic errors and confusions that might lead an audiologist to form an erroneous diagnosis.   —Eds.

HISTORICAL BACKGROUND

The deaf have been misunderstood and maligned throughout the history of mankind. The Romans drowned babies born deaf. Aristotle was of the opinion that the deaf were lacking in ability to learn because they lacked the capacity to hear. In consequence of this philosophy, little effort was made to evaluate deafness or to treat it. The hearing impaired were neither hard-to-test nor easy-to-test. They were persecuted, ignored, or cursed. (The one exception is contained in the Law of Moses: Lev. 19:14.)

In medieval times loss of hearing was often seen as a direct affliction of the Creator and that man was therefore impotent to help— only a miracle could cure the sufferer. Even when treatment was contemplated, it was bizarre. Hildegard of Bingen in A.D. 1115 suggested that deafness could be remedied by cutting off the ear of a lion and holding it over the deaf person's ear while chanting an invocation such as; "Hear, O Publius, by virtue of the living God and the keen virtue of a lion's hearing." The lion also figures in a cure suggested by a thirteenth century writer, Albertus Magnus, who claimed that "A lion's brain, if eaten causes madness, but remedies deafness if inserted in the ear with some strong oil." The Aristotlean concept was restated as late as 1873 by Schopenhauer, who opined that the deaf-mute possessed only the instincts of the animal and as such was not worthy of consideration as a human being. In consequence, there was neither need to educate him nor to try and understand the disability.

Fortunately, more enlightened individuals saw that the deaf were normal human beings but deficient in one of their senses. Ernaud in 1761 demonstrated increased auditory perception in deaf children as a result of training and practice in listening. He expressed the belief that there was no such thing as total deafness. At about the same time, the first school for the deaf was opened in Edinburg by Thomas Braidwood. His enrollment at commencement in 1760 was one pupil! The number of pupils increased and the reputation of the establishment spread such that by 1773 the number of pupils was 12 and one at least was from the New World. It is of passing interest that the grandson of Thomas Braidwood established the first school for the deaf in the United States in Virginia in 1815 (Bass, 1949).

As the realization of the educability of the hearing impaired grew, so did the need for better evaluation of the auditory capabilities of the hearing-impaired child. Assessment with the human voice was the earliest method and is, of course, still a valuable diagnostic procedure. More frequency specific and quantified information became possible with the advent of the tuning fork. This, originally known as the pitch fork, was invented in 1711 by John Shore, trumpeter to King George I, as a means of bringing the band to a uniform pitch. It was not until the nineteenth century that the otological potential of the tuning fork was discovered. Huizing (1975) shows that in 1842 Polanski gave a complete account of the test that now bears the name of Rinne. His description seems to have been overlooked or ignored, as indeed was the report of Rinne until Schwabach (1885) confirmed the value of the test, which is now one of the basic tuning fork tests. Hartmann (1878) devised an "acoumeter" which used a telephone receiver for testing hearing. This was the forerunner of the electric audiometer. An interesting application of this instrument with a hard-to-test population was that of General Korting (1879) in testing for malingering in recruits for the German army.

A major advance was made with the production of the first commerical audiometer, the Western Electric 1A in 1922. Audiometric standards soon followed, as did the ability to quantify hearing impairments in adults and children and to make differential diagnosis. As late as 1944, however, the Ewings, who pioneered the education of very young hearing-impaired children, thought it was not possible to perform pure tone audiometry before the age of 5 years. This is not to say that hearing of these children was not measurable—there are other methods of assessment than pure tone audiometry—but these children would probably have then been regarded as hard-to-test. Advances in understanding and in testing techniques are such that these children are now regularly tested with pure tones, with great success. The hard-to-test cases of 30 years ago have become routine subjects now. However, children with additional handicaps beyond hearing impairment, who then might have been regarded as untestable, are now being evaluated. In the last few decades there has probably been a real increase in the number of children with multiple handicaps. Such children would not have survived but for advances in medicine, and they present considerable difficulties in total evaluation. Differential diagnosis and assessment at the earliest possible age are vital if the child is to be provided with the most suitable environment to maximize his abilities. Evaluation of the multiply handicapped child means much more than the attachment of diagnostic labels and measurements. It means the full assessment of the child's potentials and weaknesses so that the potentials can be exploited to maximum advantage and the weaknesses minimized.

With children, it is probably among multiply handicapped that the largest number of hard-to-test subjects are found at present. Myklebust (1954) produced the first detailed discussion of differential diagnosis in children with auditory disorders. He postulated that to acquire a language a child must have both adequate hearing and an intact central nervous system. Impairment of the peripheral hearing mechanism, brain damage that interferes with the interpretation of sounds, emotional disturbances, or mental deficiency could all prevent a child from acquiring speech, and these were the four basic conditions that Myklebust suggested as requiring differential diagnosis. It is the task of the diagnostician to determine which of these conditions exist and to what degree they are affecting the child's acquisition and use of language. A fifth category might also be added to the four proposed, that of the blind child. Within a few months of birth, the normal baby develops the ability to locate sounds and to associate the sound and its source. By this means environmental sounds are given meaning. Blind children, even though having normal hearing, are not able to develop the association between sound and source unless a tactile contact can be made. In consequence, blind children may react abnormally to environmental sounds and give the impression of hearing impairment. When the vision defect is coupled to a diminished intellectual capacity the problem of differential diagnosis is both more difficult and more important.

The situation is somewhat different with respect to the adult population. Brain damage may occur as a result of head injury or stroke affecting both receptive and expressive communication ability.

Mental deficiency still poses diagnostic problems with the adult hearing impaired, although within a few years we hope to be able to make the differential diagnosis before the subjects reach adulthood. There are very specific problems in evaluation of the adult subject who was born deaf and educated in a non-oral environment. Evaluation of these individuals requires special skills on the part of the audiologist, such as signing or finger spelling. The type of psychometric tests employed have to be selected with great care so that the poor language sophistication of the subjects does not substantially bias the test conclusion.

In the very old, as in the very young, there may be difficulties in the assessment of hearing. Both tend to fatigue quickly and have short attention spans. Response times tend to be slower and particular difficulties may be encountered in the presence of a masking noise. Tinnitus can present considerable difficulty in tone testing. Pure tone tests alone may grossly underestimate the degree of handicap for speech in the presbycusic. Pestalozza and Shore (1955) found that the discrimination scores for subjects over 65 were poorer than for persons below age 40 even when the pure tone audiograms were of the same degree and type.

In both adults and children the conscientious diagnostician will be aware of and alert for the possibility of functional hearing loss. Although perhaps not strictly in the realm of hard-to-test, ignorance of the relatively common presence of functional hearing loss may result in serious misdiagnosis and in unsuitable or even harmful advice and action. Where there exists a conscious effort on the part of the subject to exaggerate his hearing loss there may be appreciable difficulties in testing, and especially in determining the true nature of the hearing loss, if any.

History shows that yesterday's hard-to-test patients have become the routine subjects for today, and no doubt many of todays hard-to-test patients will be routine evaluations tomorrow. This can only come about if the test team—not merely the individual responsible for the evaluation of hearing—are aware of the changing patterns of impairment both of hearing and the other disorders that may be associated with it and are flexible enough to adapt to these changes. The flexibility must be based on knowledge of the mechanisms that underlie the disorders, whether these be of the hearing mechanism alone or of other aspects of human development. Multidisciplinary cooperation is vital to the evaluation of the hard-to-test subject.

CURRENT HARD-TO-TEST POPULATION

The Mentally Retarded

Myklebust (1954) reported that about 9% of the children referred to the Children's Hearing and Aphasia Clinic in 1 year were mentally deficient (IQ lower than 70) and, because of this retardation, were not acquiring speech normally. The rate of occurrence agrees well with the 7–8% reported by Schein (1974) based on the Annual Survey of Hearing Impaired Children and Youth (Rawlings and Gentile, 1970; Rawlings, 1971). A higher rate was indicated in the report of the Chief Medical Officer of the Department of Education and Science (United Kingdom) based on a survey of 359 children in schools for the deaf in England. However, this may be attributable to the criterion employed: an IQ lower than 80. At this level, 20% of the children with hearing impairment were "retarded." This constitutes a high prevalence of hearing impairment among the mentally retarded (Jordan, 1972). In group comparisons the incidence of hearing defect tends to increase as the intelligence level declines.

Complicating the diagnostic problem is the fact that, in addition to any organic hearing impairment, many retardates seem superficially to be hearing impaired because of the general intellectual retardation.

The abnormal or inadequate auditory behavior of the mentally retarded is a manifestation of the general intellectual retardation. The response of the retardate to stimulation is at the level of his mental development rather than at the level associated with his chronologic age, and this must be a major consideration in the audiologic evaluation.

The Emotionally Disturbed

Fisher (1965) studied the social and emotional adjustment of children with impaired hearing attending ordinary classes with normal hearing children. The hearing losses ranged from 20–65 dB and were of a conductive type in 60% and sensorineural in 40%. There was a considerably greater amount of maladjusted behavior in the hearing-impaired children than in normal hearing children. The behavior patterns might be demonstrative (more common in boys), withdrawing, or of a mixed nature. Thomson and Brenner (1967) show that similar problems are encountered with the more severely deaf child and that these behavior patterns may be severely disabling. Children may become completely withdrawn from reality, detached from the environment. Childhood schizophrenia and autism are extreme, although fortunately rare, examples of this type of emotional disturbance that can easily be mistaken for profound deafness. Some of these children seem to have no comphrension for speech and fail to use speech as a means of communication. Occasionally however, perhaps at play, they will produce good clear speech, but without any relevance to the activity in which they are engaged, thus indicating that the hearing mechanism is at most only marginally impaired.

With somewhat older children, functional hearing loss is by no means uncommon. As already noted, there is no real difficulty in testing the child with functional hearing loss. However, the audiologist should be constantly on the alert for the possibility of functional hearing loss.

There is evidence that these children are not being discovered and so they may be justifiably classified as difficult-to-detect. Doerfler (1951) surveyed 30 leading audiology clinics in the United States and found that in the majority, functional hearing loss was being detected in less than 1% of children examined. In other centers where alertness to the possibility of functional hearing loss was maintained, as many as 5% of the children were found to have a functional component to their hearing loss. The importance of finding children with this type of hearing problem lies in the realization that the child is unconsciously expressing a need for help. Although it may not lie within the province of the audiologist to give that help, it is his responsibility to observe the distress call of the child.

The situation with the adult who has functional hearing loss is usually quite different. The apparent loss of hearing may be consciously and deliberately feigned for purposes of financial gain or to avoid some unpleasant course of action (e.g., conscription to the armed services). Such subjects truly merit the classification as hard-to-test.

The Cerebral Palsied

According to Löwe (1968) 15-20% of all cerebral palsied children have hearing losses of significant magnitude that speech and language development will be affected. Morris (1973) pointed out that the rate of occurrence of educationally significant sensorineural hearing loss in the cerebral palsied was dependent on whether the cerebral palsy was of the athetoid or nonathetoid type and, in the athetoid group, on the age of the subject. In nonathetoid cerebral palsy the incidence ($N = 224$) was 11%. In the atheloid group comprising ages 4 years or less, only one child of the six examined had sensorineural loss, but in the 26 children between ages 5 and 15, 13 (50%) were sensorineurally hearing impaired. Morris comments "The steady decline in perceptive hearing impairment over the years can be attributed to improved medical care, especially improved prevention of haemolytic disease....By the use of D positive rhesus serum it is now possible to prevent kernicterus due to rhesus incompatibility which is the commonest cause of kernicterus. Therefore the number of children afflicted with athetosis should continue to decrease and consequently so should the number of deaf athetoids. As it is difficult to prevent cerebral damage of children, and if improved medical care results in the saving of damaged infants, the incidence of perceptive deafness among spastic children is not expected to decrease further."

The difficulty involved in testing the child with cerebral palsy is largely related to the degree of physical handicap, but many other factors complicate the evaluation of the true hearing capability. Moderate or severe degrees of spasticity may prevent the child from performing the movements normally employed to indicate hearing. With the athetotic child the involuntary movements make judgment of response difficult, and these movements tend to be exacerbated in situations of stress such as a hearing test.

In addition to these more obvious motor problems, the child may have forced responsiveness characterized by high distractability to any environmental stimuli. The child may perseverate or take an abnormally long time to respond. Mental deficiency compounds the testing difficulty in a substantial proportion of cerebral palsied children and there may be further difficulties caused by visual abnormalities such as strabismus and nystagmus.

The Hyperkinetic Child

These children pose test difficulties because of their inability to cease all motor activity. They cannot stop and listen and may therefore seem hearing impaired. Restraint merely causes distress to the child, the parents, and the tester.

The Blind-Deaf Child

The normal infant develops the ability to locate the source of a sound within a few months of birth. This enables the developing child to give meaning to environmental sounds, to associate source and sound. However, Morris (1976) regards the orientating reflex as a relatively weak mechanism that requires constant reinforcement. The blind baby will initially attempt to localize sound, but because of the lack of association and reinforcement, may cease to turn towards the source. Consequently, when tested by the standards of children characterized by normal development, blind children may seem to have defective hearing.

The blind-deaf child with a severe degree of auditory handicap may never naturally develop localization. Taylor (1964) describes two such children and shows that with training, turning toward sound and feeling for the source developed.

CNS Disorders

Children may sustain brain damage either before, during or after birth as the result of trauma, chronic infection, or a toxic condition. Such children may show disorders of auditory function not necessarily accompanied by a decrease in threshold sensitivity. Many different terms have been used to describe these problems of auditory perception and integration: aphasia, congenital auditory imperception, auditory agnosia, central auditory imperception, etc. These terms do not contain any real explanation of the underlying disorders, although they may assist the determinations of the best course of action to be pursued in the management of the child. What is of more relevance in the context of audiologic evaluation is the differentiation of children with brain injury from those with uncomplicated peripheral hearing loss or functional loss. The responses of these children to sounds may be most inconsistent. Uncomfortably loud stimuli may be ignored, yet a definite response may be made to a minute sound that coincides with a moment of interest. Adults who have had cerebrovascular accidents may also present as hearing impaired. With some there may be true hearing loss, but with others the problem may be aphasia. The importance again lies in the differentiation of the two possibilities so that correct rehabilitation procedures may be instituted.

Geriatric Patients

Increasingly large numbers of geriatric subjects are being seen in audiology clinics as a result of the increasing longevity of the population. As far back as 1947, Wilkins (1948), using a random sampling technique, showed that among those older than 74 years, more than one-quarter of those surveyed had hearing difficulties. In the decade before age 74, the prevalence of hearing difficulties was 1 in 8. Another survey carried out in 1962 (Government Social Survey) indicated that in persons 65 years old or over, almost 28% admitted difficulty in hearing and another 3.8% were considered by the interviewers to have difficulty in hearing that was not admitted by the subject. In the geriatric subject, the lesion may be specific to the cochlea, but is more likely to be of a generalized nature having additionally a conductive component and a central component. The ability to process complex acoustical information such as speech, particularly in the presence of competing background noise, may be poorly demonstrated by pure tone audiometry, which assesses only the sensitivity of the system. Furthermore, even with the simple pure tone test there may be difficulties attributable to reduced attention span and poor motivation.

Probably the main reason for assessing hearing impairment in the geriatric patient is to determine the possibility of assistance through either electronic or nonacoustic hearing aids. In this context speech testing is more relevant than pure tone testing. The difficulty experienced by the elderly may be considerably greater in unfavorable acoustic situations. However, although tests of speech reception in noise may be more suited to the evaluatory purpose, these may be of too great complexity for the elderly person to handle. A fine balance has to be drawn between increasing the complexity of the test to enhance its relevance and increasing the difficulty of the test to the point where it goes beyond the limited capabilities of the subject.

The Non-oral Deaf

With the severely and profoundly deaf adult evaluation may be rendered difficult by the basic problem of communication. There is the initial difficulty of explaining to the subject the nature of the stimulus and of the response desired. Because of the high intensities required there is a real possibility of confusion occurring in the lower frequencies between true auditory response vibrotactile sensation. An ingenious approach to masking out the vibrotactile element with young severely deaf children has been employed by Boorsma and Courtoy (1974). Comprehensive "evaluation" of the non-oral deaf adult is a problem much more in the sphere of the psychiatrist than the audiologist. In this context, the remarks of Denmark (1966) are particularly appropriate. He says, "The inability of the deaf to express dissatisfaction or anger in the normal way, or quickly enough by emotionally toned verbalisation, often leads to the physical display of such feelings. To those without a knowledge of deaf persons these reactions, at times explosive in character, are incomprehensible and may be mistaken for the manifestations of mental illness. They have on occasion resulted in admission to psychiatric units." A specific example of this confusion and misdiagnosis is described by Wolff (1973). "Sam" was born in 1928 and the indications are that he has always been severely hearing impaired (80–90 dB over the speech range). Apparently because of his "erratic" behavior, at the age of 12 he was committed to a hospital for the mentally subnormal and has remained there as a high grade patient for 31 years. Recently it was recognized through nonverbal intelligence tests that he is, in fact, of about normal intelligence. It would be reassuring, but probably unrealistic, to believe that such a situation could not happen today.

Other Causes of Difficulty in Testing

The child with atresia of the external auditory meatus may present special difficulties in assessment. If the hearing loss is dominantly conductive, then a bone conduction hearing aid from an early age will ensure that the "period of readiness for listening" will be employed to best effect. However, Gill (1969) suggests that even with the bone conductor aid these children do not develop anything approaching normal fluency of speech. In certain types of congenital atresia he recommends surgery at 12–18 months of age, especially in certain cases where infection in the mastoid process is suspected. It is valuable to know before the surgery the degree of cochlear function, but this poses considerable difficulties in children so young. After surgery, even with older children, the accurate assessment of hearing is difficult because masking presents particular problems in these situations. The operated ear may have a degree of sensorineural loss and the unoperated ear a large conductive loss. With the physically normal subject adequate masking may be obtained by the use of an insert, but this is not possible in the child without a meatus.

A small group of subjects require special care during evaluation. Precautions must be taken with patients having discharging ears or infective skin disorders so that other patients are not put at risk. The tester needs to take special measures when working with patients with infective illness such as tuberculosis. Mention should also be made of the (fortunately) rare patient with claustrophobia. The distress occasioned by being placed in a small enclosed space to victims of this disorder may be such as to totally invalidate any audiometric or audiologic investigations (D'Andrea, 1967). Even at the risk of sacrificing some degree of accuracy, the solution rests in testing outside the confines of the acoustic booth or room.

PRESENTING PROBLEM

The most common presenting symptom that arouses suspicion of hearing loss in young children is absent, delayed, or abnormal speech. Although there were earlier reports in the literature on differential diagnosis of the causes of delayed speech, it was Myklebust (1954) who produced the first comprehensive and detailed treatise on the subject. He suggested that there were four principal conditions that might lead to disordered communication: lesions in the peripheral auditory mechanism, involvement of the central auditory system, emotional disturbance (psychic deafness), and mental deficiency.

A substantial proportion of the uncomplicated peripheral hearing losses are now being detected at a fairly early age, but with the multiply handicapped child diagnosis may well be delayed for months or even years because of the difficulties involved in determining the extent to which each factor of the handicap is involved in the communicative disorder. Some of the problems are outlined or illustrated below.

Physical/Psychologic Problems

Physical handicaps may make a person seem hearing impaired: "Rachel" is a 12-year-old in a unit for the severely physically handicapped as a result of cerebral palsy. Her mental age is assessed as about 4 years. When her hearing was tested for the first time by the audiologist, Rachel was sitting in her wheelchair. Because she is almost totally unable to maintain her equilibrium, even sitting in her chair imposes a substantial degree of stress on Rachel. The threshold obtained at this hearing test was at about the 40 dB level. The test was repeated a few days later, but on this occasion Rachel was lying on her bed. The responses this time were rapid, consistent, and within the normal range of hearing. Another test, undertaken when Rachel was standing with support on either side from the physiotherapists, produced responses that were very slow and inconsistent and tended to indicate a functioning level of about 60–75 dB. Other children in the unit were tested under similar situations of low and high stress and frequently reacted in the same manner, the apparent threshold of hearing deteriorating as the degree of difficulty of the task increased. Even such simple tasks as crayoning on a sheet of paper required such concentration from some of the children that their hearing levels fell dramatically both to pure tones and occasionally even to speech (Robinson and Hendley, 1976). These observations seem to indicate that although the auditory systems of these children are capable of functioning at normal or near normal levels, inhibition may occur in certain stressful situations. The tester's lack of awareness of this possibility may well lead to the erroneous conclusion that there is a moderate or severe hearing loss. This has important implications in structuring the learning programs for these children.

The motor impairment of some cerebral palsied children may pose a problem. A normal child can usually be conditioned quite rapidly to indicate that he has heard the stimulus. He may do this by dropping a brick (block) in a box, by putting a peg in a hole, by banging with a pencil or stick on the table, by raising a hand, or by some similar physical action. The child with poor motor control may find this task, if not impossible, then certainly very difficult and time consuming. Repeated failure in the chosen motor activity brings with it emotional difficulties—frustation and rage—and the validity of the test is soon destroyed unless the response is selected with great care to be within the capabilities of the child.

Another complicating factor with some of the cerebral palsied is the delayed response characteristic. The delay may occur at different stages of the signal-response process: in the awareness that the signal has been presented, in the interpretation of the signal, or in the initiation and carrying out of the motor response. Combination of the motor handicap and the delayed response characteristic may result in several seconds elapsing between presentation of the signal and completion of the response. With these children it is vital that ample time be given for the response if one is not to confuse and frustate the efforts of the subject.

Functional hearing loss has already been noted as a possible cause for apparent hearing loss, and in children stress may be the root cause. "Jane" was a schoolgirl of 12 when she was treated for a furunculosis (painful nodule formation) in the auditory meatus. A hearing test at that time indicated a loss of about 20 dB. A year later her mother brought her to the hospital with the complaint of deafness, and on testing Jane produced a pure tone audiogram of a flat sensorineural pattern at the 50-dB level. Retesting a month later elicited a similar pattern, but at the 70-dB level. More detailed testing clearly indicated that the loss was dominantly functional, but the consultant in charge of the child elected to fit her with a low gain hearing aid. Jane was well suited with this, being able to "switch off" when it suited her purpose.

Approximately 1 year later mother and daughter reappeared at the hospital requesting a repeat hearing test on the basis that the hearing had "recovered." Pure tone testing confirmed that threshold was now within 10 dB of normal. Questioning the mother brought out the facts of the situation. Jane had been very unhappy at school and also at home, so unhappy that she had run away. She was returned home by the police in the early hours of the morning and there had been a tearful but frank confrontation between mother and daughter. Within a week Jane was transferred to another school and reconciliation between mother and daughter took place. It was very shortly after this that Jane's hearing was restored!

There is an interesting sequel to this episode. In their discussion of functional hearing loss, Chaiklin and Ventry (1963) pose the question of whether functional hearing loss recurs in those children in whom the problem seems to have been resolved. In the case of Jane, the answer is yes. After a lapse of more than 10 years she returned recently to the hospital, again complaining of loss of hearing. She is now a young lady of 28. The consultant referred her for hearing tests and, as on the previous occasion, the pure tone audiogram was of a sensorineural nature and at about the 60-dB level, although speech tests indicated a very much lower deficit. Middle ear muscle reflexes were also present at about normal levels, and to all intents and purposes it looked as if the functional hearing loss had returned. On questioning Jane it emerged that she had very recently become engaged to be married. As with many brides, she was anxious and uncertain. Fortunately few young ladies in this position react in this way, but with Jane it seems that hearing loss is a simple and convient shield from stress. Once again she gladly accepted a hearing aid with which she claimed to hear well. It will be interesting to see if the "hearing loss" recovers this time.

CNS Problems That Necessitate Test Modification

In some cerebral palsied children there may be cortical inhibition of auditory response caused by the high distractability of the child. Any visual or tactile stimulation with these children may compete for their attention and reduce their ability to perform the listening task. With this type of child, it is therefore advisable to minimize the decoration of the testing room and to limit the stimulation to the acoustic modality as much as possible.

At the other extreme is the child who is almost or completely disinterested in his surroundings and who does not seem to respond to any type of stimulation, be it acoustic, olfactory, tactile, or visual—the autistic child or the juvenile schizophrenic. This very lack of response to any stimulus in an otherwise healthy and physically normal child should alert the tester to the possibility that the problem is more deep seated and extensive than simple hearing loss.

With both types of child, conventional pure tone testing is likely to be unrewarding and more basic procedures are therefore advocated. The child may respond to a stimulus in a reflex manner perhaps by a stilling of activity in the distractable child, or by startle or turning in the otherwise unresponsive child.

Careful observation of the child during the test session or at play may enable the audiologist at least to decide that the hearing is not the major problem. If even such a fundamental conclusion is not possible, then some type of objective testing might be considered.

Cautions for Testing Patients Who Have Had Head and Aural Surgery

To be efficient the headbands of both earphones and bone conductors have to exert a substantial pressure. After head surgery this pressure may be both undesirable and painful to the patient.

If hearing evaluation is vital so early after operation, then the phones should be detached and hand-held; similarly with the bone conductor. Masking obviously presents problems under these circumstances, particularly if the patient has a dressing in or on the ear.

Another situation in which masking presents particular problems and special caution is necessary is in the testing of subjects who have undergone successful surgery for otosclerosis on one ear and are having the other ear evaluated. Masking is required on the good ear to evaluate the bone conduction threshold on the poorer ear, which may have a maximal air-bone gap. There is a possible hazard of using masking levels that are too high. The stapedius muscle on the operated side will probably have been sacrificed at operation, and it has been suggested that the operated ear is consequently at greater risk of noise damage. Some modification of bond conduction testing such as the Rainville (1955) technique might overcome this difficulty. Impedance testing is now a routine part of evaluation of the difficult-to-test, but caution should be employed in testing patients after middle ear surgery. Impedance instruments are capable of producing uncomfortable and, in these circumstances, possibly hazardous pressures on the tympanic membrane. It is wise not to use greater pressure differentials than 200 mm H_2O. If it is necessary to perform air conduction tests on an ear that is actively discharging, it is advisable to protect the earphone with a disposable cover. Should any discharge, blood, or pus come into contact with the muff, this should be swabbed off and the muffs disinfected. Similar cautions apply to the testing of children with skin conditions such as eczema or impetigo, and indeed to any subject with contagious diseases. A study by Talbott (1969) showed that the three most common bacteria can be 98% deactivated in a 90-sec sterilization cycle of a special earphone sterilizer. (One of the commercially available models is produced by Allison Laboratories in Austin, Texas.)

THE TEST

The procedures used in the assessment of the difficult-to-test subject are, if not exactly the same as those used in normal subjects, then certainly based on normal hearing tests. Pure tone audiometry is the basic audiologic test that provides information about the function of the auditory system in terms of frequency and intensity. Data obtained from pure tones alone can assist in gross differential diagnosis of the site of auditory impairment. However, complex stimuli may be more valuable and more relevant in the assessment of communication disorders, speech being the most important of these stimuli.

It is relevant in considering tests for the hard-to-test to first review the conventional clinical hearing tests as employed from infancy to adulthood.

In the newborn child the responses to auditory stimuli are purely reflexive, the Moro and auropalpebral reflexes being the best known and most frequently observed and employed. Additionally or alternatively, "objective" means may be employed to assess the auditory function by measuring changes in an autonomic function such as the heart rate (Butterfield, 1962; Bartoshuk, 1964), respiration pattern or rate (Bradford and Bradford, 1975), skin resistance (Barr, 1955; Bordley, 1956), or brain activity. By the age of 18–20 weeks the normal child has adequate neck and head control and is sufficiently mature to localize sounds and may be tested with sounds that have roughly quantifiable dimensions of loudness and pitch. When performing this type of test and interpreting the responses the state of arousal and interest of the child are factors of great importance (Fisch, 1967).

During the 2nd year of life cooperative testing may be possible, the child responding to simple verbal requests such as, "Show me your teddy bear" or "Where is mummy?". A little later, around 30 months, the average child will be capable of performance testing, making a specified response to a test sound. The sound may at first be loud and complex, such as a drum or xylophone, but later softer and simpler sounds may be employed, such as pitch pipes. From this point the child can usually be transferred to pure tone stimuli—first in free field and then headphone listening. Pure tone audiometry may be employed at an earlier age through such techniques as conditioned orientation response audiometry (Suzuki and Ogiba, 1960). Until recent times, the air-bone gap has been the main audiologic procedure for determining the presence of conductive lesions. Impedance audiometry has in many respects superseded air-bone audiometry in that it not only indicates the presence of a conductive lesion, but to a large degree also indicates the nature of the lesion and its site in the middle ear. In difficult-to-test patients impedance measurement is particularly valuable as the test is not dependent on the cooperation of the subject. Provided the patient is not actively hostile, much valuable information can be obtained by impedance testing, not only as to the nature of impairment in the mechanical conduction system, but also regarding lesions higher in the auditory tract.

Common Diagnostic Errors/Confusions

Confusion between true auditory and nonauditory responses   It is possible to fail to recognize severe hearing loss in infants by misinterpreting responses to nonacoustic stimuli as acoustic reflex responses. This may happen if, for instance, the shadow of the tester or assistant is visible to the child (Martin, 1971). Not only visual clues but olfactory stimulation, such as might occur if the tester or assistant wears perfume, may cause the child to produce nonauditory responses.

Assumption that response to acoustic stimulation indicates hearing Response to sound indicates that certain parts of the auditory system are functioning but not necessarily that the subject is hearing, if by hearing we mean perception and not merely reflex reaction. A neonate may produce a strong Moro reflex but later be shown to have severe deafness. Hardy and Bordley (1973) reported that of the 27 rubella infants who had auditory screening in the neonatal period and were later identified as having significant hearing defects, only one failed to respond to a stimulus of 65–70 dB intensity in a test applied on one or more occasions in the nursery. Coleman (1972) reports the case of a child who at 18 months had good localizing reflexes and was thought to hear normally. The child had further tests on several different occasions including apparently normal audiometric responses at 4 years and 10 months. However, because of delayed language she was re-evaluated at 6½ years of age and found to have a severe high tone loss. The localizing responses undoubtedly mislead the examiners into thinking hearing was normal over the whole auditory range. The "normal" audiometric responses are more difficult to explain, but a possible explanation lies in the string of previous reports of normal hearing although there is also the possibility that the child was responding to some nonauditory clues involuntarily provided by the tester.

Assumption that absence of response to sound indicates deafness It is perhaps obvious that the test employed to assess the hearing of a child (or even in some cases the hearing of an adult) must be related to the developmental level of the subject. If an inappropriate test is employed, a test requiring a higher degree of sophistication than is appropriate to the age or developmental level of the subject, then response may be totally absent or present at markedly reduced levels. Myklebust (1954) in discussion of the auditory capabilities of the mentally deficient writes that auditory stimuli that entail abstractedness and experiential associations beyond the patient's level of capacity are ignored; therefore such stimuli are unsuitable for evaluation of auditory capacities. Central factors may also produce inhibition of response despite an intact auditory system, functional hearing loss and autism being illustrative of this phenomenon. Hardy and Bordley (1973) comment on rubella children who fail to respond to neonatal screening tests but who later may be shown to have no detectable hearing loss.

Assumption that lowest response is threshold of hearing Some children through immaturity cease to respond to stimuli of an abstract nature at levels well above their true threshold of hearing. Usually these are young children, but occasionally the same effect is observed in older children. Children 12 or 13 years old have been examined who responded to pure tones at levels of approximately 50 dB. With narrow band noise as a stimulus, the responses improved by some 10–20 dB and improved again with broad band noise. If speech was employed as the test medium, normal hearing was indicated. Such children are sometimes classified as having a functional hearing loss, but the term "artefactual" as used by Coles and Priede (1971) may be more appropriate. The same response pattern has been observed in the mentally subnormal and in brain-injured children, and the use of narrow band noise in testing advocated by Sortini (1960). Excessive visual stimulation will, even with normal babies, produce auditory inhibition and lead to suprathreshold responses that may be misinterpreted as hearing impairment.

Decisions on Tests to Administer

The pure tone audiogram is generally regarded as the most fundamental of the hearing tests and in consequence is the first objective in assessment. However, if the patient is mentally subnormal to such a degree that pure tone audiometry is not possible, or if the age of the subject is such that the use of pure tone stimulation is unrealistic, then one may have to accept assessment in different and possibly less precise terms. If the subject will not tolerate the wearing of headphones, some form of freefield testing with its inherent problems has to be employed.

Regardless of the information obtained by this kind of test, acoustic impedance testing is now virtually mandatory. Provided that the subject is not actively hostile, a great deal of valuable information can be obtained in a relatively short time by this method of examination and in subjects ranging in age from infancy to extreme old age. Originally, impedance testing was employed by Metz (1946), the Danish otolaryngologist who pioneered its clinical use, as a means of differentiating between conductive and "perceptive" deafness. In the majority of subjects it will certainly perform this function and indeed much more. Whereas pure tone audiometry gives merely an indication of the degree of conductive impairment, tympanometry, absolute impedance measurement, and observation of the threshold and pattern of middle ear muscle reflex responses will to a large extent resolve the degree and nature of a conductive impairment. This is particularly valuable in mentally subnormal subjects. Conductive hearing disorders seem to be particularly common in subjects with Down's syndrome (Fulton and Lloyd, 1968; Brooks et al., 1972). Much of the impairment seems to stem from middle ear effusion and hence is a remediable condition. Early detection is particularly important in this group. In children of normal intellectual ability, even mild hearing losses can be educationally handicapping (Hamilton, 1973). The combination of mental subnormality and hearing loss is potentially disastrous and all possible steps should be taken to minimize the handicap. Acoustic impedance testing from infancy is advocated in children with Down's syndrome.

Profoundly deaf children in residential schools, many of whom are now in the multiply handicapped and difficult-to-test category seem to be much more prone to middle ear effusion than normal hearing children in normal schools (Brooks, 1975). This may considerably reduce the efficacy of the hearing aids used by the children apart from being medically undesirable. Additionally, impedance testing is of assistance in differentiating between sensory and neural impairment. The presence of recruitment that indicates sensory involvement (although not necessarily the absence of neural involvement) can often be detected by the Metz test (Metz, 1952). Neural impairment may be indicated by abnormal decay of the reflex response to low frequency stimulation to the involved ear (Anderson et al., 1970). Identification of sensorineural hearing impairment by observation of the acoustic reflex relaxation pattern has been advocated by Norris and colleagues (1974). It may be possible in some children to get a reasonably accurate estimate of their hearing status using the differential thresholds of the middle ear reflexes to pure tone and broad band noise stimuli (Niemeyer and Sesterhenn, 1972; Jerger et al., 1974). More accurate evaluation of hearing levels at individual frequencies, possibly comparable in accuracy with conventionally achieved pure tone thresholds, may be possible by preactivation of the stapedius muscle with a high frequency tone (Sesterhenn and Breuninger, 1977). The acoustic reflex is also helpful in the differential diagnosis of functional hearing loss both in children and adult subjects. However, all these techniques depend on the ability to elicit a stapedius muscle reflex, and in a substantial percentage of children and adults this may not be possible (Brooks, 1977). Indeed, so much information is attainable from the acoustic impedance evaluation that it would now be unthinkable to contemplate the evaluation of hard-to-test infants, children, or adults without employing impedance testing.

In subjects with suspected functional hearing loss, speech audiometry is invaluable. In a series of 53 cases, Coles and Priede (1971) found speech audiometry to be the best detector of functional hearing loss in a battery of six tests (pure tone audiometry, speech audiometry, delayed speech feedback, Stenger, acoustic reflex test, and Békésy audiometry). Only five subjects gave both a good correlation between speech audiometry and pure tone average, and normal patterns of speech response. Atypical responses seen were: a) intelligibility scores dropping from near 100% to near 0% within an intensity range of 5 dB; b) always responding incorrectly to the first or second consonant of the CVC words employed in the test; c) giving alternatives to the test word such as "men" or "pen" d) only responding to every second or third word consistently. Where formal speech audiometry is not possible, informal testing may still be valuable.

A great deal of information is contained in the simple act of a child turning towards the tester when his name is spoken softly. It gives indications not only of the hearing level, but also of the integrity of the whole auditory system.

Where none of the conventional hearing tests may be employed a range of other tests are possible, subject to availability of time, expertise, and equipment. Fulton (1974) has shown what can be achieved with the difficult-to-test severely retarded subjects employing operant procedures. These may be developed to obtain not only pure tone thresholds, but also to perform such sophisticated tests as the short increment sensitivity index, threshold tone decay and even frequency difference limena. Psychogalvanic skin resistance measurement has already been mentioned. It has been employed by many researchers and clinicians but this method of testing has never achieved widespread acceptance. Fundamentally, the electrical conditioning stimulus has to be unpleasant to produce the desired change in skin resistance and many audiologists feel that this type of test should therefore be reserved for adult patients only. Shimizu and his colleagues (1957) tried to avoid the unpleasantness of the electrical shock and condition with either bright light flashes or momentary glimpses of a lantern slide that would appeal to the child. They comment, "These two trials were both satisfactory in that they did not cause the patient any pain or fear, but were unsatisfactory in that the stimulation was weak and difficulty was experienced in conditioning because it was impossible to change properly the intensity of the stimulation during the test. In this respect electrical stimulus was better than the other two ... only this had the disadvantage of creating fear in the child." Electrical response audiometry has also been proposed as an "objective" method of assessing auditory function. Early optimism about cortical response testing has been abated by the realization that the patients who are difficult-to-test by the conventional methods of behavioral observation are also the difficult-to-evaluate by cortical response measurement. The young, the brain-injured, and the mentally retarded may produce such aberrant responses that conclusions about the subjects' hearing capacities are not possible. Technical sophistication may overcome some of the difficulties but there still remains the major problem that cortical responses do not directly correlate with the subjects ability to use hearing in a meaningful way.

Electrocochleography seems to have greater potential in the area of differential diagnosis of sensorineural impairment, but it is still in the research and development stage. There are two basic approaches to obtaining the electrical activity of the auditory system. One approach employs an electrode placed on the promontory anterior to the round window and the other, a noninvasive technique, employs an electrode placed in the external meatus. With the former technique the difficult-to-test subject will require anesthesia. A local is sufficient for adults, but with children a general anesthetic is usually required. With the external electrode method anesthesia is probably not necessary, although sedation may be required with the hyperactive child. The disadvantage of the noninvasive technique is that the potentials to be recorded are reduced by at least an order of magnitude and more powerful signal detection systems are required. Thornton (1976) asserts that for accurate evaluation of hearing thresholds and a measure of the activity of the auditory system both surface recording and transtympanic methods are required, being complementary in the information that they give. Transtympanic recording is of most value in the measurement of cochlear and cochlear nerve responses. By means of the surface recording technique information about the brain stem may be obtained, thus assisting in differential diagnosis in neurologic and retrocochlear pathologies.

HOW TO MODIFY STANDARD TESTS/TECHNIQUES

The Mentally Retarded

The retarded subject performs at the level of his intellectual maturation. If hearing impairment is suspected, the type of hearing test employed must be related to the mental and not the physical age of the patient. With the severly subnormal child there may be a generalized lack of awareness of the environment, a lack of response to all stimulation that may mislead an observer into thinking that the child is hearing-impaired. One approach to this type of child is to touch the child from behind on the pinna with a cold spoon to see if there is response to tactile stimulation. Objects are moved into and out of the visual field to see if the child will respond to visual stimulation. If the child does quickly respond to these tactile and visual stimuli, then one can proceed to distraction testing. With children who do not respond to either tactile or visual stimuli, a first resort may be to the reflex test—Moro, auropalpebral, or stapedius muscle with acoustic stimulation. Taylor (1964) describes how the "auditory attention" of such a child might be augmented by stimulating first the visual or tactile sense—by shining a torch (flashlight) onto the child's hand or holding the hand and gently moving the arm up and down—and then on withdrawal of that stimulus, substituting an auditory stimulus. St.James-Roberts (1976) has developed this method of cross-modal facilitation of response in behavioral audiometry. Although he did not employ mentally retarded subjects, it seems likely that the technique would be effective with this group.

With less severely retarded patients play audiometry may be employed. Ewing and Ewing (1944) pioneered this method, which involves the child in some play activity such as putting brightly colored blocks in a box, or rings on a stick. The tester attempts to condition the child to perform the activity on reception of a sound.

With adequate time, knowledge, and equipment it is possible to test even the most severely retarded subjects (Fulton, 1974). The value and importance of acoustic impedance testing with the mentally retarded should again be mentioned because of its simplicity, objectivity, and sensitivity in detecting middle ear abnormalities, which occur frequently in the retarded population. If the subjects will not tolerate the headset of the instrument it may still be possible to obtain useful information by holding the probe to the ear under test (a capability now possible with a number of instruments) and by the use of ipsilateral reflex stimulation.

The Emotionally Disturbed/Functionally Hearing Impaired

Fortunately, the truly autistic child is uncommon. His behavior is, however, quite distinctive, and is at the root of the testing difficulty. Autistic children are withdrawn, totally lacking in communication, devoid of any apparent emotion, and interested in objects rather than in other people. Observation of the child when engrossed in some personally satisfying activity may yield clues as to the hearing ability, interest occasionally being shown in some quiet sound although louder sound may be ignored. "Objective" hearing tests (electric response audiometry, acoustic impedance testing, etc.) may indicate that the hearing mechanism is organically intact and that the child's apparent disinterest in sound is not the result of deafness, but is of psychic origin.

Functional hearing loss in children can usually be evaluated by careful application of standard subjective audiometric tests. Speech audiometry will often yield an articulation curve that is normal or near normal both in pattern and in sensitivity. Narrow bands of noise or frequency-modulated tones may produce more sensitive thresholds than pure tones, and ascending stimulus presentation rather than the descending mode may also elicit a lower threshold of hearing. Békésy audiometry with continuous tone stimulation generally yield a more sensitive threshold than with pulsed stimulation (Jerger type V). The adult with functional loss may be considerably more difficult to assess. Determining the functional nature of the apparent loss may be fairly straightforward, but the determination of the real hearing status is generally much less simple. Psychogalvanic skin resistance measurements and electrical response audiometry seem to be the evaluatory methods of choice, but delayed auditory feedback is also being considered (Beagley and Knight, 1968; Coles and Priede, 1971).

Cerebral Palsied Children

Cerebral palsied babies and children suffering from severe hypotonia or hypertonia have great difficulty or even total inability in turning to localize acoustic stimuli. As a consequence they do not develop human orientation reflexes and may wrongly be judged as hearing impaired when tested by distraction methods. If visually involved, these children may not respond to acoustic stimulation and consequently testing must be designed to reduce visual involvement to an absolute minimum.

The uncontrolled involuntary movements of the athetotic child complicate the assessment of response. A period of time must be first devoted to determining the best way in which the child can respond and then in conditioning the response.

Further complication may arise if the child is mentally deficient. Behavioral testing, acoustic impedance evaluation, and possibly electrical response testing are methods thay may be employed with these hard-to-test subjects.

The CNS Disordered

The tests employed in testing children with CNS disorders are basically no different from those used for testing other children except that a wider range of acoustic stimuli may be valuable. Tape recordings of familiar sounds such as animal cries, the laughing, cooing, and distress cry of a baby, domestic sounds, and rhythmical music may be valuable, occasionally producing a response where other simpler stimuli fail. The principal requirement in testing these children is that the tester should be completely adaptable, ready to switch from an apparently unsuccessful approach to another that it is hoped will yield more information. The tester must also be an alert observer, quick to detect a fleeting response and ready to capitalize on any interest displayed.

Some aphasic children pay little or no attention to pure tones under test conditions nor do they respond to speech, but other sounds such as music might elicit a definite response. Unusual or bizarre sounds may also give evidence of hearing, and in this category band-pass noise is particularly useful in that it can be calibrated with some degree of precision and hence gives more frequency- and intensity-specific information than squeaker toys, percussion instruments, and rattles.

Ames et al. (1970) report that children with auditory imper-ception may respond normally or near normally to pure tones, but when speech is employed as a stimulus the response is at a much reduced level. Indeed, a common feature of many children with CNS disorders is inconsistency of response within one type of stimulus or more especially between different stimuli. The child may express interest the first time a new sound is presented, but on the second and subsequent presentations shows no further interest. The diagnosti-cian must be alert to these features of the child with CNS disorders and seek for valid responses in every possible way.

The Geriatric Patient

With the geriatric subject, it frequently takes a longer time to per-form even the basic pure tone audiogram as the ability and readiness of the patient to make decisions regarding the presence or absence of the tone tends to be impaired. Not infrequently, as in young children, the patient ceases to respond to the presentation of the tone not at true threshold, but at some arbitrarily determined level where the tone is no longer easily audible. The tester must be alert to this pos-sibility and constantly encourage the patient to pursue the tone down to true threshold. Tinnitus will often add to the difficulties of tonal recognition and for this reason the use of pulsed tones is strongly recommended.

A not uncommon observation in the elderly is that discrimination for speech is worse than would be expected from the pure tone audi-ogram. If audiologic testing is being carried out with a view to re-habilitation of the patient with a hearing aid, then the hearing for speech is more relevant than the pure tone data. With the geriatric patient the testing procedures for speech may need modification. Speech audiometry using taped material can be difficult because of the rather short intervals normally allowed between word presentations. Live voice may be preferable, or a tape with longer interword pauses may be prepared or the pause button on the recorder may be held down after each word has been presented to allow adequate time for the response. The word lists themselves need careful consideration, and with some patients it may be desirable to use a forced choice method with the words illustrated by pictures as one does with children. The audiologic examination may have to be performed over a number of sessions if the patient shows a sign of tiredness or lack of interest.

The assumption has been made that before commencing audiologic examination, the patient has been otologically investigated. This is important because obturating cerumen may be present in a substantial number of elderly persons. In examining 117 patients between 64 and 94 years of age, Kronholm (1968) found 43 with this condition and 22 had a considerable improvement in hearing when the obstruction was removed.

IMPORTANCE OF EXTRA-AUDIOLOGIC DATA

In evaluation of "hard-to-test" children and adults, a number of disciplines may be involved. An obvious member of the team is the otolaryngologist, preferably one with knowledge and understanding of child development and of the problems of the infant and child. A complete history is an important step in reaching a differential diagnosis. In children, this should include details of prenatal, birth, and postnatal conditions and illnesses. Developmental landmarks are noted and compared with those of normally developing children, particularly features related to language development. The child's behavior and emotional adjustment are also relevant factors and, particularly in the multiply handicapped child, psychologic assessment is vital. Indeed, with these children the psychologic assessment and the audiologic assessment must go hand-in-hand. Without a knowledge of the capabilities and limitations of the child, the audiologic evaluation may be meaningless or even misleading.

The evaluation of the visual sense may be important where there is any suspicion of impairment. The aberrant behavior of some blind children has already been commented on. Lesser degrees of visual impairment than total blindness may be relevant to the overall assessment of the child's capabilities and also to the actual audiologic evaluation. Functional hearing loss is said to occur frequently in blind children (Harper, 1971).

In adult differential diagnosis, vestibular function testing is often of considerable value. With children, the value seems to be greatly reduced. Arnvig (1955) tested a substantial number of children who were severely or profoundly deaf and found that the vestibular function tended to be within normal limits where the hearing impairment was genetic, but was frequently abnormal or absent in acquired hearing loss cases. Rosenblüt, Goldstein, and Landau (1960) tested 164 children who were either deaf or aphasic using a modification to the Fitzgerald-Hallpike test. They concluded that vestibular tests had little value in the differential diagnosis of auditory disorders in young children. Undoubtedly much of the reason for the poor diagnostic value of vestibular testing lies in the fact that although the hearing and equilibrium organs are an organic whole, they are functionally quite distinct and disorders of one part do not necessarily affect the other part. However, many ear, nose, and throat specialists are of the opinion that vestibular testing could be of more assistance if a suitable stimulus-response procedure could be developed. Groen (1963) demonstrated that babies as young as 9 days old could be tested with the aid of rotational stimulation and was further able to show the development of normal inhibitory mechanisms. It is possible therefore to obtain information both on the peripheral mechanism and on the central aspects of the vestibular portion of the cochlea. Little work has been carried out in this area with the multiply handicapped child where such information might be especially helpful. Rotation testing seems to be a more suitable stimulus than caloric testing, which may be distressing to the young.

TEST-RETEST COMPARISON

With normal hearing subjects, there is a learning effect in audiometric testing that is greater between the first and second test than between the second and subsequent tests. Overall the threshold change is not normally greater than 10 dB, and ±5 dB is the normal variability in the midfrequency range with intelligent, cooperative subjects of mature disposition. With children, the test-retest variability is higher and rises as the age diminishes. In 5-year-old children the test-retest difference in thresholds obtained by conventional pure tone audiometry exceeded 15 dB in 20% and exceeded 10 dB in 36% in a study reported by Goto (1964). Even higher figures were reported for children of 3 and 4 years of age, but numbers in these ages were too small for reliable statistical treatment, because of the fact that few children of such tender years could perform conventional pure tone autiometric tests.

Children as young as 2 years were tested, with peep-show testing, but successful results were obtained in only 10% of the 2-year-old children tested. By 3 years of age the percentage of successful cases was 60% and in these children 55% had a test-retest difference not greater than 10 dB. Greater test-retest differences were observed in children with moderate degrees of hearing loss than in either children with normal hearing and mild losses or children with severe hearing loss. Sato (1962) performed startle response audiometry and conditioned orientation reflex audiometry or play audiometry with 21 hearing impaired children and the difference between the two thresholds was within ±5 dB in 57%.

Fulton et al. (1975) tested nine infants (median age, 14 months) using an operant procedure. Test-retest differences of 5 dB or less were obtained in 74% of the threshold measurements. In older children and adults, large test-retest differences (greater than ±10 dB) are probably indicative of some disorder in addition to loss of auditory sensitivity.

Aphasic children and those with other CNS disorders tend to respond inconsistently to sounds and in consequence exhibit large test-retest differences. This is particularly noticeable in children who have severe multiple handicaps. Stresses associated with the test situation may very considerably affect the threshold as measured, as reported by Robinson and Hendley (1976) in the cerebral palsied.

Mentally retarded children may respond more consistently to stimuli that are more meaningful than pure tones. Sanders and Josey (1970) tested 10 mentally retarded subjects with both pure tones and narrow bands of noise and obtained consistently lower test-retest differences with the narrow band noise stimulus. In older children and adults test-retest differences larger than ±10 dB should alert the tester to the possibility of a functional element in the hearing loss.

Among geriatric patients, repeatability of pure tone testing is poorer than in the younger population, and ±10 dB may be accepted here as normal rather than indicative of functional loss.

FORMING THE DIAGNOSIS

The ultimate aim of the evaluation of the difficult-to-test subject is a definitive statement of the factors involved in the presenting problem (communication handicap) and the degree to which each is involved. It is essential that all disciplines involved are aware of and conversant with the contributions that the other disciplines can and do make to understanding the problem. Audiologic assessment should contribute to the total picture both qualitative and quantitative measures of auditory responses. It should indicate not only the deficits in the auditory system, but also, especially with the hearing-impaired child, the potential remaining capacity. It will probably fall within the province of the audiologist to give guidance on methods of ameliorating the handicap through amplification, again an area where a cooperative approach is essential. It will be the responsibility of the teacher of the deaf to further the education of the child, but the audiologist can offer much assistance in the selection and fitting of the auditory prosthesis.

REFERENCES

Ames, M. D., Plotkin, S. A., Winchester, R. A., and Atkins, T. E. 1970. Central auditory imperception: A significant factor in congenital rubella deafness. JAMA 213:419-420.

Anderson, H., Barr, B., and Wedenberg, E. 1970. Early diagnosis of VIII nerve tumours by acoustic reflex tests. Acta Otolaryngol. 263(Suppl.): 232-237.

Arnvig, J. 1955. Vestibular function in deafness and severe hardness of hearing. Acta Otolaryngol. 45:283-288.

Barr, B. 1955. Pure tone audiometry for preschool children. Acta Otolaryngol. 121(Suppl.):5-82.

Bartoshuk, A. K. 1964. Human neonatal cardiac responses to sound: A power function. Psychon. Sci. 1:151-152.

Bass, A. R. 1949. History of the education of the deaf in Virginia. Virginia School for the Deaf and Blind, Staunton, Virginia. Cited by Burr, H. 1963.

Beagley, H. A., and Knight, J. J. 1968. The evaluation of suspected non-organic hearing loss. J. Laryngol. Otol. 82:693-706.

Boorsma, A. and Courtoy, M. 1974. Hearing evaluation with hearing impaired children. Br. J. Audiol. 8:44-46.

Bordley, J. E. 1956. An evaluation of the psychogalvanic skin resistance technique in audiometry. Laryngoscope 66:1162-1185.

Bradford, L., and Bradford, M. 1975. Neonatal auditory testing. II. Respiration audiometry. Maico Audiol. Lib. Serv. 13:Report 10.

Brooks, D. N. 1975. Middle ear effusion in children with severe hearing loss. Impedance Newsletters. (Am. Electromedics) 4:6–8.

Brooks, D. N. 1977. Use of acoustic impedance in hearing aid evaluation. Problems and Pitfalls. Paper presented at the XIth World Congress of Otorhinolaryngology, March, Buenos Aires.

Brooks, D. N., Wooley, H., and Kanjilal, G. C. 1972. Hearing loss and middle ear disorders in patients with Down's syndrome. J. Ment. Defic. Res. 16:21–29.

Burr, H. 1963. The first school for the speech and hearing handicapped in the New World. J. Speech. Hear. Assoc. Va. 4.

Butterfield, G. 1962. A note of the use of cardiac rate in the audiometric appraisal of retarded children. J. Speech. Hear. Disord. 27:378–379.

Calearo, C., and Lazzaroni, A. 1957. Speech intelligibility in relation to the speed of the message. Laryngoscope 67:410–419.

Chaiklin, J. B., and Ventry, I. M. 1963. Functional Hearing Loss. In: J. Jerger (ed.), Modern Developments in Audiology. 1st Ed. Academic Press, New York.

Coleman, R. O. 1972. Delayed identification of hearing loss in a six and one half year old child: A case study. J. Commun. Dis. 5:368–372.

Coles, R. R. A., and Priede, V. M. 1971. Non-organic overlay in noise induced hearing loss. Proc. R. Soc. Med. 64:194–199.

D'Andrea, G. A. 1967. Audiology vs. claustrophobia. Audecibel 16:198, 200–201.

Denmark, J. C. 1966. Mental illness and early profound deafness. Br. J. Med. Psychol. 39:117–124.

Dix, M. R., and Hallpike, C. S. 1947. The peep-show: a new technique for pure tone audiometry in young children. Br. Med. J. 2:719–723.

Doerfler, L. G. 1951. Psychogenic deafness and its detection. Ann. Oto. Rhino. Laryngol. 60:1045–1048.

Ernaud. 1761. Cited in Goldstein, M. A. 1939. The Acoustic Method. Laryngoscope Press, St. Louis.

Ewing, I. R., and Ewing, A. W. G. 1944. The ascertainment of deafness in infancy and early childhood. J. Laryngol. Otol. 59:309–333.

Fisch, L. 1967. The physiology of children's reactions to test sounds in free field. Int. Audiol. 6:121–126.

Fisher, B. 1965. The social and emotional adjustment of children with impaired hearing attending ordinary classes. M. Ed. dissertation. University of Manchester.

Fulton, R. T. 1974. Auditory stimulus-response control. University Park Press, Baltimore.

Fulton, R. T., Gorzycki, P. A., and Hull, W. L. 1975. Hearing assessment with young children. J. Speech Hear. Dis. 40:397–404.

Fulton, R. T., and Lloyd, L. L. 1968. Hearing impairment in a population of children with Down's syndrome. Am. J. Ment. Def. 73:298–302.

Gill, N. W. 1969. Congenital atresia of the ear. J. Laryngol. Otol. 83:551–587.

Goldstein, M. A. 1939. The Acoustic Method. Laryngoscope Press, St. Louis.

Goto, S. 1964. Audiometric tests of young children. Nagoya University School of Medicine, Nagoya, Japan.

Government Social Survey. 1962. Older people in Lewisham. King Edward VII Hospital Fund, London. p. 43.

Groen, J. J. 1963. Postnatal changes in vestibular reactions. Acta Otolaryngol. 56:390–396.

Hamilton, P. 1973. Reading and language skills in children with impaired hearing in ordinary schools: some recent research findings and discussions of educational provision. Occasional Paper No. 6. North Regional Association for the Deaf, Manchester.

Hardy, W. G., and Bordley, J. E. 1973. Problems in diagnosis and management of the multiply handicapped deaf child. Arch. Otolaryngol. 98:269–274.

Harper, F. W. 1971. Recognition of functional hearing loss by a speech therapist in a residential school for the blind. Educ. Visually Handicapped. 3:87–90.

Hartmann, A. 1878. Ueber eine neue Methode der Horprufant mit Hulfe elektrischer Ströme. Arch. Anat. Physiol. (Physiol. Abt):155–158.

The Health of the Schoolchild, 1962 and 1963. Report of the Chief Medical Officer of the Department of Education and Science. Her Majesty's Stationary Office.

Huizing, E. H. 1975. The early descriptions of the so-called tuning fork tests of Weber, Rinne, Schabach, and Bing. II. The Rinne test and its first description by Polansky. ORL (Basel) 37:88–91.

Jerger, J., Burney, P., Mauldin, L., and Crump, B. 1974. Predicting hearing loss from the acoustic reflex. J. Speech Hear. Dis. 39:11–22.

Johnson, K. O., Work, W. P. and McCoy, G., 1956. Functional deafness Ann. Oto. Rhino. Laryngol. 65:154–170.

Jordon, O. 1972. Mental retardation and hearing defects. Scand. Audiol. 1:29–32.

Korting, G. E. 1879. Ueber Telephonische Hörprüfung. Deutsche mil-artz. Z. 7:337–000. Cited in Glorig, A. and Downs, M. 1965. Introduction to Audiometry. In: A. Glorig (ed.), Audiometry: Principles and Practices. The Williams & Wilkins Company, Baltimore.

Kronholm. A. 1968. Auditory problems in a home for the aged. In: G. Liden (ed.), Geriatric Audiology, pp. 58–62. Almquist and Wiksell, Stockholm.

Löwe, A. 1968. Pädoaudiologische Massnahmen in her Frühbetreuung cerebral bewegungsgestörter Kinder. Neue Bl. Taubst. 22:371–322.

Martin, J. A. M. 1971. Problems of diagnosis of hearing loss in the young child. Proc. R. Soc. Med. 64:571–574.

Metz, O. 1946. The acoustic impedance measured on normal and pathological ears. Acta Otolaryngol. 63(suppl.):11–254.

Metz, O. 1952. Threshold of reflex contractions of muscles of middle ear and recruitment of loudness. Arch. Otolaryngol. 55:536–543.

Morris, T. 1973. Hearing-impaired cerebral palsied children and their education. Public Health (London) 88:27–33.

Morris, T. 1976. Personal communication.

Myklebust, H. R. 1954. Auditory Disorders in Children. Grune & Stratton Inc., New York.

Nash, M. M., and Wepman, J. M. 1973. Auditory comprehension and age. The Gerontologist 13:243-247.

Niemeyer, W., and Sesterhenn, G. 1974. Calculating the hearing threshold from the stapedius reflex for different sound stimuli. Audiology 13:421-427.

Norris, T. W., Stelmachowicz, P. G. and Taylor, D. J. 1974. Acoustic reflex relaxation to identify sensorineural hearing impairment. Arch. Otolaryngol. 99:194-197.

Pestalozza, G., and Shore, I. 1955. Clinical evaluation of presbycusis on the basis of different tests of auditory function. Laryngoscope 65:1136-1163.

Rainville, M. J. 1955. Nouvelle Méthode d'Assourdissment pour le Relevé des Courbes de Donctive Osseuse. J. Fr. d'Otorhinolaryngol. 4:851-858.

Rawlings, B. 1971. Summary of selected characteristics of hearing impaired students—United States 1969-70. Gallaudet College, Office of Demographic Studies, Washington D.C.

Rawlings, B., and Gentile, A. 1970. Annual survey of hearing impaired children and youth: Additional handicapped conditions, age at onset of hearing loss, and other characteristics of hearing impaired students—United States 1968-69. Gallaudet College, Office of Demographic Studies, Washington D.C.

Robinson, A., and Hendley, M. 1976. Some aspects of the effect of stress on the performance of brain injured children. J. Chartered Soc. Physiotherapists. In press.

Rosenblüt, B., Goldstein, R. and Landau, W. M. 1960. Vestibular responses of some deaf and aphasic children. Ann. Oto. Rhino. Laryngol. 69:747-755.

St. James-Roberts, L. 1976. Cross-modal facilitation of response in behavioural audiometry with children. J. Acoust. Soc. Am. In press.

Sanders, J. W., and Josey, A. F. 1970. Narrow band noise audiometry for hard-to-test patients. J. Speech Hear. Res. 13:74-81.

Sato, I. 1962. Studies on startle response audiometry. Jap. J. Otolaryngol. 65:755-801.

Schein, J. D. 1974. Education and rehabilitation of deaf persons with other disabilities. School of Education, New York University. p. 7.

Schwabach, D. 1885. Ueber den Werth des Rinneschen Versuches für die Diagnose des Gehörs-Krankheiten. Z. Ohrenheilk. 14:61-147.

Schimizu, H., Sugano., T., Segawa, Y., and Nakamura, F. 1957. Study in psychogalvanic skin resistance audiometry. Arch. Otolaryngol. 65:499-508.

Sesterhenn, G., and Breuninger, H. 1977. Determination of hearing threshold for single frequencies from the acoustic reflex. Audiology 16:201-214.

Sortini, A. J. 1960. Hearing evaluation of brain-injured children. Volta Rev. 62:536-540.

Suzuki, T. and Ogiba, Y. 1960. A technique of pure tone audiometry for children under three years of age: Conditioned orientation reflex (C.O.R.) Rev. Laryngol. 1:33-45.

Taylor, I. G. 1964. Neurological mechanisms of speech and hearing in children. University Press, Manchester.

Thomson, R. E. and Brenner, L. O. 1967. The emotionally disturbed deaf child. Proceedings of the International Congress on Oral Education of the Deaf. A. G. Bell Association for the Deaf, Washington D.C.

Thornton, A. R. D. 1976. Electrophysiological studies of the auditory system. Audiology 15:23-8.

Waldon, E. F. 1973. Testing hearing of subnormal children. J. All India Speech Hear. 4:44-48.

Wilkins, L. T. 1948. The prevalence of deafness in the population of England, Scotland, and Wales. Central Office of Information, London.

Wolff, J. G. 1973. Language, Brain, and Hearing. Methuen & Co. Ltd., London. [Distributed in the United States by Harper and Row, New York.]

Recommendation of Hearing Aids

Jeffrey L. Danhauer

CONTENTS

The traditional approach to the fitting and recommendation of hearing aids has been the subject of considerable controversy during recent years. This controversy has resulted from technologic advances, redefinition of professional roles, and increasing demands from consumers for better services. Dr. Danhauer sees the audiologist as the hub of the hearing health team. The relevance of the current trends he discusses are supported by the literature; with 56% of the references chosen from publications appearing during 1975 or 1976. Factors such as the three types of aids available and their basic components remain constant while the method of evaluation is controversial. More prescriptive approaches using electroacoustic, KEMAR(Knowles Electronic Manikin for Acoustic Research), narrow band noise, most comfortable listening and threshold of discomfort measures are recommended with the procedures of Victoreen (1960, 1973a, b), Wallenfels (1967), Berger (1976a, b), Shapiro (1976) and others explained in some detail. Criteria for choosing monaural, binaural, or bilateral (use of a Y-cord) amplification are discussed. The trend in the fitting of hearing aids is toward better quantification of measures to make recommendation an objective process.   —Eds.

Because the historical development and technical specifications of amplification devices for the hearing impaired have been iterated and reiterated quite adequately in other texts by other authors (e.g., Briskey, 1972; Lybarger, 1972; Carver, 1972; Kasten, 1972; Berger, 1974; Donnelly, 1974; Pollack, 1975), the purpose of this section is to focus more specifically on the procedures involved in the recommendation of hearing aids. This chapter deals with the hearing aid recommendation service in terms of four main issues:

1.   Who provides the service
2.   What is provided
3.   How are services provided
4.   Who are the services provided for

In addition, several special considerations are presented regarding the issues.

    Because space does not permit it, much in-depth coverage and corresponding references to areas of the hearing aid recommendation procedure that have been elaborated upon by numerous qualified authors in other texts have been omitted. Instead, the aim is to reorganize some of the vital information, and to present a coverage of comparatively newer ideas and approaches to the hearing aid recommendation along with up-to-date references. One of the goals in this chapter is to present a current trend in the hearing aid-recommendation procedure. The hearing aid and procedures for its recommendation have seen considerable changes even within the past 5 years, therefore much of what is presented in this chapter is also certain to meet with modifications in the future; many will be welcomed.

WHO PROVIDES THE RECOMMENDATION

Before discussing actual procedures, it is important to know who is involved in making the recommendation.

    In the past few years we have observed considerable evolution in both evaluative and referral procedures for the recommendation of hearing aids. These changes have stemmed largely from an increased concern by those involved with the process of providing improved services for the hearing aid user. In addition, public consumer protection agencies and governmental legislators have also become interested in the hearing aid-recommendation process (Berger, 1974; Rubin, 1976). The professional team involved with the recommendation of hearing aids still basically includes the hearing aid manufacturer and dealer, the otologist, and the audiologist, but their respective roles and the extent of their participation in the process have seen modifications.

Each team member's role in the hearing aid-recommendation process may be generally defined as follows.

Hearing aid manufacturer—designs, constructs, and wholesale dispenses hearing aid instrumentation including hearing aids and auditory trainers; promotes research and development in hearing aid technology.

Hearing aid dealer—retail dispenses hearing instrumentation, primarily the hearing aid; provides some testing, proper fitting, adjustment, and servicing of instrument; supplies batteries, cords, and accessories; often initiates maintenance and hearing aid-usage programs.

Otologist—responsible for medical diagnosis of hearing loss and related problems; provides medical and surgical treatment when appropriate; often refers to the audiologist for hearing testing and hearing aid recommendation.

Audiologist—studies in-depth the hearing process and problems and needs of the hearing impaired; clinically provides full audiometric and hearing aid evaluations and their follow up via aural rehabilitation, habilitation, and counseling; conducts research in various areas of audiology.

In the early years of the hearing aid, instrumentation and engineering limitations restrained the manufacturer in hearing aid development. However, recent advances in these areas have permitted improvements in hearing aid design such as compression amplification, frequency emphasis, directionality, increases in power and fidelity capabilities, and decreases in distortion characteristics and size (for cosmetic appeal). These manufacturer improvements, as well as more in-depth understanding of hearing aid and earmold characteristics, have enabled the hearing aid dealer to provide better services for the hearing impaired. Increased liaison with the audiologist and the other professionals on the team, the advent of hearing aid dealer licensure bills, 30-day trial periods, and greater concern for clients are having an impact on the quality of services provided by the hearing aid dealer.

The role of the otologist in the recommendation of hearing aids has also increased in recent years. Many otologists have become more familiar with the capabilities and limitations of hearing aids. They have also shown increased interest in impedance audiometry, electronystagmography, and other special tests, as well as their usual diagnostic test battery. Professional referrals and close contact with other team members have resulted in a greater percentage of "true" sensorineural fittings. That is, fewer patients are fitted with hearing aids when their losses indicate a conductive component that could be treated either medically or surgically. The otologist has increasingly become a vital part of the hearing aid-recommendation process. A few, like some audiologists, have even become actively involved in hearing aid dispensing.

The audiologist's participation in hearing aid recommendation has expanded considerably in recent years from just assisting in the selection of proper amplification to the point of actually prescribing a specific hearing aid in many cases. Although the audiologist is not usually the "sole" determiner of what amplification is to be used, he has acquired much of the responsibility for the recommendation of hearing aids and is usually the "hub" to which other team members report. A possible working model of this relationship is depicted in Figure 1. Because of his contact with and knowledge of the hearing process and the hearing-impaired individual, the audiologist is often the coordinator of the audiologic evaluation, referrals to the otologist and the hearing aid dealer, and follow-up procedures. This follow-up usually includes the periodic evaluation of the hearing aid, both electroacoustic and physiologic, and the therapeutic management of aural rehabilitation and speechreading procedures (Blood and Danhauer, 1976; Roeser, Campbell, and Brown, 1976). Additionally, the audiologist is often responsible to others involved with hearing health including the family, family physician, educators, and social workers and funding agencies such as the Bureau of Vocational Rehabilitation, the Veteran's Administration, and the Bureau of Crippled Children.

In the ideal hearing aid recommendation, all members of the team are aware of and responsible to each other for proper referrals. They are all usually involved in counseling the client in some way regarding their respective findings. Although the status of the "ideal" team approach to hearing aid recommendations may not yet be at its optimum, we are seeing a trend in the direction of higher quality ser-

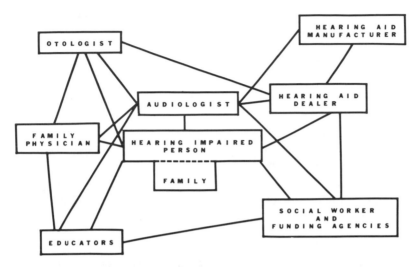

Figure 1.   Model of the hearing health team.

vices for the hearing impaired. However, regarding the fitting and distribution of hearing aids, it should be pointed out that many controversies still exist concerning how and by whom the hearing aid recommendation should be conducted. This is exemplified by the increasing number of audiologists, otologists, and private clinics who have included some form of hearing aid dispensing as yet another of their services. The pros and cons of the dispensing issue have been discussed in other sources (e.g., Pollack, 1975; Rubin, 1976), and it soon becomes clear that the controversy will not be settled for quite some time.

WHAT IS RECOMMENDED

Regardless of who accomplishes the hearing aid evaluation or what procedure is employed in achieving it, the end result for the hearing-impaired person is typically a recommendation for some form of amplification. Although various interim or alternative modes of amplification (i.e., auditory trainers) may be advised, this recommendation usually takes the form of a wearable hearing aid.

Berger (1974) stated "the purpose of a hearing aid is to bring sound more effectively to the ear, primarily by making it louder." In his excellent introduction to a current text entitled *Amplification for the Hearing-Impaired*, Carhart (1975) posited the following four main goals in the selection of a hearing aid:

1) restore to the user an adequate sensitivity for the levels of speech and of other environmental sounds he finds too faint to hear unaided;
2) restore, retain or make acquirable the clarity (intelligibility and recognizability) of speech and other special sounds occurring in ordinary, relatively quiet environments;
3) achieve the same potential insofar as possible when these same sounds occur in noisier environments; and
4) keep the higher intensity sounds that reach the hearing aid from being amplified to intolerable levels. (p. xxiv)

With these goals in mind the audiologist or person making the recommendation has a wide range of possibilities for wearable amplification devices from which to choose.

Wearable Amplification Styles

Perusal of the various hearing aid journals and trade magazines, as well as the lengthy list of members of the Hearing Aid Industry Conference (published in Volume 29, 1976, of the *Hearing Aid Journal*), should lead one to believe that there must be a model of hearing aid available for virtually any type and degree of hearing loss imaginable. It is true that the past 25 years have brought about numerous hearing aid manufacturers, all with complete lines having the potential to service most hearing-impaired individuals. However, additions to the basic types of wearable amplification have not been seen. The three main types of wearable amplification still include: 1) body-borne aids, 2) ear-borne aids, and 3) in-the-ear-borne aids. The basic hearing aid styles are shown in Figure 2. Most of these aids come in either air conduction (most often used) or bone conduction versions, and provide numerous options for modifying input and output characteristics of intensity, frequency, and time (e.g., microphones; on/off, tone, and volume controls; telephone switches; compression circuitry; and earmolds), as well as for size and price.

Body-borne aids   The rectangular shaped body aid shown in Figure 2A is probably the largest of the wearable aids used today. The separation of the microphone and receiver by a wire cord allows for increased output with fewer acoustic feedback (squeal) problems. It is usually reserved for individuals with more severe hearing losses because it provides more output than the other types. Because of its size, this aid is usually worn on the body in a shirt pocket or in a special harness positioned on the wearer's chest or back. The case is constructed of durable plastic or metal, so this aid has been found useful for active young children and mentally retarded persons who have trouble taking care of an aid.

Ear-borne aids   Figure 2, *B* and *C* shows two basic types of ear-borne aids. The first is described as an ear-level aid, also called post-auricular, behind-the-ear, or over-the-ear. This aid is considerably smaller than the body type and therefore has more cosmetic appeal to many users. The aid is constructed of durable plastic molded to fit the contour of the pinna on which it is worn with a plastic tube leading to the ear canal. Because of its size, the microphone and receiver are considerably closer together than in the body aid, thus in some cases resulting in less power capabilities. For increased power and less feedback, a modification of this type employs an external receiver connected to the aid by a short wire. A properly fitting ear mold is critical

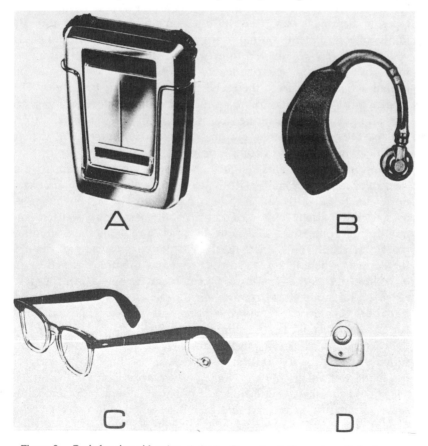

Figure 2.   Basic hearing aid styles, *A*, body; *B*, ear-level; *C*, eyeglass; *D*, in-the-ear.

for increased power capabilities in the ear-level aids. Studies have shown that, in the past 10 years, the ear-level fitting has become by far the most common type.

Another type of ear-borne aid is the eyeglass fitting. This type possesses many of the advantages and disadvantages of the ear-level fitting. With the aid located in the frames of the glasses and increased separation of the microphone and receiver, some improvements in power output and feedback are noted over the ear-level fitting. Although having some advantage for persons who must wear eyeglasses, it also presents problems by having to use one's glasses for vision and hearing aid for audition simultaneously. Obviously, this situation is not always desirable, especially when one must relinquish the prostheses for both senses when either device is in need of repair.

Many variations of the ear-level fitting are available for specific types of hearing losses. Most of these modifications fit within the family of contralateral routing of the signal (CROS) type hearing aids, which can easily be adapted to eyeglass fittings. A CROS fitting entails positioning the microphone on the poorer ear with the signal routed across the head to the receiver situated in the better ear. This type of fitting has been found useful for many unilateral and some high frequency type hearing losses (Matkin and Thomas, 1972). Pollack (1975) has adequately described and evaluated the various modifications within the CROS family.

In-the-ear-borne aids   Figure 2D depicts the other main style of wearable amplification, the in-the-ear aid, which is also somewhat misleadingly called the all-in-the-ear type. This type is much smaller in size and initially possessed considerably less power output and modification potentials, and more feedback problems than the other types described. This aid is typically custom constructed and fits into the earmold where it is worn in the concha of the user's ear. Because of its size, the in-the-ear aid has great cosmetic appeal. In the past, its power limitations restricted its usefulness for much of the hearing-impaired population (its widest market was probably the individual with a slight to mild hearing impairment who would be considered a "borderline" candidate for use of an aid). However, because of consumer demand for its small size, increased manufacturer's research has made and will continue to make it a widely used aid in the future. Many clinicians have found this type of fitting adequate for moderate to severe hearing losses and feel that it is superior to other types of fittings because of its potentials for localization.

Hearing Aid Design and Basic Components

Regardless of the hearing aid style, there are four main components housed within the unit. These include the: 1) microphone, 2) amplifier, 3) battery or power supply, and 4) receiver. Depending on the particular model, some aids possess additional features such as tone controls, volume controls, and telephone circuits. Another component very important for optimal functioning is the coupling device used to direct the sound from the aid to the ear. This is usually either a custom earmold or fitted-plastic tubing. The basic hearing aid components are depicted in Figure 3.

Microphone The microphone is a vital part of the hearing aid because it picks up acoustic energy and converts it into electric energy, thus fitting the definition of a transducer (a unit converting one form of energy to another). The various types of microphones include: crystal, ceramic, magnetic, carbon, condenser, and the new, more durable and widely used electret condenser. Traditional fittings have one non- or omnidirectional microphone, with only one port (inlet or opening) through which sound can enter. Now, through technical advances, a larger segment of the hearing-impaired population is receiving improved service with the various "directional" microphones, having two ports. These microphones have been found to provide better sound localization and understanding by attenuation of environmental noise from the rear, thus emphasizing reception from the front. The advantages of directional microphones have been treated by other authors (e.g., Lentz, 1972; Frank and Gooden, 1974; Carlson, 1976; Preves, 1976).

Amplifier The amplifier, perhaps the major component in the hearing aid, provides the acoustic gain needed for the aid to function. Most of the changes resulting in modifications of the basic output of the aid are made in this stage. Today most amplification is provided by a series of small transistors. The amplifier has been discussed in detail by Truax (1974), and Hogg (1976) and Goldberg (1976) have covered linear, limiting, and compression systems. Other components affecting the amplifier include: the volume control, tone control, and on/off switch. These too are described by Truax (1974). The volume control, a variable resistor allowing for manipulations of the gain or loudness settings, is available on many aids in the form of a manually operated dial. Other forms of volume control used to protect the user from noises above his tolerance level include two basic methods built

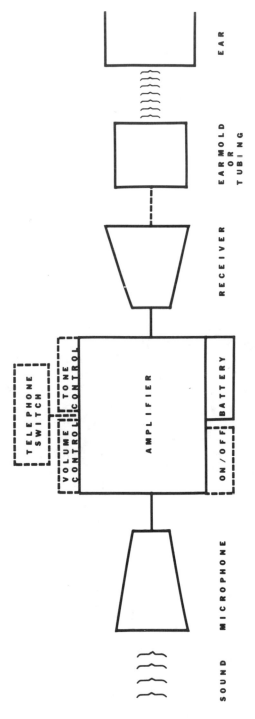

Figure 3. Block diagram of a typical hearing aid showing basic components.

into the aid to limit its output: 1) peak clipping, and 2) compression amplification or automatic gain (volume) control (AGC, AVC). The first allows the signal to be amplified to some maximum level, but beyond that point the peaks of the incoming sound waves are clipped (usually resulting in some distortion, but not enough to affect intelligibility greatly). The second, a more sophisticated method, operates by a feedback circuit, which either limits (beyond a certain level) or compresses (at all levels) the input signal. The latter method has been found beneficial to users who have tolerance problems or who spend time in irregular noise levels (Berger, 1974; Vargo, 1974; Jorgen, 1974; Truax, 1974). The tone control, available on many aids as a user-manually operated switch or as a dealer-adjustment inside the aid, provides manipulations of the frequency spectrum. Composed of condensors and resistors, the tone control allows for base and treble or low frequency and high frequency emphasis. Telephone and on/off switches are optional accessories on many aids. The telephone pick-up allows the user to hear on some telephones through use of a telecoil instead of the hearing aid microphone. The on/off switch permits the user to turn the aid off when not in use, as opposed to having to remove the battery to prohibit voltage drain.

Battery   Another important component is the battery or power supply. The battery, usually either mercury or silver oxide, provides the small electric current (about 1.5 volts) used to drive the amplifier. It is usually housed within easy access of the hearing aid case. Historical development and the advantages and disadvantages of the various types of hearing aid batteries have been discussed by Berger (1974) and by several authors in a recent issue of *Hearing Aid Journal* (Broderick, 1976; Cook, 1976; Kelley, 1976; Smith, 1976; Spar, 1976; Wiltse, 1976).

Receiver   The receiver is the second transducer in the hearing aid and serves the reverse purpose of the microphone. That is, it converts the amplified electric energy back into acoustic energy to be passed on to the ear. Hearing aid receivers are usually either bone conduction vibrators, or the type more commonly used in air conduction units composed of magnetic coils through which the electric currents pass causing movements of a diaphragm and resulting in sound waves. In ear-level type aids the receiver is usually internal (housed within the hearing aid case) and the sound waves are passed on to the ear through a molded plastic tube. Body aids typically use the external button type receiver, which snaps into the user's earmold. As mentioned earlier, some ear-level aids may be fitted with an external receiver for increased power output with less acoustic feed-back.

Earmold   The earmold, coming in various types and made of several materials, is a vital part of the hearing aid and can often mean the difference between a successful satisfactory fitting, or failure. Basically, it is a custom-made plastic insert or earpiece into which the receiver or tubing of an aid is fitted and through which the sound waves are sent to the user's ear. Although its purpose may range from modifying the basic frequency response of the aid by venting (drilling an additional channel in the mold) to just structural support for an ear-borne aid, the earmold should be considered vitally important in the hearing aid fitting. Because the earmold is one of the major sources of acoustic feedback, its proper fitting is essential in the young child, whose pinna size changes rapidly in the first few years. Excellent coverage of earmolds and the effects of acoustic couplers on the performance of hearing aids has been presented by several authors (e.g., Nielsen, 1971; Lybarger, 1972; Berger, 1974; Briskey and Wruk, 1974; Caine, 1974; Green, 1974; Hastings, 1974; Konkle and Bess, 1974; Langford, 1975; Berger, 1976a; Coogle, 1976; Frank and Karlovich, 1976; Hocks, 1976; Kaplan, 1976; Kolb, 1976; Morgan, 1976; Sheeley, 1976).

Manufacturer's specifications   In order to determine the potential use of a specific hearing aid and to be sure that each hearing aid is being used with the proper components, the audiologist should obtain copies of the manufacturer's specification sheets before attempting the hearing aid evaluation. Figure 4 is an example of such an information sheet. The specification sheet should detail how the aid should be used and should include information about such characteristics as: size, weight, batteries, and potential power outputs and frequency responses. Although the audiologist should use the specification sheet as a guide, it should be pointed out that the actual performance of a particular aid may not match the manufacturer's statements. Therefore, each aid should be evaluated electroacoustically by the audiologist before fitting. This topic is discussed, subsequently.

Knowing who provides the hearing aid recommendation and what may be recommended, we may now move to the evaulation procedure itself.

HOW SERVICES ARE PROVIDED

An investigation of the hearing aid evaluation would probably reveal that about as many different types or modifications are performed as

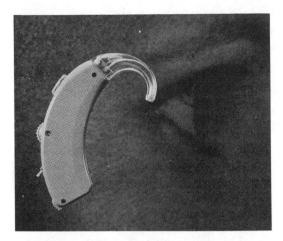

The Widex A3 Directional Microphone facilitates individual voice selection in group conversation and improves speech discrimination.

•

Compression Circuit: Exclusive distortion-free, function-perfect compression circuit reduces attack time to nil. Continuously adjustable control granting a dynamic extension up to 30 dB without distortion.

•

Output-control may be preset over a full 14 dB range from 111 to 125 dB SPL with corresponding battery economy.

•

The Widex Variable Rheostat Tone Control permits fine accurate adjustment through a wide band of low frequencies.

•

A3 H version
incorporates Noise Suppressor Switch: Pure gold, moisture and perspiration-resistant external bass-cut switch.

A3 T version
incorporates an improved induction pickup coil. Much greater efficiency due to max. extension of special numetal core.

The WIDEX A3 – a most advanced and versatile earlevel hearing aid development

Directional Hearing ■ Adjustable Compression/Output and Tone ■

The specially constructed directional Electret microphone incorporates a time delay element which has its effect on rear entry sounds. Sounds from the front are thus more pronounced and the direction from where the sound emanates can therefore be identified.

The directional effect of the Widex A3, as measured in a free field in the anechoic chamber at the Widex factory, is illustrated in the graph below.

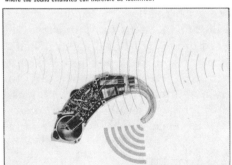

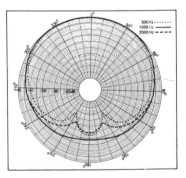

Figure 4. Sample of a manufacturer's hearing aid specification sheet. (Courtesy of Widex Hearing Aid Co., Inc.)

there are audiologists who perform them. As pointed out earlier, how the evaluation is to be performed is still a major source of controversy (Johnson, 1972). In this section are presented various forms of the traditional evaluation. However, before any hearing aid evaluation

(HAE) there are several tests that should be administered to determine:
1) if there is a need for amplification, and 2) whether or not an individual is a candidate for amplification.

Tests Preceding Hearing Aid Evaluation

Although the tests to be administered before the hearing aid evaluation have been covered thoroughly in earlier chapters of this text, it is worthwhile to mention them briefly again here. These preliminary tests would be administered in a thorough diagnostic hearing evaluation (HE) usually conducted at a separate time before the HAE. The acquisition of a complete case history including the client's otologic records and prior medical and audiometric results become important to the HAE. The HE should include at least cursory otoscopy to ensure otologically normal ear canals and tympanic membranes. Abnormalities of the external ear system such as atresia (blockage) or stenosis (narrowing) of the canals, impacted cerumen, or otitis (infections of the external or middle ear) could possibly prevent the acquisition of accurate test results, let alone satisfactory impressions for earmolds in air conduction hearing aid fittings; bone conduction fittings might prove beneficial in such cases (Miller, 1967).

Depending upon the person conducting the HE, tests with tuning forks might be administered before electronic audiometric evaluations. These are often administered by the otologist, as well as the audiologist, and can give insight to the integrity of both the conductive and the sensorineural systems before the audiometer is ever turned on.

Audiometric tests administered in the HE should include acquisition of complete air and bone conduction pure tone thresholds with appropriate masking if necessary; speech reception thresholds (SRTs); and speech discrimination scores in both quiet and noise conditions. These tests should be accomplished for each ear independently under earphones. Additional information is gained by testing both ears in the sound field condition.

As a preliminary to the HAE, it is advisable to determine independent ear scores for tolerance and comfort levels respectively measured as the "uncomfortable loudness" (UCL) or "threshold of discomfort" (TD), and the "most comfortable listening" (MCL) levels. The "dynamic range" can be computed as the difference between the UCL and the SRT. This information is especially helpful for the client with recruitment, an abnormal sensitivity to loud sounds often seen in clients with high frequency sensorineural hearing losses. The dynamic range gives an indication of how much amplification the client can use, and is therefore useful in determining what type of aid to try.

The above tests should be administered as a minimum before the HAE, and should be accompanied by any of those from the special test battery when necessary. Special tests might include: the short increment sensitivity index (SISI), alternate binaural loudness balancing (ABLB), or monaural loudness balancing (MLB) tests for recruitment; tests for tone decay (the inability for the ear to hold the perception of a tone for a normal length of time; this abnormal fatiguing often indicates a retrocochlear lesion involving the auditory nerve); and the Stenger, Lombard, or Doerfler-Stewart tests for functional or nonorganic losses. Other preliminary evaluations should include impedance and acoustic reflex testing (to be discussed in more detail later) which assess both the middle and inner ear systems.

Compiling Results of Preliminary Testing

The audiologist should be cautious against recommending amplification for clients with conductive hearing losses such as otospongeosis (otosclerosis), which could be treated successfully by the otologist, retrocochlear lesions such as tumors that could endanger the client's life, functional or feigned hearing losses and those associated with special diseases such as Meniere's or labrynthitis, which cause serious illness as well as problems in speech discrimination. For these reasons it behooves audiologists to keep in close contact with the other professionals on the hearing health team. The best policy is always to obtain medical clearance from the otologist before recommending amplification (Miller, 1967; Winchester, 1967). The information gleaned from the HE and consultation with the hearing health team should allow the audiologist to diagnose the status of the client's hearing, especially as to type and degree, pure tone configuration, amount, discrimination, and tolerance of speech, and otologic background of the hearing loss.

Berger and Millin (1971) posited the following as a determiner of hearing aid candidacy based on the contour or configuration of the pure tone thresholds:

1. Most favorable: flat, gradually rising, or gradually falling.
2. Less favorable: steep falling, deep saucer-shape, or irregular dips and peaks.
3. Least favorable: sharp drop at any lower frequency, islands of hearing only, or a remnant of hearing at lowest frequencies only.

They further indicated that based on pure tone thresholds (re: dB
ISO 1964) the expected benefits from amplification would be as
follows:

0–30: usually no aid needed
30–40: borderline
40–55: good benefit from an aid
55–85: profit most from an aid
85–100: probably will give some benefit
100–110: aid seldom useful

Berger and Millin (1971) also used the following unaided speech discrimination scores as predictors of user success with amplification:

90% or better: probable good results with amplification
70–90%: mild difficulty
50–70%: substantial difficulty
50% or poorer: amplification probably not entirely successful

They did point out, however, that even poor speech discrimination
scores may be improved to useful levels for the severely impaired individual receiving little other auditory stimulation.

Also, from in-depth counseling with the client, the audiologist
should know the client's subjective feelings about his hearing and the
possibility of wearing personal amplification. In compiling these data,
the audiologist should have an accurate picture as to whether or not
the client would be a good candidate for a hearing aid evaluation. If
positive, the next step is the hearing aid evaluation.

Traditional Hearing Aid Evaluations

In this section some of the basic concepts of the traditional hearing
aid evaluation are presented, followed by a few step by step examples
and critiques of such approaches. In the traditional hearing aid evaluation the audiologist's goal has been mainly to help the client select
the proper type of amplification. Because the audiologist is usually
not directly concerned with the sale of the instruments he evaluates,
he is free to sample objectively many different types of aids in his
attempt to provide the best amplification possible for his client. As
noted earlier, this has become a source of controversy since many
audiologists have become actively involved in the hearing aid dispensing process. Nevertheless, as an objective third party, the audiologist in the traditional evaluation goes about his business of compar-

ing various makes and models, and frequency and gain (loudness) settings among the hearing aids tested, thus, the essence of the traditional HAE. In this procedure it is common for the audiologist to make several comparisons among many aids (usually at least three) and settings for unaided versus aided SRT, speech discrimination, and tolerance level scores, both in quiet and in various competing noise situations. Typically, the client is also permitted to experience the aids in various informal communication settings such as the clinic waiting room, offices, on the street, in a cafeteria, and in conversations with one or more persons. Obviously, to experience all aids tested in the same informal settings would require considerable time and would be a difficult task to control. Such exposures should allow the client to provide some subjective input as to what aid he prefers, conceivably an influencing factor in the evaluation. Once the audiologist has determined the type of aid from which the client should derive the most benefit, he traditionally sends him with a general recommendation to a local reputable hearing aid dealer who selects the specific aid the client will try. The client then purchases the aid from the dealer and is told to return to the clinic for follow-up testing at a later date. An obvious disadvantage of this approach is that there is no guarantee that the client will receive the exact same type of aid employed in the HAE, let alone whether or not he will return for the follow-up services. These are yet other reasons why the audiologist has become more involved with the specific recommendation of aids.

The *Carhart Method*, one of the first hearing aid evaluation procedures used by the audiologist, was described in a series of publications in 1946 by Carhart and his associates at the Deshon General Hospital (Carhart, 1946a–d). This has been called the traditional or conventional hearing aid evaluation procedure and its basic steps were summarized by Ross (1972) as follows:

1. The subject's unaided sound field SRT, tolerance limit, and discrimination score (PB-50s at 25 dB SL) were measured. These scores served as the reference for comparison with aided performance.
2. The gain control of the first instrument was adjusted until the subject reported that a 40-dB hearing threshold level (HTL) speech signal was at the MCL level. An aided SRT and TD were then measured.

3. The aid was set on maximum gain and the aided SRT and TD were again measured.

4. The gain control was adjusted to permit the subject to reach an MCL level with a 50-dB HTL input speech signal. Two signal-to-noise ratios were obtained, one with white noise and the other with sawtooth noise. The intensity of the noise was alternately increased and decreased until a point was reached where the subject could barely repeat several test words. The difference between the speech and the noise levels at this point defined the signal-to-noise ratios.

5. The aid was again adjusted to permit the subject to reach an MCL level, this time with a 40-dB HTL input speech signal. The SRT was again measured for a reliability check against step 2. A 50-word intelligibility test was administered at a 25-dB SL.

These basic steps were repeated for all aids tried in the evaluation. These steps allowed aids to be compared and selected on the basis of 1) best SRTs, 2) best dynamic range, 3) best tolerance of noise in speech discrimination, and 4) best speech discrimination scores. Although some of these measures have been changed (e.g., SRTs and TDs are not routinely assessed at maximum gain settings, and speech discrimination is measured under different types and levels of competing noise and no noise conditions), most are still the basis of the traditional HAE.

Berger and Millin (1971) have summarized another of the early traditional approaches by Wiener and Miller (1946) as follows:

A. Monaural tests without the aid.
    1. Pure tone thresholds.
    2. Thresholds for speech.
    3. Tolerance for pure tones.
    4. Tolerance for speech.
    5. Discrimination tests.
B. Free field tests without the hearing aid.
    1–5. Same tests as listed under A.
C. Free field tests with the hearing aid.
    1. Pure tone threshold(s).
    2. Threshold for speech.
    3. Tolerance for loud speech.
    4. Discrimination test(s).
    5. Judgments of quality.

6. The effect on speech thresholds or discrimination when annoying sounds and various background noises are present.

As with the Carhart method, all aids are tested with steps C 1-6 and are compared for their performances.

Yet another typical traditional HAE was presented by Berger and Millin (1971) who, after preselecting several aids for testing, employed the following evaluation based primarily on patient performance:

1. With the speech audiometer at 40 dB (i.e., 62 dB SPL) a recording of cold running speech is played, or the audiologist reads informative but nonemotional speech materials. With the aid in place the patient experiments with the volume or tone controls to find a comfortable listening level. Once this level is obtained, he is told not to touch the controls until he is told to do so.
2. An aided free field SRT is obtained by either recordings or monitored live voice (MLV).
3. Aided discrimination testing is done at SRT plus 40 dB (or 25 dB SL, or MCL, or any other constant level that approximates normal conversational speech) by recordings or MLV.
4. Speech-in-noise tests are administered: a) SRT in white noise—speech and noise from separate speakers (find amount of noise needed to alter SRT); or b) obtain a speech discrimination score for a predetermined signal-to-noise level (e.g., +10, +5, or 0).
5. Determine tolerance for cold running speech.
6. After completion of tests, aid is removed and settings are noted and recorded on a hearing aid evaluation form.
7. Some clinics add or substitute a step for steps 4 and 5 (i.e., obtain discrimination and tolerance scores for the aid set at full volume).

This procedure would be repeated for all aids tested. Only after testing all aids are patient's subjective ratings sought and relative costs of the hearing aids discussed. Criteria for selection of an aid would include: 1) improvement in SRT, 2) improvement or maintenance of speech discrimination scores, and 3) client's preference.

It should be noted that improvements in the SRT do not necessarily imply improvements in discrimination.

Compiling Results of Hearing Aid Evaluation

Following the evaluation, the client should be thoroughly counseled regarding the test results and various aspects of amplification. He should be made aware of the advantages and disadvantages of a hearing aid (i.e., although an aid may help, it will not restore hearing to normal; some discrimination problems may still be noticed from distortion). The client should be informed of adjustment periods; control settings; tolerance of the earmold, the aid, unfamiliar sounds in the environment; and follow-up in the form of aural rehabilitation or counseling.

Regardless of the hearing aid evaluation procedure employed, each clinic should have a hearing aid evaluation form on which to enter the results of each aid tested. Figure 5 is an example of such a form used in our clinic. This form has spaces in which the specific aid, various settings, and corresponding test results should be recorded. Other important information includes type of earmold, ear fitted, and recommendations. Once an aid has been selected (or the choice has been narrowed to a few in the case of a general recommendation), a hearing aid recommendation form should be completed and forwarded to the hearing aid dealer. Such a form is shown in Figure 6. Some clinics prefer not to recommend a specific dealer, but to supply the client with a list of several reputable dealers in his area, and let him choose one. In this case the form should accompany the client to the dealer.

Criticisms of Traditional Hearing Aid Evaluation

It should be noted that these traditional methods did not stand without criticism. In a publication known as the "Harvard Report," Davis et al. (1946; 1947) questioned the idea of selective amplification and criticized the use of lengthy fitting procedures for most cases, with the exception of the "hard-to-fit" patient. They proposed a testing program in which identification of spondees was tested at 20 or 40 dB, and 60 or 70 dB (re: speech audiometric zero), and tolerance was assessed at 100 dB. From these values the dynamic range was computed and used to estimate user success and to predict a certain pattern of amplification.

Later Shore, Bilger, and Hirsh (1960) questioned the value of making comparative measures of SRT and speech discrimination in noise and quiet conditions for patients wearing many different types of hearing aids having differing acoustic characteristics. Because such measures had low test-retest reliability, they found them un-

Name _____ Tester _____ Date _____ Earmold Used _____

AUDIOMETER: _____

	Date
	Ear
	Make & Model
	Receiver
	Tone Setting
	Volume Setting

	UNAIDED		
	R	L	SF
SRT			
UCL			
PB Quiet			
PB Level			
PB Noise			
Noise Level			

Recommendations _____

Remarks _____

dB: American Standard

Figure 5. An example of a hearing aid-evaluation worksheet used at the Bowling Green State University Hearing Clinic.

Speech and Hearing Clinic

HEARING AID RECOMMENDATION

Dealer:

Name:
Address:

Phone:
Age:

The follwing hearing aid was recommended for this person.

Make:

Model:

Ear:

Mold:

Gain:

Tone:

The above hearing aid dealer will contact you. If you have any difficulty adjusting to your hearing aid after you get it, call us at (419) 372—2223 to arrange for further consultation.

_____

Supervising Audiologist

Figure 6. An example of a hearing aid-recommendation form used at the Bowling Green State University Hearing Clinic.

warranted for the large amounts of clinical time invested in their administration. In essence, they felt these tests did not show distinguishing differences among listener performances with several aids.

Although Resnick and Becker (1963) also advocated discontinuing the elaborate comparisons among aids in the traditional evaluations, they supported greater emphasis on client counseling regarding possible benefits and problems with amplification. They felt this would better prepare the client to select an appropriate aid from a reputable dealer.

More recently, Berger and Millin (1971) posited issues pertaining to the following, which need to be resolved in order to better predict how an individual will perform with amplification.

1. The problem of the validity in comparing a user's performance with an aid in the clinic sound room versus outside in the problem environments of everyday life.
2. The problem of predicting from short duration tests how a user will adjust to an aid after prolonged experience with it.
3. The problem of finding suitable competing noise stimuli that adequately reflect those encountered by the user in everyday life.
4. The problem of testing the aid in a reasonably nonreverberant sound room and predicting how the aid will perform in hard-walled rooms such as offices, kitchens, schoolrooms, and living rooms.
5. The problem of testing and recommending a specific aid in the HAE, but fitting the user with an instrument of the same model from the dealer's stock, which may vary in acoustic performance from the aid tested.
6. The problems regarding the user's psychologic adjustment to amplification.

Carhart (1975) has also criticized the traditional HAE procedures. He pointed to the inadequacies of its methods for speech audiometry as a serious deficiency of contemporary audiology. Carhart further stated:

> The fact is that speech audiometry as practiced clinically for hearing aid selection is relatively archaic and unrevealing. It needs improvement in several ways if its results are to be of greatest help to hearing aid users. For one thing we are still awaiting a definitive validational study of the relationship between formal scores obtained via speech audiometry and work-a-day hearing aid efficiency. (p. xxix)

According to Carhart, there are problems with current tests and how they are administered (e.g., much time is wasted on words contained on the W-22 test that are easily discriminated by most people and thus contribute little to critical differences in discrimination). He discouraged use of the PB "half-list" procedure of measuring speech discrimination, especially in evaluating hearing aid performance, because it tends to reduce credence in the results. Like Berger and Millin (1971), Carhart questioned whether speech audiometry as currently employed by many clinics truly simulates everyday listening situations. This becomes critical when evaluating hearing aid performance in unrealistic conditions of steady state noise (e.g. white noise); "multitalker" noise composed of several human speakers is probably a better indicator of real life situations.

By now it should be obvious that the use of speech stimuli is a major part of predicting and assessing success with amplification in the traditional hearing aid evaluation (Kasden, 1975). Much of this testing is performed in quiet environments and at sub-MCL levels (Ross, 1976). Because many hearing aid users require considerable gain and they do not routinely employ their aids for listening to very quiet sounds (i.e., near threshold), it would seem logical that other test measures might give more realistic results. Even Carhart, undoubtedly one of the "fathers of audiology and the hearing aid evaluation," has challenged the subjective aspects of current hearing aid evaluation procedures. For increased objectivity and quantification many audiologists have moved to more prescriptive approaches, many employing electroacoustic, narrow band noise, MCL, and TD measures in order to reduce the subjectivity in the hearing aid recommendation.

Electroacoustic Measurements

One avenue of research and development that has enhanced objectivity in clinical aspects of the hearing aid recommendation is electroacoustic measurements. Regarding hearing aid dispensing, Libby (1975) has referred to these measurements as "the arrival of a new era"; a giant step toward reducing the "art" in hearing aid fittings, and replacing it with a "science." He indicates that these physical measures are important because they provide for routine electroacoustic testing of aids, quantitative analysis as opposed to qualitative (human ear performances), maintenance of standardization and reproduciblity, determination if an aid meets manufacturer's specifications, and facilitation of repair by pre- and postrepair measures.

The history, development, procedures, and rationale for electroacoustic hearing aid measurements and their standards have been elaborated upon by several authors (e.g., Carver, 1972; Lybarger, 1974; Pollack, 1975; Rubin, 1976). The pros and cons of electroacoustic measurements have been covered in a number of recent publications, which should be of interest to the avid reader (e.g., Libby, 1975; Schneider, 1975; Curran, 1976; Ely, 1976; Fradkin, 1976; Heide, 1976a,b; Sinclair, 1976; Teter, 1976). Therefore, these issues are presented in considerably less detail here. The standards used for such measurements include those proposed by the American National Standards Institute (ANSI S3.3, 1960; S3.8, 1967) and the Hearing Aid Industry Conference (HAIC, 1961). These standards have been described in the sources listed above. In addition, a new revision of the ANSI standards (ASA STD 7-1976; ANSI S3.22-1976) has been accepted and has been described and summarized by Lybarger (1976) and Lilly (1976) and in Rubin (1976). It should be noted that the revised standard is completely voluntary and discretionary for hearing aid manufacturers and suppliers.

Basically, the electroacoustic measures and standards provide a uniform method for making evaluations between and among different hearing aid makes, models, and settings that should be reproducible from one test situation to the next. These measurements are made without the aid being worn by a hearing aid user, but in a fashion representing a "normal" communication situation in which a user might typically find himself. That is, in a sound field setting, at intensity levels approximating average conversational speech (60–70 dB SPL), and at usual speaker-listener distances (3–15 feet). For the purposes of these measurements, the sound field becomes a commercial hearing aid test box (such as those available by Bruel and Kjaer Instruments) or an anechoic chamber; the human speaker becomes a signal emitted from an audio oscillator (either discrete or sweep frequency) and directed to a loudspeaker situated within the test room; and instead of evaluating the aid on an actual user, it is connected to an artificial ear (2-cc coupler). From the artificial ear the response of the aid is directed to various meters (e.g., sound level meter, distortion meter, voltmeter) and finally printed out on a graphic level recorder. The oscillator must have a relatively constant output from 200–5,000 Hz. Its total harmonic distortion (THD) cannot be greater than 0.2% for frequency response measures, nor greater than 0.5% for distortion measures. It should be noted that an additional oscillator and mixer are needed for intermodulation distortion measures. Figure 7 is a block diagram of a commercially available electroacoustic measurement system. It should be realized that the hearing aid test chamber depicted in the figure may be replaced by an anechoic-type room meeting the ANSI standards. Two basic methods are described in the standards for maintaining a constant signal sound pressure level (± 1.5 dB from 200–3,000 Hz and ± 2.5 dB from 3,000–5,000 Hz) within the test chamber. Both methods are accomplished with a condenser microphone (situated inside the test room) and compressor amplifier (placed outside in the control room). The first is the "substitution" method in which the hearing aid and the

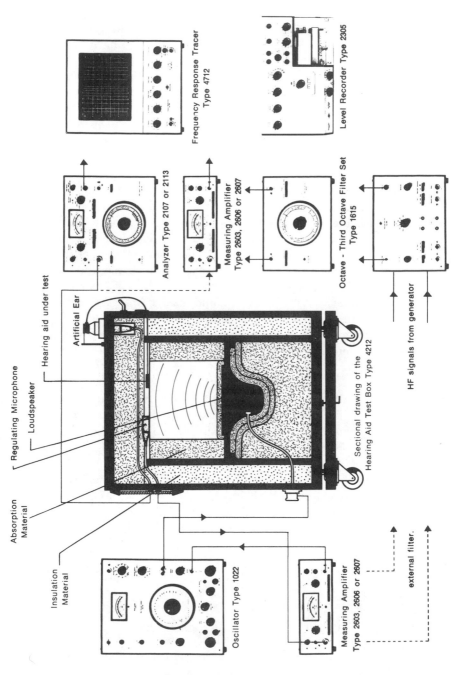

Figure 7. Block diagram of a Brüel and Kjaer hearing aid measurement system. (Reprinted by permission of Brüel & Kjaer Precision Instruments.)

condenser microphone are placed alternatively at the same test point in the sound room. The second is the "comparison" method in which the hearing aid and the condenser microphone are placed at two different points in the sound room. Both serve to regulate the noise levels within the sound chamber.

Before making electroacoustic measurements the audiologist should realize that he may not be able to reproduce the manufacturer's specifications for a particular hearing aid. This could be attributable to actual differences among aids, but is more likely because of differences in test equipment and procedures. It is also important to note all volume and tone control settings, as well as battery type and life. Many manufacturers make their measurements at "full-on" gain settings; that recommended in the new ANSI standard is a lower setting more representative of that actually employed by the user. Also, in the new standards the harmonic distortion measures are made at a level close to the maximum output capability of the hearing aid; some manufacturers might use a lower setting that tends to improve the looks of these data. The power supply to the aid could also be the source of differences among measures. That is, if the manufacturer tests the aid with a new battery, these measurements probably will not closely approximate those made on the aid containing a battery that has been used for several hours, thus suffering from more drain.

The electroacoustic methods typically provide measures of a) gain; b) saturation sound pressure level; c) frequency response; d) frequency bandwidth or range; e) distortion such as harmonic, intermodulation, frequency, and transient; and f) battery drain. The actual step by step procedures for each of these measurements are listed in the published standards.

Gain—Gain is measured in dB and is the difference between the signal entering the hearing aid (input) and that leaving it (output). For example, gain would equal 70 dB if the input were 50 dB and the output were 120 dB. "Average gain" was measured by averaging the output at 500, 1,000, and 2,000 Hz in the earlier standards. The new ANSI standard varies in this computation by taking the average of 1,000, 1,600, and 2,500 Hz, and is thus called the high frequency average (HF average). This measurement is made with the aid at the full-on setting and with an input signal of 60 dB SPL (a 50-dB SPL input may be used if the aid reaches saturation at the higher level). Both the earlier HAIC and ANSI standards used an input of 50 dB SPL, but the new

ANSI level of 60 dB SPL corresponds more closely to that used by most hearing aid manufacturers. "Peak gain" provides the dB level and the frequency at which the highest gain is reached. This measure could be of importance in special fittings (e.g., cases of recruitment) where the peak gain may be several dB higher than the average gain, thus causing tolerance problems before an adequate average gain setting is reached. It should also be noted here that the new standard and Federal Trade Commission (FTC) and Food and Drug Administration (FDA) legislation will deem that any aid providing outputs in excess of 130 dB SPL shall enclose a warning to the fact that it may damage residual hearing in the hearing-impaired user.

Saturation sound pressure level—Saturation sound pressure level (SSPL), also called "acoustic output" or "maximum power output" (MPO), is the most output SPL the aid can produce, regardless of the amounts of gain and input. This is the saturation point where the aid no longer produces a satisfactory corresponding increase in output for increases in input, and where beyond this level considerable distortion will result. The new ANSI standard calls for a full-on setting, measures the same frequencies as in the HF average, and employs an input signal level of 90 dB SPL. Measures are also taken across the frequency range from 200–5,000 Hz with the above setting and input. This measure is referred to as $SSPL_{90}$. These measures must have a tolerance within plus or minus a certain number of decibels of the manufacturer's specified value for that model. Pollack (1975) has pointed out that these measures are of particular importance in hearing aid evaluations to be sure an aid is providing an SPL sufficiently above the user's threshold to be maximally useful, but that it does not exceed his threshold of discomfort. An additional measure called for in the new standard is the "reference test gain control position," measured with a 60-dB SPL input and resulting in an average output that is 17 dB less than that noted for the HF average $SSPL_{90}$ value. (If the gain available does not reach this level, the full-on setting can be considered the reference test gain control position). This setting allows measurements to be taken at levels closer to those typically used by the hearing aid user, and is employed in measurements of frequency response, harmonic distortion, and equivalent input noise level.

Frequency response—The frequency response in the new standard is measured using the reference test gain control position, and depicts the relative amount of gain provided by the aid at each frequency. This response is either automatically or manually recorded across the frequencies 200–5,000 Hz.

Frequency bandwidth—The frequency bandwith or "range" in the new standard expresses the upper and lower limits of frequencies of usable amplification available from the aid. The manufacturer's average of 1,000, 1,600, and 2,500 Hz is found; 20 dB is subtracted from this value; and a line parallel to the abscissa is drawn at that level. The range indicated by the crossing of the parallel line and the lower and upper frequency limits is the frequency bandwidth. The old standards used the average for the frequencies 500, 1,000, and 2,000 Hz and a line 15 dB below that level. This measure seems to provide little additional information to that already gained from the complete frequency response curve.

Distortion—In an "ideal" hearing aid the signal reproduced by the aid should be identical to the input signal. The hearing aid, unfortunately, is not ideal, and therefore produces some distortion on the signal. The most common type measured and reported by hearing aid manufacturers is "harmonic distortion." This type results when the aid generates additional frequencies that are whole number multiples of the input signal fundamental. Usually, the higher the gain setting, the higher is the resulting harmonic distortion. This becomes an important factor when selecting an aid. If the aid only provides the user with satisfactory amplification near its maximum gain setting, distortion will probably also occur and possibly cause a reduction in speech intelligibility. In the new standard, harmonic distortion is measured in the reference test gain control setting and at 500, 800, and 1,600 Hz with an input of 70 dB SPL. The resulting values are recorded in percentage of total harmonic distortion (%THD). "Intermodulation distortion" results as sum and difference frequencies in the output when the input signal is composed of two or more frequencies. "Transient distortion" arises whenever the aid is unable to handle sharp rise and decay times in a signal causing a lingering or "ringing" wave form that interferes with transients within the speech signal. "Frequency distortion" relates to fidelity and distortions resulting from differences in the frequency response and bandwidth between the input and output signals. All the various types of distortion can interfere with an aid's functioning and cause a reduction in speech intelligibility.

Battery drain—In the new standard, battery drain is measured by
setting the aid in the reference test gain control position. Battery
current is measured in milliamperes (mA) with a 1,000-Hz input
signal at 65 dB SPL.

It should be noted that although these electroacoustic measurements are available only for air conduction hearing aids (no standards
or measures have been proposed for bone conduction units), they represent a sophisticated scientific supplement to the traditional hearing
aid evaluation procedure. A positive point is the recommendation
that the new standards be reviewed every 5 years in order to update
procedures that will undoubtedly be needed to meet with changes in
hearing aid and instrumentation design, and increases in our understanding of electroacoustic measures. It should be remembered that
these electroacoustic measures only evaluate the hearing aid in and
according to the test conditions specified in the standards and may
not truly represent how the aid will function when worn on a human
ear. With respect to this problem, current research is being conducted
with manikin measurements that more closely approximate the real
ear conditions.

Knowles Electronics Manikin for Acoustic Research

Carhart (1975) pointed out some of the problems with the "test box"
electroacoustic measures. A main concern is the fact that the measurements taken in the closed 2-cc coupler may not represent how the
aid would function when worn in a user's ear canal (because of resonance effects) in real life. When the aid is not worn on the body or
head, normal diffraction and "baffle" effects, which modify the signal
intensity reaching the hearing aid microphone, are not accounted for.
In an attempt to account for such effects, the Knowles Company
devised the Knowles Electronics Manikin for Acoustic Research
(KEMAR) depicted in Figure 8. KEMAR's development, dimensions,
and construction have been described in several sources (Burkhard
and Sachs, 1975; Knowles and Burkhard, 1975; Burkhard, 1976;
Radcliffe, 1976) as well as at the Manikin Measurement Methods
Conference held in Washington, D.C. on April 5, 1976. Burkhard
and Sachs (1975) described the body baffle effect and cited earlier
investigators who attempted, but failed, to account for it with various
head and body model "dummies."

KEMAR, according to Burkhard and Sachs (1975), Burkhard
(1976), and Knowles and Burkhard (1975), provides the following advantages for electroacoustic measurements:

1. Average anthropometric dimensions of an adult human
2. Ear canal and eardrum to match real ears in open, partially closed, and closed ear use. All sound pressures are measured at the eardrum
3. Acoustically and dimensionally average pinna
4. By using a statistically sized manikin, a good estimate of a given parameter for a population is immediately available

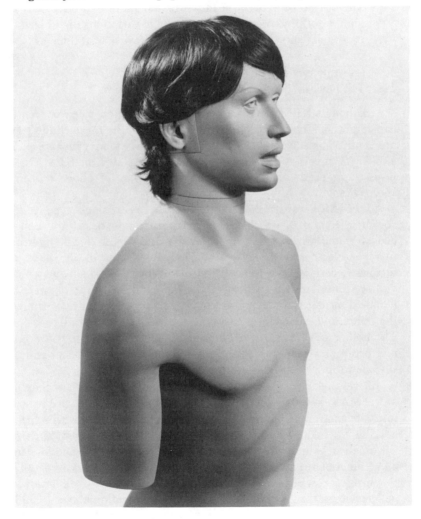

Figure 8.   Knowles Electronics Manikin for Acoustic Research (KEMAR). (From Burkhard and Sachs, 1975, reprinted by permission.)

5. The contribution of sound diffraction around a wearer is included in the gain and other parameters
6. The subject's physical size is always the same. It is a completely reproducible test person. The subject can be positioned repeatedly in the same way
7. Easily exchangeable pinna to permit study of ear size effects
8. The subject is stationary. It stays in place for a test indefinitely. There is no time limit on measurements attributable to any of a number of physiologic and psychologic variations of subjects
9. It does not show changes of response because of fatigue or health status
10. Its responses can be readily calibrated
11. The pay and overhead rates are very attractive

Although KEMAR is currently used at many research centers, two requirements may prohibit its routine use in most clinics. They are: 1) the initial expense of purchasing KEMAR and its accessories, and 2) for precision measurements of hearing aids on KEMAR, the investigator needs an anechoic-type sound room of about 3 m in its shortest length.

KEMAR's eardrum is modeled with a Zwislocki-type coupler shown in Figure 9, which seems to approximate better the real ear acoustics and dimensions than does the traditional 2-cc coupler used in other electroacoustic systems. The dimensions of the head and torso were derived from the average size of over 4,000 men and women, and are reported to be within 4% of the combined average male and female dimensions. Although based on a smaller number of subjects, the pinna and ear canal measures were derived in a similar fashion. The hollow head and torso are constructed of fabricated fiberglass-reinforced polyester; the easily removable ears are soft, tear-resistant silicone rubber.

Several electroacoustic aided-ear and unaided-ear gain measures on KEMAR have demonstrated its likeness to the true change in sound intensity an average hearing aid wearer might anticipate with a specific hearing aid fitting. Terms used in the literature to denote such true ear relative gain include "orthotelephonic gain," "etymotic gain," and "functional gain." According to Knowles and Burkhard (1975), the need for KEMAR became clear 1) in order to eliminate the deficiencies of the 2-cc coupler for receiver calibration above 4,000 Hz, when receivers with responses at higher frequencies were proposed; 2) because no valid means were available for proper measure and

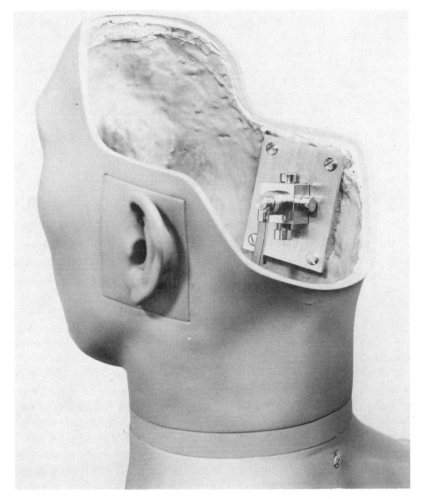

Figure 9.   View of KEMAR's hollow head and Zwislocki-type coupler. (From Burk-hard and Sachs, 1975, reprinted by permission.)

specification of open ear canal (e.g., CROS, BICROS, and IROS) and vented mold fittings; and 3) in order to gain a meaningful mea-surement of the directional properties of hearing aids when worn by the user. One of the more important of these uses is the measurement of the directionality of hearing aids (Knowles and Burkhard, 1975; Causcy, 1976; Prevcs, 1976). Causcy (1976) described the procedure for such measurements. Knowles and Burkhard (1975) presented results of polar plottings from KEMAR for both directional and non-directional hearing aids, which revealed that a non- or omnidirectional aid worn by KEMAR or, it is supposed, a real person was no longer nondirectional. That is, Figure 10 shows that when a nondirectional aid is measured in a standard 2-cc coupler and anechoic chamber it is equally sensitive to sound pressure from all directions, because the hearing aid and the 2-cc coupler are the only things causing diffraction of the sound. The figure shows that the same aid worn by KEMAR exhibits a "head shadow" effect (regions of higher gain when sound source and aid are on the same side and regions of lower gain on the opposite side), thus it is no longer nondirectional. Figure 11 shows that similar findings were noted for directional aids, which were found to function directionally in standard laboratory free field conditions. But when placed on KEMAR, the figure shows that the directionality of this aid is disturbed by the presence of the head, thus making it more sensitive to sounds coming from the same side on which the aid is worn and less sensitive to those on the opposite side. The head shadow again causes this aid to be more sensitive "slightly forward and to the side," as opposed to "straight ahead" as seen in the measurements without KEMAR. Knowles and Burkhard (1975) state, "in actual use, then, a hearing aid must be considered a directional instrument.... Directional microphones only alter the details of directionality." These findings help to quantify more accurately how such aids will perform when fitted on a real hearing-impaired user and should be considered by the audiologist in his recommendation. Obviously, as KEMAR becomes more widely employed, the electro-acoustic measurement procedures and standards will have to be modified to account for its use. The following is a preliminary outline for an ANSI proposal regarding requirements and procedures for making hearing aid measurements with a manikin (Knowles Industry, M. Burkhard, April, 1974; revised, January, 1976). It should be clearly understood here that these are not yet standards; they are merely critical issues for discussion and consideration by knowledgable parties.

1. The uniformity of the sound field will be measured. A suggestion now is that the eight corners of a cube centered on the head, without the head, will have a specified maximum range of sound pressure, front to back, side to side, and up-down. Diagonal lengths of this cubic space would be 20 cm.
2. The measurement conditions will be specified relative to free

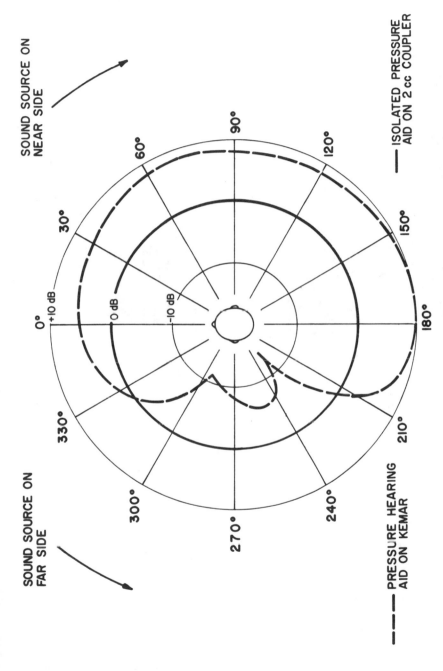

Figure 10.   Polar plotting of a nondirectional hearing aid with and without KEMAR present. (From Knowles and Burkhard, 1975, reprinted by permission.)

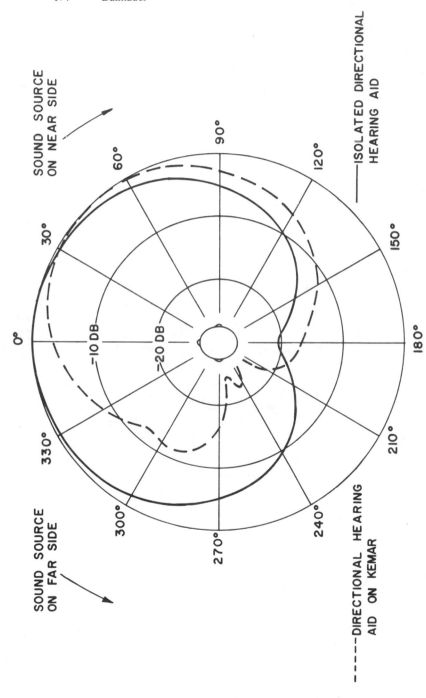

Figure 11.   Polar plotting of a directional hearing aid with and without KEMAR present. (From Knowles and Burkhard, 1975, reprinted by permission.)

field at the location in the sound field that will be the center of the head. The center of the head will be defined as being the center of a line between the ears.

3.   The distance to the source will be 1 m.

4.   The source size will be restricted tentatively to less than 8 inches in diameter. It will be a single simple loudspeaker source, i.e., no multiple loudspeaker or vented boxes (unless the vent is concentric with the speaker).

5.   Horizontal for the manikin has been defined (see Burkhard and Sachs, 1975, p. 217). The effective center of the source will be 6.4 cm below this horizontal on the manikin, with the manikin centered on the source axis in all other aspects.

6.   In reviewing the requirements here, it was decided that reference marks should be placed on the manikin.

7.   Some attention to room size or possible definition of absorption in the room may be necessary. This must be evaluated.

8.   The manikin KEMAR is supplied with two mounting positions. We will specify the recommended mounting position as the most forward one.

9.   Clothing will be used on the manikin. The suggested clothing is a T-shirt and a lab coat or equivalent.

10.   For head-worn hearing aids using acoustic tubing, the hearing aid will be mounted on the manikin as it is expected to be worn on a person. Then the tube will be cut to a length that connects the hearing aid directly to the earmold in a conventional manner. This is a departure from ANSI standard practice permitting arbitrary specification of tube length. The tube length should be stated.

11.   For open ear and vented earmold calibrations, the measurement should be made with gain depressed (a certain number of decibels, to be verified by the experimenter) relative to the acoustic feedback gain level, if observable.

12.   For open earmold calibrations, the depth of insertion of the tube will be specified. Tentatively, it seems that this should be at the entrance of the ear as defined by the junction between the rubber-molded ear and the brass fitting to which it connects.

13.   For body aids, a harness will be used that will support the hearing aid in the center of the front, below the neck junction of the manikin (exact distance to be established).

14.   There will be a note added about precautions in using control

microphone signals with KEMAR, probably in connection with specification of the room, distance to source, etc.

15.   Coordinates for directional measurements would be a clockwise rotation, with 90° indicating that the active ear is closest to the sound source.

16.   Provision to be made, by means of standard corrections, for converting nonmanikin data to manikin equivalents. This could permit reporting of data obtained in sound boxes to be compared with data obtained on manikins with the increased tolerance or increased uncertainty pointed out.

Clearly, the advent of KEMAR and the standard electroacoustic measurements permit considerable objectivity and quantification of hearing aid evaluation procedures, which should lead to more successful recommendations and fittings. These procedures also lend themselves to various prescriptive type hearing aid fittings.

Prescription Hearing Aid Fittings

In this section, some prescriptive methods that have been presented for the clinical recommendation of hearing aids are described. The electroacoustic measurements just discussed play an important part in this type of recommendation. One of the first of these methods is the Victoreen Method (Victoreen, 1960; 1973a, b). In this method, and those that follow, each patient is to have had thorough otologic and audiologic evaluations before the hearing aid evaluation. These methods are based on the assumption that sufficient gain must be provided for satisfactory amplification, but that it is illogical to fit a hearing aid at gain settings beyond an individual's tolerance levels. In this method, threshold of discomfort and most comfortable listening levels for speech and pure tones under earphones are equated to hearing aid performance. Therefore, the measures under earphones (obtained in dB HTL) must be converted to dB SPL. This information is plotted on a hearing aid-fitting table such as the one in Figure 12. This figure shows discrete test frequencies across the *abscissa*, decibels of sound pressure level on the *left ordinate*, and decibels hearing threshold level in the form of phon lines beginning on the *right ordinate* (the first such line begins at the bottom of the table and is seen to represent audiometric zero or normal threshold). The normal maximum tolerance pressure (MTP), otherwise known as UCL or TD, is noted on the table as a shaded area at and beyond 115 dB SPL at each frequency. Because this method employs pure tone stimuli, the tolerance levels are plotted as a curve across the frequency range as opposed to just one value as obtained with speech UCLs or TDs. Once the threshold is determined, the dynamic range for each frequency is computed as the difference between threshold and 115 dB SPL (MTP). This is also denoted as the range of residual hearing. Then MCL levels are determined at the most desirable points within this range, and are considered to be where amplification should be provided. A point at 65 dB SPL (seen as the *large circle* in Figure 12) represents the level of normal speech sounds, and is near the center of the dynamic range for most of the frequency range with the exception of those below 500 Hz. The MCL for 500 Hz is determined as being at the lower one-third of the dynamic range for that frequency, as opposed to one-half the range at the other frequencies. This is done to keep the more intense low frequency sounds from being amplified to the point where they mask out the highs.

The fitting of amplification at the MCLs should provide adequate hearing without going over the client's tolerance levels. This method relies heavily on pure tone stimuli, and places less emphasis on speech. Northern and Downs (1974) point to this as an advantage for young children, because fitting an aid requires "only the audiometric threshold points, which can be obtained by estimates from observations of behavioral responses or by conventional audiometric techniques, including play audiometry." In an examination of five different hearing aid-evaluation procedures on speech discrimination, Kemker and Johnson (1972) found that the fittings of amplification characteristics to the MCL as determined by Victoreen was among the more desirable methods. Their findings indicate that although the use of pure tone audiometry for hearing aid evaluations is sometimes looked upon somewhat negatively, its ability to predict the adequacy of suprathreshold discrimination performance and tolerability is important criteria against which hearing aid users can measure satisfaction (Kretschmer, 1974).

Another of the prescription methods is the Wallenfels Method (Wallenfels, 1967). Wallenfels pointed out that the prescription of hearing aids involves both "arriving at" and "filling" the prescription. His definition of prescription entails arriving at "a written set of specifications for a definite sound pattern, plus the request to provide a specific amount of amplification for each of the important frequencies within the speech range." As well as relying on complete otologic and audiometric data, this method places considerable emphasis on electroacoustic measurements that are valuable in the "filling" stage of the prescription.

Wallenfels pointed out that it is an unsuccessful effort to try to match or "mirror" amplification to the pure tone audiometric thresholds, because a patient probably hears differently at his actual lis-

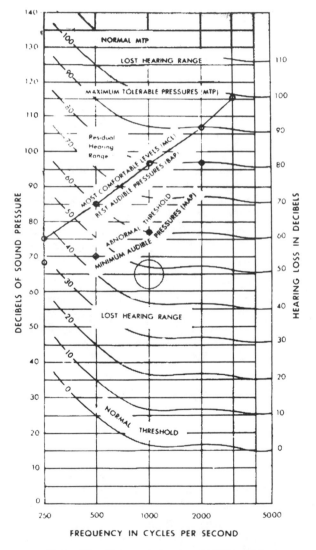

Figure 12.   Victoreen's hearing aid-fitting table.

tening level than he does at his threshold of hearing. This method also requires the conversion of dB HTL values to dB SPL, the first step in working out the prescription. Figure 13 shows that an audiogram or hearing fitting table similar to that used by Victoreen is employed and also plots normal audiometric zero as a curve near the bottom of the *abscissa*. An uncomfortable level curve is plotted as a curve at each frequency rather than as a straight line as in the Victoreen Method. This curve is said to provide a visual picture of recruitment or tone decay if they are present. In other words, a person with good tolerance in the low frequencies, may not necessarily have it for the highs. This noise sensitivity study is performed with narrow band noise calibrated to an output of 120 dB of white noise (re: 0.0002 dyne/cm^2) centered at the following frequencies: 500, 1,000, 2,000, 3,000, and 4,000 Hz. The UCL at each frequency is determined by simply turning the noise up and down until the patient complains, or "until the muscles around the eyes are seen to twitch" (a measure helpful for young children or geriatric patients unable to respond otherwise). These values are plotted as the tolerance curve that marks the upper limit of the patient's remaining useful hearing, and the level at which amplification must stay safely below. Wallenfels stated that violation of this UCL level is the "greatest single cause of dissatisfaction with hearing aids."

Next, the optimum hearing level curve is drawn; this is unique for each patient. It is accomplished by finding the center point between the threshold of hearing and the UCL at 1,000 Hz, and drawing a line bisecting the remaining hearing between 1,000 and 4,000 Hz. Exact location depends upon the size of the dynamic range, and less amplification is usually provided below 500 Hz for the same reason noted by Victoreen. Thus, the prescription and the amount of amplification needed at each frequency are then read off as the difference between the level of normal conversational speech, 65 dB SPL (also indicated by a large circle in the figure), and the optimum hearing level. The optimum hearing level should be very close to MCL. For the example in Figure 13, it can be seen that the prescription values listed on the right are derived from the differences between the large circle at 1,000 Hz and the optimum level. The reference point is 1,000 Hz.

As a follow-up measure, an actual listening level is determined by having the user return to the clinic after a trial period, removing the aid (without disturbing any of the controls), and performing an electroacoustic check on it. Wallenfels reports that a successful user will always wear his aid one-half the distance between his threshold of hearing and UCL at 1,000 Hz (Figure 13 would indicate such a user), whereas the unsuccessful user cannot run his aid at this setting without at the same time violating his UCL. He also pointed out the advantage of quantifying the amount of amplification provided by this procedure over the nebulous method used by many audiologists of turning an aid to one-half or one-quarter on, for instance, and guessing at what the output may be.

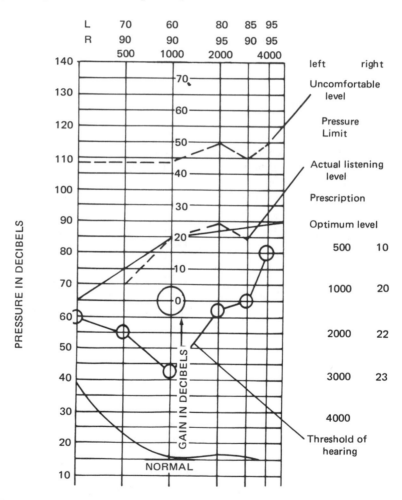

Figure 13.   Wallenfels' hearing aid-fitting table. (From Wallenfels, H., Hearing Aids on Prescription, 1967, Courtesy of Charles C Thomas, Publisher, Springfield, Illinois.)

The Shapiro Method provides for yet another prescriptive approach (Shapiro, 1976). The rationale Shapiro provided for this procedure was basically as follows:

1. A user will not wear an aid whose maximum power output exceeds his TD
2. The user will set the gain of the aid to his MCL
3. He will achieve his best speech discrimination at or near his MCL
4. Hearing aid manufacturers can closely match specifications provided by the audiologist

After having clinically employed the Wallenfels method, Shapiro found that many users were not receiving sufficient gain because the midpoint measures between threshold and UCL were not adequate indicators of MCL. He found that measuring MCL directly from the narrow band noise resulted in higher levels of SPL needed to reach actual MCL. Although being basically similar to the Wallenfels method, the Shapiro method consists of the following:

1. Obtain complete otologic and audiologic evaluation. Convert dB HTL measures to dB SPL. Plot pure tone air conduction values on a graph similar to Victoreen's, but with the center column of members indicating gain relative to 60 dB SPL for normal speech.
2. Determine TD for pulsed narrow bands of noise centered at 250, 500, 1,000, 2,000, 3,000, and 4,000 Hz. Plot the values on the graph. For TD, the patient is instructed to indicate the level where he would not want the sound to be made any louder. The MPO of the aid should not exceed these values.
3. Determine MCL for pulsed narrow bands at the same frequencies. Plot the values on the graph. The client is told that MCL is the level at which the noise would be most comfortable for long term listening. One would probably fit the ear with greatest range between MCL and TD.
4. Subtract 60 dB (equal to signal input) from MCLs at 1,000, 2,000, 3,000, and 4,000 Hz to find gain needed at each frequency. For gain at 500 Hz, subtract 10 dB from that needed at 1,000 Hz (for same reason indicated in other methods).
5. Add 100 dB to the values obtained above for additional gain reserve, thus equaling the full-on gain frequency response of the aid. Averaging the TDs for 500, 1,000, and 2,000 Hz gives the MPO of the aid.

6. From the selection of stock aids, choose one that matches the frequency response, gain, and MPO desired. The aid is fitted and the user adjusts it to MCL for cold running speech at 50 dB HL.
7. At that level, a speech articulation function is accomplished with half-list W-22s at 35, 50, and 65 dB HL, representing low, normal, and loud levels of speech.

Shapiro's criteria for appropriate amplification entails speech discrimination at 50 dB HL within normal limits; equals or exceeds unaided discrimination; and no decrease in discrimination at 65 dB HL. The score at 65 dB HL is thought to represent both the patient's tolerance for loud sounds and presence of distortion within the aid. A discrimination score at 65 dB HL better than 8% of that at 50 dB HL indicates a need for more gain, whereas one of less than 8% indicates distortion and a need for an aid with less gain. User satisfaction is also considered. Shapiro reported that over one-half his fittings were acceptable with the first aid selected and that few required more than one modification. The patient is thoroughly counseled regarding the results and amplification, and is sent to a reputable dealer with the general prescription. A follow-up evaluation is also performed after a 2- to 3-week trial period.

Shapiro also pointed out the fact that the pure tone audiogram predicts little about suprathreshold auditory function as it relates to hearing aid use, a point noted earlier by others including this author (Fry, 1966; Danhauer and Singh, 1975a, b). Shapiro described several advantages of his procedure over the traditional HAE technique.

1. This method helps to decide which ear to fit (when both ears have relatively equal hearing) by pointing out more differences between them.
2. This evaluation requires only about 30 min to complete, as opposed to traditional HAEs, which require up to 2 hr or longer. Counseling time remains the same, however.
3. Because only a general prescription is made, problems of recommending a specific make and model aid and finding the user fit with one having different response characteristics are eliminated.
4. User-specific amplification parameters are described with relatively clearly defined test measures relating directly to hearing aid specifications.
5. By aiming at socially adequate discrimination of speech at normal

conversational levels, users require considerably less gain than previously supposed.

6. It permits a professional liaison between the audiologist and the dealer, allowing each to perform the duties of his own expertise.

The following are some disadvantages cited by Shapiro.

1. These earphone measures may not be exact regarding the same SPLs at the eardrum after the sound passes through the aid, tubing, and earmold.
2. The method may not work with all patients (i.e., small, nonverbal children, or for those not understanding the concepts of UCL or MCL).
3. The frequency response from the MCL data may not provide the best speech articulation curve, thus requiring some modifications on the aid.

Still another of the prescription methods is that recently proposed by Berger (1976b). As the first step, this method also uses SPL values to record results, requires otologic and audiologic evaluations before testing to determine if an aid is appropriate, and relies heavily on electroacoustic measurements. After determining which ear to fit and whether to fit with air or bone conduction, the heart of the prescription begins. This next step involves prescribing the appropriate Saturation Sound Pressure Level (SSPL) or MPO, gain by frequency, and earmold characteristics. The following is a basic summary of these measures with the Berger Method.

1. Determine the SSPL, which is defined as the output obtained at full-on gain control with an input of 90 dB SPL at each test frequency. The SSPL is a measure of UCL determined with narrow band noise centered at each frequency. The desired SSPL at each frequency =

	250	500	1000	2000	3000	4000	Hz dB SPL
UCL +	2	8	4	6	5	6	

The correction values at each frequency serve as a margin between UCL and hearing aid amplifier cutoff (a low SSPL at the low frequencies is desirable for the same reason as in the earlier methods). For UCLs not reached by the limits of the audiometer, an arbitrary 5 dB may be added to the dial reading at each test frequency. An additional 2 dB may be added for each 10 dB of air-bone gap. For use of conventional amplifiers, 45 dB dynamic range at 500 and 1,000 Hz is recommended, otherwise compression amplification should be considered.

2. Establish gain and frequency response requirements. The gain-frequency response determined is based on:
   a. average listening level for speech is between 55 and 75 dB SPL,
   b. the aided signal should improve speech intelligibility,
   c. the desired gain will have an average magnitude slightly more than one-half the user's pure tone hearing level,
   d. amplification of low frequency ambient noise detracts from intelligibility,
   e. less amplification is needed at and below 500 Hz than at the frequencies more important for speech,
   f. frequencies above 4,000 Hz contribute little to speech intelligibility,
   g. less amplification is required at the frequencies suffering greatest damage,
   h. overamplification can lead to poor speech intelligibility, even if aided sensitivity is better than unaided,
   i. the aid should have a smooth frequency response, i.e., without spurious peaks.

Gain-frequency response is computed in HL rather than MCL and the formula assumes that electroacoustic measurements are made at full-on with a 50 or 60 dB SPL input. Based on the air conduction pure tone audiogram, the formula is:

$$\left(\frac{\text{HL at 500 Hz}}{2} + 10 \right):$$

$$\left(\frac{\text{HL at 1,000 Hz}}{1.6} + 10 \right):$$

$$\left(\frac{\text{HL at 2,000 Hz}}{1.5} + 10 \right):$$

$$\left(\frac{\text{HL at 3,000 Hz}}{1.7} + 10 \right):$$

$$\left(\frac{\text{HL at 4,000 Hz}}{2} + 10 \right).$$

These denominators were chosen to provide amplification slightly greater than one-half of the hearing level, and to mirror the long interval spectrum of speech between 500 and 2,000 Hz (and to a lesser degree at 3,000 and 4,000 Hz). A 10-dB arbitrary reserve gain at each frequency is built into the formula for ear-level aids for several reasons stated by Berger. He also presents several qualifications for specific cases.

The prescription for gain-frequency response can be made by expressing the maximum gain at specific frequencies, or the maximum gain at 500 Hz can be reported with a specified rise in decibel gain per octave. For mixed and conductive losses the following insertion should be made to the formula just before the +10 dB reserve at each frequency: $+(AC - BC)/4$. A 15-dB reserve gain per frequency is used for body aids instead of the 10 dB used for ear-level aids. Also, the denominator values at 500 and 2,000 Hz should be changed to 2.2 and 1.4, respectively, in order to correct for body baffle effects. No correction is suggested for Y-cord fittings. For in-the-ear aids the denominator values at 2,000 and 3,000 Hz should be changed to 1.6 and 1.9, respectively, to account for the pinna effect.

3. Choose proper earmold characteristics. These will vary depending upon the type of fitting and whether an open or closed mold is used.

After the prescription has been made and a reasonable trial period has been allowed, the user should be seen for a recheck to ensure that the prescription was accurate. At that time electroacoustic measurements should be performed on the aid itself for operating gain, full-on gain, and SSPL. Also important are aided versus unaided free field comparisons with pulsed warbled pure tones, narrow band noise, and speech discrimination at 65 dB SPL. Any adjustments and counseling should be made at this time. Berger pointed out that traditional hearing aid-selection procedures involve mainly intuition based on experience and a more or less trial and error comparison of selected aids. The prescription, on the other hand, embraces electroacoustic recommendations as well as a prediction of performance while using the chosen factors; it also provides a means of testing them. It implies that the prescriber is not limited in the number and type of aids available, but that he can obtain these from close cooperation with the manufacturer. According to Berger, the "prescription moves from a choice of what is available to enumerating rather specifically and precisely what should be provided for in a given loss."

Recently, Crouch and Pendry (1975) reported on a project geared to implement otometry (the shaping of loudness sensation magnitudes in audition relative to environmental sound pressures) into a clinical hearing aid-dispensing program. Their purpose was to establish otometry as an alternative method to the traditional HAE for selecting and fitting hearing aids on hearing-impaired persons, especially those incapable of responding to standard speech and pure tone hearing test signals. They found traditional HAE procedures to be predictive in nature, dependent largely on the intuition and experience of the examiner, and limited in data logic. Their definition of otometry includes: dealer responsibility, classical physics, sensory psychophysics, use of residual hearing, prescription of sound pressures, shaping loudness sensations, relevant instrument analysis, demonstrated achievement of a predefined objective in aided hearing, and dispenser responsibility. Although desiring direct observation measures of "comfortable" loudness sensations, they found pure tone and speech stimuli inadequate, and thus employed a "damped wavetrain" (DWT signal generator/attenuator system) as the test signal. The DWT signal frequencies used were 250, 500, 750, 1,000, 1,500, 2,000, 2,500, 3,000, 4,000, and 6,000 Hz. Their procedure also included electroacoustic and audiometric measurements. The otometric procedures resulted in a series of otometric graphs similar to the hearing aid tables used by Victoreen (1960). They found use in the bisecting method for determining probable MCL for young, nonverbal children, but stated that it suffers from lack of direct observation. In determining MCL, they instructed clients to gesture when the sound was "just dectably loud" (+JTL) and also when it was "just detectably low (−JTL). These values were graphed and bisected to find MCL. Normal subjects consistently judged MCLs to be 70 dB SPL for the DWT signal across the frequencies tested. Hearing-impaired patients were tested in sound field with an aid fitted on one ear and the other ear occluded. MCLs for the DWT signals at 70 dB SPL were obtained at each frequency by adjusting the volume control of the aid to the MCL determined by the subject. MCL sound pressures were ascertained by bisecting +JTLs and −JTLs at each frequency. The aid was then analyzed at the volume control settings used for the MCL observations. The hearing aid output sound pressures with 70 dB SPL tone input were plotted at each frequency across the amplification range of the aid. The differences between the MCL and 70-dB levels were applied to the response curve of the test aid to establish that of the desired aid. The authors indicated that this approach would be desirable for hard to test clients including young children, the nonverbal, and non-English speaking persons.

The foregoing methods are prescriptive approaches that serve to remove as much subjectivity as possible from the hearing aid recommendation. Although none of the methods may be "perfect" or hold all the answers, they are a step in the right direction.

Other Nontraditional Approaches

In this section a few other nontraditional approaches are presented. Although they do not involve prescription fittings directly enough to be discussed along with the prescriptive methods, they are relatively new procedures that further attempt to quantify the hearing aid recommendation, and thus seem to be more objective than traditional in nature.

Garstecki and Bode (1976) further explored the use of narrow bands of noise for determining sound field thresholds in hearing aid evaluations. Because the use of narrow band noise (NBN) stimuli is becoming commonplace in HAEs, they felt a need to explore the relationship between NBN thresholds in aided and unaided conditions with normal and sensorineural hearing-impaired subjects. They pointed out that the advantages of narrow band noise stimuli include:

1. They are more flexible for repeated measures than are speech stimuli when learning is a factor.
2. Presumably, they, unlike speech, are not dependent upon the integrity of the listener's central auditory system.
3. They are promising for HAEs, because they reduce the problem of standing waves, which can occur when pure tones are used in sound field.

They compared: a) pure tone and NBN thresholds obtained under phones, b) NBN thresholds under phones and in sound field, and c) aided and unaided NBN thresholds in sound field using standard, low, and high frequency emphasis hearing aid settings. From their results, Garstecki and Bode reported that NBN stimuli seem to be capable of distinguishing differences among hearing aids in their abilities to improve thresholds, and that they should serve as a guide for proper hearing aid selection. They also indicated that this approach is valuable for cases in which traditional methods involving voluntary verbal responses from the hearing aid candidate cannot be obtained.

Jerger and Hayes (1976) have presented a hearing-aid evaluation procedure in which they revived the use of the Synthetic Sentences Identification (SSI) test and speech competition in varying message-to-competition ratios (MCRs). They stated that the main problems of the traditional HAE were that it: a) employs basically only two conditions, PB words in quiet and in noise; thus, it is often incapable of delineating substantial differences among hearing aids; b) it suffers from lack of face validity because single word stimuli do not sufficiently represent a user's social adequacy for continuous real life speech; and c) it provides little useful information upon which to initiate a rehabilitation process.

The Jerger and Hayes method was directed towards: a) determining the most suitable hearing aid arrangement for a user, b) defining differences among aids in real life listening conditions, c) providing information on realistic expectations of hearing aid use for client counseling, and d) making rehabilitative recommendations to users. Their recorded stimuli consisted of ten synthetic sentences (third order approximations of normal English sentences, containing normal English phonology and syntax, but lacking semantics; e.g., "go change your car color is red") on one channel of a dual channel magnetic tape, and continuous discourse (competing message) on the second channel. The MCRs were determined by holding the sentences constant at 60 dB SPL (representing normal conversational speech levels) and varying the intensity of the competing message between 40 dB SPL and 80 dB SPL. This resulted in five MCRs representing different levels of listener difficulty, namely: $+20$ = very easy; $+10$ = easy; 0 = average; -10 = difficult; and -20 = very difficult. The client's performance is assessed at various MCRs under both unaided and aided conditions, and different aids are evaluated at the same varying MCR conditions. Results are reported in %SSI scores and plotted on an articulation function showing the percentage of correct as a function of the various MCRs.

In an evaluation of this procedure in comparison to PB and PTA data, they found that neither the PB Max nor the PTA related strongly to user satisfaction with amplification in that neither adequately differentiated satisfied from unsatisfied users. They also found that, contrary to popular opinion, users with sloping audiometric configurations were more satisfied than those with flatter configurations; and that satisfaction was a function of age (increase in age led to a decrease in satisfaction). They demonstrated that although traditional audiometric measures were unable to depict these differences, the SSI test was.

Jerger and Hayes posited the following advantages to the SSI procedure:

1. Use of real life-like listening conditions helps to determine the most suitable aid for the user.
2. Varying the difficulty of the MCR conditions clearly defines differences among aids.
3. User counseling is more realistic from comparisons of both aided and unaided conditions to normal listeners' performance.
4. Potential user satisfaction is more predictable based on the SSI-MCR data.
5. It can be used with almost any degree of hearing loss. It is also useful in CROS and BICROS fittings because the head shadow effect can be assessed by changing the patient's seating arrangement within the test room.
6. It is adaptable to almost any language.
7. It is open-ended and flexible to change, e.g., adding video stimuli to assess the contribution of speechreading to amplification and vice versa.

The authors stated that they find this procedure substantially better than the traditional HAE. Although the authors did not mention it, clinically we have found that this procedure requires considerable amounts of time in order to complete an evaluation in which several aids and settings are employed. However, this may not be much more than that required for the less objective "hit or miss" aid selection and gain setting procedures often used by many audiologists. In practice, the audiologist may desire to initiate the test at lower MCRs, and once he determines where the subject's scores begin to deteriorate, he may wish to continue in smaller steps. Also, although this approach does not terminate in a prescription of specific gain at each frequency, it has obvious potentials and should be considered by the audiologist as an additional quantitative pre- and postprescription measure.

Another nontraditional type of evaluation involves the use of impedance and acoustic reflex measures in the fitting of hearing aids. In the past 5 years there has been considerable interest in the value of using acoustic reflex (AR) and loudness discomfort levels (LDLs) for such purposes (e.g., Niemeyer, 1971; McCandless and Miller, 1972; McCandless, 1973; Olson and Hipskind, 1973; Shallop, 1973; Blegvad, 1974; Tonisson, 1975; Holmes and Woodford, 1976; Snow and McCandless, 1976).

Although not directly related to the use of hearing aids, Niemeyer (1971) determined that the acoustic reflex threshold (ART) for the stapedius muscle is normally about 10-20 dB lower than the threshold of discomfort. He also found that "the peripheral receptors remain sensitive to strong noise exposure even though they have long ago lost their subjective discomfort, which is elicited primarily in the cochlea." These findings are relevant to hearing-impaired persons and generated concern about fitting hearing aids at LDLs.

McCandless and Miller (1972) reported that many hearing aid users fail to succeed in wearing amplification because the MPO of the aid often violates their TD. They also discussed the variations in results for TDs, which related to the different ways in which they are determined. Most LDLs are determined for the upper limit of the TD (i.e., the level at which one more increment would be "too" loud). Their preference was to define the LDL as a "just uncomfortable level" or a "threshold of beginning discomfort" because the lower level would result in fitting hearing aids with lower MPOs. They stated that many hearing aids are fitted under the theory that the user can learn to tolerate sounds up to about 130 dB SPL. Their findings indicated the contrary and may be summarized as follows:

1. A TD defined as "just comfortably loud" is an appropriate measure for the upper limit of usable loudness. This level equals approximately 100 dB SPL for both normal and cochlear loss ears.
2. The TD and AR occur at the same sensation levels.
3. Most patients refer to discomfort as the reason for failure in hear-aid satisfaction.
4. Almost all hearing aid candidates with losses up to 70-80 dB should be able to use ear-level aids, because they actually require less gain than traditionally thought.
5. Both tolerance and AR measures are constant over time, therefore, sounds that initially annoy the user will probably continue to bother him. That is, he will not "get used to them."

Based on similar findings, McCandless (1973) recommended the use of greater power limiting in hearing aids, with MPOs of less than 105 dB SPL for mild losses. In a study comparing LDLs and ARTs in a deaf population, Holmes and Woodford (1976) pointed out that many clinicians arbitrarily add 15-20 dB to the ART as a means of determining MPO fittings. Their results indicated that because of individual differences among deaf subjects, indiscriminate use of such criteria might result in many fittings exceeding the subjects' LDLs.

Use of impedance measures was adequately reviewed in a recent publication by Snow and McCandless (1976), who have found such procedures to be enlightening as to the function and integrity of the peripheral auditory system.

Impedance measures have recently been used in determining output, gain, and frequency response parameters in hearing aids. Snow and McCandless (1976) reported that these measures are especially helpful in evaluations of young children and hard-to-test patients because they require little patient cooperation and no subjective responses. They reiterated the fact that the MPO of an aid should not exceed the ART where speech or pure tone stimuli just becomes uncomfortable because sustained usage at this level could result in temporary threshold shifts or tonic contraction of the AR, a condition not tolerated well by most subjects. They describe two uses of the impedance method in determining MPOs for persons unable to report voluntarily subjective discomfort levels.

1. Present speech, pure tones, or narrow band noise to one ear with an impedance probe in the contralateral ear. Find ARTs, convert these levels to SPL, and use as the MPO.
2. Place a hearing aid or master aid in one ear with an impedance probe in the contralateral ear. Introduce free field stimuli calibrated to average speech levels, and adjust the MPO of the aid to settings just below the point where the middle ear muscle is in constant contraction.

For determining gain, Snow and McCandless concur with the results of Tonisson (1975) who used the differences between aided and unaided ARTs to one-third octave noise bands in sound field as an indication of real ear gain. He also pointed out inadequacies of the standard 2-cc coupler for determining actual use because it does not account for such factors as ear canal size, earmold and tubing parameters, and microphone placements. Real ear measures using the AR were found to be effective for objectively determining gain requirements in young children and infants. Snow and McCandless suggest placing an aid on the child and obtaining the AR for the contralateral ear. The gain setting is determined as the point just below which the reflex is barely observed for signals corresponding to average speech levels. However, this method is ineffective if the loss is so severe that the AR is not present. Here, the authors were unclear as to the difference between gain and MPO (i.e., where gain ends and MPO begins).

In the future the AR may be used for determining real ear frequency response needs, by obtaining the reflex in the contralateral ear to the hearing aid and comparing thresholds to pure tones and narrow bands of noise with various aids. This may be useful for pointing out quality differences among aids for candidates unable to make such judgments themselves.

Several other procedures and modifications of traditional discrimination tests are available that attempt to quantify the patient's responses to auditory stimuli (e.g., monosyllabic rhyme tests and synthetic sentence identification tests). Recently, more emphasis has been placed on analyzing a client's errors to stimuli as opposed to simply indicating whether his responses are just right or wrong. One such procedure involves the construction of "feature-gram" profiles based on a distinctive feature information transmission analysis of a subject's perceptual errors to consonant (or vowel) stimuli (Danhauer and Singh, 1975c). This approach takes into consideration the productive and perceptual parameters of speech and allows the clinician to see what aspects of the signal the hearing-impaired individual uses in his perception of it. The resulting feature-gram also provides a basis for beginning aural rehabilitation therapy, making comparisons among a client's performance with different aids, and assessing the contribution of speechreading to amplification and vice versa.

As indicated earlier, many of the tests and hearing aid-evaluation procedures presented here will likely see modifications in the next few years. However, the important trend to note from the methods covered in this section is that there is a movement toward providing better services for the hearing aid user by improving our ability to quantify our measures and to make the HAE a much more objective process. In other words, the concerned audiologist no longer seems to be satisfied to just fit a hearing aid on a "magical hunch" or an "educated guess." He is indeed trying to move the art to a science.

WHOM THE SERVICES ARE PROVIDED FOR

This section discusses for whom the services are provided, as well as some postevaluative services for the hearing-impaired client; in so doing it is hoped to tie together some of the issues and concepts presented in the earlier sections.

Various definitions have been presented as to who the hearing impaired person is, but probably the one most used is that determined by the Committee on Nomenclature of the Conference of Executives of American Schools for the Deaf (Committee on Nomenclature, 1938);

1. The deaf: Those in whom the sense of hearing is nonfunctional for the ordinary purposes of life. This group is made up of two distinct classes based entirely on the time of the loss of hearing.
   a. The congenitally deaf: those who were born deaf.
   b. The adventitiously deaf: those who were born with normal hearing but in whom the sense of hearing becomes non-functional later through illness or accident.
2. The hard-of-hearing: those in whom the sense of hearing, although defective, is functional with or without a hearing aid.

Although these definitions have been around for some time, they are still the basis of classifying hearing-impaired persons. The important thing to remember, however, is that a hearing impairment is not an all-or-none phenomenon; there are various degrees of hearing loss and just because an individual has such a handicap, it does not mean that he is "totally deaf and dumb." Experience has shown that even individuals with highly similar audiometric data may perform very differently from one another. Although somewhat categorical, hearing loss is a very individualistic phenomenon; this should be taken into consideration by all members of the hearing health team as they go about providing their respective services for each hearing-impaired person.

Although some of the basic criteria for determining what amplification to use and possible determiners of user success have been discussed in the previous sections, of further importance are criteria for 1) what ear to fit, 2) use of monaural or binaural amplification, and 3) what basic type of aid to recommend.

Binaural versus Monaural

Berger (1976b) provided the following as guidelines for determining whether the right, left, or both ears should be fitted with amplification.

1. If the average hearing level in the worst ear is 35 dB or less at 1,000 and 2,000 Hz fit monaurally, unless binaural fitting can be shown to provide localization where monaural fitting will not.
2. If the thresholds differ by no more than 15 dB at any of the speech frequencies and are roughly parallel, if the dynamic range of each ear is about the same, and if at the same hearing level speech discrimination scores are approximately alike, fit binaural. With audiometrically similar ears, localization will be provided by the binaural fitting.
3. Financial considerations should not be the determiner of monaural

or binaural amplification, although practically they must be dealt with.

Berger provided further guidelines for monaural fittings.

1. Fit the ear with the best speech discrimination. Differences in scores of 8% or less in quiet conditions with commonly used word lists are insignificant.
2. If the PTA for 1,000 and 2,000 Hz in the better ear is no worse than 40 dB and the average in the poorer ear is no worse than 60 dB, fit the poorer ear to permit unaided participation by the better ear.
3. Fit the ear with the largest dynamic range. This relates to fewer problems with output limitations of the hearing aid. The UCL or recruitment, as isolated factors, are not important in choosing the ear to be fitted (some audiologists might disagree with the latter).
4. Fit the ear with the largest air-bone gap, assuming there is no chronic drainage or anatomical problems. This assumes that conductive losses have larger dynamic ranges and better speech discrimination.
5. If both ears have approximately the same audiometric scores, fit the one with the flattest or smoothest threshold contour. Consideration should be given in this case to fitting the opposite ear employed for telephone use.

The question of whether to fit monaurally (one aid to one ear) or binaurally (two aids—one to each ear) has been and continues to be a problem that perplexes the audiologist, and is one of the main issues of controversy in hearing aid fittings. Although hearing aid manufacturers and dealers have consistently advocated the use of binaural amplification, the audiologist has been more cautious in doing so. The problem for the audiologist is that although the hearing aid user often subjectively feels greater success with two aids, he is rarely able to measure significant contributions made by the addition of the second aid. That is, "if the audiologist cannot measure it, he does not believe it"; this inability may be attributable, however, to the inefficiency of current clinical tests (such as speech discrimination in quiet) to measure such differences. The basic advantages of binaural amplification relate to a more faithful reproduction of the incoming signal with regard to intensity, time, and spectrum differences of the auditory signal arriving at each ear for better sound localization;

speech discrimination in noise, ease in listening; sound quality; and spatial balance. Binaural amplification also provides approximately a 3-dB increase in signal intensity over the monaural fitting. Another advantage relates to the "squelch effect" or the ability to pick out the speech signal from the ambient background noise; in other words, improvement in auditory figure-ground discrimination. Binaural amplification has been discussed in greater detail in other texts (e.g., Katz, 1972; Donnelly, 1974; Northern and Downs, 1974; Pollack, 1975; Rubin, 1976). The importance of interaural phase differences on binaural hearing aid fittings was discussed by Zelnick (1974). Recently, Nielsen (1976) reported on the effect of monaural versus binaural hearing aid use by patients in Denmark. From results on a Social Hearing Handicap Index, he found that binaural amplification was equal or superior to monaural amplification for persons of different ages with various types and degrees of hearing loss. He also reported that hearing aid users did not seem to feel any greater cosmetic disadvantage with binaural than with monaural eyeglass-type hearing aids. Nielsen stated that the objective of a rehabilitation program must be an optimum hearing aid treatment, and this is usually binaural.

The literature suggests that the true advantages of binaural amplification are better gained via two ear-level-borne instruments than with two body-borne aids. This is attributable to the spatial separation and location of the instruments. That is, two body aids worn on the chest have a microphone separation of only about 2–3 inches, as compared to about 7–8 inches when aids are worn on the ears; also important is the head shadow effect noted when the aids are worn on the ears. The information cited earlier in this chapter would indicate that most hearing-impaired individuals could benefit from the ear-level fittings.

Besides the true binaural fittings (two separate aids with two microphones, amplifiers, and receivers—one to each ear), a pseudo-binaural or Y-cord fitting is available from most body type aids. This Y-cord arrangement uses one aid (one microphone and one amplifier), but two receivers, one to deliver the sound to each year. Lybarger (1973) presented the advantages of the Y-cord over the monaural fitting.

1. Both ears are receiving auditory stimulation.
2. Although not as good as with true binaural, speech discrimination is better.

3. Lower initial cost than binaural.
4. Lower operating cost (i.e., less battery consumption than with binaural).

The limitations Lybarger presented relate to:

1. Not all body aids are designed to work with Y-cords.
2. Y-cord may cause distortion. It works best when the difference between ears is about 10–15 dB.
3. There is about a 3-dB loss in signal intensity with the Y-cord fitting. However, most aids have enough reserve gain to offset this problem.

Pollack (1975) pointed out that an adjustment period is a key factor in a person's acceptance of binaural aids; (although this issue is also controversial) both aids should be fitted at the same time; and they should meet the needs of the patient. They are beneficial to persons who work in conditions frequently requiring binaural hearing (e.g., business meetings; academic and social settings), but may not be needed by someone whose communication demands are less. Pollack stated that binaural aids are questionable for most asymmetrical losses having more than a 15-dB difference between ears in the speech range because a) either the better ear can compensate satisfactorily, or b) the poorer ear may cause increased distortion that could interfere with the better ear's performance. He also stated that CROS amplification may be advisable in such cases.

Ross (1975) cited an increased usage of binaural amplification for children at the Willie Ross School for two reasons: a) most of the children were eventually found to have bilateral, symmetrical losses, with differences between ears of about 10–15 dB at each frequency; and b) parents were more receptive to binaural amplification when the child was first fitted with aids as opposed to such a fitting at a later date. His rationale for recommending two aids was also based on the assumption that if two aids are superior to the use of one for adults who can be objectively tested, then the same should be true for young children who cannot respond objectively and for whom the superiority is harder to demonstrate. He also reported the superiority of binaural aids on deaf children as determined by subjective ratings by parents and teachers. The superiority of binaural aids was also shown by Yonovitz (1974) who obtained responses from 20 hearing-impaired children wearing both monaural and binaural aids. They listened to recorded stimuli under various signal-to-noise (S/N) ratios and in different noise sources. His results clearly demonstrated a binaural advantage under all S/N ratios.

Recently, Griffing (1976) advocated the use of binaural in-the-ear aids for both adults and children, and stated that too many audiologists just automatically think only of body aids when it comes to amplification for children. He further noted that the in-the-ear aid offers more cosmetic appeal and equal or better freedom of activity than do either the ear-level or body types, and that these aids can be custom-designed to meet each user's needs. The recent literature indicates that the time has come when more children may be able to benefit from ear-level or in-the-ear aids rather than just the traditionally used body type (Blood, Blood, and Danhauer, 1977). Peterson (1976) stated that infants who are not walking are usually fitted with binaural body aids in front and to the sides to allow for crawling and other "on the tummy" activities, but that when the child is sitting or walking well, ear-level aids are used to avoid problems of weight and dangling cords. However, the body aid still may be useful for geriatric and mentally retarded populations who have manual dexterity problems.

Time of Acquisition of Hearing Loss

Probably the most critical factor for the future of the hearing-impaired person is what time in his life he acquires his hearing loss. As mentioned earlier, the congenital loss occurring at birth or soon after is usually the most devastating type. If such a loss occurs before the acquisition of normal speech and language development it is called prelinguistic. Depending upon the severity of the loss, amount of early stimulation, amplification and training, and luck, the individual with a prelinguistic loss may or may not be capable of acquiring speech that is adequate for communicating socially. Recently, early diagnosis of hearing loss (through neonatal hearing screenings, high risk registers, and preschool and school hearing screenings) has enabled the hearing health team to provide amplification and training for many prelinguistic hearing-impaired children at a much younger age. Northern and Downs (1974) and Ross (1975) advocate early fitting with amplification for such individuals to give them a better chance to learn speech and language. The critical stages for speech and language are approximately between 2 and 7 years of age. Northern and Downs (1974) indicated having fit infants as young as 1 month old with hearing aids. Although this may be a controversial practice, such early fitting and training programs are vitally important for such children.

These individuals will often have to spend much of their lives in aural habilitation clinics in order to obtain and maintain their speaking and listening skills. Aural habilitation instruments such as auditory trainers and multisensory approaches such as the Verbotonal Method are not covered in this chapter, but have been in other sources (e.g., Sanders, 1971; Guberina, 1972; Katz, 1972; Donnelly, 1974; Staub and O'Gara, 1974; Pollack, 1975). Realistically, some of these individuals may never learn speech and may have to rely on some form of manual communication.

Northern and Downs (1974) posited specific hearing aid-selection procedures for the nonverbal child, 2–16 years old; and the verbal child, 3–16 years old. One of the main problems with the prelinguistically handicapped, as with the hard-to-test patient, is his inability to respond to conventional auditory test batteries. This increases the difficulty of arriving at an exact diagnosis, let alone an adequate recommendation for amplification. For these individuals, the non-participatory methods discussed earlier in this chapter become invaluable. The impedance and acoustic reflex tests provide a means for determining what type of amplification to use. Once appropriate amplification has been provided the postfitting services are of vital importance. These are discussed later.

The adventitious type of loss implies that the person has acquired his hearing impairment postlinguistically, that is, after the normal acquisition of speech and language. Obviously, this type is usually the easier of the two to deal with, but can vary in difficulty depending upon time of acquisition and severity of the loss. Often this individual can be helped by amplification, but because of the loss of the auditory feedback loop, may have to spend much of his life in aural rehabilitation programs that focus on auditory training, speechreading, and speech production and perception. This person may also benefit from multisensory stimulation to supplement his lack of auditory sensitivity. If the loss occurs later in life, chances are the individual will retain usable speech and may only need minimal aural rehabilitation for speech maintenance. Obviously, if the loss occurs earlier, more time will be spent in therapy. As with the congenital loss, amplification becomes an important part of this person's life. Because this person usually is able to provide subjective responses to auditory stimuli, most of the diagnostic tests and hearing aid-evaluation procedures presented in this chapter can be used. Because of his responsiveness, the hearing aid recommendation should be achieved fairly easily for this person, but again as for the congenitally impaired, the postfitting services are vitally important for successful communication and hearing aid use.

Postfitting Services

I have often told my students that I would rather fit an aid on one person successfully than to fit aids on 10 persons unsuccessfully with the aids winding up in their dresser drawers. The successful fitting should be the goal of every fitting because the aid will do the user no good unless he uses it. The part of the hearing aid fitting process upon which user satisfaction is probably most dependent is that of the postfitting services. These services include: a) trial periods, b) counseling, c) hearing aid orientation, d) rehabilitation or habilitation, and e) periodic hearing and hearing aid re-evaluations.

Trial period—No matter what type of loss is fitted or what type of aid is used, a trial period should be employed. This is a set amount of time (usually 2-6 weeks) during which the user can wear his newly fitted aid. During this time he should adjust to amplification and become acquainted with the aid. This provides a better indicator of long range success than does the short duration testing administered in the original HAE. Usually the hearing aid dealer will provide this on a money back guarantee basis, although a slight fitting fee may be charged if the aid is not purchased.

Counseling—This is probably one of the most vital parts of the fitting process. This counseling should include the user and as much of his immediate family as possible, and may require several sessions to complete. Psychologic and social adjustment problems of both the user and his family may be necessary; this may be a long range problem. In this setting the user and his family should also be educated on topics including: proper care and use of the aid, need for habilitation or rehabilitation, potentials and limitations of the aid, volume and tone control settings, batteries, earmold care and insertion, use of telephone, the connection between speech production and speech perception, wearing times and places, conversations and possible problems. Dye (1976) has suggested some points to be covered with the user's family or friends, which include: getting the user's attention before attempting to converse with him; speaking slowly and distinctly, but not shouting; articulating clearly and using normal gestures; taking extra care when talking in noisy environments; rephrasing the question or statement if the user fails to comprehend the first time. This counseling should also be directed to the school teacher if the child is of school age. She too should be made aware of the possibilities and limitations of the hearing aid. Many teachers fail to realize that there are various degrees of hearing impairment and think that because the child wears an aid he is deaf. Also some have misconceptions regarding the benefits of an aid. Whereas many teachers think a child is completely deaf, they are often just as unrealistic in thinking that an aid can bring his hearing back to normal. This is not a criticism of the teacher, for most lay persons make the same assumptions because of lack of contact with hearing-impaired individuals. Also, the teacher should be aware of "preferential seating," speaking so she can be easily lipread, writing out or rephrasing lengthy instructions, and the effects of ambient room noise.

Hearing aid orientation—This includes the trial period and counseling, but also is a way of providing the user or his family with a plan for getting used to amplification. Various wearing adjustment programs have been presented and this seems to be an area of controversy. Northern and Downs (1974) presented "A Primer for Parents of a Hearing-Aided Child" in which they detailed a week-by-week home program geared to get the child to gradually accept the aid. This program initiates with short 10-min periods of use for the 1st week, gradually working to longer periods of use. This method does not force the aid on the child and retreats until another time if the child rejects the aid the first time. Ross (1975) presented the opposite viewpoint, namely that the person initiating the wearing program should be knowledgable, authoritative, confident, competent, and somewhat forceful. The child should be made to accept the aid in the same way he is for being changed, fed, dressed, and so on because amplification is also a way of life for this person. Ross criticized the short 10–15 min daily use programs because they bring too much attention to the aid itself. He prefers to view the aid as an integral part of the child and this should be transmitted to the child and his family. He stated that he would not put the child in the position where he has the option to wear or not wear the aid, "for what if he said no?" Ross suggested that the younger the child, the easier is his acceptance of the amplification.

Troubleshooting—This should also be a vital part of the counseling and orientation process for both the user and his family, and the teacher. Items to be covered should include: the aid's proper operation, demonstrate how to check battery voltage and to replace when necessary, examination of the aid, battery terminals, receiver, cord, and earmold for physical damage. Parents might be fitted with their own earmold or could use a commercial hearing aid stethoscope to notice proper functioning of the aid. The effects of covering the aid with layers of clothing resulting in "clothing noise" should be explained. Also, reasons for feedback or squeal should be covered. The earmold fitting is often the cause and the parents should be informed of the need for periodic refitting of the mold for young children. Randolph (1976) devised a method of checking the operation of a hearing aid via a cassette recorder. He described how to construct such a device, which could be used by interested, knowledgable parents. Roeser, Gerken, and Glorig (1976) recently described a hearing aid-malfunction detection unit (HAMDU), which electrically checks for proper hearing aid operation. HAMDU is a miniature add-on device providing a check of the aid every half-hour. It checks battery voltage, gain, distortion and noise, integrity of the receiver cord, and whether the aid is "on or off." A malfunction is indicated by a bright electrically tripped light. They described HAMDU as small, low in cost, and easily adaptable to most body aids. Obviously, such a device would be highly beneficial for parents and teachers of young children.

Habilitation or rehabilitation—As indicated earlier, most hearing-impaired persons will probably spend much of their lives in some form of special training. The extent depends upon the capabilities of the individual and his communication needs. Lerman (1976) stated that variation in the linguistic competence within the deaf population is much greater than that among the normally hearing. He remarked that some deaf children become good enough speakers and excellent lipreaders to keep their language skills commensurate with their normal hearing peers, whereas others cannot, and remain illiterate. The reasons why some achieve while others do not have not been determined, but the earlier the training process begins, the better is the prognosis. Lerman found that teaching the parents how to work with their children was highly beneficial, especially in the acceptance of the hearing aid and its use. The rehabilitation or habilitation process should be individualistic and flexible to meet the needs of each client.

Periodic hearing and hearing aid re-evaluation—This is another of the important postfitting services. The re-evaluation is necessary to: monitor the client's loss; further assess the hearing in the case of the young child or hard-to-test individual for whom exact thresholds were not yet obtained; evaluate user performance with the aid; ensure that the proper aid was recommended; monitor the functioning of the aid; and evaluate progress in therapy. Both electroacoustic and physiologic measurements should be included in the re-evaluations.

In order to accomplish, ensure, and maintain the proper hearing aid recommendation, the whole hearing health team must work to see that the user is adequately serviced and satisfied. This then, brings us in full circle to where we began this chapter, thus demonstrating the total dependency of each of the steps and components of the hearing aid recommendation process on the other.

CONCLUSION

In this chapter I have discussed the hearing aid recommendation as a total process involving many interested parties and various clinical procedures. In discussing who provides the services, the roles of the respective members of the hearing health team were defined. Regarding what services are provided, various hearing aid types and characteristics were covered. In describing how the services are provided, a current trend toward more objective recommendations was presented by discussing on a continuum the traditional HAE and its criticisms, nontraditional methods, and newer approaches that quantify the recommendation by including electroacoustic and manikin measurements, and various prescription methods. Then, who are the services provided for was discussed in terms of the different types of losses, children versus adults, and postfitting services.

In summary, we have seen many changes in the ways in which hearing aids are recommended. The older traditional HAE relied heavily upon the audiologist's experience and "chance" in testing and making comparisons among many different aids on the client. The newer prescriptive approaches, relying heavily on electroacoustic measurements of hearing aid parameters, allow the audiologist to use fewer aids in his selection. Although as many aids from different brands and models may still be employed, only aids with appropriate characteristics based on the prescription are tried. The newer approaches still provide much flexibility because the selection can be either an "exact" prescription in which the audiologist tells exactly what aid and earmold characteristics are to be used, or a "general" prescription in which the parameters of the aid are determined by the audiologist, but the actual selection of the specific aid meeting the prescription is left up to the hearing aid dealer. Either way these procedures should give the audiologist more confidence in his recommendation. As I have indicated, the hearing aid recommendation process has seen considerable change in the past few years; unfortunately the same cannot be said for the postfitting services. The modes of therapy (either habilitation or rehabilitation) used today are basically unchanged from when they were developed. It is time for the audiologist and the other members of the hearing health team to take a greater interest in what happens to the user after the fitting. The statistics showing the large disparities in educational and communication achievements between the hearing impaired and the normally hearing speak for themselves. We, as concerned audiologists, must become as involved with follow-up as we have with diagnosis. After all, that is a major part of servicing the hearing-impaired client. I am sure that if we can direct some of the same energies to finding new approaches to follow-up services that we have toward improving our diagnostic and hearing aid recommendation procedures, we will be better able to serve our hearing-impaired patients. Only time will tell.

ACKNOWLEDGMENTS

Acknowledgment is due Ingrid Blood, Les Goldstein, Brad Edgerton, Lee McLeod, Dixie Hawes, Ed Cohill, Dave Klodd, and Becky Tunis, my students and colleagues who read and criticized this work. Appreciation is also given to Janet Watson, Gerri Nagy, and Marilyn Slatton for their excellent typing skills. This chapter is dedicated to Susan and Tatum who have given up so much to let me be me.

REFERENCES

American National Standards Institute, 1960. Electroacoustical Characteristics of Hearing Aids. American Standard S3.3—1960, New York.
American National Standards Institute, 1967. Methods of Expressing Hearing Aid Performance. American Standard S3.8—1967, New York.
American National Standards Institute, 1976. Specifications of Hearing Aid Characteristics. ASA STD7—1976 (ANSI S3.22—1976), New York.
Berger, K. 1974. The Hearing Aid: Its Operation and Development. The

National Hearing Aid Society, Detroit.

Berger, K. 1976a. The earliest known custom earmolds. Hear. Aid J. 29:10–35.

Berger, K. 1976b. Prescription of hearing aids: A rationale. Presented at Ohio Speech and Hearing Association Convention, Columbus, Ohio.

Berger, K., and Millin, J. 1971. Hearing aids. In: D. Rose (ed.), Audiological Assessment, pp. 471–517. Prentice-Hall, Inc., Englewood Cliffs, New Jersey.

Blegvad, B. 1974. Clinical evaluation of behind-the-ear hearing aids with compression amplification. Scand. Audiol. 3:57–60.

Blood, G., Blood, I., and Danhauer, J. 1976. The "hearing aid effect." Hear. Instr. 28:12.

Blood, I., and Danhauer, J. 1976. Are we meeting the needs of our hearing aid users? Asha 18:343–347.

Briskey, R. 1972. Binaural hearing aids and new innovations. In J. Katz (ed.), Handbook of Clinical Audiology, pp. 590–601. The Williams & Wilkins Company, Baltimore.

Briskey, R., and Wruk, K. 1974. Acoustic influence of insert vents. Hear. Instruments. 25:12–14.

Broderick, T. 1976. Trends of the future. Hear. Aid J. 29:11.

Burkhard, M. 1976. Considerations for use of KEMAR. Presented at Manikin Measurement Method Conference, Washington, D.C.; and Personal communication.

Burkhard, M. 1976. KEMAR, a tool for hearing aid evaluation. Audecibel 25:126–134.

Burkhard, M., and Sachs, R. 1975. Anthropometric manikin for acoustic research. J. Acoust. Soc. Am. 58:214–222.

Caine, M. 1974. Plastics and materials utilized in earmolds. Hear. Instruments. 25:17.

Carhart, R. 1946a. A practical approach to the selection of hearing aids. Trans. Am. Acad. Ophthalmol. Otolaryngol. 50:123–131.

Carhart, R. 1946b. Selection of hearing aids. Arch. Otolaryngol. 44:1–18.

Carhart, R. 1946c. Tests for selection of hearing aids. Laryngoscope 56:680–794.

Carhart, R. 1946d. Volume control adjustment in hearing aid selection. Laryngoscope 56:510–526.

Carhart, R. 1975. Introduction. In: M. Pollack (ed.), Amplification for the Hearing-Impaired, pp. xix–xxxvi. Grune & Stratton, Inc., New York.

Carlson, E. 1976. Hearing aid transducers. Hear. Aid J. 29:6–29.

Carver, W. 1972. Hearing aids—a historical and technical review. In: J. Katz (ed.), Handbook of Clinical Audiology, pp. 564–576. The Williams & Wilkins Company, Baltimore.

Causey, G. 1976. Current developments in hearing aids. In: M. Rubin (ed.), Hearing Aids—Current Developments and Concepts, pp. 7–19. University Park Press, Baltimore.

Committee on Nomenclature. 1938. Conference of executives, American Schools for the Deaf. Am. Ann. Deaf 83:3.

Coogle, K. 1976. NAEL's standard terms for earmolds. Hear. Aid J. 29:5.

Cook, R. 1976. Remarkable hearing aid batteries. Hear. Aid J. 29:8–41.

Crouch, J., and Pendry, B. 1975. Otometry in clinical hearing aid dispensing. Parts I and II. Hear. Aid J. 28:12–48, 18–32.

Curran, J. 1976. Problems in measuring harmonic distortion in hearing aids.

Hear. Instruments 27:13-32.

Danhauer, J., and Singh, S. 1975a. A multidimensional scaling analysis of phonemic responses from hard of hearing and deaf subjects of three languages. Lang. Speech 18:42-64.

Danhauer, J., and Singh, S. 1975b. Multidimensional Speech Perception By the Hearing Impaired: A treatise on distinctive features. University Park Press, Baltimore.

Danhauer, J., and Singh, S. 1975c. A study of "Feature-Gram" profiles for three different hearing impaired language groups. Scand. Audiol. 4:67-71.

Davis, H., Hudgins, C., Marquis, R., Nichols, R., Peterson, G., Ross, D., and Stevens, S. 1946. The selection of hearing aids. Laryngoscope 56:85-115, 135-163.

Davis, H., Stevens, S., and Nichols, R. 1947. Hearing Aids. Harvard University Press, Cambridge.

Donnelly, K. 1974. Interpreting Hearing Aid Technology. Charles C Thomas, Publisher, Springfield, Illinois.

Dye, B. 1976. Counseling the family and friends of the hearing-aid wearer. Hear. Aid J. 29:7.

Ely, W. 1976. The art and technique of hearing aid performance testing. Hear. Instruments 27:20-21.

Frádkin, M. 1976. Hearing aid testing equipment—a new plus for clients. Hear. Instruments 27:12.

Frank, T., and Gooden, R. 1974. The effect of hearing aid microphone types on speech discrimination scores in backgrounds of multitalker noise. Maico Audiol. Library Ser., 11:19-23.

Frank, T., and Karlovich, R. 1976. Ear-canal frequency response and speech discrimination performance as a function of earmold type. Hear. Aid J. 29:12-30.

Fry, D. 1966. The development of the phonological system in the normal and the deaf child. In: F. Smith and G. Miller (eds.), The Genesis of Language: A Psycholinguistic Approach, pp. 187-206. The MIT Press, Cambridge.

Garstecki, D., and Bode, D. 1976. Aided and unaided narrow band noise thresholds in listeners with sensorineural hearing impairment. J. Am. Audiol. Soc. 1:258-262.

Goldberg, H. 1976. Electroacoustic amplification. Hear. Aid J. 29:8-46.

Green, S. 1974. The "JH" earmold. Hear. Instruments 25:20-21.

Griffing, T. 1976. ITE hearing aids for children and adults. Hear. Aid J. 29:6-7.

Guberina, P. 1972. Case studies in the use of restricted bands of frequencies in auditory rehabilitation of the deaf. Department of Health, Education and Welfare, Zagreb, Yugoslavia.

Hastings, L. 1974. The earmold—a first hand look. Hear. Instruments 25:22-23.

Hearing Aid Industry Conference, 1961. HAIC Standard Method of Expressing Hearing Aid Performance. HAIC, New York.

Heide, J. 1976a. Electroacoustic testing of hearing instruments. Hear. Instruments 27:10-11.

Heide, J. 1976b. Hearing aid testing, performance and standards. Hear. Aid. J. 29:10-35.

Hocks, B. 1976. Guidelines for taking earmold impressions. Hear. Aid J.

29:6–30.

Hogg, D. 1976. Putting compression into perspective. Hear. Aid J. 29:11, 36–39.

Holmes, D., and Woodford, C. 1976. Acoustic reflex threshold and loudness discomfort level relationships in deaf children. Presented at the Acoustical Society of America Convention, Washington, D.C.

Jerger, J., and Hayes, D. 1976. Hearing aid evaluation. Arch. Otolaryngol. 102:214–225.

Johnson, E. 1972. The hearing aid evaluation—a point of view. Maico Audiol. Library Ser. 10:5–7.

Jorgen, H. 1974. Output limitation. Hear. Instruments 25:26–28.

Kaplan, S. 1976. Fitting earmolds to children. Hear. Aid J. 26:7–35.

Kasden, S. 1975. Speech discrimination and hearing aid use. Audiol. Hear. Educ. 1:45–46.

Kasten, R. 1972. Body and over the ear hearing aids. In: J. Katz (ed.), Handbook of Clinical Audiology, pp. 557–589. The Williams & Wilkins Company, Baltimore.

Katz, J. 1972. Handbook of Clinical Audiology. The Williams & Wilkins Company, Baltimore.

Kelley, K. 1976. Quality control in battery manufacture. Hear. Aid J. 29:7–30.

Kemker, F., and Johnson, R. 1972. The effect of five different hearing aid evaluation procedures on speech discrimination. Presented at the American Speech and Hearing Convention, San Francisco.

Kolb, W. 1976. Professional earmold lab services. Hear. Aid J. 29:9.

Konkle, D., and Bess, F. 1974. Custom earmolds in hearing aid evaluations. Maico Audiol. Library Ser. 22:17–21.

Knowles, H., and Burkhard, M. 1975. Hearing aids on KEMAR. Hear. Instruments 26:19–41.

Kretschmer, L. 1974. Evaluation Procedures for Adults. In: K. Donnelly (ed.), Interpreting Hearing Aid Technology, pp. 124–158. Charles C Thomas, Publisher, Springfield, Illinois.

Langford, B. 1975. Coupling Methods. In: M. Pollack (ed.), Amplification for the Hearing-Impaired, pp. 81–113. Grune & Stratton, Inc., New York.

Lentz, W. 1972. Speech discrimination in the presence of background noise using a hearing aid with a directionally-sensitive microphone. Maico Audiol. Library Ser. 10:34–38.

Lerman, A. 1976. Early training of infants and their parents. Hear. Aid J. 29:10.

Libby, E. 1975. Electro-acoustic hearing aid measurements at the dispensing level. Hear. Instruments 26:16–17.

Lilly, D. 1976. Electroacoustic measurement of hearing aids with the new standard. Presented at Ohio Speech and Hearing Association Convention, Columbus, Ohio.

Lybarger, S. 1972. Ear molds. In: J. Katz (ed.), Handbook of Clinical Audiology. pp. 602–623. The Williams & Wilkins Company, Baltimore.

Lybarger, S. 1973. Advantages and limitations of the "Y" cord. Hear. Aid J. 26:6–34.

Lybarger, S. 1974. Electroacoustic measurements. In: K. Donnelly (ed.), Interpreting Hearing Aid Technology, pp. 40–84. Charles C Thomas, Publisher, Springfield, Illinois.

Lybarger, S. 1976. New hearing aid specification standard. Hear. Aid. J. 29:12.

Matkin, N., and Thomas, J. 1972. The utilization of CROS hearing aids by children. Maico Audiol. Library Ser. 10:29–33.

McCandless, G. 1973. Hearing aids and loudness discomfort. Presented at Oticongress 3, Copenhagen.

McCandless, G., and Miller, D. 1972. Loudness discomfort and hearing aids. Hear. Aid J. 25:7–32.

Miller, M. 1967. Clinical hearing aid evaluation. Maico Audiol. Library Ser. 3:24–33.

Morgan, R. 1976. Why a custom earmold? Hear. Aid J. 29:6–32.

Nielsen, T. 1971. New thinking in the world of earmolds. Hear. Dealer.

Nielsen, H. 1976. Effect of monaural vs. binaural hearing aid treatment. Hear. Aid J. 29:8–29.

Niemeyer, W. 1971. Relations between the discomfort level and the reflex threshold of the middle ear muscles. Audiology 10:172–176.

Northern, J., and Downs, M. 1974. Hearing in Children. The Williams & Wilkins Company, Baltimore.

Olson, A., and Hipskind, N. 1973. The relation between levels of pure tones and speech which elicit the acoustic reflex and loudness discomfort. J. Auditory Res. 13:71–76.

Peterson, B. 1976. Fitting hearing aids to young children. Hear. Aid J. 29:5–28.

Pollack, M. 1975. Amplification for the Hearing-Impaired. Grune & Stratton, Inc., New York.

Preves, D. 1976. Directivity of ITE aids. Hear. Aid. J. 29:7–32.

Radcliffe, D. 1976. KEMAR. Hear. Aid J. 29:10–40.

Randolph, K. 1976. Checking hearing aid operation using a cassette recorder. Audiol. Hear. Educ. 2:28–40.

Resnick, D., and Becker, M. 1963. Hearing aid evaluation: A new approach. Asha 5:695–699.

Roeser, R., Campbell, A., and Brown, B. 1976. The hearing health team... A one way street? Audiol. Hear. Educ. 2:8–11.

Roeser, R., Gerken, G., and Glorig, A. 1976. A hearing aid malfunction detection unit (HAMDU). J. Acoust. Soc. Am. 59:S16.

Ross, M. 1972. Hearing Aid Evaluation. In: J. Katz (ed.), Handbook of Clinical Audiology, pp. 624–655. The Williams & Wilkins Company, Baltimore.

Ross, M. 1975. Hearing Aid Selection for Preverbal Hearing-Impaired Children. In: M. Pollack (ed.), Amplification for the Hearing-Impaired, pp. 207–242. Grune & Stratton, Inc., New York.

Ross, M. 1976. Introduction and review of hearing aid evaluation procedures. In: M. Rubin (ed.), Hearing Aids—Current Developments and Concepts, pp. 143–148. University Park Press, Baltimore.

Rubin, M. 1976. Hearing Aids—Current Developments and Concepts, University Park Press, Baltimore.

Sanders, D. 1971. Aural Rehabilitation. Prentice-Hall Inc., Englewood Cliffs, New Jersey.

Schneider, A. 1975. Acoustical evaluation of hearing aids. Hear. Instruments. 26:14–16.

Shallop, J. 1973. Some relationships among speech reception, the dynamic range of intelligible speech and the acoustic reflex. Scand. Audiol. 2:119–122.

Shapiro, I. 1976. Hearing aid fitting by prescription. Audiolgy 15:163–173.

Sheeley, R. 1976. Principles of adapter for earmold venting. Hear. Aid J. 29:7–35.

Shore, I., Bilger, R., and Hirsh, I. 1960. Hearing aid evaluation: Reliability of repeated measurements. J. Speech Hear. Disord. 25:152–170.

Sinclair, J. 1976. You must be wrong...our measurements don't agree. Hear. Instruments 27:16–28.

Smith, E. 1976. Marketing hearing aid batteries. Hear. Aid J. 29:9–32.

Snow, T., and McCandless, G. 1976. The use of impedance measures in hearing aid selection. Hear. Aid J. 29:7–33.

Spar, H. 1976. Today's battery "aids." Hear. Aid J. 29:10–27.

Staub, W., and O'Gara, E. 1974. Auditory training systems for the hearing impaired. Hear. Instruments 25:12–24.

Teter, D. 1976. Electroacoustical evaluation of hearing aids. Hear. Instruments 27:8–9.

Tonisson, W. 1975. Measuring in-the-ear gain of hearing aids by the acoustic reflex method. J. Speech Hear. Res. 18:17–30.

Truax, R. 1974. Amplifier to Prosthesis. In: K. Donnelly (ed.), Interpreting Hearing Aid Technology, pp. 3–39. Charles C Thomas Publisher, Springfield, Illinois.

Vargo, S. 1974. Compression amplification and hearing aids. Maico Audiol. Library Ser. 12:5–8.

Victoreen, J. 1960. Hearing Enhancement. Charles C Thomas Publisher, Springfield, Illinois.

Victoreen, J. 1973a . A Guide to Applied Otometric Procedures. Vicon Instrument Co., Colorado Springs.

Victoreen, J. 1973b. Basic Principles of Otometry. Charles C Thomas Publisher, Springfield, Illinois.

Wallenfels, H. 1967. Hearing Aids On Prescription. Charles C Thomas Publisher, Springfield, Illinois.

Wiener, F., and Miller, G. 1946. Hearing aids. In: Combat Instrumentation II, pp. 216–232. NDRC Report 117, Washington, D.C.

Wiltse, V. 1976. Batteries: 1906 to 1976. Hear. Aid J. 29:6–31.

Winchester, R. 1967. When is a hearing aid needed? Maico Audiol. Library Ser. 1:36–39.

Yonovitz, A. 1974. Binaural intelligibility: Pilot study progress. Speech and Hearing Institute, Texas Medical Center, Houston.

Zelnick, E. 1974. The importance of interaural phase differences on binaural hearing aid fittings. Hear. Instruments 25:12–15.

Hearing Screening

J. C. Cooper, Jr.

CONTENTS

Screening is atypical of diagnostic routines in audiology because it is imposed upon individuals who are usually not concerned about their hearing. Screening implies the use of a technique that permits probabilistic statements to be made about a hearing loss so that adverse consequences can be prevented or reduced. The rationale underlying screening has serious economic considerations; if cost were no consideration, hearing loss might be most effectively identified by complete audiologic evaluation. Because cost is a consideration, a formula for computing the cost of screening each individual is included. Professor Cooper indicates that the definition of hearing loss is crucial to selection of the screening technique. Traditional audiometric and otoscopic techniques adapted for screening have proved practically useless in detecting conductive losses

(Cooper et al., 1975; Eagles et al., 1963). The implications of conductive loss are primarily health related. Sensorineural loss affects communication efficiency, and during the language acquisition period, losses averaging no more than 20 dB may be involved in educational retardation. Professor Cooper provides specific criteria for audiometric screening to detect sensorineural losses and techniques for screening with an electroacoustic impedance bridge to detect conductive losses. Finally, a discussion of the management of a screening program is included.   —Eds.

Screening is atypical of the diagnostic and rehabilitative routines that dominate the practice of audiology. For that reason, it may be useful to recall a unique aspect of the screening process, examine the steps that make up a comprehensive hearing conservation program, and present a rationale for conducting screening. The reader should proceed with two things in mind: first, that the present discussion focuses on the identification of hearing loss in individuals older than 6 years of age; second, that the rationale developed for conducting screening is based upon economic considerations. The reader is under no obligation to assume this rationale. Subsequent sections compare available screening techniques independent of economic considerations.

ATTITUDES

Screening is a process that is imposed upon individuals who are unlikely to be concerned about any hearing loss. If they were, they would present themselves for evaluation. The intrusive nature of the process generates at least two types of problems. First is the degree of cooperation that can be expected from the person being screened. Particularly if the outcome of screening can be detrimental to the individual (as in the case of an airplane pilot who may lose his job on the basis of hearing loss), that cooperation can be less than expected had he presented himself for evaluation. Second, because the person is unlikely to be concerned about hearing loss, recommendations for evaluations to determine the nature of any possible hearing problem may not be followed. Such issues are not raised to discourage screening. The point to remember is that the person screened comes to the screening with a different set of attitudes than encountered in routine clinical practice.

HEARING CONSERVATION

Much of the controversy surrounding hearing conservation programs and their effectiveness results from a failure to clearly distinguish among the four steps that make up a program. These are: defining hearing loss, screening, evaluating failures, and taking corrective action. Defining hearing loss and distinguishing between screening and evaluation bear comment.

Hearing Loss

Defining a hearing loss is basic to the development of any screening program and particularly important for the selection of screening technique. Unfortunately, asking concerned individuals to define hearing loss can produce a wide variety of responses. The man in the street might say that "passing" means there is no hearing problem for social, vocational, or health purposes. An educator would be more specific. To him, "passing" might mean that hearing acuity is unlikely to interfere with a student's educational progress. Neither of the two is likely to make the physician's distinction between health-threatening conditions requiring medical attention and those losses, however severe, that pose no threat to the patient's health. Lastly, there is the lawyer who is concerned with possible litigation resulting from hearing loss and who is dealing with numbers from statutes generated as a by-product of compromises reached in the legislative arena.

Fortunately, the definitions of hearing loss suggested above and others can be reduced to two major targets based upon the types of ear disease that can be reliably detected. These are conductive and sensorineural hearing losses. To briefly review: conductive impairments involve malfunction of the auditory system between the external canal and the footplate of the stapes. Although a variety of audiologic and medical tests can distinguish among cochlear, VIIIth nerve, and central auditory lesions, for screening purposes the coarse category "sensorineural loss" is here used to describe a reduction in hearing sensitivity as a result of malfunction somewhere between the footplate of the stapes and the brain. The impact of these two types of hearing loss can be examined in terms of their prevalence and their medical and educational/communicative consequences.

Conductive hearing loss Estimates of the prevalence of conductive loss have been clouded by the limitations of the techniques available for its detection. Until recently, only audiometric and otoscopic techniques were widely used. The technical requirements and time factors involved in reliable audiometric determination of conductive hearing loss preclude its use with large numbers. Variations of such techniques for screening have been shown to be practically useless in the detection of conductive hearing loss (Cooper et al., 1975; Eagles et al., 1963).

Although otoscopic techniques seem to be reliable in the extremes, there is only some 60% intersubjective agreement in those transitional states between outright disease and normalcy. This is particularly true in cases where the tympanic membrane may be characterized as being retracted or having reduced mobility (Eagles et al., 1963; Roeser, Soh, Dunckel and Adams, 1977). Nonetheless, McEldowney and Kessner's review of the epidemiology of otitis media (1972), the most likely cause of conductive hearing loss, suggests that age, race, seasonal fluctuations, and socioeconomic status are major parameters. The effects of the age and seasonal fluctuations seem to be most clearly delineated with younger children at higher risk and the highest incidence occurring during winter months. The effects of race and socioeconomic background are less understood. Although American Indian and Eskimo populations have significantly higher prevalences than white populations, these findings may be confounded by the low socioeconomic status associated with such groups. Indeed, McEldowney and Kessner find no consistency among reports purporting to investigate socioeconomic status alone. In short, precise definition of the prevalence of conductive hearing loss is impossible. At worst, Cooper et al. (1975) report that 38% of children in preschool classes have conductive hearing impairments requiring medical attention and Eagles et al. (1963) suggest that middle ear disorders are the fourth most frequent complaint in the medical histories of children.

The health hazards associated with conductive hearing loss are well documented (Glasscock, 1972). These range from mastoiditis and facial nerve paralysis through intracranial complications such as meningitis, encephalitis, and brain abscess. It is clear that such health-threatening conditions cannot be ignored.

Aside from the health hazards, there is a less extensive body of evidence suggesting that chronic conductive hearing losses will lead to educational retardation. These reports are difficult to interpret for several reasons. Aside from a clear definition of chronicity, there are fluctuations in conductive hearing loss, which make specification of the degree of loss difficult. The second factor is the nature of its correlates, which cloud the effect of hearing loss alone. For example, disease may cause absence from school, which is in itself detrimental to educational progress. The low socioeconomic level ambiguously associated with conductive hearing loss may prejudice educational progress. Last, as suggested earlier, many mild cases may simply be undetected in school hearing conservation programs. With these qualifications in mind, there remains a trend that indicates that some degree of educational retardation is associated with conductive hearing loss. On a purely academic level, this includes retardation of performance on mechanical reading and arithmetic tasks (Ling, 1972) and more generalized retardation in language skills extending as far as the production of verbal responses (Forcucci and Stark, 1972; Holm and Kunze, 1969). However, conclusions regarding educational effects are not unanimous. In reporting the effects of mild hearing loss, Steer et al. (1961) found no generalized academic retardation in children. They did find that social adjustment and generalized teacher and parental ratings of impaired children were lower than those of normal children. Interestingly, the impaired children were judged to be more easily angered than their normal hearing counterparts.

Sensorineural hearing loss   The age pattern of sensorineural hearing loss prevalence is the reverse of that of conductive hearing loss. That is to say that the prevalence of congenital sensorineural hearing loss is low, estimated at some 0.05% (Northern and Downs, 1974, p. 97). Of school children sampled during the National Speech and Hearing Survey (Hull and Mielke, 1971), only some 4% of the children sampled had thresholds poorer than 25 dB (ISO, 1964) at 4,000 Hz, the highest rate of the frequencies tested. This figure would provide a ceiling for the incidence of significant sensorineural loss. The rate of sensorineural hearing loss among working adults varies widely on the basis of kind of employment. In vocations that have high levels of noise, prevalence may reach some 100%. More generally, it has been estimated that at least 25% of the geriatric population have a hearing loss sufficient to impair communication (National Advisory Neurological Diseases and Stroke Council, 1969, p. 15). As opposed to the situation with conductive hearing losses where methodological techniques for its detection have been called into question, the major problem in estimating prevalence in adult populations is not the validity of technique, rather that systematic sampling has not occurred. Thus, as in the case of conductive losses, figures are less precise than might be hoped for.

At this time, the health-related consequences of sensorineural hearing loss are less important than those associated with conductive hearing loss. Although some conditions can pose a very real threat to life (such as acoustic neuroma), the overwhelming majority of sensorineural hearing losses are neither a health threat nor amenable to medical intervention. Their major effect is to reduce communication efficiency. The issue of relating the degree of sensorineural hearing loss to the degree of communication impairment is not clear. As suggested earlier, it would seem that during the language acquisition phase of an individual's life, even mild hearing losses averaging no more than 20 dB may be involved in educational retardation. For communication purposes in a language-capable adult, average speech frequency thresholds of 20 dB seem to be satisfactory for communication. In this industrial society where noise is a significant hazard, a qualification must be added. Even though speech frequency averages remain in the 20-dB range, high frequency threshold shifts typical of noise-induced hearing loss do result in complaints of impaired communication (Cooper and Owen, 1976).

Screening and Evaluation

Failure to distinguish between the act of screening and the act of evaluation is at the root of most criticisms of screening programs. That criticism is generated when screening techniques fail to identify individuals with hearing loss and is most vocal when individuals suspected of having a hearing loss based on failing a screening test are found to have normal hearing. The position taken here is that the act of screening is not intended to produce a definitive statement about the presence or absence of a hearing loss. Screening is simply the use of a technique that permits probabilistic statements to be made about the presence of a hearing loss and permits conclusions to be drawn regarding the necessity for evaluation. To set the stage for hearing screening, it should be noted that only 80% of vision screening failures are found to have vision defects (Hatfield, 1967). Although it is always desirable to improve the efficiency of screening techniques, it is unlikely that their efficiency will ever reach 100%. This fact must be accepted as a current reality by all individuals who come in contact with a screening program, both those involved in screening and those being screened.

RATIONALE FOR SCREENING

If there were no adverse consequences of hearing loss, there would be no need for screening, nor would screening be practical if nothing could be done to ease the disability. The premise underlying screening is that adverse consequences can be prevented or reduced by detecting the hearing loss, and that a substantial savings in money and/or personal hardship can result. The problem becomes one of detecting the disability. In some diseases, screening and diagnosis can be joined into a single act or event. This is not the case in hearing loss. Moreover, a full hearing evaluation of every individual would be an economic impossibility. Thus, screening reduces to the abbreviation of some technique so that the probability of detection is maximized and the cost associated with detection is minimized.

The category of individuals likely to be screened is also related to the economics of the situation. As a practical matter, an age dimension is involved in most hearing conservation programs. The breakdown normally follows the various categories of structured activities appropriate to various age groups. In the United States, these typically begin at birth, hence hospital neonatal screening programs. Formal gathering then disappears to make preschool screening programs costly and difficult to implement outside of physicians' offices, day care centers, and well baby clinics. Educational settings provide the most encompassing opportunity to detect hearing loss. The next institution of formal gathering is a vocational setting, followed by a second diffusion of the population into retirement. Like the preschool population, the retired are difficult to screen outside the artificial communities generated by various agencies or the spontaneous groupings that occur for social and political purposes. The advantage of using groupings is the economy with which screening can be conducted. Neonatal wards, schools, and vocational settings all imply a degree of control over the individuals involved, which permits "mass production" techniques to be employed.

Costs

The economic ramifications of a hearing conservation program can be viewed as the cumulative effects of five major cost factors. The first is the personnel costs associated with the operation of the program. These derive from the time necessary to conduct screening and the salaries necessary to employ the screeners. A second major factor is equipment costs. These include not only the initial purchase price but all maintenance costs associated with the equipment over the probable lifetime of the particular device. The third factor is the number of people to be screened. Taken together, these factors permit estimation of the cost necessary to screen one individual. Because a goal of any screening program is to refer persons with suspected hearing loss for evaluation, the efficiency of such a process becomes the fourth major factor in determining the economics of screening. These costs must be related to the cost associated with not screening. That is the fifth major factor, the cost of rehabilitation. There would be little reason to go to the trouble of detecting hearing loss if it turned out that such detection were more costly than the overall costs associated with the disability. Implicit in this factor is the fact that some sort of rehabilitation technique can prevent or at least ameliorate the effects of hearing loss. Thus, it is the bottom line on the accountant's ledger that is likely to determine the longevity of any hearing conservation program.

The costs of screening can be looked at in a number of different ways. The most useful is the cost per accurate referral of a hearing-impaired individual, because rehabilitation is the end point of a hearing conservation program and such rehabilitation cannot occur without accurate referrals. The example of cost analysis that follows is basic and takes into consideration only the major cost variables. Depending upon the situation, the formula can be amplified as needed.

An Example

Taking the cost to screen one person as a starting point, the following basic equation applies:

$$\text{Cost/person} = \frac{S}{R} + \frac{C + (M \times L)}{(N \times L)}$$

In this formulation, the personnel costs are represented by S/R, the salary per hour of the screening personnel divided by the number of individuals who can be screened per hour. Equipment costs are based on four factors: C, the cost of initial purchase of equipment; M, the maintenance costs per year; L, the expected lifetime of the equipment before replacement is required; and N, the number of individuals to be screened per year. The cost to screen a person might be calculated as follows. Assume that the salary is $10 per hour, that 10 individuals can be screened per hour, that the cost of the screening device is $1,000 and its lifetime 10 years, that maintenance costs are $100 per year, and that there are 4,000 individuals to be screened per year. Thus:

$$
\begin{aligned}
\text{Cost/person} &= \frac{\$10}{10} + \frac{\$1,000 + (\$100 \times 10)}{4,000 \times 10} \\
&= \$1 + \frac{\$1,000 + \$1,000}{40,000} \\
&= \$1 + \frac{\$2,000}{40,000} \\
&= \$1.05
\end{aligned}
$$

The large effect of the salary component should be noted as well as the influence of the rate of screening on that salary component.

The next step in calculating cost per accurate referral is the efficiency with which children are referred. That efficiency is reflected in the accurate referral rate.

$$\text{Accurate referral rate} = \frac{\text{Number of accurate referrals}}{\text{Number screened}}$$

The establishment of this accurate referral rate requires some independent judgment of the number of confirmed hearing losses among all who failed the screening test. Assume that screening is for conductive hearing loss with a prevalence of 25% and that the technique identifies 90% of such cases. Of the 10,000 cases of conductive loss (40,000 × 0.25) expected over a period of 10 years, the technique identifies 9,000 (10,000 × 0.90).

$$\text{Accurate referral rate} = \frac{9,000}{40,000}$$

$$= 0.225$$

To obtain the cost per accurate referral, divide the cost to screen one person by the accurate referral rate.

$$\text{Cost per accurate referral} = \frac{\$1.05}{0.225}$$
$$= \$4.67$$

Remembering that the effect of chronic conductive hearing loss of educational progress needs to be more extensively documented, the following development attempts to estimate the rehabilitation costs associated with such losses. Ling (1972) suggests that educational retardation approximates 18 months and that no spontaneous recovery can be expected without educational intervention. If it is assumed that the time necessary to make up the 18-month retardation requires some special educational assistance of equal duration, rehabilitation costs can be estimated in the following way. At least one state in the union will contribute an additional $450.00 per year per student receiving special educational support. The rehabilitation costs would then be 1½ years times $450.00 or $675.00 per child. However, only approximately 20–25% of conductive hearing losses are likely to become chronic (Gunderson and Tonning, 1976; Lowe, Bamforth, and Pracy, 1963). Continuing with the example assuming the occurrence of 10,000 conductive losses and a chronicity of 25%, the costs to a school for not screening would be $1,687,500 ($675.00 × 10,000 × 0.25) over a 10-year period. [1] Screening will have cost $42,030 ($4.67/ accurate referral × 9,000 referrals) to detect 9,000 cases, only 2,250 of which would have become chronic. One thousand would not be detected, of which 250 would become chronic and need rehabilitation. The cost of that rehabilitation would be $168,750 ($675.00 × 250). Now, to get to the bottom line:

Cost of not screening		$1,687,500
Cost of screening		
Direct	$ 42,030	
Rehabilitation of undetected	168,750	
		(–)210,780
Savings from screening		$1,476,720

What has not been taken into account are two additional categories of costs. The first is the cost of medical remediation of the conductive hearing loss. This would reduce the degree of savings by the amount of such medical costs. The second factor would increase the savings by the amount of whatever value one attaches to the discomfort and possible long term health hazards associated with an unattended conductive hearing loss.

The preceding formulation and values for the various constants in the equations are presented only for the purpose of demonstration of a technique that can be employed to justify hearing conservation programs. The basic equations presented here must be tailored to the particular situation and viewpoint of the agency or individuals who are considering a hearing conservation program. Many of the costs that have been referred to cannot be accurately determined. However, one by-product of such an analysis is a rather specific means for comparison of alternate screening techniques. The most near-sighted way to make such a comparison is simply to look at the cost

---

[1]Of course, if the school administration were willing to graduate these children in an educationally retarded state, there would be no costs. In spite of whatever feelings the reader may have about administrators, it is unlikely that they would admit to doing so.

to screen per individual. That goal is readily attainable in any screening situation. The more farsighted view would include the cost per accurate referral. However, recalling that one of the major problems that may be encountered in a hearing conservation program is the failure of individuals screened to take the step between screening and evaluation, data for the establishment of an accurate referral rate may be difficult to come by. The broadest perspective on the efficiency of a screening program can be obtained by taking into account the costs that accrue by failure to conduct screening. These costs, because they involve not only direct expenditures but varying degrees of human suffering, are almost impossible to generate with any degree of precision.

SCREENING TECHNIQUES: HISTORICAL PERSPECTIVE

Four major types of tests have been used for the detection of hearing loss: variations of a person's response to speech, tuning fork tests, audiometric techniques, and electroacoustic impedance bridge measures.

Speech Tests

It might be assumed that hearing loss would be disclosed by extended interaction between two individuals. Unfortunately, such extended interaction, as in the case between a teacher and her students, has been shown to be a poor indicator. Geyer and Yankauer (1956) report that teachers were able to identify only some 62% of children who were found to have a hearing loss. Moreover, 88% of those suspected of having a hearing loss in fact did not have one. The lack of reliability of such indices can be understood by recalling the various factors that contribute to the understanding of speech. These include, among others, the hearer's familiarity with the message and his language sophistication, the length of the utterance, the nature of the speaker's voice, and signal-to-noise ratio associated with the communication situation. Nonetheless, it is noted that a formalization of tests involving one person's responses to another person's speech are still sanctioned by the federal government's Standard Form 88. In this instance, the examiner is asked to judge a person's hearing on the basis of a ratio between the distance from an individual for minimal understanding of speech and the distance necessary for a normal person. Thus, 20/20 indicates that an individual hears at 20 feet what the normal person would hear at the same distance. 10/20 would indicate that the individual must be at 10 feet from the screener to hear what a normal person would hear at 20 feet. Another formalization of responses to speech as a screening technique is the Verbal Auditory Screening Test for Children (VASC) developed by Griffing, Simonton, and Hedgecock (1967). A comparison of the VASC test to pure tone screening (Mencher and McCullough, 1970) indicated that some 50% of children who passed the VASC test failed a pure tone test. They concluded that "mild losses of 30–40 dB (ISO) in the speech range and even greater at other frequencies are not adequately detected by the VASC." In spite of the face validity of using speech as the acoustic signal for screening and the greater responsivity of young children to speech in comparison to pure tones, there seem to be no reliable techniques for screening with speech.

Tuning Fork Tests

Tuning fork tests remain a useful, if qualitative, index of hearing with reliable persons who are able to understand the judgments required. In children, however, Wilson and Woods (1975) report that the Bing tuning fork test correctly identified conductive hearing losses only some 60% of the time. They found the Rinne test correctly identified 100% of conductive hearing losses if the air-bone gap was 40 dB or greater. The correct identification rate gradually diminished to a low 0% for 10-dB air-bone gaps. In an unpublished examination of its efficiency, Cooper and Gates found that the Weber correctly identified only 58% of first grade children in need of otologic management. The Schwaback test for estimation of sensorineural loss is seldom used and reports of its efficiency were not uncovered.

Audiometric Techniques

Audiometric screening is based upon the presence or absence of the behavioral response to a tonal representation by air conduction. Recommendations for screening have ranged from a single 4,000-Hz presentation to each ear (House and Glorig, 1957) to five tonal stimuli (Darley, 1961). Minimum levels (corrected to ANSI standards) at which a response must occur for the person to pass have ranged from 20 dB at 4,000 Hz to as high as 30 dB at 500 Hz. Fortunately, for the purpose of this chapter and in the context of current professional consensus and governmental regulations, the details of this cursory summary are not relevant. The important issues in audiometric screening revolve around its capability to detect conductive hearing loss and its reliability in estimating overall hearing sensitivity.

With respect to the detection of conductive hearing losses, audiometers are categorically worthless. As early as 1963, Eagles et al. concluded that "audiometric testing, however complete it may be, cannot identify all children with physical abnormalities which may have predictive value, or who may need medical treatment." A variety of recent studies have indicated that audiometric screening techniques detect between 61% (McCandless and Thomas, 1974) and 24% (Cooper et al., 1975) of otoscopically confirmed conditions requiring medical attention.

From a different point of view, audiometric screening techniques seem to be a valid estimate of hearing sensitivity, hence sensorineural hearing level in the absence of conductive impairments. Melnik, Eagles and Levine (1964) indicate only 2% of those who passed an audiometric screening test failed a threshold test. This value could be reduced to less than 0.5% if a second screening were interposed between the first and a threshold test. Thus, in children at least, audiometric screening can be taken as a reliable estimate of overall hearing sensitivity. With adults, no large scale studies have been uncovered that address themselves to the reliability of audiometric screening. A small scale study by Gosztonyi, Vassallo, and Sataloff (1971) suggests that there may be a difference in reliability between hourly-wage and salaried personnel. Nineteen of 25 hourly-wage subjects failed to produce reliable audiograms based on test-retest comparisons of automatic audiometry. On the average, these responses were some 10 dB poorer than those obtained by manual threshold audiometry. In reviewing the circumstances of each case, the authors uncovered the fact that more than half of the subjects were receiving or were applying for compensation based upon noise-induced hearing loss. These findings reinforced the fact that screening adiometry is not equivalent to diagnostic examinations and re-emphasized the need to separate the two in a hearing conservation program.

The superficial inconsistency between an audiometer screening technique's inability to detect conductive losses and its reliability in estimating thresholds can be accounted for on the basis of three factors: the small air conduction threshold shift associated with many conductive pathologies, the failure to obtain bone conduction thresholds for comparison to air conduction, and the typical levels of noise in audiometric screening situations, which force screening levels into the 20–25 dB range.

Impedance Bridges

In the last 5 years or so, the electroacoustic impedance bridge has increasingly demonstrated its value in the detection of conductive hearing losses and its ability to economically evaluate large groups. Using the schema for describing otoscopic findings presented in *Otitis Media* (Glorig and Gerwin, 1972, pp. 276–277), there are five major indicators of middle ear disease based on observation of the tympanic membrane: perforations, mobility, retraction or bulging, scarring, and color. The impedance bridge provides concrete data regarding three of the five parameters and may provide information regarding the fourth. Perforations are reflected by the large compliance values associated with the volume of the external and middle ear combination. Mobility and bulging or retraction are quantified in the tympanogram, although in infants this indicator has come under question (Paradise, Smith, and Bluestone, 1976). Factors such as the membrane's elasticity, scarring, or surface tension effects attributable to the presence of small amounts of liquid in the middle ear may affect the tympanometric peak, normally taken as an indicator of middle ear pressure. Scarring, alone, may find expression in the shape of the tympanogram, particularly if the probe tone is higher than 220 Hz.

As early as 1968, Brooks suggested that the impedance bridge is a more efficient device for the detection of conductive hearing loss than the audiometer. Using an abbreviated impedance technique with only middle ear pressure equal to or more negative than -100 mm H_2O and absence of an acoustic reflex as criteria for failure, both McCandless and Thomas (1974) and Cooper, et al. (1975) demonstrated that an impedance bridge detected in excess of 90% of otoscopically confirmed conductive losses. The reservations expressed about such criteria involve the over-referral rate, which was 24% in the latter study. More than half of the over-referrals involved indications of negative middle ear pressure in excess of -100 mm H_2O. The effect of negative middle ear pressure bears further examination.

In an examination of that effect on air-bone gap, Cooper et al. (1977) found that the Pearson product movement correlations of negative middle ear pressure with air-bone gap range between approximately 0.3 and 0.4 for the frequencies of 250–4,000 Hz. Of particular interest was the fact that the mean air-bone gap in the speech frequency range approximated 15 dB for middle ear pressures between -100 and -150 mm H_2O. Since Forcucci and Stark (1972) have associated 15 dB hearing losses with language retardation, such minimal deviations in middle ear pressure may be educationally significant.

Indeed, negative middle ear pressures of as little as -50 mm H_2O have been implicated in the existence of middle ear disease (Alberti and Kristensen, 1972). At the other extreme, Brooks (1968) has suggested that middle ear pressures more negative than -200 mm H_2O are necessary before serous otitis media may be reliably inferred. As an alternative, Lewis et al. (1975) have suggested that as many as four successive tests may be necessary to reach a responsible referral decision. Increased efficiency in detecting middle ear fluid can also be had by examining the compliance and slope of the tympanogram (Paradise et al., 1976). Unfortunately, the results of that investigation are not readily convertible to other models of impedance bridges.

Criteria for making the decision that a conductive loss exists are in a state of flux. Suggestions range from using only the presence or absence of a stapedial reflex (Brooks, 1976) to using a combination of otologic history, audiometry, and tympanometry (Berry, Bluestone, and Cantekin, 1975). One reason for the range of criteria which have been proposed is the poor understanding of middle ear disease, particularly its natural history. One of the few studies to provide longitudinal data regarding the natural history of middle ear disorders (Brooks, 1976), suggests that one-third of school children will have no more than two episodes of middle ear disease during a period of 7-8 years. One-sixth will have recurrent disease for periods of up to two years, after which the disease will permanently resolve. Only one-twentieth will demonstrate persistent middle ear disorders extending over more than 2 years. Depending on the relationship between the time of screening and the onset of both transient and persistent disease, one-half of all children might fail a single screening. Should they be referred? The answer is "no" if the screening target is limited to chronic conductive hearing loss and the consequence is the necessity for rescreening over periods of months, if not years. The answer is "yes" if the presence of disease alone is the screening target and is supported by Herer's (1976) report that the optimum point for referral, which will be confirmed by otoscopy, is negative middle ear pressure in the range between -100 and -160 mm H_2O. As of autumn 1977, no consensus regarding screening criteria had been reached. Nonetheless, a practical judgment must be made on the basis of current information and is presented in the section of recommendations. The reader has the obligation to revise his thinking on the basis of reports that will undoubtedly be published after this chapter has gone to press.

Because of the nature of the measurements made, it is obvious that the tympanogram simply does not provide any information about sensorineural function. This limitation of impedance bridge technique is, in part, compensated for by measures of an acoustic reflex. Whether by the ipsilateral or contralateral technique of elicitation, the reader will recall that an VIIIth nerve response on the side of stimulation is required for the stapedial contraction to occur. Measures of the threshold of elicitation of the stapedial contraction to a variety of acoustic signals have been used to predict sensorineural function (Jerger, Burney, Maulding, and Crump, 1974). However, the steps involved would seem excessive for the present definition of screening technique. Returning to a screening criterion that involves the simple observation of an acoustic reflex, it seems that its maturation is, in part, a function of age (Jerger, 1970; Jerger, Jerger, and Mauldin, 1972; Jerger, Jerger, Mauldin, and Segal, 1974). It may also be a function of the frequency used to elicit the reflex, with responses to 4,000 Hz seemingly having no pathological significance. Taken together with tympanometric results indicating no hearing loss, it would seem that as many as 5% of such cases in children would fail to produce an acoustic reflex. With this degree of variability inherent in normal hearing individuals, it is judged that impedance bridge screening alone is insufficient to the task of detecting sensorineural hearing loss. The experience of Brooks (1973) and Cooper et al., (1975) have led them to recommend a combined bridge-audiometric technique when both conductive and sensorineural hearing losses may be present in the population to be screened.

Related Factors

Environment An adequate acoustic environment depends on which technique, impedance bridge or audiometric, is being used. For impedance bridge techniques alone, ambient noise is not critical in any practical sense. However, the levels of noise are critical in the employment of audiometric techniques.

To review, recall that responses to auditory stimulation are a function of ambient noise and the true auditory threshold. In one sense, the effects of noise are indistinguishable from hearing loss. In noise sufficient to prevent a normal hearing person from hearing presentations of less than 30 dB, both a person with normal hearing and a person with a 30-dB hearing loss will produce 30-dB thresholds. The person with normal hearing is responding at 30 dB because the noise interferes with his hearing of less intense signals. He is hearing both the signal and the noise. The person with a 30-dB hearing loss may be unaware of the bulk of the noise occurring and only hears the

Table 1. Maximum octave band levels for ambient noise, in dB SPL

Band width (Hz)	Test frequency	Level for screening	Level for threshold testing
300–600	500	46	26
600–1,200	1,000	50	30
1,200–2,400	2,000	58	38
2,400–4,800	4,000	76	51

signal. In the absence of noise, the normal hearing person would produce thresholds on the order of 0 dB and the hearing-impaired person's threshold would remain at 30 dB. Reduction in the noise level is the only way to distinguish between the two individuals. Guidelines for the maximum levels of noise permissable for screening are reproduced in Table 1 (American Speech and Hearing Association, 1975). The levels in the third column are for screening levels of 20, 20, 20, and 25 dB for the octaves from 500–4,000 Hz. If, as is the case in some screening programs, threshold measurements are used as a follow-up to failure of screening, then the fourth column figures should be used to evaluate ambient noise.

As a matter of comparison, the proposed Department of Labor standards for ambient noise in a test environment are 40, 40, 47, 52, and 62 dB SPL in the bands surrounding octave intervals from 500–8,000 Hz. Although the Department of Labor advocates threshold testing rather than screening, the figures in Table 1 make it clear that "screening" is occurring in the sense that 0 dB hearing is unlikely to be measured at such noise levels.

The degree of quiet achieved at the tympanic membrane is a function of the distance of the tympanic membrane from the source of the noise and the attenuation of noise as it passes through the various media between the noise and the tympanic membrane. To achieve a quiet environment, the test site may be located at a distance from sources of noise or be surrounded with sound insulation and absorbing materials. These may be as simple as acoustical tile, rugs, and heavy drapery or as sophisticated as special sound rooms located at the test site. A questionable alternative is the use of sound attenuating covers for earphones. Such special headsets are, in effect, being advertised as portable sound booths. A variety of studies, the most recent being Roeser, Seidel, and Glorig (1975), disclose that some models of sound-attenuating headsets produce poorer thresholds than standard sets when used in quiet, i.e., their use would suggest the presence of a threshold shift when one did not actually exist. Even in noise, one model tested was found to be no more efficient than standard headsets. In the case of the model that seemed to attenuate ambient noise and still maintain appropriate calibration, thresholds representative of those obtained from quiet could only be maintained in noise that did not exceed 40 dB per octave band. A review of Table 1 indicates that 40-dB ambient noise is acceptable for screening with standard headsets. If noise levels are above 40 dB, then even these headsets are likely to distort threshold measures of hearing. The net effect of research in this area is that the use of sound-attenuating headsets must be considered with some hesitancy and, if necessary, used only after careful exploration of their particular capabilities and limitations.

Cooperation by the person screened   The nature of impedance bridge function requires only that the person being screened remain relatively still so that bodily noise will not be detected by the bridge and mask results. This is not the case in audiometric screening where the person screened is required to produce a behavioral response when he hears an acoustic stimulus. It must be presumed that the bulk of people undergoing audiometric screening will cooperate in the task. As suggested earlier, this may not be true in certain vocational groups, nor may it be true in certain disadvantaged groups brought up in high levels of noise (Goldman and Sanders, 1969). More generally, the attention and cooperation of young children are suspect. It is difficult to believe that a group of 6-year-olds herded into a single room and forced to wait while each one undergoes a hearing screening test will keep their minds on the problem of detecting the tone. The better part of valor would lead to the isolation of the child from visually distracting elements in the environment as well as the acoustic interference discussed above. One last comment about the visual environment is that there should be no visual clue to the person being screened as to when the tone is being presented. The need to ensure that a response is contingent solely upon the acoustic stimulus, and not upon other factors, is obvious.

Equipment calibration   A detailed examination of calibration techniques is beyond the scope of this chapter. That incorrect calibration distorts results is obvious. What is not generally realized is the magnitude of the problem. Thomas et al., (1969) report that only 2% of audiometers meet strict calibration standards. If this report represents the condition of equipment in the typical program, screening results must bear no more than a random relationship to the occurrence of hearing loss. The reader is referred to the various professional and governmental calibration standards for details. Among others, Wilbur (1972) provides a summary of audiometric calibration techniques with appropriate references. Of particular interest to those who are involved in daily use of audiometers is her discussion of listening and visual examinations easily completed without specialized equipment. Recent models of electroacoustic impedance bridges have built-in calibration adjustments designed for operator use. Particularly if screening observations are limited to middle ear pressure and presence of an acoustic reflex, such adjustments are adequate. Any audiometric stimuli included as part of the screening bridge should be subject to the same scrutiny as audiometers.

SCREENING TECHNIQUES: RECOMMENDATIONS

The initial problem faced when selecting a screening technique is the definition of hearing loss. Three practical targets can be isolated in terms of the groups that lend themselves to economical screening and the type of hearing loss (sensorineural or conductive), which constitutes the major threat to hearing. These are children with conductive losses, teenagers and adults who may develop a sensorineural hearing loss as a result of noise exposure, and presbycusic losses in older adults and geriatric populations.

Sensorineural Hearing Loss

Because of the remoteness of the structures involved and short of the employment of electrophysiologic techniques, audiometric screening remains the only viable way to detect sensorineural hearing loss. Although a variety of specific techniques have been used in the past, the current consensus is best reflected in the American Speech and Hearing Association's *Guidelines for Identification Audiometry* (1975). The *Guidelines* acknowledges the inability of audiometric techniques to detect conductive losses and was designed for the identification of "persons who have a hearing impairment that interferes with or has the potential of interfering with communication." To pass, a person must hear 20 dB (ANSI, 1969) presentations at 1,000 and 2,000 Hz and a 25-dB presentation at 4,000 Hz. The use of 500 Hz is not recommended because such information contributes little insight into possible sensorineural hearing problems with the exception of rare conditions such as Meniere's disease, certain VIIIth nerve and brain stem lesions, and hereditary low frequency hearing loss (Vanderbilt University Heredity Deafness Study Group, 1968). The *Guidelines* does not recommend the use of 6,000-Hz screening tone because of the variability of the earphone to ear coupling at frequencies above 4,000 Hz (Villchur, 1970). Nonetheless, 25-dB screening at 6,000 Hz is here judged to be mandatory in any situation where noise constitutes a hazard to hearing. Hearing loss is likely to first become evident above 4,000 Hz.

It should be noted that there is not unanimity among standards of serviceable hearing in adults. For example, the Department of Defense has concluded that responses at 30 dB (ANSI, 1969) at 500 and 25 dB at 1,000 and 2,000 Hz are required for admission to pilot training. The criteria are more lenient at higher frequencies. The arithmetic sum of thresholds at 3,000, 4,000, and 6,000 Hz for both ears cannot exceed 260 dB. The variability of adult criteria for passing is evident when it is noted that the American Academy of Opthalmology and Otolaryngology's method for estimation of hearing would attribute a 1% loss to an individual who just met the criteria for pilot training. For the purpose of detecting hearing loss before it becomes a detriment for communication, the American Speech and Hearing Association standards are judged to be the most reasonable.

The *Guidelines* recommends that screening be done on an individual rather than a group basis, primarily because of problems associated with the maintenance of calibration in audiometers with more than one pair of earphones and the sheer cumbersomeness of such group equipment. There is the additional problem of simultaneously maintaining the attention of the group, particularly with young children. Manual rather than automatic audiometry is recommended for two reasons. First, the increased complexity of responses to automatic audiometry may decrease its reliability in children. More obviously, automatic audiometry requires the person to respond at threshold rather than the dichotomous response implicit in the hearing or not hearing a particular tone at a particular level. Because of the difference in the task faced by the individual being screened, a practice effect amounting to no more than 5 dB has been noted for the first two tonal presentations by automatic audiometry (Thomas, Royster, and Scott, 1975).

Instructions must be tailored to the individuals screened and it should be emphasized that a response should occur even though the stimulus seems to be very soft. These instructions can be reinforced by presenting the initial tone at 50–60 dB followed by successively softer presentations in approximately 10-dB steps until the criterion level is reached. At this point, the succession of tones may be pre-

sented at the appropriate screening level. The typical automatic audiometer requires a person to press a button when he hears the tone
and release it when the tone becomes inaudible. This operation should
be made clear to the person screened, and the tracing monitored
initially to ensure instructions have been followed. The threshold response is taken to be the midpoint of the excursions during the course
of a single tonal presentation. In some cases, particularly during the
first several tones, the practice effect mentioned above can be seen in
the form of an ascending track. The last few excursions should then
be taken as threshold.

All individuals should be screened on entry into the institution
conducting screening. The frequency of rescreening is governed by
the hazards to the integrity of the sensorineural hearing mechanisms
generated by belonging to the institution or those inherent in the age
of the individual, such as noise exposure in high school students. In
the absence of intramural hazards, the frequency of rescreening reduces to the moral obligations assumed by the institution for the overall health of its members. This position is less stringent than the recommendation of the American Speech and Hearing Association with
respect to rescreening children. The Association suggests screening
each year during the period from nursery school through the third
grade. The rationale for such rescreening is undoubtedly based upon
the devastating effects of hearing loss during the first years of the
educational process. As it turns out, the technique involved in screening for conductive hearing loss (the major threat to hearing during
the first years of school) is readily adaptable to the detection of sensorineural loss. There is good reason to pair the two targets in screening
young children.

The above recommendations for screening are applicable to most
hearing conservation programs with the following notable exception.
Institutions subject to Department of Labor regulations are required
to take two additional steps not included above. The first is that
threshold measures by air conduction are required for the frequencies
500, 1,000, 2,000, 3,000, 4,000, and 6,000 Hz. These may be obtained
by either manual or automatic audiometry. Second, average retest
threshold responses at 2,000, 3,000, and 4,000 Hz must be compared
to initial results. The employee must be notified if that average is
poorer by 10 dB or more. No explicit pass or fail criteria are proposed.
It should be added that the regulations go beyond threshold testing
and include the range of topics from measurement of noise levels
through maintenance of records. At the time of this writing, the

department has not yet acted upon proposed revisions to the regulations (Federal Register, October 24, 1974, pp. 3773-3778). The reader involved in industrial hearing conservation should be certain to consult the most recent regulations.

Conductive Hearing Loss

It is clear that the only reasonable technique for the detection of conductive hearing loss is based upon electroacoustic impedance bridge measures. What is not clear are the criteria for passing. The following is based upon this writer's judgment of the evidence at this time. The reader is warned that the almost daily publication of new insights into both conductive hearing loss and impedance bridge technique is likely to modify what follows. Furthermore, because of the small amount of additional effort involved, the recommendations include the use of behavioral response to an audiometric presentation for the purpose of detecting sensorineural hearing loss in the absence of indications of a conductive loss.

Although the information display of different bridges varies, two dimensions are relevant to screening. These are middle ear pressure as inferred from the tympanogram and the presence or absence of an acoustic reflex resulting from stapedial contraction in the vast majority of cases. Ideally, the acoustic reflex should be elicited by ipsilateral stimulation to avoid complications in interpretation, which are possible in the use of contralateral stimulation. A reflex is most likely to occur in response to stimulation in the speech frequencies, suggesting that a 1,000-Hz tone be used for its elicitation.

Pressure variation during tympanometry should be no more positive than that required to ensure that an adequate seal has been obtained, generally no more than + 100 mm H_2O. Variation in the negative direction should not exceed − 200 mm H_2O. Criterion for middle ear pressure is the presence of a tympanometric peak at pressures no more negative than − 100 mm H_2O. Failure occurs when that tympanometric peak occurs at a pressure more negative than − 100 mm H_2O or when no peak is observed. Acoustic reflex thresholds are not obtained, rather, the presence or absence of a reflex is noted for a presentation of 110-dB, 1,000-Hz tone. Thus, two pieces of data that bear on the existence of conductive pathology are collected on each ear:

1. Tympanogram type in three categories following Jerger's (1970) nomenclature: type "A," where the peak occurs at pressures

more positive than -100 mm H_2O, type "C," where the tympano-metric peak occurs at pressures between -100 and -200 mm H_2O, and type "B," where no tympanometric peak is observed.

2.   Presence or absence of an acoustic reflex is recorded by a plus sign when present or a minus sign when absent.

The addition of an audiometric presentation of a 25-dB (ANSI, 1969) 4,000-Hz tone requiring a behavioral response can easily be integrated into the above procedure by including an earphone on the headset generally used to hold the bridge's probe. The earphone will already be a part of the bridge's components if contralateral stimulation is used to elicit an acoustic reflex. As reflected in Newby's concise review (Newby, 1964, pp. 218–220), reservations have been expressed about the efficiency of detecting hearing loss with so limited an audiometric exploration of an individual's hearing. The reservations, however, dealt with the fact that a single frequency check would fail to detect conductive impairments. The use of a single frequency for the detection of sensorineural loss was generally assumed to be adequate. The present recommendation for the employment of a single frequency audiometric presentation is made on the basis that, following initial passing of an audiometric screening, rescreening for sensorineural loss can be effectively accomplished by single frequency presentations to each ear. When so used, the third piece of screening datum is the presence (+) or absence (−) of a response. Passing is then A, (+), (+) for both ears.

The opportunity of those awaiting screening to observe the screening process is helpful in allaying any apprehensions that those individuals may have, particularly in the case of young children.

Instruction sufficient to indicate that the person to be screened will feel some pressure variations in his ear and hear both loud and soft sounds is sufficient and can be given at any time before screening. A point to be emphasized is that the individual should remain as physically quiet as possible so that body movement or vocalization will not interfere with the obtaining of a tympanogram or observation of the acoustic reflex. The instruction to respond to the 1,000-Hz tone can be readily handled just before its presentation because the individual has already been exposed to the presentation of sound. With young children, it may be necessary to begin with a 50-dB presentation and reduce it to 25 dB to ensure the child's cooperation and a reliable response. To avoid confusion, the probe tone of the impedance bridge must be turned off during this portion of the examination.

Although new to many individuals engaged in hearing screening, impedance bridge technique is not difficult to master. The major problems are the development of appropriate motor patterns and the accumulation of sufficient experience to judge quickly the correct size of probe tip. The typical sequence of events is to set up a table to hold both the impedance bridge and at least seven tip sizes in sufficient quantity to sustain a day's screening. A total of some 250 tips is not inappropriate. A sterile ear tip should be used for each ear to prevent any possibility of cross-infection. The proportions of sizes depend on the population screened. For younger children it is easiest for the person screening to be seated so that he is able to have his eyes at a level roughly approximating a standing child's ears. It will be more convenient to stand when examining adults. All known cases of middle ear disease, cases under medical management, or with pressure equalization tubes in place are excluded. The first step after the individual has approached the screening site is to visually inspect the mouth of the external auditory canal. Any indication of disease such as foul smell or discharge disqualifies the person for screening and, obviously, qualifies him for immediate referral to a physician. Similarly, any evidence of debris other than cerumen qualifies the person for referral. Whether or not the presence of cerumen excludes a person from screening must be decided on an individual basis by observing its amount and correlating this amount with the screener's previous experience. The problem with cerumen is that it clogs the probe and generates results that reflect its presence in the probe passages rather than the condition of the conductive mechanism. At this point the headset is mounted, an ear tip selected and put upon the probe, and the probe is inserted into the mouth of the external canal. External canal pressure is increased to $+100$ mm H_2O and briefly held to insure that a seal has been achieved. If no seal has been achieved, an alternative tip is selected and the ear canal repressurized. The air pressure in the external canal is then reduced while the person screening observes variations in compliance. The reversal of compliance values is taken as the indicator of the peak and air pressure at that point is noted. Air pressure in the external canal is maintained at approximately this pressure and the stimulus for elicitation of the acoustic reflex is presented. The presence or absence of the acoustic reflex is noted and the probe tone turned off. This is followed by the presentation of the 4,000-Hz tone and the presence or absence of a response is noted. The headset is reversed and the procedure repeated.

Processing of Failures

The initial decision that must be made upon an individual's failure in screening is whether to retest or refer the individual for a complete evaluation. The decision must be made upon several factors which include the reliability of behavioral responses, nature of the suspected disorder (which will dictate the urgency associated with the referral), and the demonstrated efficiency of the technique used to screen.

For whatever reason and by whichever technique, the referral of an individual from the screening stage of hearing conservation to the evaluation stage is made in the absence of any certainty of hearing loss and is made on the basis of probabilities that certain outcomes indicate hearing loss. For this reason the phrasing of the statement of failure is critical to the credibility of any screening program. The statement should reflect:

1. The probability that some hearing impairment is present. With proper monitoring of a particular program, numerical values may be assigned to that probability.
2. The program's conclusion that a definitive statement with regard to the presence or absence of a hearing loss is necessary for the individual's continued progress in school, for his continued health, etc.

The statement should be addressed to whoever is legally responsible for the individual screened.

Audiometric failures   There seems to be no overwhelming reason to rescreen audiometric failures except in those cases where responses are judged to be unreliable. The bulk of such cases will involve young children or those who, for whatever reason, seem not to be able to follow instructions. As indicated earlier, rescreening can improve the efficiency of audiometric technique with children. If reliable results cannot be obtained during the first rescreen, it is unlikely that continued struggles to obtain more reliable results will shed any light on possible auditory problems. Something is wrong and the skills of persons involved in audiologic evaluation are undoubtedly required to come to a reasonable conclusion about the nature of possible disorders.

It is not uncommon to encounter programs where the threshold measures are obtained following any failure. Such efforts are commendable, although this writer can uncover no rationale for the procedure. In a very practical way, no useful purpose is served by knowing that a given individual's thresholds are 25, 30, and 40 dB at 1,000, 2,000, and 4,000 Hz. Is discrimination of conversational speech affected? Are ototoxic drugs, progressive hereditary hearing loss, or any other of the several possible etiologies involved? It is difficult to believe that the typical person screening has either the experience or equipment to make an adequate judgment. It is this writer's conclusion that a failure deserves an evaluation.

If hearing conservation is conducted under Department of Labor jurisdiction, and if any test indicates an average threshold shift of 10 dB or more (2,000–4,000 Hz), retest within 1 month is required in the proposed regulations. If the shift persists, the employee must be notified.

Impedance bridge failures   Failure to obtain an "A" tympanogram, observe an acoustic reflex, or obtain a behavioral response to the audiometric presentation constitutes a failure. The current level of understanding of conductive disorders permits distinguishing between failures that require screening and those that warrant referral. The tympanogram type forms the basis for the distinction. Type "B" tympanograms warrant medical examination, if only to remove impacted wax, a task judged to be beyond the competency of the person likely to be screening or the individual screened. To confirm their validity, the probe tip should be examined for occlusion of the ports and the screen repeated immediately. Type "C" tympanograms may indicate either a temporary or resolving problem as well as being the forerunner of more serious disease. These cases should be retested in 6–8 weeks, a period over which the typical isolated case of middle ear disease revolves.

Any absence of an acoustic reflex warrants failure. No reflex is expected with "B" tympanograms and may or may not be present with "C" tympanograms, depending upon the severity of the involvement. "C" tympanograms with reflexes present support the assumption that the condition is transitory, particularly when middle ear pressure is more positive than -150 mm H_2O. The absence of a reflex in the presence of an "A" tympanogram suggests one of three things: an anatomical abnormality that may have no effect on day to day auditory function, reduced auditory sensitivity in the ear presented with the eliciting stimulus, or conductive pathology, although the height of the tympanometric peak is generally lower as well. In the absence of an acoustic reflex, audiometric screening is recommended. If the individual passes audiometric screening, no further action is necessary.

The absence of a behavioral response to a 4,000-Hz tone in an otherwise cooperative individual warrants referral. A summary of these recommendations is presented in Table 2.

PERSONNEL

A wide variety of different professions have been involved in hearing conservation. Speech pathologists, safety engineers, physicians, other health professionals, the new category of hearing conservation technicians, and volunteers have played a part in screening programs as well as the expected involvement of audiologists. In determining the propriety of any individual's involvement, a distinction must be made between overall program management and the act of screening itself.

Screening

Historically, screening has been conducted by audiologists, nurses, specifically trained technicians, and volunteers. Because screening itself is relatively simple, it is judged that any properly trained, employable individual should be able to conduct screening without difficulty. The basic issue is proficiency in the task rather than any professional or paraprofessional category of nomenclature. However, some consideration of the status of volunteers is appropriate. Such individuals are in a unique position in that conventional motivators of performance, such as continued employment and wages, do not function. In my experience, volunteer performance is sufficiently uneven to make regularly employed individuals preferable. Because proficiency is the basic issue, a brief review of some of the resources

Table 2. Recommended action for various tympanometric screen results

Outcome			Action
Tympanogram type	Reflex	4,000-Hz response	
A	+	+	Pass—no action
A	−	+	Fail—audiometric screen
A	+ or −	−	Fail—refer
C	+ or −	+ or −	Fail—rescreen in 6-8 weeks, refer if refail
B	+	+ or −	Malfunction—outcome is not logical
B	−	+ or −	Fail—refer

for training material is appropriate. At least three organizations have developed training outlines for audiometric screening:

1. United States Department of Health, Education and Welfare
   United States Office of Education
   Division of Manpower Development and Training
   (Audiometric Assistant Trainees Workbook)
2. American Association of Industrial Nurses
   79 Madison Avenue
   New York, New York 10016
3. Council for Accreditation in Occupational Hearing Conservation
   1619 Chestnut Avenue
   Haddon Heights, New Jersey 08035

Because the techniques and criteria for electroacoustic impedance bridge work screening remain in a state of flux, there are no widely used training outlines in this area. Because a behavioral response to a 4,000-Hz tone is included in the present recommendations for tympanometric screening, the information and experience necessary to adequately conduct audiometric screening need to be included in the training of anyone using an impedance bridge. In addition, the following topics should be included:

1. The anatomical basis for distinguishing between conductive and sensorineural hearing loss.
2. The energy transfer characteristics of the middle ear.
3. The physical basis for the operation of an impedance bridge.
4. The capabilities and limitations of such measurement techniques.
5. The mechanics of the techniques of screening.
6. The criteria for passing, failing, rescreening, and referral.

The student should also demonstrate his proficiency in an ongoing screening situation.

A set of problems beyond training arises in the case of the growing number of individuals specifically employed for screening. These include the complicated issue of opportunities for vertical mobility and development of consistent training programs that will provide an employee with horizontal mobility. The recent certification of screening personnel by the Council for Accreditation in Occupational Hearing Conservation has done much to increase the possibility of horizontal mobility. As the parameters for impedance bridge screening become clearer, uniform training programs in this area of screening should develop. It is not unreasonable to expect that the next 5 years will bring adequate horizontal mobility for all screening personnel. The opportunity for vertical mobility is contingent upon a clarification of the hierarchy among those involved in hearing conservation. At present no such clear hierarchy exists. The reader interested in such issues is referred to papers by Moll (1974) and, particularly, Yantis (1975).

Management

At least two disciplines have logical involvement in the management of hearing conservation programs. These are audiology and medicine. Ignoring the issue of professional preogative and examining the manager in terms of the skills he will require, it becomes evident that any manager must be able to define the likely hearing hazards and the screening target, select a screening environment and the technique for screening, supervise the ongoing screening process, and evaluate and monitor results. For these functions, individuals trained and experienced in psychoacoustics, auditory pathology and its consequences, and process evaluation are required. Audiologists are likely to be qualified in the first and second areas and can easily acquire competence in the third. It is judged that, at minimum, audiological consultation is necessary to the establishment of screening programs and their ongoing monitoring. With such input and with appropriate consultation with physicians, any intelligent and motivated individual can assume the responsibility for the screening portion of an overall hearing conservation program. In educational settings, and within the context of any hearing conservation program that includes rehabilitation, the need for the services of a person qualified in the education of the hearing impaired is obvious.

RECORDS

The specific format of record keeping is not critical. Because the material contained in such records is, this general overview of record keeping will focus on content. In certain circumstances, governmental regulations may dictate the exact format as well as additional content not mentioned below. Obviously, statutes should be consulted wherever applicable. Two minimum categories of information must be maintained. The first deals with a historical record of the performance and maintenance of equipment. The second deals with the individuals screened and the screening outcomes. Two additional categories of information will prove useful to any comprehensive screening program.

The first includes descriptors of program efficiency such as the cost of operation, proportion of failures in both sensorineural and conductive categories, and the results of the evaluation of such failures. The second optional category deals with the broadest meaning of hearing conservation program effectiveness. Such records would include estimates of the degree of rehabilitation or habilitation achieved as a result of detecting hearing loss.

Equipment

Monitoring and documentation of the state of equipment calibration are more important to screening than to clinical programs because of the stressful kind of use the equipment receives. This is particularly true if the equipment is moved from site to site. An individual historical log should be maintained on each piece of equipment from the day of purchase. The initial entry should show the results of a complete calibration and check-out of the equipment before it is placed in service. After this, two subsequent levels of entries regarding calibration and maintenance should be recorded. The first level is the annual calibration and preventive maintenance procedure that is the minimum necessary to an adequate program. In addition, a quarterly electroacoustic calibration check should be conducted for audiometers and audiometric functions of impedance bridges. Second, an informal user check-out should be conducted daily. Any discrepancies should be recorded and appropriate corrective action initiated. All costs associated with calibration and maintenance should be recorded.

When dealing with audiometric screening techniques, ambient noise levels at each screening site should be checked and recorded before used for screening, including monitoring of levels over periods of time typical of those during screening. Remeasurement should occur at any time when the acoustic environment is suspected or known to have changed.

Aside from being able to document the status of equipment, important by-products of such records are the evaluation of particular pieces of equipment and determination of costs of screening. Knowledge of the reliability and stability of various pieces of equipment gained from calibration records will permit more intelligent decisions regarding the replacement of equipment. Knowledge of overall costs will permit more precise estimates of cost factors and assist in comparing various screening techniques.

Individuals Screened

Records of an individual's performance on screening tasks should be maintained at at least four levels. These should include all individuals screened, all individuals who failed, all individuals who are eventually referred for evaluation, and those individuals whose hearing loss is confirmed by evaluation. Because the use of a single form for all four purposes can be confusing and create difficulties in access to specific records, it is suggested that four separate formats be used. A convenient way to handle this is by the use of a single document or card for each individual involved.

Every individual screened should have a document that permits chronologic entries in the event that screening occurs more than once. For each date the following information should be available: the name of the person screening, the instrument used, the results of each step of the screening process, and a conclusion as to whether or not the individual screened passed or failed. A last entry should indicate whether or not the person was referred for evaluation or for rescreening. The second category of records includes all those individuals who failed. If rescreening is a part of the program, the results of such rescreening should be recorded and, when appropriate, the date the decision to refer was made. The third category of records, all those who are referred, is a subset of the second category. This record should include the date a referral decision was made, the person or agency to whom referral was made, and the outcome of the evaluation. This file is of particular value because it represents those individuals who have left the realm of hearing conservation control. As mentioned at the beginning of the chapter, a major problem in the maintenance of a hearing conservation program is the cooperation of those individuals who may have a hearing loss. Follow-up on the recommendation for evaluation may simply not occur. Regular review of records of individuals referred for evaluation will quickly disclose whether or not the evaluation has occurred and will permit the screening organization to take whatever steps are appropriate to ensure that evaluation does occur. The last category of information is comprised of those individuals who were referred and have a hearing loss. It should include recommendations coming out of the evaluation and the specific steps actually taken in their implementation. As rehabilitative measures are completed, estimates of the effectiveness of such measures should be recorded. This file serves two different purposes: The first involves those who have a temporary or correctable hearing loss and who must be followed with subsequent screenings until the hearing loss is corrected. The second is to ensure that those with permanent hearing loss receive appropriate habilitation or rehabilitation. Although the actual process may occur outside of the control of the hearing conservation program, knowledge that it is occurring and knowledge of the results are important in gauging the overall program effectiveness.

Program Descriptors

In addition to those records described above, other information can be valuable in estimating the effectiveness and cost of a hearing conservation program as well as providing data needed for the more precise understanding of the magnitude of hearing problems. This can be done by statistical abstraction of some of the data from the first two sets of records. The resulting data can provide information regarding the prevalence of various categories of hearing loss, particularly if carefully correlated with the results of evaluation of those referred. Review of financial records associated with equipment and personnel can provide more precise estimates of the cost of hearing conservation. It should be remembered that personnel costs go beyond time spent in screening. They also include time for review of screening outcomes as well as time spent in following up those individuals who are referred. A comprehensive cost analysis would include office space, supplies, furniture and telephone costs, among other possible categories.

Rehabilitation Effectiveness

The goal of any hearing conservation program is the rehabilitation of those with hearing losses. Of prime importance in school settings is the increased academic progress achieved by rehabilitation. To implement an adequate data bank for such investigations requires at least two major categories of information. The first is some estimate of the academic potential of the individual with hearing loss. The second is a periodic estimate of the academic achievement of the same individual. Because of the vagaries associated with estimates of "intelligence quotients" and the variety of parameters that may be used to gauge actual level of function, the phrases "academic potential" and "academic achievement" are used in a common sense way. The details of measurement must be left to qualified psychologic and educational consultants. Although almost impossible to achieve in any precise way, estimates of the degree of rehabilitation and its cost are critical to the long term justification of hearing conservation.

SUMMARY

Screening for hearing loss is different from evaluating known or possible hearing impairments. First, the person being screened is unlikely to be concerned about any hearing loss. He comes to the screening with a different set of attitudes than a person presenting himself for evaluation. More importantly, screening can never be taken as unequivocal evidence of hearing loss. Rather, screening techniques permit no more than a probabilistic statement regarding the likelihood that some hearing impairment exists. Confirmation of the existence of a hearing loss is the task of evaluative procedures that should follow any failure in screening. Errors will be made with all screening techniques. The major problem in the selection of a hearing screening technique is to achieve a balance between errors and cost of screening. An outline of an economic rationale for evaluating screening costs and for comparing screening techniques was developed.

A historical review of screening techniques was based upon two categories of hearing loss, conductive and sensorineural. Audiometric screening can only be considered adequate for the detection of sensorineural hearing loss. Responses at 20 dB (ANSI, 1969), to 1,000- and 2,000-Hz tones and at 25 dB to 4,000- and 6,000-Hz tones are recommended as criteria for passing. If conductive hearing losses are a screening target, electroacoustic impedance bridge techniques are necessary for their detection. Because the application of bridge techniques to screening is relatively new, and because of the relatively poor understanding of the course of conductive impairments, criteria for passing are in a state of flux. Nonetheless, such criteria are recommended and include the presence of an acoustic reflex and middle ear pressure no more negative than -100 mm H_2O. Continual refinement of pass/fail criteria can be expected and the reader has the obligation to review reports that undoubtedly will be published subsequent to this text. In most cases it is convenient to include the audiometric presentation of a 25 dB (ANSI, 1969), 4,000-Hz tone as part of screening for conductive loss. This was recommended as a continued monitoring of sensorineural function where conductive and sensorineural losses may be present, and after a given individual has passed an audiometric screening.

The personnel that should be involved in screening programs was discussed as well as recommendations for record keeping, both for the equipment and the individuals screened. Within the context of a comprehensive hearing conservation program, the need for collecting information regarding postfailure evaluation and rehabilitation was emphasized. Although difficult to come by, such information is necessary to the further understanding of the effectiveness of various screening techniques and, more broadly, the effects of rehabilitation of those individuals found to have hearing losses. The literature is scant in these areas and it is hoped that the suggestions will provide data for further research into the problems of selecting screening technique, criteria for referral, and the effectiveness of rehabilitation.

REFERENCES

Alberti, P. W., and Kristensen, R. 1972. The compliance of the middle ear. In: D. Rose and L. W. Keating (eds.), Impedance Symposium, pp. 159–167. Mayo Clinic-Mayo Foundation, Rochester, Minnesota.

American Speech and Hearing Association. 1975. Guidelines for identification audiometry. Asha 17:94–99.

Berry, Q. C., Bluestone, C. D., and Cantekin, E. I. 1975. Otologic history, audiometry and tympanometry as a case finding procedure for school screening. Laryngoscope 85:1976–1985.

Brooks, D. N. 1968. An objective method of detecting fluid in the middle ear. J. Int. Audiol. 7:280–286.

Brooks, D. N. 1973. Hearing screening: A comparative study of an impedance method and pure tone screening. Scand. Audiol. 2:67–72.

Brooks, D. N. 1976. School screening for middle ear effusions. Ann. Otol. Rhinol. Laryngol. 25(Suppl. 85): 223–228.

Cooper, J. C., Jr., Gates, G. A., Owen, J. H., and Dickson, H. D. 1975. An abbreviated impedance bridge technique for school screening. J. Speech Hear. Dis. 40:260–269.

Cooper, J. C., Jr., Langley, L. R., Meyerhoff, W. L., and Gates, G. A. 1977. The significance of negative middle ear pressure. Laryngoscope 87:92–97.

Cooper, J. C., Jr., and Owen, J. H. 1976. Audiological profile of noise induced hearing loss. Arch. Otolaryngol. 102:148–150.

Darley, F. L. (ed.). 1961. Identification audiometry. J. Speech Hear. Dis. Monogr. Suppl. 9.

Eagles, E. L., Wishik, S. M., Doerfler, L. G., Melnick, W., and Levine, H.S. 1963. Hearing Sensitivity and Related Factors in Children. Laryngoscope, St. Louis, Missouri.

Forcucci, R. A., and Stark, E. W. 1972. Hearing loss, speech-language and cystic fibrosis. Arch. Otolaryngol. 96:361–364.

Geyer, M. L., and Yankauer, A. 1956. Teacher judgment of hearing loss in children. J. Speech Hear. Dis. 21:482–486.

Glasscock, M. E., III. 1972. Complications of otitis media. In: A. Glorig and K. S. Gerwin (eds.), Otitis Media, pp. 221-227. Charles C Thomas, Springfield, Illinois.

Glorig, A., and Gerwin, K. S., (eds.). 1972. Otitis Media. Charles C Thomas, Springfield, Illinois.

Goldman, R., and Sanders, J. W. 1969. Cultural factors and hearing. Except. Child. 35:486-489.

Gosztonyi, R. E., Vassalo, L. A., and Sataloff, J. 1971. Audiometric reliability in industry. Arch. Environ. Health 22:113-118.

Griffing, T. S., Simonton, K. M., and Hedgecock, L. D. 1967. Verbal auditory screening for preschool children. Trans. Am. Acad. Ophthalmol. Otolaryngol. 71:105-111.

Gunderson, T., and Tonning, F. 1976. Ventilating tubes in the middle ear. Arch. Otolaryngol. 102:198-199.

Hatfield, E. M. 1967. Progress in preschool vision screening. Sight Sav. Rev. 37:194-201.

Herer, G. 1976. Use of impedance in pediatrics and screening (workshop B). Third International Symposium on Impedance Audiometry, October 1, New York.

Holm, V. A., and Kunze, L. H. 1969. Effect of chronic otitis media on language and speech development. Pediatrics 43:833-839.

House, H. P., and Glorig, A. 1957. A new concept of auditory screening. Laryngoscope 67:661-668.

Hull, F. M., and Mielke, P. W., Jr. 1971. The national speech and hearing survey: Preliminary results. Asha 13:501-509.

Jerger, J. 1970. Clinical experience with impedance audiometry. Arch. Otolaryngol. 92:311-324.

Jerger, J., Burney, P., Mauldin, L, and Crump, B. 1974. Predicting hearing loss from the acoustic reflex. J. Speech Hear. Dis. 39:11-22.

Jerger, J., Jerger, S., and Mauldin, L. 1972. Studies in impedance audiometry: I. Normal and sensorineural ears. Arch. Otolaryngol. 96:513-523.

Jerger, S., Jerger, J., Mauldin, L., and Segal, P. 1974. Studies in impedance audiometry: II. Children less than 6 years old. Arch. Otolaryngol. 99:1-9.

Lewis, N., Dugdale, A., Canty, A., and Jerger, J. 1975. Open ended tympanometric screening: A new concept. Arch. Otolaryngol. 101:722-725.

Ling, D. 1972. Rehabilitation of cases with deafness secondary to otitis media. In: A. Glorig and K. S. Gerwin (eds.), Otitis Media, pp. 249-253. Charles C Thomas, Springfield, Illinois.

Lowe, J. F., Bamforth, J. S., and Pracy, R. 1963. Acute otitis media: One year in general practice. Lancet 2:1129-1132.

McCandless, G. A., and Thomas, G. K. 1974. Impedance audiometry as a screening procedure for middle ear disease. Trans. Am. Acad. Ophthalmol. Otolaryngol. 78:ORL98-102.

McEldowney, D., and Kessner, D. M. 1972. Review of the literature: Epidemiology of otitis media. In: A. Glorig and K. S. Gerwin (eds.), Otitis Media, pp. 11-30. Charles C Thomas, Springfield, Illinois.

Melnick, W., Eagles, E. L., and Levine, H. S. 1964. Evaluation of a recommended program of identification audiometry with school-age children. J. Speech Hear. Dis. 29:3-13.

Mencher, G. T., and McCullough, B. F. 1970. Auditory screening of kindergarten children using the VASC. J. Speech Hear. Dis. 35:241–247.

Moll, K. L. 1974. Issues facing us, supportive personnel. Asha 16:357–358.

Newby, H. A. 1964. Audiology. Appleton-Century-Crofts, New York. 1969.

National Advisory Neurological Diseases and Stroke Council. Human Communication and Its Disorders. 1969. National Institutes of Health, Bethesda, Maryland.

Northern, J. L., and Downs, M. 1974. Hearing in Children. The Williams & Wilkins Company, Baltimore.

Paradise, J. L., Smith, C. G., and Bluestone, C. D. 1976. Tympanometric detection of middle ear effusion in infants and young children. Pediatrics 58:198–210.

Roeser, R. J., Soh, J., Dunckel, D. C., and Adams, R. 1977. Comparison of tympanometry and otoscopy in establishing pass/fail referral criteria. J. Am. Audiol. Soc. 3:20–25.

Roeser, R. J., Seidel, J., and Glorig, A. 1975. Performance evaluation of two noise-excluding earphone enclosures for threshold audiometry. Sound Vibration 10:22–25.

Steer, M. D., Hanley, T. D., Spuehler, H. E., Barnes, N. S., Burk, K. W., and Williams, W. G. 1961. The behavioral and educational implications of hearing loss among elementary children. Purdue Research Foundation and U.S. Department of Health, Education and Welfare. Cooperative Research Project No. 492. Lafayette, Indiana.

Thomas, W. G., Preslar, M. J., Summers, R., and Stewart, J. L. 1969. Calibration and working condition of 100 audiometers. Public Health Rep. 84:311–327.

Thomas, W. G., Royster, L. H., and Scott III, C. E. 1975. Practice effects in industrial hearing screenings. J. Am. Audiol. Soc. 1:126–130.

Villchur, E. 1970. Audiometer-earphone mounting to improve intersubjective and cushion-fit reliability. J. Acoust. Soc. Am. 48:1387–1396.

Vanderbilt University Hereditary Deafness Study Group. 1968. Dominantly inherited low-frequency hearing loss. Arch. Otolaryngol. 88:40–48.

Wilbur, L. A. 1972. Calibration: Pure tone, speech and noise signals. In: J. Katz (ed.), Handbook of Clinical Audiology, pp. 11–35. The Williams & Wilkins, Baltimore.

Wilson, W. R., and Woods, L. A. 1975. Accuracy of the Bing and Rinne tuning fork tests. Arch. Otolaryngol. 101:81–85.

Yantis, P. A. 1975. Audiology, the association and occupational hearing conservation. Asha 17:835–836.

LANGUAGE

Introduction

Donald M. Morehead

The appearance of transformational linguistics in the late 1950s produced the most far reaching impact—save possibly that of Piaget—on behavioral and applied sciences since Darwin and Freud. Not only did this linguistic revolution revise our thinking about the nature of language and language acquisition but it also has resulted in one of the most productive periods of research in language and language behaviors (see Abrahamsen, 1977, for a complete listing of references). One of the benefits of this productivity has been a wealth of information for those interested in the study and habilitation of both children and adults with linguistic deficiencies. For example, during the last few years there have appeared a number of excellent full length sources on language deficiency in children (Schiefelbusch and Lloyd, 1974; Lenneberg and Lenneberg, 1975; Morehead and Morehead, 1976; Crystal, Fletcher, and Garman, 1976; Ingram, 1976; Bloom and Lahey, 1977; Lahey, 1977) and in adults (Goodglass and Blumstein, 1973; Prucha, 1976; Whitaker and Whitaker, 1976). Because of the complexities of fully developed human language—including its disturbances—many more studies have appeared on children than on adults.

Even though there is a large amount of information now available on linguistic behaviors, we are still confronted with the central problem of the precise ways in which this information is useful in the understanding and treatment of language dysfunctions. As a case in point, Brown (1973) proposes a law of cumulative complexity, which states that the number of relations in a sentence—rather than the number of words—is a good measure of how complex the sentence is. This proposal suggests that a relational measure may be more useful than mean-length-of-utterance in terms of words to establish linguistic level, but the ways in which relations—as opposed to words or sentences—can be taught are not at all obvious. A second and related problem is the effect that new information has on applied disciplines.

The demands of theory construction and revision are often very different from the demands of assessment and habilitation. To assess linguistic dysfunctions and to develop viable training programs, the clinician needs a broad informational base that includes fields as diverse as neurology and family counseling. The clinician, then, becomes a generalist who must keep abreast of many disciplines at one time; when one of these areas explodes with new information, he may restrict the informational base, taking a single approach such as behaviorism or linguistics. The work of de Ajuriaguerra et al. (1976) on dysphasic children is an excellent example of the benefits of considering the whole child even when the disability seems to be primarily linguistic.

The chapters in this section also provide excellent examples of taking the broader view of linguistic deficiencies in children and adults. The chapters on bilingual children by Burt, Dulay, and Hernández-Chávez give important cultural information necessary to determine first language from second language deficiencies. The chapter by Lynch puts linguistic disorders in the general context of learning disabilities in children, demonstrating that the early language-deficient child becomes the dyslexic in the primary school years. Finally, the chapter on adult aphasia by Halpern provides the necessary distinctions between intellectual versus linguistic impairment and separates these impairments from those involving motoric difficulties such as dysarthria and apraxia.

REFERENCES

Abrahamsen, A. A. 1977. Child Language: An Interdisciplinary Guide to Theory and Research. University Park Press, Baltimore.

de Ajuriaguerra, J., Jaeggi, A., Guignard, F., Kocher, F., Maquard, M., Roth, S., and Schmid, E. 1976. The development and prognosis of dysphasia in children. In: D. M. Morehead and A. E. Morehead (eds.), Normal and deficient child language. University Park Press, Baltimore.

Bloom, L., and Lahey, M. 1977. Language development and language disorders. John Wiley & Sons Inc., New York.

Brown, R. 1973. A first language. Harvard University Press, Cambridge.

Crystal, D., Fletcher, P., and Garman, M. 1976. The grammatical analysis of language disability. North-Holland, Amsterdam.

Goodglass, H., and Blumstein, S. 1973. Psycholinguistics and aphasia. The Johns Hopkins University Press, Baltimore.

Ingram, D. 1976. Phonological disability in children. North-Holland, Amsterdam.

Lahey, M. (ed.). 1977. Readings in language disorders. John Wiley & Sons Inc., New York.

Lenneberg, E. H., and Lenneberg, E. (eds.). 1975. Foundations of language development, Vol. II. Academic Press, New York.

Morehead, D. M., and Morehead, A. E. (eds.). 1976. Normal and Deficient child language. University Park Press, Baltimore.

Prucha, J. (ed.). 1976. Soviet studies in language and language behavior. North-Holland, Amsterdam.

Schiefelbusch, R., and Lloyd, L. (eds.). 1974. Language perspectives: Acquisition, retardation, and intervention. University Park Press, Baltimore.

Whitaker, H., and Whitaker, H. 1976. Studies in neurolinguistics, 2 volumes. Academic Press, New York.

The Process of Becoming Bilingual

Heidi C. Dulay, Eduardo Hernández-Chávez,
and Marina K. Burt

CONTENTS

One of the more difficult challenges in diagnostics is the evaluation of the bilingual child. Most examiners lack practical as well as theoretical knowledge of the process of second language learning and consequently feel unsure of what constitutes normal development for the bilingual child. Because of the significance of understanding normal language development in such children and the paucity of available information, the section on evaluation of bilingual children has been expanded to two chapters with the first chapter focusing entirely on the steps that constitute normal acquisition of a second language and the following chapter presenting procedures for evaluating the child who has been exposed to two languages.

In this chapter Professors Dulay, Hernández-Chávez, and Burt discuss the need for specification of what constitutes normal development for a child acquiring a second language. They present a clear and thorough treatise for the determination of the factors of second language acquisition. Absence of this information has led to some tragic problems. This chapter not only describes the existing problems and related questions but also presents valuable evidence that will begin to answer these questions. There is pertinent insight into the sequence of second language acquisition, first language maintenance and loss, and the use of two languages in bilingual speech. The language clinician will be very interested in the information brought forth in this chapter involving systematic errors that are evident in the child's construction of rules. The discussions and models set up by Professors Dulay, Hernández-Chávez, and Burt on the similarities and differences of their research on second language acquisition with the present research on first language acquisition are invaluable for a language clinician. The speech pathologist will certainly benefit from their discussion of simultaneous acquisition of two phonologies. This chapter is a much needed step in organizing the existing research on L2 phonological, syntactic, and semantic acquisition. Dissemination of this knowledge may help prevent the dual tragedies of labeling normal children who happen to speak two languages as "abnormal," while neglecting to refer for remediation those bilingual children who have a true linguistic disorder.

—Eds.

In the United States the school age population living in homes where first languages other than English are spoken exceeds 7.6 million and continues to grow dramatically every year (National Center for Education Statistics, 1975). Many of these students, who are still in the process of learning English, have begun to appear in increasing numbers in the caseloads of language, speech, and hearing specialists throughout the country. Such students are often referred to the school speech clinician because they do not yet demonstrate the fluency or proficiency in English or the verbal initiative demonstrated by their agemates who learned English as natives.

Take an example of a child who has been in the United States about 2 years, who uses some English phrases while playing, but in class rarely offers verbal responses, or at best uses one-word or short, ungrammatical sentences. Such a child is very likely to be referred by a classroom teacher to the speech therapist, especially if the classroom teacher is not a bilingual education specialist, or if a teacher of English as a Second Language (ESL) is not available. If the therapist tests the child in English, that child is likely to exhibit characteristics typical of aphasic or oral language handicapped monolingual children.

According to the California Administrative Code, for example, criteria to determine aphasia or severe oral language handicaps include the following: "when a spontaneous language sample of at least 50–100 utterances can be obtained, [the child] shows development judged clearly inadequate for the minor's age in at least two of the following areas of language development: syntactic, semantic, morphologic, phonologic" (California Administrative Code (Section 3600 (g) of Title 5)). Yet it is normal for a child from a language background other than English who is still in the process of acquiring English to exhibit exactly those characteristics in English. Moreover, if children notice that their native language is denigrated by schoolmates or teachers, or that English is clearly the prestige language in school, they often become reluctant to use their native language, even if they speak it freely and fluently at home.

This is but one example among many that illustrate the potentially misleading superficial similarities between the verbal performance of children who are becoming bilingual—who are still learning English as a second language—and that of monolingual English speakers who truly suffer a communicative disorder. The temporary inability to speak English proficiently, or perhaps a reluctance to speak at all, may cause normal children who are in the process of acquiring English to be mistakenly classified as aphasic or as having some other severe language disorder.

Paradoxically, however, in the attempts to avoid just these problems of misclassifying children of non-English language backgrounds, another problem may occur: all the children may be considered normal second language learners and consequently, real communicative disorders may go unnoticed and untreated.

As educational psychologists and speech pathologists know, a certain percentage of any given population of children is likely to fall outside of the category of linguistically normal children. It is estimated that about 9% (or more than 3,000,000) of the children in the United States suffer from communicative disorders of various types (National Institute of Neurological Diseases and Stroke, 1967). A substantially smaller or larger percentage for a particular group of children would lead us to inspect very closely either the factors that might contribute to such a deviation, or else the criteria used for classification.

In groups of bilingual children, we should expect to find that the proportion of children who genuinely suffer some communicative disorder is substantially the same as that found in monolingual groups. Often, however, we find instead that the majority of children in a speech clinician's caseload are bilinguals, although bilingual children are a minority in a school's overall population. Because bilingual children are no more likely to suffer from linguistic abnormalities than are monolingual children,[1] such situations present genuine difficulties; the speech specialist must find ways of distinguishing normally developing bilinguals from those developing abnormally.

As is the case for English monolinguals, the determination of ab-

---

[1] In fact, Feldman and Shen (1971) demonstrate that bilingual Head Start children consistently exhibit functioning in the use and linguistic manipulation of new words that is superior to their monolingual counterparts. See Dulay, Burt and Zappert (1976) for a summary of research findings on effects of bilingualism and bilingual education on student performance.

normality in a bilingual's language functioning entails a specification of what is "normal." Specifically, it entails what is normal for second language (L2) development at a given age and with a given type of exposure to the second language; what is normal for first language (L1) development given the onset of and the sociolinguistic circumstances surrounding second language acquisition; and finally, what the normal interaction is between a bilingual's two languages in everyday conversation. As important as such questions are to education in the United States, it is only in the last decade that we have seen research literature concerning systematic efforts to deal with these topics. Although much has been written about how to teach children English as a second language or how to use the child's dominant language as a medium of instruction in school, the independent socio- and psycholinguistic processes relevant to becoming and being bilingual have only recently begun to receive serious attention. These are the focus of this chapter. Three major processes involved in normal bilingualism are discussed: 1) second language acquisition, 2) first language maintenance and loss, and 3) the use of two languages in the speech of bilinguals.

SECOND LANGUAGE ACQUISITION

Second language acquisition refers to the process of learning a new language by children or adults who have already acquired a substantial amount of a first language. A distinction is usually made between "host" and "foreign" language acquisition. In the former the language being acquired is one that is spoken in the region or country in which it is being learned; for example, English would be acquired as a "host" language by a Mexican child living in the United States, whereas it would be acquired as a "foreign" language if the child were living in Mexico. This distinction becomes important, for example, when one realizes how much more easily English is learned in an English-speaking country than in a classroom in a non-English speaking country.

Another distinction must be made between the simultaneous acquisition of two languages and their sequential acquisition—what we have elsewhere called, respectively, bilingual acquisition and second language acquisition. In the former, the child receives input from two languages from infancy so that both are being learned together and their development is essentially parallel. In the latter, one of the languages is relatively well established before the child is exposed to a second language. As the title of the section indicates, we will focus primarily on sequential second language acquisition.

One of the primary processes responsible for a child's acquisition of a second language is the "creative construction" of the new language by the child. Creative construction refers to the process by which learners gradually reconstruct rules for speech they hear, guided by innate mechanisms that cause them to formulate certain types of hypotheses about the language system being acquired. The process continues until the learner's rule system is consistent with that of native speakers in the child's environment. The child's construction of linguistic rules is said to be creative because no native speaker of the target language—whether peer, parent, or teacher—uses many sentences of the kind produced regularly by children who are still learning the basic structures of the language. For example, utterances such as *No wipe finger* (Klima and Bellugi, 1966), *Where daddy go?* (Brown, 1973), *He say father buy him car* (Dulay and Burt, 1974a), or *I no scare ghost* (Hernández-Chávez, 1972) are not typically produced by proficient native speakers of English, although they are typical of both first and second language learners.

Such observed "deviations" from well formed sentences are not haphazard lapses of memory or poor attempts at imitation. Rather, the occurrence of systematic errors comprises "...the best evidence we have that the child possesses construction rules" (Brown, 1973). Positing a creative construction process to account for language acquisition is, therefore, to recognize the independent contribution made by the learner to the language acquisition process. Creative construction does not view the acquisition process as one of filling up the child's (presumably empty) head with sentence patterns, vocabulary, etc., but one in which the child's mental mechanisms may be said to interact with the available linguistic environment. Creative construction assumes, therefore, a certain degree of learner independence from external input factors such as the exact form of utterances modeled, their frequency of occurrence, or rewards for correctness. Experienced speech therapists and ESL specialists who have worked with second language learners know only too well, for example, that error correction is often useless and that learners sometimes produce utterances and structures that have not been taught in class yet.

This is not to imply that language learning can take place independently of the available linguistic environment. Rather, that the acquisition process is guided in important respects by certain developmental forces that regulate input in a manner that is consistent with the learner's own developmental level of English proficiency. When the learner is developmentally ready, then certain learning environments and training procedures will have maximum benefits for language learners.

Given the myriad conscious and unconscious internal factors interacting with input to produce learner speech, it may not be possible to isolate these entirely. Nonetheless, given the data presently available, it seems we may attribute certain discrepancies between input and learner output to at least five very general but distinct sources: a socio-affective filter, a cognitive organizer, a monitor, personality, and past experience (the first language).

The socio-affective filter refers to conscious or unconscious motives or needs, attitudes or emotional states of the learner. As the term suggests, these filter the input and affect the rate and quality of language acquisition. Among other things, the socio-affective filter contributes to: 1) individual preferences for certain input models over others, 2) prioritizing aspects of language to be learned, and 3) determining when language acquisition efforts should cease. For example, depending on various criteria, a learner will "tune in" more to certain speakers of the language than others.

Preference for certain models is clearly demonstrated by learners acquiring one of two dialects to which they are exposed in daily communication. Milon (1975) reports that a 7-year-old Japanese-speaking child who had immigrated to Hawaii learned the Hawaiian Creole English of his agemates rather than the Standard English of his teachers during his 1st school year. When he moved to a middle class neighborhood the following year, however, he quickly picked up Standard English, which his new friends spoke. In explaining this phenomenon, Milon states that "there is no question that the first dialect of English these young immigrant children learn is the dialect of their peers, and that they learn it from their peers. If they learn productive control of the dialect of their teachers it is not until later..." (Milon, 1975, p. 159). [2] Similarly, Benton (1964) reports that Maori children learn the English dialect of their own group rather than standard New

---

[2]It is interesting to note that one cannot explain the early acquisition of Hawaiian Creole here by appealing to the idea that its syntactic structures are somehow a "simplification" of Standard English. Compare several Hawaiian Creole structures produced by Milon's subject to their Standard English equivalents: HCE: "Over here got one." SE: "There's one over here." HCE: "How come no more any of those?" SE: "Why are those all gone?" The differences in the forms of the corresponding utterances cannot be described by any notion of "simplicity" advanced to date in the L2 literature.

One teacher reported that a Maori child had told her: "Maoris say *Who's your name,* so that's what I say." Maori English is often an important sign of group membership and a source of security for these children. (Benton, 1964:93 in Richards, 1974:169)

Zealand English. In some cases this model preference is consciously articulated:

In addition to learning from certain models rather than from others, learners acquire certain types of verbal routines or vocabulary items rather than others, and some stop acquiring the target language at a point before they reach native-like proficiency. All these types of behaviors may be attributed to affective factors interacting with external sociolinguistic factors. These delimit to a significant extent the input data that are made available to the cognitive organizers.

The importance of taking into account the possible effects of socio-affective filter of input on child verbal performance cannot be overemphasized. When child speech is not entirely consonant with that of the speakers to whom the child is being compared (say the teacher or certain other children in the community), one may not simply assume that the discrepancy is the result of delayed or incorrect learning; it is entirely possible that because of certain sociolinguistic circumstances, the child prefers to acquire forms other than those used as the norm. This very important distinction between *cannot* learn and *prefers not* to learn must be made before it is justifiable to conclude that the child's speech is the result of learning disabilities.

The cognitive organizer refers to the internal data-processing mechanisms responsible for the construction of the grammar we attribute to the learner. It is what Chomsky has referred to as the "Language Acquisition Device," and what others have called the "black box." It contributes, among other things, to: 1) the error types that occur systematically in developing speech, 2) the progression of rules that learners use before a structure is mastered, and 3) the order in which structures are acquired.

Slobin (1971), for instance, provides a classic example of the development of the past tense morpheme in English: the past tense of *break* and *drop* are first expressed as *broke* and *drop*; then when the child acquires the *-ed* rule for past tense formation, the forms *breaked* and *dropped* are used. As the child learns that the long form of the past tense ending *-ed* is used with words ending in *t* or *d*, the two words are further regularized to *breakted* and *dropted*, and only in the final stage are the correct forms sorted out. These examples, as well as others discussed later, make it obvious that children do not learn their language by successive approximations to the adult norm through a process of more and more correct imitations. Rather, they actively and creatively build up the rules of the emerging grammar, constructing hypotheses about the form that it should take. This is discussed in a later section.

A third source of creative activity is the "monitor" (Krashen, 1977; in press), which may be defined as the conscious editing of one's own speech. The degree to which speech is edited depends upon individual criteria as well as the nature and focus of the task being performed. Concern over grammatical correctness is an individual criterion operating in many individuals. This concern often results in a great deal of editing, as seen in numerous hesitations or constant self-correction. On the other hand, tasks that cause speakers to focus on communication tend to bring on less self-editing, whereas tasks whose focus is linguistic analysis (such as fill-in-the-blank or translation) seem to invite more editing.

It seems useful to think of internal processing of language input as the successive operation of the socio-affective filter, the cognitive organizer, and the monitor, in that order, with personality factors and first language experience influencing the operation of all three. For example, persons with outgoing, uninhibited personalities have been observed to monitor their speech infrequently, while self-conscious, introverted persons are more likely to overmonitor their speech (Krashen, in press).[3] Similarly, the past experience of having learned one's first language is integrated into some of the organizing strategies used by a learner to acquire a second language. This is evident, for example, in certain aspects of the acquisition of phonology and the use of code alternation as a second language learning device. (See "L2 Phonology" and "Code alternation," below).

Although our current knowledge of the L2 acquisition process is far from detailed or complete, it is sufficient to begin to sketch the general outlines suggested by available research. The operation of internal factors in the language acquisition process just discussed is illustrated in Figure 1. As indicated in the figure, learners delimit the linguistic input to which they are exposed, and organize the input they "tune in" to into a system of rules that gradually evolves as the learner continues to be exposed to natural speech in the target language. From their developing rule systems, learners generate the

---

[3]For further discussion of personality factors in second language acquisition, see Carroll (1977) and Naiman, Frolich, and Stern (1975).

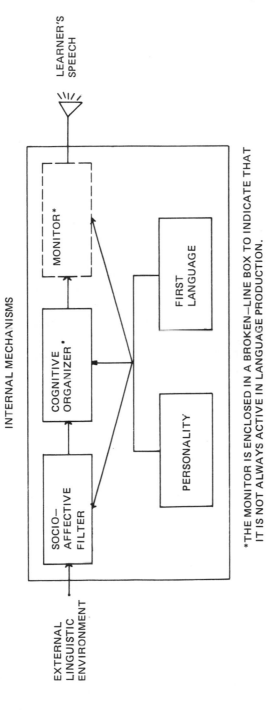

INTERNAL MECHANISMS

*THE MONITOR IS ENCLOSED IN A BROKEN—LINE BOX TO INDICATE THAT
IT IS NOT ALWAYS ACTIVE IN LANGUAGE PRODUCTION.

Figure 1.   Working model for some aspects of creative construction in language acquisition.

utterances that we study, diagnose, and hope will soon give way to the grammatical sentences of proficient speakers.

In the sections below we present the major observations that researchers have accumulated to date on the characteristics of developing L2 utterances. As most of the work has focused on syntax and morphology, these receive the most comprehensive attention here. In addition, some recent provocative work on the acquisition of a second phonology and semantic system is presented.

L2 Syntax and Morphology

Three aspects of L2 syntax and morphology are especially revealing of the L2 acquisition process: a) error types, b) steps in the acquisition of particular structures, and c) acquisition sequences. Each is discussed below.

Error types   The study of errors in L2 research has been one of the most productive types of analyses undertaken. Perhaps the major significance of the study of children's L2 errors to date has been the discovery of a striking similarity between the errors made by children learning a second language and those made by first language learners. The observed similarities provided the first inklings that a process of creative construction, which had been posited to explain much L1 speech behavior, also accounts for major aspects of L2 acquisition.

In the earlier stages of first language development, children produce primarily content words (nouns, verbs, and adjectives), and omit functors (also called grammatical morphemes) (articles, prepositions, and morphological elements) as adults do when they compose telegrams: *He throw marble* (child) or *Send money urgent* (adult). The systematic omission of functors in early "telegraphic" utterances is also a characteristic of L2 learners' speech.

Over-regularization—or "overgeneralization," as it is often referred to—is another error type that occurs in both L1 and L2 speech. For example, forms such as *mans* and *feets* (the over-regularization of the English plural -*s*) are typical occurrences in L1 and L2 speech protocols.

The similarities observed in L1 and L2 error types do not imply, however, that all rules and resulting utterances are identical for first and second language learners. The second language learner at, for example, age 4 or 5 is older and as a consequence is cognitively more mature than an infant beginning to learn to talk. The L2 learner's knowledge of the world and level of conceptual organization is already quite advanced; there are qualitative differences in the child's approach to all sorts of learning; and there is, of course, the experience of having learned a language once before. Moreover, the L2 learner's acousticoarticulatory system is relatively highly developed, which, as we shall see later, has important consequences for L2 phonological development. We should therefore expect the use of some developing constructions that are more varied and, in some ways, more sophisticated than those used by L1 learners. For example, the overuse or misuse of some functors during intermediate stages of L2 acquisition is not typical of L1 acquisition. Utterances such as *He nots eats* or *She's dancings* found in L2 speech protocols (Dulay and Burt, 1975a) have not been reported for L1 learners.

Therefore, as we shall also see for acquisition orders, although the general creative characteristics are the same for L2 and L1 utterances, specific details differ, attesting to the differences in cognitive sophistication, affective focus, acousticoarticulatory ability, and experience.

Most of the errors children make while acquiring a second language are creative. They are the necessary result of the child's gradual organization of the linguistic input received. The majority of creative errors in L2 acquisition may be grouped into six types: over-regularizations, omissions, use of archi-forms, the alternating use of the members of a class, double markings, and misorderings. These are described in detail below.

Over-regularization   The overextension of a rule to items where it does not apply is a common phenomenon in the learning of both first and second languages. Whenever there are both regular and irregular forms and constructions in the language, the rules used to produce those that are regular may be overextended to those that are irregular, resulting in error types such as those presented in Table 1.

Table 1. Errors of over-regularization in child L2 production

Construction	Regular rule	Example of error
Simple past tense	Addition of *-ed* to verb stem, e.g., walk*ed*	She *eated/ated*. It *breakted*.
Present indicative tense	θ ending on verb (only 3rd person requires *-s* ending) e.g., I/you/ we/they see it.	She *see* herself in the water. He *eat* too much.
Noun plural	Addition of *-s* or *-es* to the singular form e.g., girl*s*	tooths, teeths mans, mens mouses

In the comprehension of grammar, exceptions to pervasive rules of English are also common sources of error. Chomsky (1969) for L1 acquisition and d'Anglejan and Tucker (1975) for adult L2 acquisition report that exceptional verbs like *promise* and *ask* cause miscomprehension when appearing with reduced complements, as the verbs are treated as though they were regular. Table 2 summarizes the sentence pairs that have a similar surface structure, but whose meaning (and deep structure) are quite different. The first sentence of each pair permits an interpretation that is typical for such a construction, but the second, because of the exceptional nature of the predicate, requires a different interpretation. The erroneous interpretation, given when students are still treating the exceptions as though they were regular, is given in the table beside the sentence that is misinterpreted.

The overextension of linguistic rules to exceptional items is a common phenomenon that may occur even after some facility with English has been acquired, as the pervasive principles governing the form and interpretation of more advanced and complex structures of English (complement types, for example), also have exceptions.

Omission of major constituents   In the very early stages of learning the second language, major constituents such as nouns, verbs, or adjectives may be omitted. In many cases, however, gestures offered by the children help make their intended meaning clear. For example:

Examiner: "What's he doing?" (pointing to a boy eating)
Child: "Him this" (gestures eating)

Many children, however, will not produce such one or two word constructions, preferring to wait to speak until they have acquired more

Table 2. Irregular predicates causing misinterpretation in L1 and adult L2 comprehension

Sentence pairs[a]	Erroneous interpretation
Regular: Don *allowed* Fred to stay.	
Irregular: Don *promised* Fred to stay.	Don promised Fred that *Fred* would stay.
Regular: The girl *tells* the boy what to paint.	
Irregular: The girl *asks* the boy what to paint.	The girl asks the boy what *he* should paint.
Regular: John is *eager* to see.	
Irregular: John is *easy* to see.	It is easy for *John* to see.

[a] The sentence pairs are taken from d'Anglejan and Tucker (1975).

vocabulary items. Occasionally, words and phrases from the first language may be used by the child. These differences in verbal behavior may be partially due to differences in personality styles, or to differing reactions to the sociolinguistic circumstances of the conversation.

Omission of functors (*grammatical morphemes*)   Much more typical and pervasive is the omission of functors in the speech of L2 learners. All the morphological aspects of English are candidates for omission during the learning process. Table 3 lists some of these. Other typical morphological omissions are too numerous to list here, since any grammatical morpheme may be omitted by the learner while still in the learning process. (See, for example, Venable (1974) for more examples of this sort.)

Use of archi-forms   The selection of one member of a class of forms to represent others in the class is a common characteristic of all stages of second language acquisition. We call the form selected by the learner an "archi-form." For example, of the demonstrative adjectives *this, that, these,* and *those*, a learner may temporarily select just one to do the work for several of them: *that dog*; *that dogs*. For this learner, *that* is the archi-demonstrative adjective representing the entire class of demonstrative adjectives.

Learners may also select one member of the class of personal pronouns to function for several others in the class. For example, *Give me that*; *Me hungry*; illustrate the use of *me* as an archi-pronoun.

In the production of certain complex sentences, the use of the infinitive as an archi-form for other complement types, (e.g., gerunds and that-clauses) has also been observed[4]: *I finish to watch TV*; *She*

Table 3. Errors of functor omission

Functor		Example of error
Noun endings:	Plural -s/-es	three girl; two house
	Possessive 's	the king food
Verb endings:	Present indicative (3rd person singular -s)	She sleep there every night.
	Simple past -ed/irregular	Yesterday we walk around the yard.
	Progressive -ing	They are sing.
Auxiliaries:	*do, be, have*	We not like him. They swimming.
Copulas:	*be*	They hungry. She a girl.
Articles:	*the, a, an*	This is king food. We have dog.

[4]For further discussion of L2 errors involving complements, as well as other error types made by adult L2 learners, see Burt and Kiparsky (1972).

suggested him to go. The particular form selected for such archi-use may vary for different learners. The use of archiforms, however, is a typical phenomenon in the acquisition of a new language. If a particular structure is acquired fairly early, such as the nominative-accusative case distinction, the use of the accusative as an archi-form for both nominative and accusative constructions is observed early in the acquisition process. The past irregulars and past participles, on the other hand, are acquired relatively late, and thus archi-form usage for those structures (past irregular for both simple past and past participle) is observed during the later phases of L2 acquisition.

Alternating use of members of a class   As the learner's vocabulary and grammar grow, the use of archi-forms often gives way to the apparently fairly free alternation of various members of a class with each other. Thus, we see for demonstratives: *those dog; this cats.* In the case of pronouns, we see: masculine for feminine (or vice versa), as in *he* for *she*; plural for singular (or vice versa), as in *they* for *it*; accusative for nominative case (or vice versa), as in *her* for *she*. In the production of verbs we have observed that when the past participle form (*-en,* as in *taken*) is being acquired, it may be alternated with the past irregular, as in *I seen her yesterday; He would have saw them.*

Such alternations are probably occasioned by the onset of new grammatical differentiations within the same form class, and are thus limited to the members of a given form class. Demonstratives alternate with other demonstratives, not with auxiliaries. For example, *This dog those sick* (for *This dog is sick*) is not a normally occurring substitution. Similarly for pronouns, we do not normally see verbs alternating with pronouns. *Falling is fat* for *He is fat* for example, does not normally occur, while alternations within the form class of pronouns are normal in developing speech.

Double marking   In English, some semantic features such as tense may be marked syntactically only once in most environments. For example, we say *I didn't go*, although *go* may take a past tense marker in other environments such as *They went to lunch an hour ago.* [5] Children in the process of acquiring English however, will tend to mark both the auxiliary *do* and the verb *go* for past when they occur in the same clause, as in *She didn't went.* Table 4 presents the types of double marking observed in the speech of L2 learners.

---

[5] Other semantic features may be marked more than once, however; as in *Two girls are here* where number is marked three times: in the numeral, in the noun and in the copula.

Table 4. Errors of double marking

Semantic feature	Error	Example of error
Past tense	Past tense is marked in the auxiliary and the verb	She *did*n't *went/goed*.
Present tense	Present tense is marked in the auxiliary and the verb	He do*e*sn't eat*s*.
Negation [a]	Negation is marked in the auxiliary and the quantifier	She did*n't* give him *none*.
		He do*n't* got *no* wings.
	Negation is marked in the auxiliary and the adverb	They do*n't hardly* eat.
Equational predicate	Equation is marked in two copula positions	*Is* this *is* a cow?
Object	The object is both topicalized and expressed in the object pronoun.	That's *the man* who I saw *him*.

[a]Double negatives are permissible in some dialects of English, and therefore must not be considered errors when analyzing the speech of children who speak those dialects.

Double marking is an especially good indicator that some basics have been acquired, but the refinements have not yet been made. It is a normally occurring phenomenon during the language acquisition process.

Misordering Errors in the order of major constituents in the speech of child L2 learners are among the least frequent type, although they may occur during the early stages of learning. Word order errors typically involve major constituents, such as: *Wear mitten no*; *I want all the time to do it*.

We do not normally see misordering of elements *within* major constituents, however, particularly where morphology is concerned. For example, we do not normally see *Dog the is here* or *We are ing sleep*, in which the noun and article comprising the noun phrase are misordered, or the verb and its ending are misordered. Such errors are not normal for either first or second language learners.

A note on L1 "interference" It may be surprising to some that "interference" errors are not included in this taxonomy, as it is not uncommon to be told that L2 learners will tend to use the structures of their first language when they attempt to speak a second language. Although this notion may seem intuitive—largely because of certain pronunciation and lexical differences observed in the speech of L2 learners—the current research on children's acquisition of the syntax and morphology of a second language has not borne out the influence of the first language at all. [6] Available research indicates that children do not rely on their knowledge of the surface structures of their L1 to formulate L2 utterances. Rather, they seem to treat the new language as an independent system, which they gradually reconstruct from the L2 speech data they hear. Modern L2 research has demonstrated this repeatedly. It has shown that differences between L1 and L2 structures do not predict a child's L2 errors; neither do children learn those L2 structures that are similar in both languages earlier than those that are different. (See, for example, Price, 1968; Dulay and Burt, 1972 and 1974a, b; Hernández-Chávez, 1972, 1977a, b; Ravem, 1974; Ervin-Tripp, 1974; Venable, 1974; Gillis and Weber, 1976.) These studies include samples of children from a variety of language backgrounds, including Spanish, Chinese, Japanese, and Norwegian-speaking children learning English; and English-speaking children learning Welsh or French.

For example, Spanish-speaking children learning English as a second language do not tend to say *The dog it ate* (*El perro se lo comío*) even in the early stages of English acquisition; rather, they say *Dog eat it*, omitting functors as do children learning English as a first language. Likewise, although Spanish plurals are formed like English plurals (by adding *-s* or *-es* depending on the word ending) Spanish-speaking children learning English as L2 still omit these endings during the early stages of English acquisition (cf. Hernández-Chávez, 1972). Thus, neither "negative transfer" nor "positive transfer" of specific L1 syntactic and morphological structures provides an adequate predictive account of children's L2 performance.

There are structures that are sometimes given as examples of Spanish transfer, e.g., *He no can play* or *the fat* (for *the fat man*). These constructions, however, have also been observed in the normal development of children learning English as their first language, for whom, of course, transfer from any other language is not a possible process. (For additional examples and further discussion of these topics, see Dulay and Burt, 1974a, b.)

Studies of adult foreign language learning have, on the other hand, reported that some 20–30% of the observed errors may be

---

[6]Borrowing and code alternation, terms used to refer to the interactive use of a bilingual's two languages, should not be confused with L1 interference phenomena. Borrowing and code alternation are normal and pervasive linguistic behaviors. These are discussed under "Code Alternation," below.

traced to the learner's native language. It is not clear however, whether such errors are induced by certain types of pedagogical practices (such as contrastive presentation of a structure) or speech elicitation techniques (such as translation), or whether they are the result of monitoring or some other aspect of L2 production that is characteristic of adults. More empirical research is needed before such questions can be answered adequately.

Steps in the acquisition of L2 syntactic and morphologic structures   As in the early error research in child L2 acquisition, the earliest research on steps in the acquisition of particular L2 structures focused on comparing developing structures in child L2 performance with those previously described by Roger Brown and his colleagues for L1 acquisition. Again, the major purpose for the comparison to L1 was to permit researchers to determine whether child L2 acquisition was, to a significant extent, a process of creative construction. English negation and *wh*-questions were studied in this framework. Again, as was found for L2 errors, although expected minor differences were observed, striking overall similarities obtained between the developing structures described for the L1 and L2 performance of children. The creative aspects of the L2 acquisition process are also reflected in recent studies of the L2 development of English reflexives and word order in embedded *wh*-questions. All these findings are summarized below.

Negation   Table 5 illustrates the development of English negation in first language acquisition (Klima and Bellugi, 1966), and in second language acquisition by children whose first languages include Spanish (Hernández-Chávez, 1972), Japanese (Milon, 1974; Gillis and Weber, 1976), and Norwegian (Ravem, 1974). All the studies used as a data base the natural speech protocols of children, collected longitudinally over a period of time. All reported striking similarities between the developing structures of L2 learners and those of L1 learners.

Simple wh-questions   Ravem's (1974) study of his Norwegian-speaking son and daughter over a period of 4 months and Gillis and Weber's study (1976) of two Japanese boys over a period of 5 months revealed that the developmental steps followed by the children in acquiring English *wh*-questions were similar to those reported by Klima and Bellugi (1966) and Brown (1973) for their L1 subjects. The children produced structures such as *Where Daddy go?* and *Where Daddy is going?* before producing the mature form *Where is Daddy going?* Compare, for example:

L1	L2
What the dollie have?	What you eating?
Why not me sleeping?	Why not me can't dance?
How he can be a doctor?	What she is doing?

Embedded wh-questions   The steps in the development of certain "higher level" structures—embedded *wh*-questions—have also been the subject of recent investigations. Hakuta (1975), in a longitudinal study of a Japanese-speaking child learning English, and Dulay and Burt in a recent cross-sectional study of Keres-speaking children learning English have observed similar steps in the development of these structures.

The progression of rules used by learners is particularly revealing of how the learner's reliance on previously acquired L2 rules results in certain intermediate steps when new and related L2 structures are being acquired. Table 6 illustrates the intermediate steps observed in the acquisition of these structures.

As the table shows, in the first attempt to formulate the embedded question, children use the inversion rule they have learned for the simple *wh*-question, which is of course required when these appear alone. That is, the subject and auxiliary must be inverted, as in *What are those? What's that?* and *Where is it?* which show subject-auxiliary inversions of *Those are x's; That's an x* and *It is there.*

When constructing the embedded question, children at first do not realize that the subject-auxiliary inversion rule, which characterizes simple questions, must be undone when questions are embedded in a complex sentence.

Reflexives   The development of the reflexive pronouns *herself*, *himself*, and *themselves* was investigated in a recent cross-sectional study by Dulay and Burt on the acquisition of selected complex structures of English by 175 Spanish-speaking children in the United States. The following developmental sequence was observed:

> her → herself
> him → hisself → himself
> them → theirself → themself/themselves [7]

As the illustration shows, the feminine reflexive form has but one intermediate step with *her* preceding *herself*, whereas the masculine form has two; *him* precedes *hisself*, which in turn precedes *himself*.

---

[7] In communities where *hisself* and *theirselves* are typically used, of course, children cannot be expected to acquire the standard forms.

Table 5. Intermediate steps in the acquisition of negation by children: L1 and L2

First language acquisition	Second language acquisition		
(Klima and Bellugi, 1966)	L1 = Norwegian (Ravem, 1974)	L1 = Japanese (Milon, 1974; Gillis and Weber, 1976)	L1 = Spanish (Hernández-Chávez, 1972)
Stage 1 $S \to \left(\begin{array}{c} no \\ not \end{array} \right)$ - Nucleus - $\left(\begin{array}{c} no \\ not \end{array} \right)$ Examples: no wipe finger not a teddy bear wear mitten no	Stage 1 not like it now not ready no, no like it	Stage 1 not me not dog not cold	Stage 1 no milk no sleeping
Stage 2 $S \to$ Nom - Aux ^{neg} - $\left\{ \begin{array}{l} \text{Predicate} \\ \text{Main Verb} \end{array} \right.$ Examples: I don't set on Cromer coffee He not little, he big He no bite you	Stage 2 I not this way I not like it Dolly "er" not here	Stage 2 I no queen I not give you candy I no more five	Stage 2 I no like this one I no know it I not dumb
Stage 3 $S \to$ Nom - Aux - $\left\{ \begin{array}{l} \text{Predicate} \\ \text{Main Verb} \end{array} \right.$ Aux → T - V ^{aux} - (Neg) Examples: No it isn't That was not me I didn't caught it	Stage 3 No, I didn't I haven't seen this afore You can't have this back	Stage 3 (Examples from Hawaiian Creole)	Stage 3 I'm not scare ghost

Table 6.   Intermediate steps in the L2 acquisition of embedded *wh*-questions

Intermediate steps	L1 = Spanish (Dulay and Burt, forthcoming)	L1 = Keres (Dulay and Burt, forthcoming)	L1 = Japanese (Hakuta, 1975)
Step 1 [S] + [WH-word - Aux - NP]	I don't know where's the food I don't know what are those	I don't know what's that	I don't know where is it
Step 2 [S] + [WH-word - Aux - NP - Aux]	I don't know where's the food is — [a]	I know what's that is	I don't know where is the woods is
Step 3 [S] + [WH-word - NP - Aux]	I don't know where the food is I don't know what those are	I know what that is	I know where it is

[a]No example for Step 2 involving the plural copula was found in the children's speech protocols.

The plural has two (or three) intermediate steps, as indicated by the forms connected by the arrows.

It is interesting that the developmental steps observed demonstrate that children do not simply add -self to the pronouns they have already acquired (him, her and them) even though this might seem to be the most direct way to form reflexives. Instead, they first reclassify the simple pronouns as possessive, changing their forms to his and their in order to be consistent with similarly functioning constructions already acquired (his house, their own dog, etc.). (The form her remains the same in its possessive form.) Not until later, however, do the learners realize that although reflexives express a kind of possession, possessive pronouns are not used to form them.

The previous section dealt with sequences of intermediate structures children use before they produce mature forms; this section deals with the order in which mature structures are acquired.

Acquisition order in L2 syntax and morphology Those who are conversant with the first language acquisition literature are familiar with Roger Brown's discovery that fourteen grammatical morphemes (functors) were acquired by three unacquainted children in an approximately invariant order (Brown, 1973). This finding was replicated in a subsequent cross-sectional study of 24 children learning English as a first language (deVilliers and deVilliers, 1973) and has been the source of much hypothesizing about what possible universal characteristics of human language development might be responsible for the order found. Although no firm conclusions have yet been formulated,[8] the discovery that a developmental order existed for first language acquisition provided the impetus for much of the subsequent work in second language acquisition.

The possibility that a common order of acquisition of certain structures might exist for groups of children across the country who have different learning environments and language backgrounds was indeed intriguing, to both L2 theoreticians and practitioners. A natural order of acquisition, if it existed and could be found, would aid in theory construction as well as in curriculum development and testing. Dulay and Burt thus began a series of investigations into L2 acquisition order, studying some of the functors previously studied by Brown, as well as others.

---

[8] See however, Brown (1973) for suggestions, and Dulay and Burt, (1975b; 1977) for further discussion.

The first study included three groups of Spanish-speaking children in different instructional programs: Puerto Rican children in New York City; Chicano children in Sacramento, California; and Mexican children who lived in Tijuana, Mexico and attended school across the border in San Ysidro, California (Dulay and Burt, 1973). The second study included two groups of children, one Spanish-speaking and one Chinese-speaking, both from New York (Dulay and Burt, 1974b). Finally, a national study including over 400 children in 10 states throughout the country was undertaken (Dulay and Burt, 1975b; Burt, Dulay, and Hernández-Chávez, 1976).

All the data were collected using a "structured conversation technique": cartoon-type pictures and questions were used to elicit natural utterances containing a range of syntactic and morphological structures. Anything the child offered in response to the eliciting questions was accepted. No attempts were made to encourage or prod the child to use certain structures, nor were children corrected or otherwise discouraged. The acquisition orders discovered for certain structures are illustrated in Figure 2.

The labels for the grammatical items in Figure 2 are precisely defined grammatical structures. For example, "case" here includes only nominative and accusative pronoun forms in simple sentences and within simple subjects. Sentences like *She and I are leaving* were not elicited. The *possessive* is almost always the elliptical, such as *the dog's*, rather than *the dog's food*. (See Table 7 for the definitions of the structures that appear in Figure 2.)

The figure shows that the items in Group 1 are acquired before all the items in the groups below. Items in Group II are acquired after those in Group 1, but before those in Group III and IV, etc. The reverse is also true. Namely, the acquisition of items in Group IV implies the acquisition of the items in Groups I–III.

These orderings relationships obtained for all three of our samples, including Chinese- and Spanish-speaking children, for a total of 536 children across the United States who were in the process of learning English as a second language. (It may be of interest to note here that many of the ordering relationships presented in Figure 2 have been found to be similar for adults learning English as a second language in the United States (Krashen, Maden, and Bailey, 1975).)

Word order in wh-questions   A group of related structures whose order of acquisition was studied cross-sectionally for both Keres and Spanish-speaking children are the embedded *wh*-questions. Dulay and Burt, who investigated the singular and plural forms of these

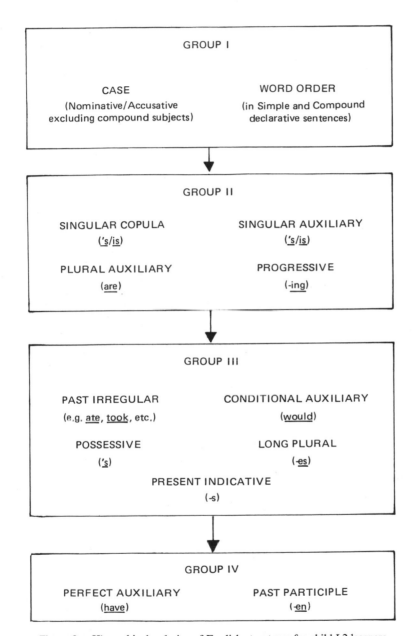

Figure 2.   Hierarchical ordering of English structures for child L2 learners.

Table 7. Definition of structures in Figure 2

Word order	The order of constituents in simple and compound declarative sentences. (Interrogatives and complex sentences are not included.)
Case	Nominative and accusative case in simple pronoun subjects or objects, excluding coordinate noun phrases such as *he and I*. Regularly elicited were the pairs *he-him, they-them,* and less frequently *she-her.*
Singular copula	The third person singular of *be*, as in *She IS a girl.*
Singular plural auxiliary	The third person singular and plural of *be*, as in *She IS dancing*; *They ARE sleeping.*
Progressive	*-ing* in any progressive tense, whether present, past, or future, as in *He is/was/will be feedING* the birds. (Gerunds are not included.)
Past irregular	The irregular past form of main verbs, such as *ate, stole,* and *fell.* Auxiliaries (*was, were,* etc.) are not included here nor are past participles such as *gone.*
Conditional auxiliary	The auxiliary *would* in simple conditional and perfect conditional constructions, e.g., *If she turned around she WOULD see them*; *He WOULD have stolen it.*
Possessive	The possessive marker *'s* on nouns, e.g., *the girl's flower.*
Long plural	All cases where the /ɨz/ allomorph is required for plural formation, as in *housES* and *nosES*
Perfect auxiliary	The auxiliary *have* in perfect conditional constructions, e.g., *She would HAVE eaten it.*
Past participle	The marker *-en* on the main verb in a perfect construction, e.g., *They have takEN the basket*; *She would have fallEN down too.*

questions in embedded contexts, report the following acquisition order for the children studied:

What's that/this

↓

What are those/these

↓

I don't know what those/these are

↓

I don't know what that/this is

The arrows indicate that the acquisition of the structure at the top of the arrow precedes the acquisition of the one at the bottom (as in Figure 2 above).

As the acquisition order illustrates, the correct form of simple questions precedes their correct form in embedded contexts, where the once correctly formed questions must take on an uninverted form. It is interesting that although *What's that* is the first learned of this group of related structures, its correct form in the embedded context is also the last to be learned. It is likely that *What's that?* is learned as one vocabulary word at first (as opposed to *What are those?*), making it difficult for the learner to segment it appropriately when required to do so. (For further discussion of structures learned as unanalyzed chunks, see Dulay and Burt, 1977 and Brown, 1973).

Reflexives The acquisition order of the reflexive pronouns for Spanish-speaking children learning standard English was also investigated in the study mentioned in the previous section. The following order of acquisition was found for the children studied:

him, her, them
↓
herself
↓
himself
↓
themselves

This order of acquisition too, as in the case of the embedded *wh*-questions just discussed, demonstrates the learners' creative restructuring of reflexive structures to make them consistent with rules and structures already acquired. As we saw under "Steps in the Acquisition of L2 Syntactic and Morphologic Structures: Reflexives," it seems that children restructure the sequence *him-self* as a possessive construction, i.e., as *his-self* at first, because they are already using basic possessive constructions such as *his basket, their food*. Because the feminine form of the possessive pronoun does not change in its possessive form, the feminine reflexive form is acquired early, obscuring its temporary misclassification into the possessive structure. The late acquisition of *themselves* results from failure to pluralize the *-self*, rather than from any characteristic inherent to the formation of reflexives.

Acquisition order in L2 semantics In a recent longitudinal study of a Spanish-speaking preschooler learning English, Hernández-Chávez (1977a, b) discovered that an orderly sequence of development also obtains for L2 semantic relations. Furthermore, all the basic semantic relations of L2 sentence structure are acquired before the onset of learning of grammatical functors. These grammatical meanings that, in adult English, are expressed through functors, the child first learned to express through basic word order. Table 8 shows the order of emergence of the major semantic relations in the first 8 months of L2 learning.

In addition, Hernández-Chávez found that grammatical categories of words also followed a well defined order of learning. Moreover, each category was first restricted to the semantic relation in which it was learned. For example, nouns were first learned as predicates in equational sentences; following this they were learned as objects of verbs; and only much later were they learned as subjects of sentences. In a similar way, personal pronouns first emerged as subjects of indicative sentences (i.e., having nonimperative verbs), then as subjects in equational sentences, and not until quite late were they acquired as indirect and direct objects.

L2 Phonology

In comparison to the work that has been done in L2 research on the acquisition of syntax, our knowledge of the development of phonology in second language learning is still in its infancy. In this section we will discuss the available empirical studies of second language phonological acquisition, as well as some of the theoretical implications of this work for our understanding of the process involved.

Table 8. Order of emergence of the basic English semantic relations

Length of exposure to English	Sentence type	Semantic relation	Example
(Months)			
2.0	Equational	Subject, predicate	This for-me
3.5	Imperative	Verb	Lookit
		Object	Gimme pa-pow (= gun)
		Locative	Please sit down here
	Indicative	Subject, verb	I make-it
3.75	Indicative	Object	I like-it this
4.0	Indicative	Negative	I no wannit
5.0	Indicative	Catenative auxiliary	I gonna push you
5.5	Equational	Locative	That mine right there
6.0	Equational	Copula	This is white
		Predicate adjective	That's blue
7.0	Indicative	Past tense	You squirt (= squirted) me!

Second language learners will often employ pronunciations that, from the point of view of monolingual learning, would be considered deviant and would require some sort of corrective intervention. Yet, as has been demonstrated also for syntax and morphology, given particular conditions and stages of learning, such pronunciations, rather than being abnormal, are the expected outcome.

Simultaneous acquisition of two phonologies   Most of the research to date on the L2 acquisition of phonology describes the simultaneous acquisition of two languages. (See "Second Language Acquisition," above.) One important finding of these studies has been that in all essential respects early simultaneous bilingualism does not differ from the acquisition of a single language. In the earlier stages of development, phonological acquisition consists of learning to make the fundamental vowel and consonant distinctions that are common to both of the languages in the child's environment. The processes involved are indistinguishable from those of L1 phonological development. For example, earlier reduplicated syllables like [kiki] "kitty" become differentiated as [kiti] (Burling, 1959); phone substitutions similar to those that occur in learning a single language are made, as for example, [t] for [s] or [d] for [l] in the Spanish forms [but] /bus/ or [dus] /lus/, respectively (Contreras and Saporta, 1971); consonant clusters are simplified, e.g., [pi ˡs] for *please* or [ʔsi] for *horsie* (Vogel, 1975); etc. These processes apply equally to words from each of the two languages of the learner.

Differentiation of the phonologies in simultaneous acquisition begins to take place somewhere around the 24th month. Major (1976) purposes that this differentiation begins with different phonetic realizations for "identical" segments at about 21 months. Thus, Portuguese /i/ is pronounced [iᵊ] in *aqui*, while English /i/ in *me* has the form [ei]. However, he also notes that as late as age 31 months, comparable segments in both languages have the same substitutions. For example, English *fly* is [fuai] and the Portuguese *flor* is [fuθh]. Vogel (1975) also notes that at 24 months the Romanian- English-speaking child she studied still had a single, undifferentiated system. Burling (1959) places the differentiation between Garo and English in his son, Stephen, as late as 31 months when previously identical vowels begin to show distinct phonetic realizations in the two languages.

Besides this variation in the timing of the divergence of the two languages, there are other differences as well. It seems very clear that the earliest phonologies in all cases combine the two input systems into a single unified output. It is as though the child does not yet realize (on some level below consciousness, of course) that it must learn two phonologies. Later, at about the end of the 2nd year, some children will split the heretofore combined system into two. Each of the two shares a "common core" of phonological elements and processes, differing principally on the basis of new learning. Other children, such as Burling's son, will begin very distinctly to favor one or the other of the two languages rather than splitting the systems. In Stephen's case, Burling reports that the phonetics of certain segments were distinctly Garo sounding. For example, the k and g type sounds were pronounced as the postvelars [ḳ] and [g] in both Garo and English words. The distribution of certain positional variants, e.g., the vowel [ɛ], which is always short in Garo, followed the Garo rather than the English pattern.

All of the studies cited above report the bilingual development of individual children, each in a unique set of learning conditions, so it is not surprising to find important differences in the time and manner of the differentiation of the two languages. For some, each of the parents spoke a different language to the child; others had, in addition, nursemaids who spoke one of the languages with the child, others did not. It is interesting to note that the Burling child, whose first development beyond the single system favored one of his languages and who did not differentiate the two until late in his 3rd year, was also a child whose principal environment language was Garo, i.e., there was an imbalance in the amount and the nature of the input he received from each of his languages.

This case is particularly instructive because in several respects the development of Stephen's English phonology is comparable to that of a child learning English as a second language, i.e., sequentially. Stephen's learning of English phonological structures began at a time when several structures specific to Garo phonology had already been learned. In fact, his phonology can be said to have been essentially Garo until approximately 31 months of age. After the beginning of the systematic differentation, Garo continued to be the child's principal language until he was taken away from the Garo-speaking environment.

Sequential acquisition of a second phonology   In sequential second language learning, children approach the task of acquiring a new language under a very different set of conditions from those that hold for L1 and for the earlier stages of simultaneous learning. Besides being older, more cognitively advanced, and with a relatively developed motor coordination, sequential L2 learners already know a substantial amount of their first language. For the vast majority of child L2 learners in the United States, L2 acquisition proceeds concomitantly with the continued development and use of L1, at least for a period of several months or even years.

Under such circumstances, we can expect that, in the beginning stages, the L2 phonology will follow closely the pattern of the first language, in a way analogous to Stephen's favoring Garo phonology rather than immediately becoming differentiated from English. The segments that have been built up in L1, together with their characteristic phonetic make-up within each of their permitted positions, form the foundation upon which the second language phonology is constructed. As the sequential learner progresses, the two phonologies will begin to diverge, first in the phonetics of some of the corresponding segments in the two languages, and later with respect to other characteristics. Stephen's earliest distinctions were in the qualities of the vowels. Thus, the lax high front vowel type, which previously had an identical pronunciation in each of the languages, by 32 months of age began to be pronounced [I] in English and [ɪ] (a somewhat backer variant) in Garo; the mid vowels *e* and *o* at this same time began to acquire for English their characteristic lax pronunciations [ɛ] and [ʔ]. In a similar way, we have observed that one of the first distinctions made by Spanish-speakers acquiring English involves the differentiation of the English diphthongized vowels from their Spanish undiphthongized counterparts, e.g., [oṵ] versus [o] and [eị] versus [e].

Thus, in order to account for the learning of phonology in sequential second language acquisition, we must be able to specify the components of at least two major factors: the child's existing L1 phonology and the process of L2 phonological acquisition. It seems very clear that the sequential second language learner begins the acquisition of L2 by using the L1 system as a starting point, gradually differentiating the two. Until the various parts of this core system are differentiated, it acts as a filter through which the production of L2 forms must pass. In this way, forms are able to be produced without depending upon the full scale acquisition of the L2 phonology, and at the same time without hindering its systematic development.

The role of L1 phonology in the acquisition of L2 phonology Many scholars have written contrastive analyses comparing various pairs of languages. Because Spanish-English bilingualism is one of the important areas of educational concern in this country and some of the most explicit contrastive analyses that exist compare these two languages, we take our examples for this section largely from the learning of English by speakers of Spanish. One of the most thorough analyses constrasting Spanish and English is that of Stockwell and Bowen (1965). There is no need to reproduce their work here, and the interested reader is asked to refer to it directly. However, a few examples show how this kind of analysis helps us to account for certain pronunciation characteristics of L2 learners (whose L1 is Spanish), which we might otherwise consider to be "problems."

Phonetic comparison   One set of differences between the languages pertains to the phonetic composition of sound types that the two languages have in common. Thus, both Spanish and English have in their inventory of consonants the sound types *p, t, k, l*, and *r*, among others, each of which shows systematic differences between the two languages. In English, *p, t*, and *k* are pronounced with a forceful expulsion of air in many positions within the word. This is referred to by linguists as "aspiration." This aspiration is not a feature of Spanish *p, t*, and *k*, so one expectation with respect to the pronunciation of Spanish-speaking children who are beginning to learn English is that words like *car, toy*, or *pin* will be produced without aspiration on the first segments. To the native speaker of English, such a pronunciation can leave an impression of "confusion" between *p* and *b* or between *k* and *g*. The differences between Spanish and English *r* and *l* will not leave such an impression, but only because there are no other English sounds with which they could be said to be confused. The English *l* has, in certain positions, a velar or "dark" quality, whereas the Spanish *l* is always alveolar or "light." Spanish has two *r*-type sounds, one a tap and one a trill; the English *r* is different from both of these in that it is retroflex.

In the vowel systems, one major difference that we noted above lies in the diphthongization in English of /o/ and /e/ and to some extent /i/ and /u/. None of the Spanish vowels are diphthongized in this way, so we would expect the Spanish-speaking child who has not acquired very much English to produce words like *go* or *say* with a short and unglided vowel.

Most of these differences, while they are not the source of any perceived "confusion," contribute to what is heard as "Spanish accent." As mentioned above in the case of the diphthongization, these kinds of differences are among the first to be learned by the L2 child. This is not to say that phonetic differences will not persist in these kinds of segments. Minute adjustments as in the amount of aspiration (cf. Preston et al., 1967) or in place of articulation between, say, alveolar and dental stops will continue to be made for some time, and certain differences from monolingual pronunciations will often become conventionalized within a bilingual community. The essential point here is that children becoming bilingual will very early learn to distinguish the salient phonetic qualities of most of the sound types that are shared by the two languages.

Phonemic comparison A second kind of difference between two languages that gives rise to differences between early L2 and native pronunciation of the target language is a phonetic difference associated with phonemically contrastive segments. Thus, English has both /ʃ/ and /tʃ/ while Spanish has only /tʃ/. A similar relation holds for the English contrasts /b/:/v/, /s/:/z/, /i/:/I/, /e/:/ae/, etc. In each of these cases, Spanish has only one of the contrasting pair: /b/, /s/, /i/, and /e/, respectively. We can expect, then, that a Spanish-speaking child learning English will pronounce [b] for /v/, [s] for /z/, [i] for /I/, etc.

The distribution of phonological segments We not only need to concern ourselves with comparing the contrasting and noncontrasting segments of the two languages, we must also take into account the distributions of those segments in words. So, for example, although both English and Spanish have the sounds *m* and *n*—and pronounce them in essentially the same way—both of these sounds may occur at the end of a word in English, but only *n* may end a word in Spanish. A word like *some*, then, will be pronounced by the neophyte in a way that sounds like *sun*. Another difference in distribution concerns consonant clusters. At the ends of words, Spanish allows no clusters; English permits a great many clusters in this position, e.g., *-ks* (box), *-ltʃ* (mulch), *-mp* (lamp), *-rst* (first), etc. Contrastive analysis will predict that the Spanish speaker learning English will either omit these clusters or else will pronounce only the portion that corresponds to one of the consonants that is permitted in final position in Spanish words.

Comparison of phonological systems Finally, in comparing the two languages of developing bilinguals, we need to take into account the productive rules that they have acquired in their first language. These operate on phonological segments in a dynamic way, adding, deleting, or modifying them such that actual pronunciations may be very different from the basic, underlying form of a word. All languages have rules of this sort that children must learn. For example, English /t/ in a word like *sit* is changed to a *d*-like flap [d] in the word *sitting*, or the [aɪ] of a word like *realize* becomes [I] in the form *realization*.

In sequential L2 acquisition, children can be expected to have learned some of these rules for L1 by the time they being to acquire the L2, and this learning may impinge upon the L2 production in a way that is quite complex. The result is that an untrained observer may be led to believe that the learner is utterly confused as to what segments to pronounce. For example, we have already noted that a final *m* may be pronounced as *n* in a word like *some*. There is a rule of Spanish phonology that interacts with a final *n* that occurs immediately before the initial consonant of a following word. The effect is essentially to assimilate the *n* to the point of articulation of the following consonant. Thus, the phrase *son perros* "they're dogs" is pronounced [sompeřos]. Given such a rule, an English phrase such as *one bird* might be pronounced [wʌmbɨrd]. We now have some *m*s pronounced as *n*s (some), and some *n*s pronounced as *m*s (one).

Both Spanish and English have a voicing assimilation rule by which certain sequences of two or more consonants become either all voiced or all voiceless. For example, the English past tense marker is either /t/ or /d/, depending on the previous consonant: *robbed* [rabd], *rapped* [raept]; Spanish has *los carros* [loskařos] versus *los gatos* [loz ɣatos]. There is a crucial difference in these two cases by which, in English, it is the second consonant that changes, whereas in Spanish it is the first consonant. These facts help us to account for a pronunciation like *froks* for *frogs* reported by Williams (1972) or for the apparent confusion between *s* and *z* when the child pronounces *z*s as *s*s in phrases like *these cats* (which we expect anyway because Spanish has only *s* and English has both sounds) but pronounces *s* like *z* when saying *this dog*.

Syllabification rules in Spanish and English also differ. These differences are most apparent with respect to the semivowels [I̯] and [u̯] (respectively, *y* and *w*). Details aside, English will tend to syllabify *after* these segments while Spanish syllabifies *before*. Thus, a form like *fire* will be pronounced [fa I̯-ər] by a native English speaker, but it will often be pronounced [fa-yər] by a Spanish speaker learning English. (We note, incidentally, that the different transcriptions [I̯] and [y] mainly reflect the different syllable boundaries.) Williams (1972) cites the example [ɹayəstʔri] for *write a story,* in which there is an apparent substitution of [y] for [t]. However, remembering the constraints on word-final consonants in Spanish, we see that *write a* has the basic form /ra I̯ #ə/ for the child (where # represents word boundary) which by the syllabification rule becomes [ra-yə].

In this same general context, it is appropriate to mention that the well known, almost stereotypic, epenthesis of the vowel *e* before such words as *school*, *spill*, *street*, etc. This is generally considered to be a curious characteristic of "Spanish accent." However, if we examine the permitted sequences of consonants at the beginning of Spanish and English words, we immediately see the source of such pronunciations. Although Spanish and English initial consonant clusters are very similar, Spanish permits no clusters of *s* plus another consonant in that position. Words that would otherwise have such a cluster epenthesize an *e*, e.g., *escribir* "to write," *estar* "to be," *escuela* "school," etc. It is interesting to note that the pronunciation of forms like [eskul] (for *school*) or [estap] (for *stop*) are not reported for young children, but only for older children and adults. This may be because this rule develops relatively late in Spanish.

From what has been said in the last several paragraphs, it should be amply evident that the developing phonology of a child learning English as an L2 is not a simple function of differences in the inventories of sounds in the two languages. Rather, the actual pronunciations are the result of a complex set of interactions among the segment inventories, the distribution of segments in words, and the phonological processes that operate in each of the learner's languages.

Acquisition order in L2 phonology   One remaining problem has to do with the specification of the expected order in which the various English phonological structures are learned. It is important to know this in order to assess the level of development in L2 and in order to distinguish those aspects of phonological development that form part of the normal developmental sequence from those that do not.

Contrastive analysis predictions   Contrastive analyses provide us with an inventory of the segments in conflict in two languages, their phonetic and distributional differences, and even the interaction of the two rule systems, although most analyses of this sort are based principally on an inventory of segments rather than dynamic processes. On the other hand, this kind of analysis does not tell us the order in which structures will be learned. Stockwell and Bowen (1965), in their comparison of Spanish and English structures cited above, do provide us with a "hierarchy of difficulty." However, this is based on the assumption that the learning of phonology involves a process of habit formation. According to this view, the level of difficulty of a given structure is then a function of the strength of an established habit. Presumably, the greater the difference between a habit in L1 and a new habit to be learned in L2, the greater the difficulty (and, presumably, the later such a form is learned).

But even a cursory examination of their hierarchy (Stockwell and Bowen, 1965, p. 16) shows virtually no relationship between the predicted difficulty and the known facts of English L2 acquisition. For example, their most difficult type involves a sound which is a positional variant (an allophone of a phoneme) in L2, but which is not found in L1. For English vis-à-vis Spanish this type will include aspirated voiceless stops or retroflex [ɹ], among others. Yet these are among the English sounds reported to be learned earliest by Spanish-speaking children (Williams, 1972). A sound type that Stockwell and Bowen consider relatively low in order of difficulty involves a phonemic distinction in L2 for an allophonic difference in L1. English /z/ fits this type because it contrasts with the voiceless /s/ although in Spanish it is a variant of /s/. But this is reported to be one of the most difficult distinctions for Spanish-speaking children (Sawyer, 1959; Williams, 1972). Moreover, many adults who have mastered other English contrasts continue to use [z] only as an allophone of /s/. Many other examples can be given that show that the Stockwell and Bowen hierarchy of difficulty makes erroneous predictions for Spanish speakers who are learning English. Although their contrastive analysis does show where two systems are in conflict, thus pointing out potential areas of difficulty, it does not adequately predict relative difficulty or order of learning.

Results of empirical investigations' A much more promising direction of inquiry for an understanding of the orders of learning is, rather than relying on a hierarchy of difficulty established by contrastive analysis, the direct empirical investigation of phonological acquisition processes in second language learners. We need to know a great deal more about the interaction of the L1 phonological system and L2 production: what kinds of L1 structures affect L2 learning? What are their effects? Which L2 structures are affected by L1 knowledge? In addition, we need to know much more about the various factors that are important for the orderly development of an L2 phonology, including amount and nature of the input, opportunities for use, attitude and motivation, etc. Crucially, we need much more information about the relationships that hold between L2 learning and the natural processes of phonological acquisition that are found in L1.

Most of the currently available evidence, meager though it is, suggests strongly that L2 acquisition follows a developmental course that is strikingly similar to that of L1. Mazeika (1971), in his study of a Spanish-speaking 27-month-old child, suggests that there is no negative transfer from English to Spanish in the learning of phonology. Some of the facts that he reports support the notion of an L2 development that parallels that of L1, e.g., /r/ is substituted by [w] in words like *cry* [kwai]. This is a commonly reported substitution for monolingual English speakers; Spanish speakers tend to substitute an [l], e.g., [glande] for *grande*. [θ], [δ], [v], and [ǰ] are very late in L2 development, as they also are in English L1 acquisition by monolinguals.

Williams (1972), too, reports that [θ] and [δ] are learned late. Furthermore, the Puerto Rican children he studied tended to substitute [t] and [d] for these two sounds. (In words like *brother* [brʌdər], this substitution is in direct contradiction to what would be predicted on the basis of a contrastive analysis). These same substitutions are noted by Moskowitz (1970) and others for monolingual English-speaking children. It is interesting in this regard that Wolfram (1972) records the substitution of [f] for /θ/ by Puerto Rican bilinguals in word-final position, which he attributes to the influence of Black English. However, Moskowitz (1970) reports this substitution for monolingual English speakers who are uninfluenced by Black English, so Wolfram's example does not necessarily reflect this influence.

Williams cites a number of other processes that are very much like those found in learning English as L1. For example, syllabic *l* is "vocalized" to [ʋ] in words like *purple*. Final consonants are often deleted as in [raI] *write*, [faI] *five*, or [wI] *with*. In the acquisition of clusters consisting of a nasal consonant plus an obstruent, he cites a number of examples that not only provide striking evidence that L2 processes parallel those of L1, but also give dynamic support for a universal of phonological acquisition reported recently (Hernández-Chávez, Vogel and Clumeck, 1975). These authors found that, in the L1 development of nasal clusters by Spanish-speaking children, clusters consisting of nasal plus voiceless obstruent (i.e., either stops, affricates, or spirants) became simplified by deleting the nasal; clusters with voiced obstruents, on the other hand, deleted the obstruent and kept the nasal. Williams' subject Clito produced [ǰap] "jump" and [sʌθi] "something," but [frɛn] "friend," directly paralleling for L2 English the findings of Hernández-Chávez et al. for L2 Spanish.

A number of writers have noted that the spirants are the class of consonants that is mastered last. We have already mentioned the stop: spirant contrast with [t,d] and [θ,ð]. Related to this is control over the affricate:spirant contrast [tʃ:ʃ]. Next to [θ,ð], the [ʃ] is one of the last spirants to attain stability in monolingual English (Moskowitz, 1970). Similarly, Benítez (1970) reports that [tʃ] and [ʃ] were two of the phonemes most frequently "missed" in testing Mexican-American seventh graders in a Texas school. Moskowitz also demonstrates that the voicing contrast between [s] and [z] is one of the very latest consonantal contrasts to be attained in English. Sawyer (1959) found that "not even the best bilinguals" consistently used [z] in the way that monolinguals do.

Finally, we have already seen that children acquiring two languages simultaneously simplify consonant clusters in the same way that children learning a single language do. For sequential learners, Heiler-Saavedra (1966) had similar results, as her subjects also reduced consonant clusters. In addition, she points out that this is not a necessary strategy because adult learners will often resyllabify a cluster or epenthesize a vowel rather than simplify it. Thus, the child L2 strategy is very similar to that found in L1.

Processes in the acquisition of L2 phonology   From the above discussion, a general outline begins to emerge of the processes that children employ in acquiring a second language phonology. Upon the introduction to an L2 phonology and the necessity of decoding and encoding the sounds of the patently new system, the child begins to operate dynamically on the new sounds and sound sequences in the environment. This involves either the simplification of the input in some way (reduction in the number of syllables, simplification of clusters and diphthongs, etc.), the substitution of a simpler sound for one that is less simple [9] or a sound that has already been learned for one that has not, or the generalization of constraints and the creation of phonological rules. These are all processes that are found also in L1 learning. The major difference between L1 and L2 learning is that in L2 learning the child uses as a base the sounds, sound sequences, and rules that have already been learned for L1. New phonetic distinctions (e.g., [p:pʰ]), phonological contrasts (e.g., /θ:t/), and sequences of sounds (e.g., /-mp#/) are learned in an orderly fashion that is fully analogous to that of first language learning.

---

[9]The matter of relative simplicity is a controversial and unresolved issue in phonology, as in all of linguistics. Here we do not mean simplicity in terms of the number of features involved, but rather in terms of an acquisitional hierarchy of features and feature complexes. "Simpler" sounds are, by definition, those that are acquired in similar contexts and under similar conditions. We will not attempt to specify such a hierarchy here because it continues to be a major concern of researchers in the acquisition of phonology.

Because the second language learner already has an L1 phonology and uses it as a foundation for further learning until new contrasts, sequences, and rules are learned, the L2 production will have a substratum of L1 sounds. In addition, because an L2 child is presumably older than the monolingual L1 child at a comparable stage of development, many of the sounds and sound combinations produced by the L2 learner will, from the point of view of a child learning the first language, seem immature or even pathological.

In this section we have attempted to demonstrate that such pronunciations are not only not immature or pathological, they are the result of completely normal and expected processes of phonological acquisition coupled with the interaction of the new learning that is taking place and the knowledge of a first language that the child already has. The L2 learner, in becoming bilingual, brings to bear on the new phonology all of the same natural language learning abilities available to the L1 child. At the same time, knowledge of a first language permits the fullest utilization of skills and abilities toward the intricate task of acquiring two distinct phonologic systems.

L1 DEVELOPMENT AND INTERACTION WITH L2

In the previous sections, we have been concerned with various aspects of learning a second language. In the total process of becoming a bilingual, second language learning is but one side of the coin; the other side involves continuing development of the first language along with the dynamic interaction between the bilingual's mother tongue and the emergent second language. Depending on such factors as the time of inception and character of L2 learning, continuity of contact with the first language, and social-psychological factors of language choice, the relationship and kind of interaction between the two languages will take different forms.

L1 Development in Bilinguals

Before the onset of learning the second language, we can fully expect that the mother tongue of the bilingual-to-be will develop normally, as for any other monolingual speaker of the language. Depending upon the sociolinguistic characteristics of the principal language models in the child's environment, the language that is being acquired may exhibit lexical, phonological, or grammatical features that differ from those found in a more standardized form of the language. However, it is important to recognize that sociolinguistic variation is indic-

ative only of social differentiation and not of inadequacies or deficiencies in the learning process.

After the introduction of the child to a second language, learning
conditions for the mother tongue necessarily change, if only in that
the time, effort, and attention that are given to the second language
are no longer available to the first language. Nevertheless, even with
a substantial amount of time devoted to the L2, there is every reason
to expect the continued normal development of the L1. It is well
known and has been reported in many places in the literature that,
given the opportunity and the appropriate exposure, young children
are fully capable of learning two, three, and even more languages
with native or near native facility. The learning capacities of the
human mind are immense and are rarely pushed to their limits. Under
sufficiently conducive learning conditions, the bilingual's languages
should develop to their fullest extent.

However, each community will exhibit its own pattern of interaction between the native language and the second language. In bilingual communities in the United States, the learning of English as
a second language typically begins in early childhood, often even
before the child enters school. Preschoolers may be exposed to large
amounts of English by older siblings, peers, and the omnipresent electronic media. Enrollment in school carries with it increased and concentrated exposure to the use of English. The result is that for most
children in the United States whose mother tongue is other than
English, the learning of the second language proceeds at a normal
rate and according to well documented processes. This is true as well
for those children who first encounter English after kindergarten
or first grade. As was pointed out in the preceding paragraph, given
the proper environment, the first language will also continue to develop normally leading to an equilibrium between the languages,
which characterizes full language maintenance.

But, under certain kinds of conditions, we may observe varying
amounts of disruptions of the child's native language ranging from
slowed development to interruption of learning and even, in extreme
cases, to retrograde development or language loss. Developing bilingualism can thus be viewed as a continuum, or perhaps better, as
a pair of sliding scales that function independently, although they
may both be affected by inter-related social and psychological influences.

Some children may be at a normal stage of development in their
native language and at a very early stage of development in their

second language. Other children may be well advanced in their second language development although not as advanced as their age-mates for whom that language is native. At the same time, development of their first language may be below that of their monolingual age-mates in their first language development. Still other children may be at a level of second language development that surpasses that of their first language, which for all practical purposes has ceased to develop further. Children who have reached the same stage of proficiency in both their first and second languages are at a stage called balanced bilingualism. [10]

Full maintenance   Most situations of stable and self-perpetuating bilingualism are characterized by the primary and full development of the native tongue of the bilingual community. It is the first language learned by all members of the community, and it continues to develop until it attains adult norms, even after the introduction of the second language. In addition to adult phonological, grammatical, and lexical norms, continued development involves the mastery of the full range of styles and registers that make up the "communicative competence" of speakers of that community (Hymes, 1972). For languages with a literacy tradition, this communicative competence will include the written medium as well as the spoken form.

In a situation of full maintenance, the community's second language, which for bilingual groups in the United States is normally English, also develops as fully as possible consistent with the needs and desires of speakers to participate in English-speaking society. (For some groups, e.g., migrant workers, the need and opportunity is limited; for most groups there is a substantial amount of sociocultural integration.) It is important to note that in most bilingual communities even relatively full development of the L2 will not necessarily mean that the variety of English used will reflect the norms of the monolingual English speakers of the surrounding community. Many studies have shown the existence in such speech communities of what Haugen (1956) calls "bilingual norms." For example, Sawyer (1959) and Phillips (1975), among others, point out the existence of stable and systematic phonological differences in the speech of Spanish-speaking

---

[10] Relative bilingualism or dominance involves a number of parameters including lexicon, structural proficiency, control of the phonologic systems, fluency, communicative skills, and so forth. Dominance in one of the parameters does not imply dominance in the others. A bilingual child may be balanced with respect to syntactic proficiency, but dominant in the lexicon of one of the languages. Or a child may be dominant in one aspect of the first language and be dominant in another aspect of the second.

groups in the Southwest from that of local native speakers of English. Sawyer reports many consistent lexical differences as well. These variances do not represent an inability to learn the language, but rather a natural adherence to the sociolinguistic norms of one's community.

In the normal use of two languages by a bilingual community, even in those in which there is full maintenance of the native tongue and a general balance between L1 and L2, it is usual to find that each of the languages tends to serve a particular set of functions. The sets corresponding to each of the languages are complementary, although in actual situations, of course, there is considerable overlap. Thus one of the languages—in this case English—will be used for interaction with the English speaking world: in government, in business, in education, etc. The native language will be used for relationships within the family, the neighborhood, and the community. These are the minimal functions of the native language in a maintenance situation, and it is only under these or very similar conditions that we can speak of full language maintenance. Each generation learns the community's language as its mother tongue. As a completely functioning L1, it continues to develop through adulthood, and the cycle is repeated.

In a complex urban society, we find a considerable overlap in the functions of the languages of bilinguals. Often, English will impinge on many familial and community functions, especially in interaction with outsiders, but in many cases also with family members and neighbors. Thus it is that, in these kinds of urban situations, the continuance of full language maintenance requires the active counterbalancing support of those institutions of the general society that most directly affect the community. In many areas, the native language of bilingual groups are being used for an increasing number of academic, commercial, and governmental activities that were previously the exclusive sphere of English. In this way, the native language is strengthened and its maintenance, which is an important resource both for the bilingual community and for society in general, is assured.

Disruption of L1 development   In some communities, many of the functions normally associated with the native language come to be expressed by either of the two languages without distinction, or by English alone. Such situations are brought about by a number of complex sociolinguistic factors which it is not our purpose to discuss here. In general we may say that these involve the difficulty of economic and social advancement except through English and a concomitant shift in the values associated with the use of each of the languages. Often, the major relevant institutions outside of the home are strongly English-oriented—the church, the school, neighborhood organizations, etc.—with the result that learners of the native language are not only exposed to a great amount of English in early childhood, but also the amount and variety of the native language that is heard is insufficient to support the continued normal development of the native language.

Types of L1 disruption   In *slowed development,* the regular phonological and grammatical structures continue to develop, but their rate of development is slowed to a lesser or greater extent. Very advanced structures may not develop at all. So, for example, such phonological structures of Spanish as the distinction between [r] and [r] or the morphophonemic alternations [o] ~ [ue] ~ [u] in certain classes of verbs may be learned much later than normal, or may fail to develop entirely. Similarly, the grammatical forms of the conditional or of the pluperfect subjunctive may not develop until long after their emergence under more favorable circumstances.

The virtually complete cessation of structural or sociolinguistic development may occur at any point subsequent to the onset of the second language and is the consequence of the absence in the child's linguistic environment of sufficient meaningful input in the L1 and opportunities for its use. Such a hiatus in the active acquisition of the first language we have referred to elsewhere as "interrupted development (Burt, Dulay, and Hernández-Chávez, 1976).

An extreme form of disruption of the native language is possible when, under sociolinguistic pressures within the neighborhood, from the school, and from the generally pervasive and "forceful presence" of English (Ornstein, 1951), the principal language of the home becomes English with only occasional opportunities for the use of the native language. Such situations may arise when bilingual parents, having used mainly the native language with their children, switch to English as their children bring the language into the home from the school. Under these conditions, there may occur an actual language loss or deterioration of proficiency in the use of the language. Depending upon the amount of prior development, loss may be evident at any point along the natural sequence of acquisition. Because the latest learned structures are the ones most likely to be lost first, the linguistic characteristics of language loss are extremely similar to those of slowed acquisition or interrupted development.

Characteristics of L1 disruption   Except in the most extreme cases of interrupted development and language loss resulting from the major withdrawal of opportunities to hear and use the native language, the disruption of linguistic development is most evident in the productive modality (speaking). That is to say, interruption and/or loss does not usually involve either actual forgetting or the loss of linguistic competence. [11] This is evidenced by the retention, and even the continued growth, in the ability to comprehend the native language. Interruption and loss, then, often will involve only linguistic performance factors such as fluency, memory, or the planning of sentence structures.

One of the most evident features of disruption in native language development are the lexical gaps that arise. Within those language functions associated with family and neighborhood and that are normally enacted through the native language, such lexical gaps are likely to be found mainly in active production; comprehension may remain stable. In those communicative areas that are the usual domain of English, the lexical gaps are likely to be more pervasive and to occur in comprehension as well as production.

Because all of these phenomena of native language disruption are fairly directly linked to the abrupt shift in the focus of language acquisition from the native language to the second language, we can expect that the development of the second language will follow completely normal patterns of rate and sequence of learning. As was pointed out above, the structures that are required, instead of following the norms of the general society, may adhere to patterns characteristic of the bilingual community. Coupling such circumstances with the facts of disruption of the native language, bilingual children are frequently described as "not knowing either language well" or as "alingual." This is possibly true only of the language whose development has been disrupted, not of the second language in which the norms of the bilingual community must not be taken as defective or as representing a language disability. [12] Nor is the disruption of the

---

[11]Linguistic "competence" refers to the knowledge of a language internalized by a speaker. It is distinct from linguistic "performance," which involves the actual use of linguistic knowledge in comprehension or production. See Chomsky, 1965 for a full discussion.

[12]Even in such cases where native language disruption begins at an early stage before the attainment of any substantial bilingual balance, any supposed deficiency is much more apparent than real. The child will continue with normal development of L2 and will very quickly approach monolingual norms. Moreover, the child will very easily make up for any presumed, and certainly temporary, gaps by bringing to bear any number of creative communicative devices. (See the following section for a discussion of code alternation as one of these devices, and cf. Hernández-Chávez 1977a, b for a fuller discussion of several such communicative and learning strategies.)

native language to be taken as reflecting learning dysfunctions; rather, it is the direct and predictable result of powerful social-psychological processes.

Thus far, we have seen that there exist several sources for the misinterpretation of bilingual phenomena as indications of dysfunctions in the language learning capabilities of children. These sources are: 1) English second language learning begins at a later age than the learning of English as a first language; consequently, the level of proficiency attained by English second language learners at a given age will often be lower than that of native English-speaking children; 2) differences in the structural and/or sociolinguistic rules of a given language for monolingual and bilingual speakers; 3) varying degrees of disruption of the native language caused by the action of powerful sociolinguistic forces; and 4) the existence of culturally based sociolinguistic differences in the rules for when and where to speak and what and how much to say. (These will be discussed more fully in the next chapter)

The Interaction of the Bilingual's Languages

The cultural and linguistic contact inherent in societal bilingualism gives rise to two other major phenomena that are often subject to misinterpretation: "borrowing" and "code alternation." These are often erroneously believed to symptomize serious language abnormalities or, at the very least, to signal a linguistic and mental confusion that is deleterious to general learning. In the following section, the linguistic and sociolinguistic processes involved in these phenomena are described in order to provide a clearer understanding of their structure and function.

Borrowing Linguistic borrowing, that is, the incorporation of linguistic material from one language into another, is a normal consequence of the natural contact of languages in multilingual societies. It is extremely widespread in social groups around the world, and is by no means exclusively characteristic of socially and economically subordinate linguistic minorities in the United States (Weinreich, 1953; Haugen, 1953, 1956; Vildomec, 1963, among others).

The common sorts of borrowing are individual lexical items that express either cultural concepts that are new to the borrowing group, or notions that are of particular importance in a given contact situation. [13] For example, the languages of the Old World, upon coming

---

[13]Borrowing may take a number of other forms such as "loan shifts," "loan translations," and the like. See Weinreich (1953) and Haugen (1956) for discussion of these and other categories of complex lexical borrowing.

in contact with the cultures and the fauna and flora of the New World, borrowed many hundreds of words from the American languages such as *maize, tomato, igloo, skunk,* etc. The native American languages, in turn, borrowed many words from European culture. Similarly, a great many items from Spanish have come into English by way of the Southwestern cattle-raising culture, e.g., *corral, lasso, arroyo,* and many more. The extent to which borrowing can take place under conditions of culture contact is evidenced by the case of English—a Germanic language—which, as a consequence of the Norman conquest, borrowed thousands of French words, opening the doors for a virtual flood of Latin-based borrowings. It is estimated that today the latinate vocabulary of English exceeds 60% of the total lexicon.

The non-English languages in the United States today borrow considerable numbers of words from English. Some of these represent cultural concepts that were previously unfamilar to the speakers of those languages as when Spanish borrows *queque* (cake), *béisbol* (baseball), or *lonche* (lunch). A great many words, however, are borrowed mainly because of their constant and intensive use by Spanish speakers as they come into necessary contact with English-oriented commercial and educational institutions (Espinosa, 1917). Such words as *traque* (track), *cheque* (check), *espeliar* (to spell), and *juipen* (whipping) illustrate these kinds of borrowing.

As may be inferred from the examples given in the above paragraphs, words borrowed into a language maintain the general sound pattern of the original word but modify it to conform to the phonetic and phonological system of the borrowing language. Thus, the words *cake* and *lunch* in English end in obstruent consonants. Since no word in Spanish may end in these sounds, the words are modified in the process of borrowing by the addition of the epenthetic vowel *e*. In addition, the word *lunch* contains a "short *u*" ([ʌ]) which is not used in Spanish, and it is therefore changed to the phonetically similar *o*.

Words, once borrowed, are incorporated into the grammatical structure of the borrowing language. They become, in effect, new words in that language. The words *maize* and *tomato*, for example, obey the English grammatical rules for co-occurrence with articles: *tomato* may be used with the indefinite article *a*, although *maize* may not. Similarly, the Spanish word *espeliar* forms its infinitive with an ending and is conjugated like all other Spanish verbs of the same class.

Borrowed words may have such widespread use within a community that speakers of the borrowing language may learn them from each other, not needing to have a knowledge of the original in the other language. When this occurs, it is said that the words are "integrated borrowings." On the other hand, bilingual speakers commonly learn to use a set of interlinguistic rules of phonological and grammatical correspondences that permit a process of "creative borrowing" during an act of communication. If, for example, in using the native language, the speaker wishes to express a concept that is closely associated with activities or cultural values of the other language, an appropriate foreign word not usually borrowed by the bilingual community (e.g., *experienciar*) may be brought into play and incorporated into the communication by means of the productive rules of correspondence. Such creative borrowing provides an additional linguistic resource on which bilinguals may draw to enhance their communication.

Code alternation Code alternation, [14] too, is an active, creative process of incorporating material from both of a bilingual's languages into communicative acts. It involves the rapid and momentary shifting from the syntactic, lexical, and phonological system of one language into that of the other language. This alternating may occur many times within a single discourse and is not uncommon within single sentences. The rapidity and automaticity with which the alternations take place often give the impression that the speaker lacks control of the structural systems of the two languages and is mixing them indiscriminately. However, quite the contrary is true. Code alternation is most often engaged in by those bilingual speakers who are the most proficient in both of their languages. Moreover, as we shall see, code alternation itself obeys rather strict structural rules in addition to the grammatical rules of each of the component languages.

Many alternations within a single sentence involve the insertion of a word or a short phrase that makes reference to a single, unified notion. The following examples are taken from the speech of adults reported by Aurelio Espinosa (1971). Espinsoa recorded these forms using the conventional Spanish orthography for colloquial speech.

1. Ayer juimos a los *movies*. We went to the movies yesterday.
2. Comieron *turkey* pa' Chris- Did you eat turkey for Christmas?
   mas?

---

[14]This is often referred to in the literature as "code-switching." This term lacks precision, however, in that it can and does refer to a wide range of phenomena. We use "code alternation" here to refer to the alternate use of two languages by a given speaker within a single speaking turn.

3. No andes ai de *smart Alek.*   Don't go around as a smart aleck.
4. Vamos ir al *football game* y   We're going to go to the football
    después...   game, and then...

Code alternation may also involve entire phrases or clauses with a complex internal grammatical structure. For example,

5. He is doing the best he can   He is doing the best he can in or-
    pa' no quedarse atrás, pero   der not to be kept back, but
    lo van a fregar (Espinosa,   they're going to mess him up.
    1917).
6. Te digo que este dedo *has*   I'm telling you that this finger has
    been bothering me so much   been bothering me so much.
    (Lance, 1975).
7. Those are friends from Mex-   Those are friends from Mexico
    ico *que tienen chamaquitos*   who have little kids.
    (Gumperz and Hernández-
    Chávez, 1971).
8. The type of work he did   The type of work he did when he
    cuando trabajaba, he...what   worked, he...what...that I re-
    ...that I remember, *era re-*   member, he was an irrigator at
    gador at one time (Gumperz   one time.
    and   Hernández-Chávez,
    1971).

From the last example, we note that the languages may shift back and forth several times within a single sentence. Within each stretch of speech the grammatical structure is completely that of the particular language being used. (This includes forms such as *pa'* and *juimos* which, although they are nonstandard forms, adhere to monolingual adult grammatical norms). That is to say, the word orders, morphology, syntactic processes, etc., are all those of the language of the particular stretch of speech. Furthermore, the phonetic and pho-nological structure of a given unilingual segment is systematic and conforms to the structure of the language in question. At the point of alternation, the entire structure—syntactic, morphological phonologi-cal—shifts to that of the other language. Each unilingual segment thus retains an internal structural consistency that shows all of the complex grammatical and phonological characteristics of monolingual speech.

In addition to adhering to the linguistic structures of each of the component languages, code alternating utterances obey a set of inter-systemic wellformedness conditions. In essence, these refer to the fact that code alternation is not a random, uncontrolled process. Rather, alternations occur only at specific, definable syntactic junctures. For instance, in examples 5–8, above, we notice that alternations may occur at relative clause boundaries (e.g., *que tienen chamaquitas*), before adverbial clauses (e.g., *cuando trabajaba; pa' no quedarse atras*), at the beginnings of verb phrases (e.g., *has been bothering me so much*), as appositive elements (e.g., *that I remember*), etc. Alternations may also occur at other junctures: noun qualifiers, verb complements, parts of a noun phrase, the predicate portion of an equational sentence, all may be alternated (Gumperz and Hernández-Chávez, 1971).

Alternations that are made at unpermitted junctures are considered ungrammatical by persons proficient in code alternation (Aguirre, 1975). The exact specification of the restrictions on alternations will require further detailed investigation, but it is possible to make a few tentative observations. For example, constructions like the following are rejected by speakers as being ill formed, and have also not been observed to occur in natural code alternation:

que *have* chamaquitos	who have little kids
he *era regador*	he was an irrigator
cuando *did you arrive?*	when did you arrive?
lo puso debajo de *the sink*	he put it beneath the sink

Finally, we will observe that code alternation has a number of specific sociolinguistic functions. First, code alternation is used to symbolize ethnic identification. Persons who alternate languages do so only in speaking with other members of the group or to indicate (symbolic) acceptance of a nonmember into the group. Even in essentially unilingual conversations, in either language, the occasional use of such terms as *OK, you know, and then, ándale pues, ¡híjole!, digo,* etc. functions to symbolize the intraethnic character of the interaction.

Related to this usage are those situations in which code alternation functions to permit the precise expression of ethnically or culturally relevant information. For example, in the following sentences the alternations to Spanish express certain nuances of meaning that are not available to the speaker in English:

1. I got to thinking, *vacilando el punto este,* . . .   I got to thinking, mulling that point over . . .
2. And my uncle Sam *es el mas agabachado*   And my uncle Sam is the most Americanized.
3. There are no children in the   There are no children in the

<table>
<tr><td>neighborhood. Well, sí hay criaturas</td><td>neighborhood. Well, there are kids.</td></tr>
</table>

In example 1, the word *vacilando* connotes informality, the fact that the "mulling over" is the "the fun of it." *Agabachado* in example 2 not only means "Americanized," it also includes the idea of rejection of one's own *chicanismo*. And, in example 3, the word *criaturas* carries with it the implication of "Spanish-speaking children" rather than just any children.

In the last example, we see that the very act.of code alternation itself carries a potential meaning. *Criaturas*, by itself does not mean "Spanish-speaking children." But in example 3, the contrast of *criaturas* with *children* and the concomitant phrasal switch provides the term with an unmistakable nuance of meaning. The alternation from English to Spanish, then, not only functions as an ethnic marker, as described above, it also functions to symbolize those values that are most closely associated with the Spanish-speaking community. Two final examples illustrate this point.

a) In talking about who a certain friend's children play with, a speaker says, "With each other. *La señora trabaja en la canería orita*, you know." ("The mother works in the cannery now, you know.") the mother is a Spanish speaker and "working in the cannery" is a seasonal activity that is part of the local chicano community's social and economic system. Only chicana women work in this particular cannery. The switch to Spanish symbolizes all these values.

b) Reminiscing about the frustations of smoking, an exsmoker says, "I'd get desperate, *y ahi voy al basurero a buscar, a sacar,* you know." ("I'd get desperate, and there I go to the wastebasket to look for some, to get some, you know.") The juxtaposition of the two codes here is used with great stylistic effect in depicting the speaker's attitudes. The Spanish conveys a sense of personal feeling, even one of intimacy in revealing such a private act. We can compare these kinds of effects to the changes in intonation, loudness, rate of speech, vocabulary choice, etc., that occur in stylistic switching within a single language (Cook-Gumperz and Gumperz, 1976).

From all of the above examples, it becomes very clear that code alternation, far from constituting a breakdown of a bilingual's grammatical systems or being an uncontrolled and meaningless *Mischsprache*, is a systematic and meaningful mode of communication for many bilingual communities. It is not an abnormality in the speech of a child. To the contrary, code alternation represents the creative use of both of the languages by the bilingual community and by the child who is learning to become a bilingual. The learner uses code-alternation as a learning strategy (Hernández-Chávez, 1977b), and as he learns the usage norms within the community, also uses it to facilitate the total act of communication.

As we have seen in this chapter, the psycho- and sociolinguistic processes involved in becoming and being bilingual are many and intricate. These result in normally developing L2 structures that share many characteristics with those observed for first language learners, although of course, important distinctions are evident also. We have, in addition, discussed factors influencing the development of the child's native language, and have seen how the creative use by the bilingual of both languages is a normal consequence of being bilingual.

In order for such information to have maximum educational value, the knowledge acquired and the research results obtained must be incorporated into our attempts to develop appropriate diagnostic criteria, procedures, and instruments, or to evaluate existing ones. The next chapter focuses on this task, outlining briefly some important considerations in the measurement of language proficiency and language dominance in children who are becoming bilingual.

ACKNOWLEDGMENT

We are grateful to Maria Elena Sanchez of the Merced County (California) Office of Education for providing us with information and resource documents on the characteristics and needs of the population being served by hearing, language, and speech specialists in California.

REFERENCES

Aguirre, A. 1975. Judgments of grammaticality in Code-alternation by Chicano university students. Unpublished manuscript. Stanford University, Department of Sociology, Stanford, California.

d'Anglejan, A., and Tucker, G. R. 1975. The acquisition of complex English structures by adult learners. Lang. Learn. 25:281–296.

Benítez, C. 1970. A study of some non-standard English features in the speech of seventh grade Mexican Americans enrolled in a remedial reading program in an urban community of South Texas. Masters thesis, Texas A and I University, Kingsville, Tex.

Benton, R. 1964. Research into the English Language Difficulties of Maori School Children, 1963–1964. Maori Education Foundation, Wellington, New Zealand.

Brown, R. 1973. A First Language. Harvard University Press, Cambridge, Massachusetts.

Burling, R. 1959. Language development of a Garo- and English-speaking child. Word 15:45–68.

Burt, M., and Dulay, H. (eds.). 1975. New Directions in Second Language Learning, Teaching, and Bilingual Education. TESOL, Washington, D.C.

Burt, M., and Kiparsky, C. 1972. The Gooficon: A Repair Manual for English. Newbury House, Publishers, Rowley, Massachusetts.

Burt, M., Dulay, H., and Finocchiaro, M. 1977. Viewpoints on English as a Second Language. Regents Publishing Co., Inc., New York.

Burt, M., Dulay, H., and Hernández-Chávez, E. 1976. Bilingual Syntax Measure: Technical Handbook. The Psychological Corporation, New York.

California State Department of Education. 1975. California Administrative Code. Sacramento, California.

Carroll, J. 1977. Characteristics of successful second language learners. In: M. Burt, H. Dulay, and M. Finocchiaro (eds.), Viewpoints on English as a Second Language. Regents Publishing Co., Inc., New York.

Chomsky, C. 1969. The Acquisition of Syntax in Children Age 5 to 10. The MIT Press, Cambridge, Massachusetts.

Chomsky, N. 1965. Aspects of the Theory of Syntax. The MIT Press, Cambridge, Massachusetts.

Chomsky, N. 1975. Reflections on Language. Pantheon Books, Inc., New York.

Contreras, H. and Saporta, S. 1971. Phonological development in the speech of a bilingual child. In: J. Akin et al. (eds.), Language Behavior: A Book of Readings in Communication, pp. 280–294. Mouton, The Hague.

Cook-Gumperz, and Gumperz, J. 1976. Context in children's speech. In: Cook-Gumperz and J. Gumperz (eds.), Papers on language and context. Working Paper #46, Language Behavior Research Laboratory, University of California, Berkeley.

Dato, D. (ed.). 1976. Georgetown University Round Table on Languages and Linguistics. Georgetown University Press, Washington, D.C.

deVilliers, J., and deVilliers, P. 1973. A cross-sectional study of the acquisition of grammatical morphemes in child speech. J. Psycholinguistic Res. 2:267–278.

Dodson, C. J., Price, E., and Williams, L. T. (eds.). 1968. Towards Bilingualism. University of Wales Press, Cardiff.

Dulay, H., and Burt, M. 1973. Should we teach children syntax? Lang. Learn. 23:235–252.

Dulay, H., and Burt, M. 1974a. You can't learn without goofing: An analysis of children's second language errors. In: J. Richards (ed.), Error Analysis: Perspectives on Second Language Learning, pp. 95–123.

Dulay, H., and Burt, M. 1974b. Errors and strategies in child second language acquisition. TESOL Q. 8:129–136.

Dulay, H., and Burt, M. 1974c. Natural sequences in child second language acquisition. Lang. Learn. 24:37–53.

Dulay, H., and Burt, M. 1975a. Creative construction in second language learning and teaching. In: M. Burt and H. Dulay (eds), New Directions in Second Language Learning, Teaching, and Bilingual Education, pp. 21–32. TESOL, Washington, D.C.

Dulay, H., and Burt, M. 1975b. A new approach to discovering universals of child second language acquisition. In: Dato (ed.), pp. 209–233.

Dulay, H., and Burt, M. 1977. Remarks on creativity in language acquisition. In: M. Burt, H. Dulay, and M. Finocchiaro (eds.), Viewpoints on English as a Second Language. Regents Publishing Co., Inc., New York. (Reprinted in Ritchie, in press.)

Dulay, H., and Burt, M. 1978. Why Bilingual Education? A Summary of Research Findings (poster). Bloomsbury West, Inc., San Francisco.

Ervin-Tripp, S. 1974. Is second language learning like the first? TESOL Q. 8:111–127.

Espinosa, A. 1917. Speech mixture in New Mexico: The influence of the English language on New Mexican Spanish. In: H. M. Stephens and H. E. Bolton (eds.) The Pacific Ocean in History, pp. 408–428. New York. Published by the authors, (Reprinted in Hernández-Chávez, Cohen, and Beltramo, 1975, pp. 99–114.

Feldman, C., and Shen, M. 1971. Some language related cognitive advantages of bilingual five-year-olds. J. Genet. Psychol. 118:235–244.

Ferguson, C. A., Hyman, L. M., and Ohala, J. J. (eds.). 1975. Nasálfest: Papers from a Symposium on Nasals and Nasalization. Language Universals Project, Stanford University, Stanford.

Gillis, M., and Weber, R. 1976. The emergence of sentence modalities in the English of Japanese-speaking children. Lang. Learn. 26:77–94.

Gumperz, J. J., and Hernández-Chávez, E. 1971. Cognitive aspects of bilingual communication. In: W. H. Whitely (ed.), Language Use and Social Changes, pp. 111–125. Oxford University Press, London.

Haugen, E. 1953, 1956. Bilingualism in the Americas: A Bibliography and Research Guide. Publication of the American Dialect Society #26. University of Alabama Press, University, Alabama.

Heiler-Saavedra, B. 1966. An investigation of the causes of primary stress mislocation in the English speech of bilingual Mexican-American students. Masters thesis, University of Texas, El Paso.

Hernández-Chávez, E. 1972. Early code separation in the second language speech of Spanish-speaking children. Paper presented at the Stanford Child Language Research Forum, Stanford University, Stanford.

Hernández-Chávez, E. 1977a. The development of semantic relations in child second language acquisition. In: M. Burt, H. Dulay, and M. Finocchiaro (eds.), Viewpoints on English as a Second Language. Regents Publishing Co., Inc., New York.

Hernández-Chávez, E. 1977b. The Acquisition of Grammatical Structures by a Mexican American Child Learning English. Doctoral dissertation, University of California, Berkeley.

Hernández-Chávez, E., Cohen, A., and Beltramo, A. (eds.). 1975. El Lenguaje de los Chicanos: Regional and Social Characteristics of Language Used by Mexican Americans. Center for Applied Linguistics, Arlington, Virginia.

Hernández-Chávez, E., Vogel, I., and Clumeck, H. 1975. Rules, constraints and the simplicity criterion: An analysis based on the acquisition of nasals in Chicano Spanish. In: A. Ferguson, M. Hyman, and J. Ohala (eds.), Nasálfest: Papers from a Symposium on Nasals and Nasalization. Language Universals Project, Stanford University, Stanford.

Hymes, D. 1972. Towards Communicative Competence. University of Pennsylvania Press, Philadelphia.

Klima, E. S., and Bellugi, U. 1966. Syntactic regularities in the speech of children. In: J. Lyons and R. J. Wales (eds.), Psycholinguistic Papers, pp. 183–219. Edinburgh University Press, Edinburgh.

Krashen, S. D., Madden, C., and Bailey, N. 1975. Theoretical aspects of grammatical sequencing. In: M. Burt and H. Dulay (eds.), New Directions in Second Language Learning, Teaching, and Bilingual Education. pp. 44–54. TESOL, Washington, D.C.

Krashen, S. D. 1977. The monitor model of adult second language performance. In: M. Burt, H. Dulay, and M. Finocchiaro (eds.), Viewpoints on English as a Second Language. Regents Publishing Co., Inc., New York.

Krashen, S. D. Individual variation in the use of the monitor. In: Ritchie, W. (ed.). Second Language Acquisition Research: Issues and Implications. Academic Press, New York. In press.

Lyons, J., and Wales, R. J. (eds.). 1966. Psycholinguistic Papers. Edinburgh University Press, Edinburgh.

Major, R. C. 1976. One gramática or duas?: Phonological differentiation of a bilingual child. Paper presented at the LSA Summer Meeting, Oswego, New York.

Mazeika, E. J. 1971. A comparison of the phonologic development of a monolingual and a bilingual (Spanish-English) child. Paper presented at the Biennial Meeting of the Society for Research in Child Development, April, Minneapolis.

Milon, J. P. 1975. Dialect in the TESOL program: If you never you better. In: M. Burt and H. Dulay (eds.), pp. 159–167. New Directions in Second Language Learning, Teaching, and Bilingual Education. TESOL, Washington, D.C.

Milon, J. P. 1974. The development of negation in English by a second language learner. TESOL Q. 8:137–143.

Moskowitz, A. I. 1970. The two-year-old stage in English phonology. Language 46:426–441.

Naiman, N., Frohlich, M., and Stern, H. H. 1975. The Good Language Learner. Ontario Institute for Studies in Education, Toronto.

National Center for Education Statistics. 1975. Bureau of the Census Supplement to the July 1975 Current Population Survey (CPS). U.S. Government Printing Office, Washington, D.C.

National Center for Education Statistics. 1976. Bureau of the Census Supplement to the July 1975 Current Population Survey. U.S. Government Printing Office, Washington, D.C.

National Institute of Neurological Diseases and Stroke. 1967. Research Profile No. 4: Hearing, Language and Speech Disorders. U.S. Government Printing Office, Washington, D.C.

Ornstein, J. 1951. The archaic and the modern in the Spanish of New Mexico. Hispania 34:137–42. (Reprinted in Hernández-Chávez, Cohen, and Beltramo, 1975, pp. 6–12.

Phillips, N. Jr. 1975. Variations in Los Angeles Spanish phonology. In: E. Hernandez-Chavez, A. Cohen, and A. Beltramo, (eds.), El Lenguaje de los Chicanos: Regional and Social Characteristics of Language Used by Mexican Americans, pp. 52–60. Center for Applied Linguistics, Arlington, Virginia.

Preston, M.S., Yeni-Komshian, G., and Stark, R. E. 1967. Voicing in initial stop consonants produced by children in the prelinguistic period from different language communities. In: Annual Report, pp. 307–323. Neurocommunication Laboratory, The Johns Hopkins University School of Medicine.

Price, E. 1968. Early bilingualism. In: C. J. Dodson, E. Price, and L. T. Williams (eds.), Towards Bilingualism. University of Wales Press, Cardiff.

Ravem, R. 1974. The development of *wh*-questions in first and second language learners. In: J. C. Richards (ed.), Error Analysis: Perspectives on Second Language Learning, pp. 134–155. Longman Group Limited, London.

Richards, J. C. (ed.). 1974. Error Analysis: Perspectives on Second Language Learning. Longman Group Limited, London.

Ritchie, W. C. Second Language Acquisition Research: Issues and Implications. Academic Press, New York. In press.

Sawyer, J. B. 1959. Aloofness from Spanish influence in Texas English. Word 15:270–281.

Sawyer, J. B. 1970. Bilingualism in San Antonio, Texas. In: G. Gilbert (ed.), Texas Studies in Bilingualism: Spanish, French, German, Czech, Polish, Serbian, and Norwegian in the Southwest. Walter De Gruyter & Co., Berlin: pp. 18–41. (Reprinted in Hernández-Cháves, Cohen, and Beltramo, 1975, pp. 77–98.

Slobin, D. I. 1971. Psycholinguistics. Scott, Foresman and Co., Glenview, Ill.

Smith, D. M., and Shuy, R. W. (eds.). 1972. Sociolinguistics in Cross-cultural Analysis. Georgetown University Press, Washington, D.C.

Stockwell, P., and Bowen, J. 1965. The Sounds of English and Spanish. The University of Chicago Press, Chicago.

Venable, G. P. 1974. A Study of Second-Language Learning in Children. 641 M. Sc. (Appl.) II Project, McGill University. (Author now at Scottish Rite Institute for Childhood Aphasia, Department of Special Education, San Francisco State University, 1600 Holloway, San Francisco, California, 94132.)

Vildomec, V. 1963. Multilingualism. A. W. Sythoff, Leyden, The Netherlands.

Vogel, I. 1975. One system or two: An analysis of a two-year-old Romanian-English bilingual's phonology. In: Papers and Reports on Child Language Development No. 9, pp. 43–62. Linguistic Department, Stanford University.

Weinreich, U. 1953. Languages in Contact: Findings and Problems. Mouton & Co., The Hague. Seventh printing, 1970.

Whiteley, W. H. (ed.) 1971. Language Use and Social Change. Oxford University Press, London.

Williams, G. 1972. Some errors in English by Spanish-speaking Puerto Rican children. In: Language Research Report No. 6, pp. 85–102. Language Research Foundation. Cambridge, Massachusetts. (ERIC:ED 061 850).

Wolfram, W. 1972. Overlapping influence and linguistic assimilation in second generation Puerto Rican English (PRE). In: D. M. Smith and R. W. Shuy (eds.), Socialinguistics in Cross-cultural Analysis, pp. 15–46. Georgetown University Press, Washington, D.C.

Evaluation of Linguistic Proficiency in Bilingual Children

Marina K. Burt, Heidi C. Dulay,
and Eduardo Hernández-Chávez

CONTENTS

Inability to speak English proficiently is not a communicative disorder. Based upon their extensive work with bilingual individuals, Professors Burt, Dulay, and Hernández-Chávez reiterate that 7.6 million school children in the United States are affected by this discussion because they live in households in which languages other than English are spoken. This chapter discusses procedures for determining a child's language dominance and for placing the child on the normal continuum of bilingual development. Bilingual children must be assessed in both of their languages to determine language dominance. Recommended characteristics of examiners and constraints imposed by the test situation are explained. Recent significant legislation affecting the testing and placement of bilingual children is referenced (Nakano, 1977). Means of determining a home language-usage pattern (Home Language Questionnaire, 1976) are given. The authors note that this information may help explain "low" proficiency in one or the other language. Guided by results of appropriate testing, the normal bilingual child can be correctly placed in school and the child with a true linguistic deficiency can be identified. The psycho- and sociolinguistic aspects of bilingualism have only recently begun to attract widespread attention and these two chapters by Professors Burt, Dulay, and Hernández-Chávez represent a fine combination of the latest research and a practical application of that research.   —Eds.

In this chapter, "bilingual child" refers to any child who lives in a home where a first language other than English is spoken by one or more members of the household. The child's degree of bilingualism, then, may range from a point approximating monolingualism—in which a child may only comprehend the most basic syntax and vocabulary in one language but be able to speak another fluently—to a state of "balanced" bilingualism, in which the child's proficiency in both languages is equally high.

As was mentioned in the preceding chapter, more than 7.6 million school age children in the United States live in households in which languages other than English are spoken, in addition to the 17.7 million who are 19 years old or older living in such households (Waggoner, 1976). Table 1 gives the statistics for the largest language groups, as well as a combined category of "other languages."

Although the "official" number of United States bilingual households has grown exponentially in recent decades, the development of diagnostic criteria, procedures, and instruments to evaluate linguistic proficiency in bilingual children has not kept commensurate pace. Perhaps the major obstacle to this type of applied linguistic research and materials development has been the theoretical about-face in linguistics begun only 2 decades ago. The advent of transformational generative grammar, which gave creativity a central role in theories of language acquisition and language use, has necessitated an immense amount of theoretical reorientation and reanalysis. Principles of habit formation have steadily given way to notions of cognitive creativity on the part of the learner engaged in the processes of first and second language acquisition (See "Second Language Acquisition" in the preceding chapter). Consequently, most of the efforts of the last decade have focused on the basic research necessary to lay a firm foundation

Table 1. Persons in United States households where languages other than English are spoken

Household language	Number of persons (thousands)		
	Total [a]	Ages 4–18	Age 19+
	25,344	7,667	17,677
Spanish	9,904	3,803	6,100
Italian	2,836	667	2,168
German	2,269	587	1,680
French	2,259	666	1,595
Chinese	534	142	392
Japanese	524	150	374
Greek	488	137	352
Pilipino	377	143	234
Portuguese	349	103	246
Korean	246	90	156
Other languages	5,559	1,179	4,380

Adapted from Waggoner (1976).

[a] Columns may not add to given totals because of rounding.

for diagnostic procedures and educational approaches for bilingual children. The results of that research, for the most part, are not yet reflected in existing diagnostic instruments and procedures. The preceding chapter therefore summarized the basic research findings to date that seem to be most relevant to diagnosing the language and speech of bilingual children.

Despite the lack of applied research on bilingualism, demands for materials with which to test bilingual children have increased dramatically. Each year brings added legal requirements for bilingual assessment in the form of state and federal legislation or judicial decisions. In addition, the options now available to children to learn subject matter in a language other than English—an opportunity afforded by bilingual education—have necessitated new and more comprehensive techniques of linguistic diagnosis to place children at an appropriate point along a normal continuum of bilingual development.

Because so little high quality material is available on the diagnosis of normal bilingual development, and because, so often, available testing and evaluation procedures erroneously assume that English is the only appropriate language for diagnosis, normal bilingual children are often misclassified as mentally retarded or language handicapped.

Not demonstrating proficiency in English is not a communicative disorder. Only if the child demonstrates low proficiency in both languages should the child be referred for further diagnosis, and even then it is the responsibility of the diagnostician to make sure that the demonstrated low proficiency is not attributable to biased instruments, the use of inappropriate dialectal norms in scoring, or circumstances that stifle a child's verbal initiative in either language. On the other hand, we must not permit the child's bilingualism to obscure real disorders, allowing them to go by unnoticed and untreated.

In this chapter, therefore, we focus again, as in the preceding chapter, on normal bilingual development, so that the detection of abnormal development in bilingual children might be accomplished more accurately. Whereas the preceding chapter described actual characteristics of bilingual development, this chapter deals with procedures for determining where a child is along the bilingual developmental continuum.

DIMENSIONS OF BILINGUAL MEASUREMENT

Perhaps the most obvious difference in evaluating the overall linguistic proficiency of monolingual and bilingual children is that the latter must be assessed in two languages; that is, proficiency in both the native language and English must be determined. For example, when a child's oral performance is below that demonstrated by his or her agemates on a given measure of English proficiency, it does not necessarily follow that the child has a learning disorder, even if the child has lived in the United States for a number of years. Only an assessment of the child's performance in the native language as well as in English would reveal the child's overall linguistic proficiency.

"Language dominance," one of the most widely evaluated aspects of the linguistic proficiency of bilinguals, refers to the relative proficiency of a child in two languages. To determine a child's language dominance, the child must be assessed separately in, for instance, English, and the native language. Moreover, the testing instruments (or versions of the same instrument) must measure parallel aspects of the two languages: both must test, for example, syntax production or some other aspect of language. It is not valid to test for vocabulary in one language and syntax in the other, and hope to be able to determine dominance adequately. Dominance involves a number of parameters including lexicon, syntactic proficiency, control of phonological systems, fluency, communicative skills, and so forth. Dominance in one of the parameters does not imply dominance in the others. A child may demonstrate dominance in one aspect of the first language, as well as in another aspect of the second language. For example, a child's command of the phonological system of the first language may be greater than that of the second, but the child may have a larger active school vocabulary in the second language than in the first. It is important, therefore, to know which aspect(s) of the language are of interest for particular diagnostic purposes, and whether instruments are available that measure those aspects in a parallel fashion.

Language dominance information may be used for a variety of purposes by school personnel. Besides being part of census information legally required of school districts and typically reported by program evaluators, language dominance is crucial to the placement of children in appropriate classes and to the determination of further testing needs. For example, if a Mexican-American child were English dominant, that child would not be placed in a Spanish reading class, but in an English reading class; whereas a balanced bilingual kindergartener might take reading in Spanish first, then after learning the basic reading skills, continue in both languages. If a child demonstrated low proficiency in both languages, retesting or further diagnosis would be required. (See "Summary of Diagnostic Procedures and Post-diagnostic Steps" for further discussion.) Thus, dominance testing of bilingual children is a crucial first step in determining both normal and abnormal levels of language development.

It is also possible, of course, to assess the development of one language alone and put the results to good use. For example, if a child has been assessed as Spanish dominant, a teacher might want to know the child's level of English proficiency in order to place the child in an appropriate group for English instruction. Likewise, knowing the level of a child's Spanish proficiency would assist the teacher in placing the child in an appropriate Spanish instructional group.

In addition to language dominance and language proficiency, it is also extremely useful to identify "home language usage patterns," i.e., the dominant pattern of language use in the homes of students whose linguistic and cultural background is other than English. Many times, knowledge of the amount of use of English and another language in the child's home environment along with information about who uses which language, helps clarify the results obtained from dominance and proficiency testing. For example, if a child lives in a home where English is used predominantly and only the child's grandmother speaks Spanish, it is likely that the child will not be very proficient in Spanish, and will be English dominant. Likewise, if the child has no English-speaking friends or siblings, (as in the case of migrants whose transient way of life may not permit the formation of lasting school friendships), it is possible that his or her English proficiency may not be on a par with that of age-mates for whom English is also a second language and who have lived in the United States the same amount of time. Especially for speech and language specialists, therefore, information on home language usage patterns may reveal reasons for "low" proficiency in one or the other language, and may indicate how the school can best complement the child's linguistic environment at home.

In addition, information on home language-usage patterns will assist the speech therapist and other school personnel in determining which activities parents can conduct at home to help their children either progress in regular school work or overcome a communicative disorder. For example, if it is known that the child's household is a "dual language" household in which both English and, say, Cantonese are spoken in approximately equal amounts, then it would be possible to plan home assistance activities in either language. On the other hand if a child's home is found to be a predominantly Catonese-speaking household, then parental assistance might be requested for activities that can be conducted in Cantonese.

Table 2 summarizes the four dimensions in the linguistic evaluation of bilingual children just discussed, and the uses to which each may be put.

SOME GENERAL GUIDELINES FOR EVALUATING
ORAL LANGUAGE PROFICIENCY AND DOMINANCE TESTS

As we have seen in the previous sections, the psycho- and sociolinguistic aspects of becoming bilingual have just begun to attract fairly widespread attention. Because of the recency of this interest there has not been sufficient time to develop many instruments that incorporate the research findings concerning the development of the second language, the first language, and the interaction of the two described in the preceding chapter. Thus, rather than list the existing instruments to measure linguistic proficiency, most of which have been developed locally by school districts for their own use, and nearly all of which were developed before or independently of the availability of the re-

Table 2. Uses of language testing information

Linguistic dimension measured	Purpose
Language dominance (oral)	1. Placement for reading and subject matter instruction in a bilingual program. 2. Information required by the *Lau* Remedies[a] 3. Information may be required by state law, e.g., California 4. Program evaluation 5. First step in diagnosis for further testing needs of bilingual children
Home language usage pattern	1. Information required by the *Lau* Remedies[a] 2. Information may be required by state law, e.g., California 3. Provides information for teacher or speech clinician to help explain children's linguistic performance and to plan instructional or therapeutic programs
English proficiency (oral)	1. Placement in appropriate oral English instruction level 2. Determination of readiness to begin English reading instruction 3. Program evaluation
Other language proficiency (oral)	1. Placement in appropriate other language oral instructional group 2. Determination of readiness to begin reading instruction in the other language 3. Program evaluation

[a]The "Lau Remedies" are guidelines issued by the Office for Civil Rights to assist school districts in meeting the compliance standards set forth by the *Lau* versus *Nichols* decision of the United States Supreme Court (414 U.S.C. 563, 1974). See Nakano (1977) for a detailed discussion of the educational implications of the *Lau* decision.

search findings discussed, we instead offer some general criteria for evaluating oral proficiency tests or procedures used to measure language dominance. These guidelines reflect both the research results discussed in the preceding chapter and our current state of knowledge concerning oral language testing for bilingual children. We do not intend these guidelines to be exhaustive, but rather to serve as partial criteria for evaluating oral proficiency instruments.

**Parts of Language Dominance Test That
Assess Each Language Must not be Translations of Each Other**

When one compares the grammar of any given two languages, numerous differences may be observed in various surface aspects of the languages. For example, the morphology of Spanish includes gender markings on articles and adjectives: *la manzana roja* requires the feminine article *la* (as opposed to the masculine *el*) and the feminine marker on the adjective *roja* (as opposed to the masculine *rojo*), because the head noun is feminine. One of the rules to be acquired by learners of Spanish therefore, is gender agreement on articles and adjectives when these modify nouns. In the case of English, no such gender agreement for articles and adjectives exists. Thus, the question or item used to elicit a response such as *la manzana roja* that is designed to see whether a child has acquired gender agreement in Spanish would not be useful in the evaluation of English proficiency. (In *the red apple, the* and *red* do not change their form when the head noun *apple* changes to some other noun, e.g., *flower*.) Alternatively, one may wish to test a child's control of the *do/did* distinction in certain English constructions (e.g., *Yesterday she do/did not go out*). Because the *do* auxiliary does not exist in other languages, the English question used to elicit it would not yield useful information about another language were it translated.

These examples, any many others like them, demonstrate why the different language versions of a dominance test must not be simple translations of each other. The linguistic structures of languages differ, and structural distinctions made in one language may not be the same as those in another. The corresponding language sections used in a dominance test must therefore be based on the syntax (or phonology, etc.) of the particular language being tested. In some cases, of course, there will be similarities across languages for some structures, e.g., plural formation for nouns in English and Spanish (*window-s, ventana-s*). In those cases similar questions may be used to elicit analogous structures. Such similarities must be determined before construction of the test items in each language, however, so that items accurately reflect the structures and their development in a given language.

**Content of Language Measure Must not be Outside
the Child's Experience or Cultural Customs and Values**

In order not to confound linguistic proficiency and knowledge of the world, the content of a language measure (the concepts and activities depicted in the pictures or referred to in questions) must not be outside the experience of the children being tested, or inconsistent with their cultural customs and values. For example, a northern winter scene might include pictures of skis, sleds, a snowman, and a snowball fight. If such pictures are included as stimuli, children who have never experienced a northern winter would be penalized unfairly when they are unable to answer questions based on these unfamiliar things. Likewise, a green banana represents an unripe banana to some children, but to others it represents a variety of banana used for cooking. Thus, if the target descriptors to be scored for green and yellow bananas include *unripe* and *ripe,* some children would be unfairly penalized: their failure to include the desired descriptors would not be caused by a language deficiency but to a perception of bananas that is different from the test constructor's. Likewise, children who are unfamiliar with penguins will not be able to answer correctly questions such as "Do penguins waddle?". Responses to test items that rely on unfamiliar content or that assume only one of several possible interpretations do not reflect general language ability, but merely indicate the child's exposure to that particular content.

Responses Required by Test Items
Must not Violate Conventions of Natural Discourse

If a complete sentence is required (for a perfect item score), then questions to which a single word is a natural response must not be used. For example, a question such as "Who is this?" may be, and often is, answered with just a name or a simple noun phrase. Similarly, questions such as "Is this a pencil?" are typically answered by native speakers of English with a simple "yes" or "no" rather than with "Yes, this is a pencil" or "Yes, it is." Yet, many language tests require children to produce complete sentences in response to such items in order for the response to be scored as correct or to be scorable at all. Clearly, such requirements result in eliciting artificial rather than natural speech. It is unfair to penalize children for their failure to produce complete sentences when the test questions fail to elicit them naturally. Language elicitation tasks are discussed more fully under "Oral Language Elicitation Tasks," below.

Distinction Must be Made Between
Quantity and Quality of Children's Responses

The use of open-ended questions such as "Tell me all you can about this picture" tends to obscure the critical distinction between quantity and quality, because some children respond enthusiastically to such a question, spinning endless tales, while others give limited responses in order to avoid saying something wrong (Labov et al., 1968; Cazden, 1972). When children are not familiar or comfortable with the examiner, or if they are not certain of what is being asked, they will tend to give short and limited responses (often followed by a nervous "right?"). Open-ended and imprecise questions lead to rewards for superficial verbosity and to penalties for those children who are less talkative or shy (especially with strangers), or who do not understand the intent of the question. Ironically, children who are more advanced linguistically may be penalized for short but appropriate responses in these situations. "Tell me all you can" questions may confuse language proficiency with the child's comprehension of the task, attention to detail in a picture, ability to create a story, or volubility; unless, of course, these factors do not affect the scoring of a child's response. For example, an error analysis of the speech sample (rather than measures of utterance length or frequency of any given constituent) would be a valid means of assessing such a speech protocol. (See "A Note on L1 'Interference'" in the preceding chapter for further discussion of error analysis).

Age and Grade Norms Cannot Be Used in Interpreting Bilingual Test Scores

The interpretive framework of language tests for bilingual children cannot follow the norm-referenced approach of interpreting pupil performance in relation to specific age or grade reference groups, unless length and type of exposure to the target language can be incorporated into the norms. That is, neither the kind of English nor length of exposure to English a child receives is predictable by the age or grade of the child. For example, a second grader in the United States who has hardly been exposed to English cannot be expected to have reached the average level of English proficiency attained by other second graders who have been exposed to English normally all their lives. Likewise, second graders whose bilingual parents choose to speak English at home cannot be expected to maintain Spanish proficiency to the same degree as children whose parents speak to them in Spanish most of the time.

The inclusion of language exposure variables into age and grade norms would be extremely complicated, if not impossible. At present, norms including these crucial variables do not exist. The research required is extremely complex and has only recently begun. Type of exposure to a target language includes variables such as the use of the language at home by parents and siblings, interaction with peers who speak the target language fluently, use of the language in the neighborhood, and even the amount of television viewing. These factors vary from community to community as well as from child to child, making it extremely difficult to obtain meaningful norms in the traditional sense.

In view of these complex problems in establishing age and grade norms for the language proficiency of bilingual children, it seems that non-normal language functioning is most clearly indicated by a child's poor performance (low scores) on tests of proficiency in both first and second languages. For example, on the *Bilingual Syntax Measure* (BSM), a child's proficiency level may range from a low of Level 1 to a high of Level 5 in either the first or second language. A child who scores in Level 3 ("survival" level) or lower in both languages assessed is classified in the "Special Diagnosis" category, rather than in any one of the normal bilingual categories. (In most of the normal categories of bilingual development, proficiency in one language is at least one level lower than the other, "balanced bilingualism" being the only exception.)

In addition to the above discussed considerations, much rethinking has gone into the issue of what among the various aspects or parts of language should be—and can validly be—tested. The following section summarizes those considerations.

SPECIFIC ASPECTS OF LANGUAGE TO BE TESTED

In this section we focus on four aspects of language that have been most commonly assessed by language proficiency and dominance instruments, or that are usually included in second language curricula: vocabulary, pronunication, syntax (including morphology), and functional use. Advantages and disadvantages of each as indicators of general language development in bilingual children are discussed.

Vocabulary

One of the most traditional ways of measuring verbal ability is the vocabulary test. The assumption is made, either explicitly or implicitly, that children for whom vocabulary tests are appropriate will have had those experiences that provide occasions for learning certain vocabulary items, certain thinking skills, and other linguistic skills that correlate highly with range of vocabulary. Vocabulary tests are thus most appropriate for testing groups that have had homogeneous experiences.

But contemporary educational needs call for a test that is appropriate for children from heterogeneous cultural, social, and linguistic backgrounds, and whose languages have been learned in diverse environments. Because word knowledge is a function of experience, there is no assured body of vocabulary to which all these children will have been exposed. Regional vocabulary differences, for example, often include just the common, familiar lexicon that appears in elementary tests of language proficiency; and more often than not, it is just these words that are likely to differ from region to region and between the standard and the local variety. For example, in Spanish the words for *hat, jacket, banana, beans, peas, cooking, shaving, driving,* and hundreds more will find different expression depending upon the locale and the mode of use. For a heterogeneous population, therefore, the use of vocabulary as an indicator of language development penalizes some children from not having been exposed to the "right" vocabulary.

Nevertheless, the growth of a child's vocabulary is indeed a necessary part of linguistic development, and consequently, an important part of a language curriculum. In order to fairly and accurately assess a bilingual child's lexical progress, criterion-referenced instruments developed for particular groups of children would be the most appropriate assessment tool. Such tests would be school achievement tests rather than tests of intelligence or general linguistic development.

Pronunciation

Although pronunciation is a commonly measured aspect of language, it has serious drawbacks if it is used as a major indicator of normal bilingual development. There is a great deal of variability in pronunciation across idiolects and dialects, not only in the second language, but in the first as well. For example, in Spanish there are numerous variant pronunciations according to county and region. (We refer here to the standard language only. Additional differences exist when we consider variation in social dialects.) Not only do many of the individual sounds differ, there are important differences in intonational phenomena. Particularly important are pitch and rate of speech differences, as well as certain junctural phenomena such as [ʔ] (glottal stop) or velarization of /n/. (We might compare these kinds of pronunciation differences to those between Midwestern American speakers and native English speakers, from, say, New Delhi or Aukland.)

Furthermore, it is not uncommon that a bilingual maintains a "foreign accent" in the second language, even when native-like syntactic and lexical proficiency have been achieved.

Extreme care must be taken therefore, not to confound *differences* in pronunciation with *difficulties* requiring remediation. Accent is more often an indicator of regional background, socio-economic status, and ethnic or peer group affiliation than of general language proficiency. In particular, bilingual speech communities have norms of pronunciation for both languages that may differ from those used by monolingual speakers of either language. (See "L1 Development and Interaction with L2" in the preceding chapter.)

Functional Use

Another aspect of language consists of its functional uses: asking questions, giving commands, making promises or apologies, addressing superiors, etc. Although these forms are a basic part of communication, they are difficult to elicit systematically, efficiently, and naturally from large numbers of children. It is almost impossible, for example, to elicit a sincere apology without saying something artificial such as "please apologize to (somebody) for (something)." Creating situations in which almost any child would feel naturally compelled to apologize in a given way (in order for the test to measure the same speech act) is also most difficult, if not impossible. Because of differences in environment and social custom, it is not possible to construct the number of natural situations that would be required to test knowledge of such speech acts or discourse rules. Furthermore, there are many acceptable ways to execute a speech act, depending upon the speaker's culture and various features of the sociolinguistic context.

Assessment difficulties caused by intergroup variability are especially prominent in the case of a multicultural population spanning a wide socioeconomic range, such as that with which we are concerned. As was mentioned for vocabulary, however, learning the fuctional uses of linguistic structures comprises an important component of language development. This aspect of linguistic development might be assessed more fairly and accurately by criterion-referenced instruments designed for a particular locale or curriculum.

Syntax

This aspect of language is usually referred to as the structural backbone of any language. In broad terms, syntax may be defined as the system of rules for the arrangement, inter-relationship and form of words, phrases, and sentences in a language. Of the various aspects of a particular language, syntax shows the least variation among speakers of the language. For example, one does not typically find that the position of morphological endings or constituents changes in different geographical regions. For example, *The dog ate it* does not change to *Dog the ate it* or any other possible combination of those words anywhere in the United States. For most of syntax, we are assured that children have not had variable exposure. Where variation does exist, it is systematic and can therefore be incorporated into the interpretive system of language instruments.

Most research in child second language acquisition has focused on syntax. As a result, descriptions of syntactic developmental sequences that obtain across groups of children from diverse language backgrounds and learning environments are available. (See "Acquisition Order in L2 Syntax and Morphology" and "Acquisition Order in L2 Semantics" in the preceding chapter.) These, along with information on common error types, provide invaluable input for the assessment of language development in bilinguals. (*The Bilingual Syntax Measure* is the only test to date that incorporates syntactic and morphological developmental sequences into its levels of proficiency.)

For these reasons, syntax seems to be the most suitable aspect of a language to rely upon in the evaluation of general linguistic proficiency of bilingual multicultural children. Of course, in relying primarily on syntax, other aspects of language are excluded. But this may be unavoidable when one is interested in a fair and reliable indicator of general language development in normal bilinguals.

ORAL LANGUAGE ELICITATION TASKS

Of the four language skills—comprehension (listening), production (speaking), reading, and writing—production is the most commonly used mode for determining the linguistic dominance and proficiency of bilingual children. In this section, therefore, we focus on the types of tasks used to elicit oral language for purposes of assessment.

Most tasks used to elicit speech samples or verbal responses may be grouped according to the presence or absence of a communicative focus. Accordingly, we label them "natural communication" tasks and "linguistic manipulation" tasks, respectively. A natural communication task is one in which the focus of the child is on communicating something to someone else—an idea, some information, or an opinion, etc.—in a natural manner. In such situations the child unconsciously uses the grammar rules acquired to convey the message. For example, a question such as *Why do you think he's so fat?* (asked by an examiner while pointing to a fat character) elicits an opinion or idea from the child that is directed toward that specific situation. The resulting speech is produced by the child with no conscious focus on its linguistic form. The speech is only offered in order to communicate the child's opinion to the examiner.

On the other hand, in a linguistic manipulation task the focus of the child is on performing the conscious linguistic manipulation required by the task. For example, asking a child to transform *No one was here* into a *yes/no* question requires manipulation of the elements in the sentence; however, the activity in itself does not serve any communicative functions for the child. Rather, the child is consciously focusing on the linguistic rules required to perform the operation requested, an activity that is rarely part of natural communication.

In sum, natural communication tasks permit one to make statements concerning the child's normally developing (and unconscious) grammar, whereas linguistic manipulation tasks permit one to make statements concerning the child's metalinguistic awareness, i.e., the conscious knowledge of and manipulation of the rules and forms of a language.

In this section we present common examples of both types of tasks. Natural communication tasks include structured and non-structured communication (see Tables 3 and 4), while linguistic manipulation tasks include imitation, translation, substitution, completion, etc. (see Table 3 and "Linguistic Manipulation Tasks").

Table 3 provides a comparison of natural communication and linguistic manipulation tasks in terms of their definitions, and advantages and disadvantages with regard to their appropriateness and efficacy as indicators of linguistic proficiency.

Natural Communication Tasks

Table 4 compares two major types of natural communication tasks: structured and nonstructured. As the table is self-explanatory, we need not discuss it further.

Linguistic Manipulation Tasks

Generally speaking, as mentioned in Table 3, linguistic manipulation tasks share at least one major deficiency when used as indicators of general linguistic proficiency, namely, they require child behaviors

Table 3. Comparison of two major types of oral language elicitation tasks: natural communication and linguistic manipulation

	Natural communication	Linguistic manipulation
Definition	1. Taps child's unconscious use of grammatical rules to produce utterances in a conversation 2. Uses natural speech where child's focus is on communicating something	1. Taps child's conscious application of linguistic rules to perform a non-communicative task 2. Uses artificial "speech" where child's focus is on a given rule
Some types	1. Structured communication, nonstructured communication, etc. (See Table 4)	1. Imitation, translation, completion, transformation, substitution, etc.
Advantages	1. The language sample obtained represents natural communication the skill that is ultimately being assessed 2. The task is virtually free of confounding task biases	1. Target structure seem to be readily obtained
Disadvantages	1. Certain structures are extremely difficult to elicit naturally, e.g., perfect tenses (*had seen*)	1. Confounds conscious knowledge and use of grammar rules with ability to use the language normally

that are not typical of natural language use. They are therefore severely limited as general proficiency or dominance indicators. Below we briefly describe two of the most commonly used tasks, together with any particular advantages or disadvantages, if any.

Imitation The child repeats an item or sequence of words, sounds, phrases, or sentences after a model. Imitation tasks may reveal some structures the child does not yet control and may provide information about the child's short term auditory memory. On the other hand, imitation tasks do not permit inferences about what structures the child controls, because children imitate structures and forms in imitation situations that they do not control in nonimitation

Table 4. Comparison of structured and nonstructured communication tasks

	Structured communication	Nonstructured communication
Definition	Natural conversation between child and examiner in which examiner asks child specific questions designed to elicit target structures naturally and systematically	Natural conversation between child and examiner or other person where there is no intent to elicit specific structures
Advantages	Target structures may be elicited selectively and quickly; more efficient than nonstructured communication	Structures that are difficult to elicit with specific questions may be offered by subjects spontaneously
Disadvantages	Not all structures are easily elicited, e.g., *yes/no* questions	A great deal of speech must usually be collected before a sufficient range of structures is used by the child to permit assessment of linguistic proficiency One cannot make any statements about the child's control over structures not offered during the collection period (because one cannot be certain why a structure was not offered, i.e., whether the situations did not require it or whether the child did not know it)

situations. (e.g., A child may repeat something correctly in class but use it on the playground incorrectly). Imitation may also confound memory span with linguistic proficiency. For example, a proficient child may err in repeating a sequence of words (or sounds, etc.) just heard because of a short memory span, rather than low proficiency. Likewise, children with longer memory spans, but who are not yet proficient, may be able to imitate a sequence of words accurately, obscuring an actually lower level of proficiency.

Translation   The child provides another language equivalent of an utterance provided. Translation may encourage one-to-one correspondence from the child's first language to the second, which results in certain errors. This problem is especially obvious in timed translation tasks, where the first step for many words is word matching. When time does not permit the student to reorganize the translation to "sound natural," an erroneous impression of the child's proficiency in the target language is given.

Summary

The tasks presented here are merely representative, not inclusive. Our focus has been to distinguish two basic types of tasks: those that focus on natural communication and those that don't. Nearly all linguistic proficiency and dominance tasks measuring syntax production are comprised of various combinations of linguistic manipulation tasks. They are simply too numerous to list here. Among the very few that focus on communication tasks are the *Basic Inventory of Natural Language* (BINL, English and Spanish) available from Chess and Associates, San Bernadino, California, and the *Bilingual Syntax Measure* (BSM, English, Spanish and Pilipino) from Psychological Corporation, New York, New York. The BINL represents a *free communication* task (taping children in a number of sessions over several days to obtain natural speech for analysis and scoring), and the BSM represents a *structured communication* task (10–15 min of structured conversation and scoring per child).

As interest in the measurement of general linguistic proficiency and dominance grows, we may expect there to be a commensurate amount of research directed toward discovering more ways to measure a child's ability to communicate normally in diverse situations. Because we are, after all, interested in assessing normal communicative skills (rather than in predicting who might become a good linguist), this is a long overdue area of focus. Tasks required of children must be representative of the kind of knowledge and skills we attempt to measure.

EXAMINER CHARACTERISTICS

In the evaluation of bilingual proficiency, the linguistic characteristics of the examiner assume a critical role. The examiner's own proficiency in the language(s) being evaluated, knowledge of the particular variety that the child speaks, and familiarity with sociocultural values and customs of the child's community can all affect the validity of the evaluative process. On the other hand, the examiner need not possess any specific credentials or academic degrees to administer or score language proficiency or dominance tests competently. However, adequate training in the administration and scoring of the tests is required. A summary of general examiner qualifications follows:

1. Full oral proficiency in the language(s) being assessed. If more than one language is being evaluated and if testing is conducted in each language separately two different examiners may test the child: one for each language. For example, an examiner who is fluent in English would administer the English instrument while the one is fluent in, for instance, Portuguese, would administer the Portuguese instrument. However, if a dominance test requires the use of two languages during a single testing session, the examiner must be bilingual, that is, fully proficient in both languages.
2. Proficiency in reading and writing the language(s) assessed is required when the instruments incorporate those skills in administration or scoring procedures, e.g., an examiner may have to write down a child's verbal responses.
3. The dialect of the target language spoken by the examiner during the testing session must be close as possible to that with which the child is most familiar.
4. Adequate training in the administration and scoring of the instruments to be used.

SUMMARY OF DIAGNOSTIC PROCEDURES AND POST DIAGNOSTIC STEPS

1. Evaluate the child's linguistic proficiency for both of the child's languages.
2. Compare the obtained level of proficiency in each language to determine dominance.
3. If the proficiency level in both languages is below what is normal for monolingual development in either language, the child should be further diagnosed. Three steps are recommended:
   a. Diagnose for possible communicative disorders in hearing, language, and speech. If an instrument in the test battery or subtest in an instrument requires language-specific performance, it must be administered in both languages.

b. Obtain information on the home language usage pattern in the child's household (see "Dimensions of Bilingual Measurement" above) and on the child's attitudes towards speaking each language.

c. Depending on the results of a and b above, a therapeutic program may be recommended. Parents may be involved in the program, performing activities required in either English or another language depending on the child's needs and the linguistic preferences of the parents.

4. If the child falls within the range of normal bilingual development, place the child in the most appropriate educational program for bilingual children available in the school. (See *Bilingual Syntax Measure*: *Manual* for placement recommendations for bilingual children of varying degrees of linguistic proficiency in English and Spanish.)

Types of educational models appropriate to bilingual children are varied and complex. Not only must one consider the linguistic dominance of the population whose educational needs are being served, but the cultural and social values of the communities within the school district. In addition, considerations regarding available resources—qualified, well trained staff, materials, and financial resources are necessary ingredients of sound educational planning. All of these, taken together, will help determine for a given school district the types and extent of bilingual programs provided.

In this chapter we have provided a brief overview of the needs, rationale, and methods of evaluating the linguistic proficiency of bilingual children. We have presented this information in order to help prevent potential misclassification of bilingual children, as well as to inform the hearing, language, and speech specialist generally about the nature and method of assessing linguistic proficiency and dominance in bilingual children.

In the two chapters on the linguistic characteristics and assessment of bilingual children we hope to have alerted the numerous and dedicated members of the speech, hearing, and language profession to the great need for their assistance, both in accurately diagnosing speech disorders in bilingual children, and in preventing the misclassification of bilinguals by untrained personnel. We are confident that the meaningful instructional alternatives now available for normal bilingual children, provided through bilingual education, will be a welcome educational breakthrough for all those in the United

States who work closely with children who speak a first language other than English.

REFERENCES

Burt, M., Dulay, H., and Finocchiaro, M. 1977. Viewpoints on English as a Second Language. Regents Publishing Co., Inc., New York.
Burt, M., Dulay, H., and Hernández-Chávez, E. 1976. Bilingual Syntax Measure: Technical Handbook. The Psychological Corporation, New York.
Cazden, C. 1972. Child Language and Education. Holt, Rinehart & Winston, New York.
Labov, W., Cohen, P., Robins, C., and Lewis, J. 1968. A Study of the Non-Standard English of Negro and Puerto Rican Speakers in New York City. Final Report of Cooperative Research Project No. 3288, Columbia University. [Available through ERIC.]
Nakano, P. J. 1977. Educational implications of the Lau v. Nichols decision. In: M. Burt, H. Dulay, and M. Finocchiaro (eds.), Viewpoints on English as a Second Language. Regents Publishing Co., Inc., New York.
Waggoner, D. 1976. NCES' survey of languages. Linguistic Reporter 19(3): 5–7.

INSTRUMENTS REFERRED TO IN THIS CHAPTER:

Bilingual Syntax Measure (English, Spanish, and Pilipino). 1975. The Psychological Corporation, New York.
Bilingual Inventory of Natural Languages (English and Spanish). 1975. Chess and Associates, San Bernardino, California.
Home Language Questionnaire (English, Spanish, Pilipino, Chinese, Vietnamese, and Cambodian). 1976. Available from Bloomsbury West, 545 Sansome, San Francisco, Cal. 94111.

Evaluation of Linguistic Disorders in Children

Joan Lynch

CONTENTS

Until recent years there has been a paucity of procedures capable of separating children with linguistic disorders according to their primary problem as well as their language level. This has been the case in part because: 1) the linguistic theories have obtained data primarily from the normal domain, and 2) the etiologic theories have developed almost exclusively from medical and psychological research on defective populations. An application of a well substantiated linguistic theory is extremely productive for a wider appeal of the theory and a better diagnosis of the linguistic disorder. Professor Lynch's treatise on evaluation of linguistic disorders in children starts with a very informative walk through history starting from 1853 to the present. It then presents a comprehensive treatment of linguistic, psycholinguistic, sociolinguistic, and neurolinguistic factors that have become necessary ingredients of a good differential evaluation of linguistic disorders. This chapter invests major effort in presenting a much needed blend of practical information such as examiners' qualifications and test environment and theoretical considerations pertaining to test selection and development of procedures and profiles for differential assessment of linguistic disorders. The section on test selection is endowed with a comprehensive discussion of tests and the section on linguistic assessment incorporates a thorough understanding of current linguistic theory and psycholinguistic research, e.g., Brown (1973) and Crystal (1976).   —S.S.

The failure of a young child to develop language is so obvious that few adults fail to identify this as a serious problem. Identification of the primary problem, establishing a language level, a probable etiology, and then making proper recommendations for remediation remains a challenge. How great a challenge is suggested by the maze of terminology, test instruments, and remedial procedures, which increase at an ever accelerating rate.

The classic texts on diagnostic procedures in speech pathology such as the one by Johnson, Darley, and Spriesterbach (1952), which was updated by Darley (1964), focused heavily on speech problems, especially on disorders of fluency. A more recent diagnostic handbook for student clinicians in speech pathology includes counseling (King and Berger, 1971) and interviewing techniques, but all three deal only minimally with evaluations of linguistic disorders in children.

This chapter deals entirely with evaluation procedures available for use with children suspected of having linguistic disorders. A summary of some of the significant research that has influenced our current approach to this problem introduces the chapter. This is followed by a discussion of the qualifications of prospective examiners. The focus of the chapter is on obtaining objective test results and interpreting extratest data. Finally, criteria for forming diagnostic impressions are presented.

INFLUENCE OF THE PAST

Professional interest in children who fail to develop oral language dates back almost a century and a half, and may conveniently be divided into three stages. In the first stage (from 1853–1929), neurologists and physicians were concerned primarily with identification of the problem in children they examined who were "speechless." The second period (1930–1956) saw accumulation of knowledge by a variety of specialists, each working within his own area and with little inter-specialist communication. The third period (1957–present) has been enriched by the interaction of various disciplines and most clearly shows the impact of psycholinguistic studies of child language.

Identification of the Problem (1853–1929)

In 1853, as a part of the study included in his text on the treatment of the ear, an Irishman named Wilde surveyed schools for the deaf and observed children who could obviously hear but were unable to speak (1853). It was almost 30 years before this problem received attention again in the literature. In 1867 Wilbur, an American writing in the *American Journal of Insanity*, described a similar group of children and urged better diagnosis and some attempt at training them (1867).

The first person to suggest a diagnostic label for these children was Vaisse (1866). In his publication in the bulletin of the French Anthropological Society he termed the condition "congenital aphasia." The introduction of the term "congenital aphasia" by a Frenchman at that time is not surprising. Charcot had already presented his theories on cerebral localization, and in 1861 Broca presented to the Society of Anthropology his now famous lecture on a patient who had lost his speech following cerebral injury. In fact, aphasia became such a hotly debated topic that before the end of the century the Society was refusing to accept any further papers on the subject of aphasia. Although Vaisse is seldom quoted by name, his term "congenital aphasia" appeared as a diagnostic title in at least 10 articles before 1920 and was used by approximately half the authors surveyed before 1947 (Bangs, 1947). The next most common term for this condition was "word deafness," which continued to be used by half of the authors surveyed before 1947 (Bangs, 1947).

Neurologists such as Hughlings Jackson who devoted themselves to the study of adult neurological disorders made only passing comments about absence of language in children. In the 1871 edition of *Lancet*, Jackson reported on several speechless children. His observation of their "ill-tempered, mischievous, and spiteful behavior" suggests that they left his office in the type of disarray present day examiners know well (1871). Henry Head, one of the great English neurologists and a student of Jackson, published two volumes in 1926 devoted to aphasia. Head presents what is considered the first of the organized diagnostic tests for aphasia (1926, Vol. 1). Among the 26 cases described in his Volume 2, only two are of congenital defects, and both of these individuals were examined as adults (1926, Vol. 2).

A majority of authors agreed that the etiology of congenital aphasia was cerebral lesion; the analogy to acquired aphasia in adults formed the basis of the diagnostic and etiologic reasoning. In 1900, Kerr felt that word deafness was caused by bilateral damage and in 1911 Tate agreed, suggesting that the bilateral nature of the lesion accounted for the minimal results yielded by conventional education (Bangs, 1947).

Accumulation of Knowledge by Separate Specialists (1930–1956)

The interest of physicians in the problem of the congenitally aphasic child remained strong in the first half of this century. Ewing, in England, published the first book devoted entirely to this problem, *Aphasia in Children* (1930), in which he pointed out the effect of high frequency hearing loss and stressed the need of careful audiologic evaluations of these children. Another physician, Samuel Orton (1937), had spent the 10 years before the publication of *Reading, Writing, and Speech Problems in Children* at the University of Iowa studying the language acquisition of children. Orton considered language loss in adults the basis for approaching the study of language disorders in children. The aphasias included both spoken and written language, and he presented various diagnostic terms, including "word deafness," which refers to oral language dysfunction. Word deafness was said to be caused by the inability to recall the sequence of sounds, and Orton suggested as treatment the use of simple words, short sentences, and clear enunciation by the teachers training the children.

Ironically, it was the German neurologist Goldstein, with only minimal experience with children, who profoundly influenced the course of education and diagnosis of language-disordered children during the 1950s and 1960s. After some 40 years of work in adult neurology, Kurt Goldstein published *Language and Language Disturbance* (1948). Goldstein talked about a "symptom complex," taking a Gestalt or organismic approach to the problem. He put forward the distinction between "concrete and abstract behavior," pointing out the attentional problems and the difficulty these patients had in distinguishing figure from ground. He also defined "catastrophic reaction to distress" and the perseverative or excessively orderly behavior of these patients.

In 1947 Strauss, a physician, and Lehtinen, an educator at the Cove School in Madison, Wisconsin, teamed to publish *Psychopathology and Education of The Brain Injured Child*. The symptoms observed by Head and Goldstein in adults were discovered by Strauss in

children. The behavioral characteristics of hyperactivity, distractability, and catastrophic reaction were used to separate the brain-injured
child from the mentally retarded child. Strauss and Lehtinen defined
the brain-injured child as "one who as a result of injury to the brain
may display neuromotor impairment, disturbances in perception,
thinking, and emotional behavior which prevents or impedes normal
learning" (Strauss and Lehtinen, 1947). Strauss felt that those children
whom Binet had previously described as "ill-balanced," in that they
were unruly, talkative, and inattentive, were actually brain injured.
Strauss indicated that spoken and written language disturbances could
be explained on the basis of localization theory and were specific,
whereas deviations in behavior were best explained as damage to the
organism as a whole.

A second book by Strauss, coauthored this time with Kephart
(Strauss and Kephart, 1955), focused heavily on perception. They
stated that perceptions underly language, whereas motor mechanisms
make speech possible. The brain-injured child was thought to have
perceptual disturbances so that he could not organize elements into a
whole. In neither volume were specific tests presented for determining
aphasia. The incidence of hearing loss and disturbed speech was
mentioned in some cases, but never stressed nor apparently formally
evaluated. Treatment methods focused only on perceptual and behavioral problems, not on increasing verbal productivity.

In contrast to educators such as Lehtinen and Kephart, who
worked closely with physicians, other educators worked independently.
Mildred McGinnis in 1939 proposed a training method for aphasic
children in her Master's thesis. The so-called Association Method of
training formed the basis of her work with aphasic children at the
Central Institute for the Deaf (McGinnis, 1963).

Writing in the *Journal of Speech Disorders*, Nance (1946) stressed
the need for techniques of different diagnosis of aphasia in children.
At that time the only available tests were adaptations of the instruments developed by Head and Cheser for use with adults.

Breaking with a century of medical tradition in the discussion of
aphasia, Lee Travis, the pioneer speech pathologist, discussed congenital aphasia in his 1931 text on speech pathology. In 1940 Ruth Becky
(Irwin) did her Ph.D. dissertation on congenital aphasia. She analyzed
the case histories of 50 children for possible etiologies. Her conclusion
was that delayed speech was often associated with abnormal pregnancy
or labor or neonatal distress (1942).

In the 1947 edition of *The Rehabilitation of Speech*, West,

Kennedy and Carr distinguished between dysphasia and aphasia in children on the basis of how much speech the children displayed. The defect was felt to be one of symbolization, with dysphasics being unable to associate object and picture. The damage resulting in dysphasia was said to be in the association areas of the cerebrum. The aphasic child was one who was normal but had the language of an "idiot" (1947). The authors felt that training offered hope and multisensory training was suggested.

The 1947 edition of Van Riper's *Speech Correction* devoted an entire chapter to "delayed speech"; of the 13 possible causes listed, one of them was aphasia. On this subject Van Riper said that one of the more uncommon causes of delayed speech was aphasia, and that it was always necessary to rule out deafness and feeble-mindedness before aphasia could be considered. Van Riper (1947) recommended the development of a serviceable gesture language for these children. He concludes that few clinicians will ever see an aphasic child. The entire discussion was completed in two paragraphs.

Working at the same time as Orton, Dorothea McCarthy at the Iowa Child Welfare Research Station carried out her studies of normal child language development including length of utterance and sentence complexity (1954). During the same period at Iowa, Medorah Smith developed the first vocabulary test for children between 8 months and 6 years of age (McCarthy, 1954). At the Yale Clinic of Child Development, Gesell and his associates (1940–1941) recorded motor, adaptive, language, and personal-social behaviors as they emerged in preschool children (1940). The Swiss psychologist Piaget undertook the study of the fundamental intelligence of the child, asking why the child talks and what function his language serves. His book *Language and Thought of the Child* (1923) remains an important treatise on normal language development as it relates to cognitive growth.

Working apart from the other specialists during this period were the linguists who were beginning to study child language. Lewis (1936) did one of the significant early diary studies of child language. The most extensive diary study was published between 1937 and 1949 by Werner Leopold (1973). The linguist Roman Jakobson was the first to analyze the significance of these early studies in the hope of generalizing the pattern of development of a few children to certain linguistic universals that might have application for all children (1968).

Cooperative Activity (1957–Present)

Although the need for differential diagnosis had been mentioned for almost 100 years, it was not until Myklebust published his *Auditory Disorders in Children* (1954) that definite criteria were presented for distinguishing children between 1 and 6 years who failed to develop speech. Diagnostic categories included psychic deafness, deafness, aphasia, and mental retardation. At that time diagnosis and training for linguistically disordered children were limited.

By the 1960s, however, parents had become aware that children could not be excluded from school because of ability, and they began going to court to demand appropriate training for their children. This demand brought with it a pressing need for better diagnostic and remedial procedures. Penfield, in the epilogue to his volume *Speech and Brain Mechanisms* (1959), questioned why education was not geared to the evolution of the functional capacity of the brain. He indicated that before the age of 9, a child is a specialist in learning languages. It was left to Lenneberg (1967) to elegantly trace the course of language development as it relates to other aspects of growth and development and to highlight the neurological timetable for language development. This gave impetus to the movement, already underway from other sources, for early intervention and particularly for early public education of handicapped children.

In this climate of change, Johnson with her coauthor Myklebust redefined the group of children with auditory disorders whose ability did not correspond to their achievement. These writers referred to children who have generally intact motor ability, intelligence, hearing, vision, and emotional adjustment—but who are still not learning—as having a "learning disability" (1967). One type of learning disability was considered to be disorders of auditory language. Their original study was supplemented by two volumes edited by Myklebust (1968, 1971) that presented multidisciplinary research related to the diagnosis and remediation of learning disabilities.

Although a few aphasiologists such as Kurt Goldstein occasionally quoted a linguist in their discussions of language, most of the aphasia literature referred only infrequently to linguistics. Actually, only a few linguists such as Roman Jakobson and Werner Leopold seriously examined child language. In 1957, a slim doctoral dissertation entitled *Syntactic Structures* was published by the linguist Noam Chomsky (1957). His emphasis on linguistic competence and its relationship to human knowledge and the mind excited neurologists and psychologists as well as educators and linguists. In particular, the psychology department at Harvard University became intrigued with the potential that this approach to language offered. One of these psychologists, Roger

Brown, proceeded to involve himself almost totally in the study of child language.

Brown's student, Jean Berko, demonstrated in another classic dissertation that children internalized the rules of oral grammar. In her study titled *The Child's Learning of English Morphology*, she employed an original test using such nonsense words as *wug* and *nez* (Berko, 1958). She showed that little children learn more than words; they learn the rules that generate morphological markers. This insight, plus other research based on this theory, proved a serious blow to the Skinnerian theory of verbal behavior. Now Skinnerian principles are used to train the linguistically disordered, especially the retarded, but few would suggest that a human must memorize every word and sentence through conditioning in order to speak. The work of the Brickers (1970, 1972), among others, demonstrated the effectiveness of these principles and a combination of behavioral and linguistic theories now seems feasible (Lynch and Bricker, 1972).

Paula Menyuk used Chomsky's generative model of language in the study of transformations used by linguistically disordered children. She began by asking whether these children learn language differently from or in the same order as normal children (1964). This very significant question has been further explored by both Lee (1966, 1970, 1971) and Menyuk (1964, 1972, 1976), who hypothesize that there may be differences in the learning of language by linguistically disordered children.

A significant insight into the field of child language was provided by a speech pathologist/psycholinguist, Lois Bloom (1970, 1973). She observed the significance of context and environmental clues to the parents' interpretation of the function of the words used by children. Stimulated by the work of Bloom and Schlesinger, among others, the trend of research in child language shifted to semantics (Brown, 1973). The relationship of meaning and reference to the development of language is explored in volumes such as Hayes (1970) and Moore (1973). Insights into semantic development have been deepened through renewed use of the method of baby biography by Bloom (1973), Bowerman (1974), and Greenfield and Smith (1976). Currently the most fashionable topic in child language seems to be pragmatics. Pragmatics is based upon the earlier philosophical work of Wittgenstein and Morris, among others, and emphasizes speech acts by looking at the function of language as it is used (Moerk, 1977).

The richness of the psycholinguistic influence on the entire field of child language and its disorders is reflected by the commonality of terms and methods of study. It is now difficult to identify the particular discipline of authors. A sampling of many excellent books of readings and edited books that have collected significant papers includes those edited by Bar-Adon and Leopold (1971), Morehead and Morehead (1976), and Bloom and Lahey (in press). Another recent volume devotes its several hundred pages entirely to an interdisciplinary guide to the most current literature in child language (Abrahamsen, 1977).

The extent of published literature suggests that analysis of any one child can properly be the work of an entire professional life. This luxury is never available to the diagnostician. The purpose of this chapter, then, is to present certain criteria for choosing tests that will yield a differential assessment as well as linguistic assessment so that proper impressions and recommendations can be generated.

THE DIAGNOSTIC SITUATION

There are three possible variables in the diagnostic situation: the child being tested; the examiner; and the objective procedures employed during testing. In a competent diagnostic situation, the only factor that should vary is the one actually being tested, the child. It is only when the examiner's ability is of high quality and the diagnostic assessment well chosen, adequately administered, and accurately scored that it is possible to concentrate on the variable properly under study, the child. The following section will focus on the examiner's qualifications and ability. The next section will explore the objective procedures that may be used in the differential assessment and the linguistic assessment. Finally, the analysis of extratest data such as case history, examiner's impressions and supplementary reports will be considered.

Examiner's Qualifications

The qualifications of an examiner are threefold:

1. Personal qualifications
2. Ethical qualifications
3. Legal qualifications as a speech pathologist, educational diagnostician, or school psychologist

Personal requirements Evaluation of linguistic disorders involves primarily work with young children who deserve more than an examiner who is merely tolerant of children. They deserve an examiner who retains a delight in both the child and his responses; an examiner who respects not only the child and his parents but also the environment in which they live. The diagnostic session is not the time to teach discipline to the child or impart instruction on childrearing to parents.

The diagnostic session and the interview to follow require that the examiner be a highly skilled listener. A talkative examiner risks never hearing the few words the child is capable of saying, and may overwhelm the child's parents during the conference. Essentially, a good examiner is a good observer. Observation begins when the child and his parent are in the waiting room and continues throughout the assessment and conference. A good examiner is aware of his personal biases so that they will not affect test scores.

The normal child is eager to prove his competence to the examiner; however, the examiner must adapt to the linguistically disordered child. Examinations that are speeded (timed) tend to put such children at a disadvantage. It is frequently necessary for the examiner to modify the order of administration of the subtests despite the fact that this makes comparison to norms tenuous. Few children with linguistic disorders can tolerate the constant barrage of questions that are a part of the usual procedure of many objective test batteries.

Ethical considerations In a multidisciplinary field such as linguistic disorders, there is no one specialty that trains professionals to examine a child with a linguistic disorder. The serious examiner, therefore, has the obligation of imposing his own ethical requirements that go beyond those which may be required by state or local law. Since the examiner is testing for a linguistic disorder, this presupposes a sound knowledge of normal language (linguistics). To identify a disorder an examiner must understand normal child development, which includes not only language, but motor, cognitive, and personal/social development. A knowledgeable examiner is the most important diagnostic requirement. No test battery can compensate for a poorly educated examiner.

The next ethical requirement involves appropriate training in the standard procedure for giving tests selected. Once the tests and recording procedures become routine, inter- and intratester reliability checks should be made. The rationale behind test-retest comparison, on which the placement of children is often based, assumes that scores earned on the same test are equivalent. This decision presumes uniform scoring and interpreting of the same response. The wide disparity that may exist between two skilled examiners needs to be controlled by at least yearly monitoring. The careful clinic monitors its electronic equipment more frequently than that. Ideally, this comparison can be done by having two examiners score the same child at the same time or by video taping a testing session, which an entire diagnostic staff can then view and score simultaneously. Obviously the ethical examiner makes careful, consistent, and legible notations and preserves at least one segment of the language sample on audio and preferably video tape.

Legal requirements   The examiner who is employed by an established educational, psychologic, or medical clinic need only ascertain that the person who signs the summary diagnostic report has the proper qualification and licensure to make the diagnosis. For example, only a physician may give a medical diagnosis of brain injury or minimal brain dysfunction, whereas only a licensed psychologist or psychiatrist may diagnose certain emotional disorders. An examiner in private practice must be careful to make only those diagnostic statements covered by his area of certification or license.

Within recent years the largest influx of examiners has been within the public school system. The diagnostic emphasis has shifted from the medical to the educational model. With the legislation of the 1960s ensuring that educational opportunities not be denied because of race, parents of handicapped children began seeking similar rights for their children, with the result that many states are now extending evaluation and education for handicapped children into the preschool years. Michigan, the most progressive state in the nation, now provides education for handicapped individuals from birth to 25 years of age (Department of Health, Education and Welfare, 1975). Many states provide education from age 3 onward, and there is a general national trend toward providing education from birth. The Education for All Handicapped Children Act has mandated free public education for all handicapped children between the ages of 3 and 21 years by 1980 (Public Law 94-142). To secure proper educational placement, schools must obviously provide diagnostic services. Within the last few years, public schools have become a primary diagnostic facility for the child with linguistic disorders.

The federal government claims no authority in the field of education beyond collecting statistics and promoting education by providing funds and guidelines. The broad authority resides in each state and local school board (Bodenman, 1976). The guidelines for one state, Texas, are given as an example of diagnostic services and qualifications for providing those services. In Texas, diagnostic duties are performed under the category of supportive professional personnel (Texas Education Agency Bulletin 711, 1973). The following evaluations may be done. 1) Educational diagnosticians must meet certification standards. The primary purpose is the appraisal of educational functioning, intelligence factors, and analysis of data pertaining to sociologic variables. The diagnostician may not perform appraisals of emotional or behavioral factors. 2) School psychologists must meet certification standards. The primary purpose is to appraise intelligence factors and educational functioning; to analyze data pertaining to sociologic variables; and to provide a comprehensive appraisal of emotional and behavioral factors.

The speech pathologist does not appear under the heading of supportive professional personnel, but is instead listed as a separate category. The speech pathologist must meet the criteria for the individual school district, which may or may not be identical to the American Speech and Hearing Association criteria. The speech pathologist may perform appraisals of speech but not intelligence, educational functioning, or emotional or behavioral factors unless he holds supplementary certification.

In Texas, no particular specialist is assigned to evaluate linguistic ability in the school district. A speech pathologist is listed only as certifying eligibility for entrance into programs for speech handicapped.

Diagnosticians, particularly in school and educational centers, must be aware of the 1974 legislation, Protection of the Rights and Privacy of Parents and Their Children. This legislation with the accompanying Buckley Amendment specifies that parents have the right to review their child's official educational record. They have the right to challenge statements in that record that they feel may be in error, and if they can substantiate this, the record must be changed. Parents may also request copies of reports concerning their children.

Objective Procedures

Objective procedures form the core of the diagnostic situation. This section discusses test environments and presents criteria for choosing test instruments.

Test environment   No objective procedure can succeed unless the examiner creates an optimal test environment in which to elicit the child's abilities. The first several minutes of evaluation are often crucial to the ultimate performance of a child. The skilled examiner will speak first to the parent, allowing the child a moment or two to evaluate the examiner before any demands are placed upon him to perform. Any child who needs his parent with him in the examining room should be allowed to have the parent accompany him. A testing situation is not the time to increase the child's independence.

For many children with suspected linguistic disorders, it is advisable to begin the testing session with nonverbal items. This alone is usually sufficient to establish rapport with the child, and once a child offers spontaneous comment, he is ready to begin verbal testing. If the child does not offer any spontaneous comments, the examiner should begin to elicit speech by discussing objects that can be held and manipulated, thus de-emphasizing the verbal nature of the task. If the child still remains mute, it is wise to ask the parent what words the child has been heard to say and sometimes the parent can demonstrate these by asking the child the "right" question.

The work of Houston (1969) Labov (1971) has indicated the profound effect that the test environment has on obtaining verbal responses from children. Analysis of tests with black children and the urban poor reaffirmed that when such children are faced with a strange adult, a table, and several test items, they will have virtually nothing to say; or if strongly pressed, they will respond with a few monosyllables. Labov demonstrated how such silent, apparently nonverbal children could be transformed into youngsters with so much to say that they were interrupting each other for a chance to talk. This was done by turning the formal test session into an informal situation where the child was allowed to bring a friend, where potato chips or soft drinks were served, and where the children sat with the examiner on the floor "rapping" about neighborhood gossip, which included talks of street fights, name calling, and so forth. Labov makes the crucial point that "with human subjects it is absurd to believe identical stimuli are obtained by simply asking everyone the same question" (Labov, 1971).

Choice of tests   Because no examiner can observe a child in depth and at length, tests are used to sample the child's behavior. In this chapter "test" refers to an organized system of observing behavior. To have meaning, this sample of behavior must be objective in that the same tasks are given to each child in essentially the same manner. The test itself should be reasonably free from cultural contamination so that it is not biased against one particular group of children. The test must have validity and reliability. No individual tests will be recommended; instead, widely used tests will be analyzed so that the examiner can make appropriate choices.

The primary consideration in choosing a test is the reason for testing. Until the person requesting the test and the person administering the test agree on the purpose of the test, no judgment can be made about the relative merits of available tests. To attempt to choose the "best test" without knowing the reason for testing is as impractical as attempting to choose the "best vehicle," for example a jeep versus a Cadillac, without knowing where and how the vehicle is to be driven.

The purpose of testing discussed in this chapter is the evaluation of linguistic disorders in children. "Linguistic disorder" is used to designate a problem in those children who fail to comprehend or speak their native language appropriately for their chronologic age. "Linguistic" is used instead of "language" to stress that it refers to a child's first language and specifically rules out children who fail to use the language of their geographic location or school. This designation includes not only children with specific linguistic disorders, but also the hearing impaired, emotionally disturbed, and the mentally retarded who exhibit a linguistic disorder as an obvious symptom of their primary problem.

Weiner (1972) has pointed out that when standardized tests of ability are used with linguistically disordered children, surprisingly little attention is paid to the disordered language itself. On the contrary, when language assessment is discussed in the literature (Siegel and Broen, 1976), there may be no mention of how an examiner determined whether the child has a specific linguistic disorder or whether the linguistic disorder is secondary to hearing impairment, emotional disturbance, or mental retardation.

To do an initial diagnosis with a child who has been referred because he has failed to develop oral language requires two levels of diagnosis. Level 1 consists of the Differential Assessment and Level 2 consists of the Linguistic Assessment. The purpose of these assessments is to answer the following questions.

Question to be answered	Level of assessment
1. Is the child normal?	
2. If abnormal, does the child have a specific linguistic disorder or a linguistic disorder secondary to another condition?	Level 1: Differential Assessment
3. What is child's current level of linguistic functioning?	Level 2: Linguistic Assessment

It is possible that the same examiner may not perform both levels of testing, and both levels of testing need not be completed at the same test session. Yet both levels are necessary for proper evaluation. The purpose of the Level 1 assessment is to identify the child's primary problem; the purpose of the Level 2 assessment is to classify the type and specify the extent of the linguistic disorder.

Level 1: Differential Assessment   The purpose of the Differential Assessment is to ascertain the nature of the child's problem; or to establish that the child does not have a problem. Referral for testing does not guarantee that the child has a disorder. To answer the Level 1 questions, examiners choose a single test or subtests from among tests of general ability. All of these are norm-referenced tests.

Testing in the United States functions on a norm-referenced model. The first norm-referenced test to be widely used in this country was the Stanford-Binet. This scale of subtests, arranged according to difficulty, was designed to measure intelligence and introduced the terms "mental age" and "IQ" (Terman and Merrill, 1937). The purpose of the Stanford-Binet and all subsequent norm-referenced tests was to give a child's relative standing along a continuum of attainment. They were designed to rank one child in comparison to others. They were not designed to reveal the specific information any one child possessed (Popham, 1971). Teachers and clinicians often refer a child for intelligence testing because they need information about how to manage the child in class or what specific curriculum should be taught. Tests of general ability were not designed to answer such questions.

The test or battery of tests chosen for Differential Assessment must have more than the capacity to yield a score representing the child's ability in comparison to others his age: such a battery must additionally clarify the nature of his primary and secondary problems. Because many of these children will have a linguistic problem, the tests chosen must have the capacity to measure verbal ability separately from nonverbal ability. The tests should have a minimum of environmental or cultural contamination and the standardization group must make the use of the test with a particular child appropriate.

To accomplish all of this some diagnostic centers administer a lengthy battery of tests, sometimes requiring several days to complete. At the conclusion of such testing, scores are computed and reported. This often leaves the referring source, or the parent, to decide the significance of sometimes conflicting test scores. A solution to this diagnostic dilemma is to select only those tests or subtests that can generate a profile of the child's strengths and weaknesses across the spectrum of early childhood achievement (C.A.) (Bangs, 1968). The behaviors to be sampled are language abilities, including language comprehension and language expression (primarily oral, but including gestures); memory and attention, including auditory and visual memory; and various nonverbal skills, including problem solving, visual motor perceptual skills, and gross motor development.

Differential Assessment Profile

	Language skills				Memory/attention		Nonverbal skills		
	Oral language		Gesture language						
	Compre-hension	Expres-sion	Compre-hension	Expres-sion	Auditory	Visual	Problem solve	Visual motor skills	Gross motor
C.A.									
No Score									

The above profile clarifies, for both the examiner and the referring sources, the nature of the child's problem. Only the examiner must analyze standard error, standard deviation, scaled scores, IQ, etc. Such a profile clearly illustrates how appropriately a child is performing for his age. The profile makes no obvious statement regarding IQ because the purpose of this testing is not to generate an IQ.

Each facet of development sampled on the Differential Assessment should be measured apart from intratest contamination by other facets of behavior also being evaluated. For example, did the child fail a motor test because he could not understand the directions? On the Bayley Scale (1969) a child is praised for jumping and urged, "Do it again and see how far you can get this time." This command contains grammatical complexity that a physically agile but linguistically impaired child might fail to comprehend; yet his failure would be scored on a motor item.

Could the child have demonstrated by gesture a concept such as "What do you do when you are thirsty?" or "Why do we have books?" (Terman and Merrill, 1960) even though the child lacked the necessary words to answer the question? Ideally, reasoning and concept formation should be measured by additional tests that involve no speech on the part of either the examiner or the child (such as the Hiskey and the Leiter tests). An insightful examiner can note the child's correct use of gesture to express concepts on the profile. An objective score on gesture can be obtained by administering *Manual Expression* from the ITPA (Kirk, McCarthy, and Kirk, 1968). Natural gesture can be used; if a child has been exposed to Total Communication, questions can be given in Sign.

When testing language skills the reason for inadequate performance should be explored. Did the child fail because of a linguistic disorder, or because the test placed the child at a cultural disadvantage? Is it not more logical for an urban child to search for a store rather than a cow when asked to "show me the one that gives milk" (Terman and Merrill, 1972)? A more fair question is "Show me what shines in the sky at night" (Terman and Merrill, 1972). A middle class child would be more likely than a ghetto child to explain correctly why it is better to give to an organized charity rather than to give directly to a beggar on the street or what you should do if a child smaller than you were to start a fight with you (WISC-R). The middle class child might be more familiar than the ghetto child with the many electrical appliances used as stimulus pictures in the ITPA (Kirk, McCarthy, and Kirk, 1968). Cultural bias in the vocabulary definitions from the Stanford-Binet have been noted. In 1972 the first "culturally specific" vocabulary test was published. Whereas a middle class white teenager would be expected to know the meaning of *milksop* or *harpy* (Terman and Merrill, 1972), a black teenager could define *ofay* or *stone fox* (Williams, 1972).

When testing language skills, it is not necessary to test comprehension apart from expression if a child is performing at or above age level on items from a highly verbal test of general ability. When a child does poorly on such tests, then the reason for the failure must be explored, and language comprehension and language production should be compared. Can the child follow directions, point out objects and pictures (as in the Binet, Bayley, and Birth to Three Scales) even though he says virtually nothing?

Table 1 analyzes the most commonly used norm-referenced tests of general ability in this country. It gives dates of revision of the tests, the age range, the purpose of the test, the standardization sample, and finally analyzes the subtests according to whether they are verbal or nonverbal. The most widely used of these tests, the WISC-R, the WPPSI, and the Stanford-Binet, were all designed to yield an IQ or intelligence quotient. The Bayley Scale yields an age equivalent score. This scale leaves the examiner free to adapt the order of administration to the child's needs.

The two most widely used nonverbal tests are the Hiskey-Nebraska

Table 1. Norm referenced tests of general ability

Name of test	Latest revision	Age range	Analysis of subtests				Test yields	Standardization sample
			Preverbal and verbal	Nonverbal	Gross motor			
					Verbal	Nonverbal		
Bayley Scale of Infant Development (BSID) (Bayley)	1969	2–30 months	39 items (Mental Scale)	124 items (Mental Scale)	3 items (Motor Scale)	78 items (Motor Scale)	MDI or PDI or Age Equivalent Score	N = 1,262. Controlled for sex, race, location and socioeconomic status, based upon 1960 U.S. census.
Birth to Three Developmental Scale* (Bangs and Dodson-Garrett)	Forth-coming	0–36 months	46 items (Comprehension and Expression)	46 items		28	Developmental age and profile	National norms underway.
Hiskey-Nebraska Test of Learning Ability (Hiskey)	1966	3–16 years	None	All items	None	None	Learning Age	N = 1,107 Deaf N = 1,101 Hearing Random as to race. No large cities. From 10 states.
Illinois Test of Psycholinguistic Abilities (Kirk, McCarthy, and Kirk)	1968	2–10 years	7 sub-tests	5 sub-tests	None	None	Psycholinguistic Learning Age	N = 962. 4% were black. All from medium-sized towns in Midwest.
Leiter International Performance Scale (Leiter)	1949	3–18 years	None	54 items	None	None	IQ Score and Mental Age	N = 289.
Stanford-Binet Intelligence Scale (Terman and Merrill)	1960	2½–15 years	69 items	39 items	None	None	IQ Score	N = 4,498. Controlled for sex, race, location, and socioeconomic status based upon 1950 U.S. census.

Wechsler Intelligence Scale: Children Revised (WISC-R) (Wechsler)	1972	6-16 years	7 subtests	6 subtests	None	IQ Score	N = 2,220. Controlled for sex, race, location, and socioeconomic status based upon 1970 U.S. census.
Wechsler Preschool and Primary Scale of Intelligence (WPPSI) (Wechsler)	1967	4-6½ years	6 subtests	5 subtests	None	IQ Score	N = 1,200. Controlled for sex, race, location, and socioeconomic status based upon 1960 U.S. census.

*Bangs, in preparation.

Test of Learning Ability and the Leiter International Performance Scale. Both of these tests were designed to meet the pressing need of evaluating children whose oral language was so defective that it was impractical to use the verbal tests as measures of their intellectual ability.

The Hiskey-Nebraska yields a Learning Age whereas the Leiter International yields an IQ and a mental age. Neither of these tests include any verbal items requiring comprehension or expression of language on the part of either the examiner or the subject taking the test.

Another test designed to meet a specific need was the ITPA. It was originally evolved to meet the need of evaluating mentally retarded children, who are excessively penalized by the standard intelligence test, which yields no practical information that could be used by the individual training the child (Buros, 1972). The original ITPA (1961 edition) was based on Osgood's Model of Language, but the 1968 edition has less relation to that model. This test compares intra-test scores, specifically auditory and visual channels of input and output, and suggests that the information derived be used in designing a training program for the children. As the test is described and reviewed in the Buros' *Mental Examiner's Handbook* (Buros, 1972), it is considered a test of cognitive rather than of psycholinguistic ability. If the linguistic items are analyzed this fact becomes apparent: the only expressive linguistic information that the test yields about the child's verbal output is a measure of his ability to generate the morphological rules from the Grammatic Closure subtest, and to give the name and function of four isolated items, namely block, ball, chalk, and plastic.

Another test developed to meet a specific need in differential assessment is the Birth to Three Developmental Scale, which is now undergoing national standardization. This test is designed specifically to yield a developmental age or profile. The order of item presentation on this scale may be adapted to meet the needs of the child. Special efforts have been made to ensure that this instrument will be culture fair.

Level 2: Linguistic Assessment   The purpose of a linguistic assessment is to compare what a child has linguistically with what he should have at his age. A linguistic assessment is meaningful for any child who demonstrates impaired linguistic skills, whether the primary problem is one of hearing impairment, mental retardation, emotional disturbance, or a specific linguistic disorder. Clinical experience suggests that the examiner proceed with linguistic assessment for any child whose language skills are 6 months or more below his chronologic age on the differential assessment profile.

Oral language is defined as a system of symbols arranged in a hierarchy according to an organized set of rules. Language is a productive system that allows the normal speaker to use utterances he has never heard, and the normal listener to understand sentences he has never spoken. The relationship between speaker and listener or between comprehension and expression is fundamental, because each normal user of language is both a speaker and a listener. Comprehension precedes expression developmentally, and even among normal adults there is a definite advantage of comprehension over expression. It is easier, for example, to listen to a story than to tell a story.

The system of symbols that composes language refers to concepts and the words applied to these concepts. Roger Brown, in talking about first language learning, calls this "the original word game" (1958). This game requires a speaker of the language to name things and a learner of the language to form hypotheses about the categorical nature of the things named. This game is played as long as an individual continues to expand vocabulary; usually as long as he lives. Relating words to concepts constitutes the basis of the semantic system or the lexicon of the language.

The arrangement of symbols in a hierarchy constitutes the morphosyntactic system of language. Morphemes are the basic units of linguistic analysis, and are composed of *roots* (words) plus various modifications. For example, a root such as "do" or "boy" may have a prefix added such as "*un*do" or a suffix added such as "do*ing*" or "boy*s*". The addition of such affixes modifies the meaning of the roots. Syntax is defined as arrangement of words in groups to express various meanings including such basic arrangements as subject-verb-object. Comparison of the sentences "The boy ate a fish" with "A fish ate the boy" illustrates the power of word order in English. The rule-governed behavior that results in the formation of various types of construction belongs in the area of syntax.

The linguistic assessment should provide the following information:

1. How do receptive and expressive linguistic abilities compare in terms of the following:

a. Semantic system or lexicon
b. Morphosyntactic system
2. What function does the language serve?

Since the first vocabulary tests developed in the 1920s there have been an increasing number of tests designed to explore linguistic performance (McCarthy, 1954). The earlier tests focused primarily on vocabulary, whereas later tests emphasized syntax. Most of these tests are norm-referenced with items arranged on a continuum from easy to difficult and norms based upon a mean age when the children constituting the standardization group successfully responded to each item.

Several of the more recently developed tests make use of the concept of criterion reference. A criterion-referenced test is constructed to determine whether the child being evaluated has attained a certain level of proficiency in a given task (Popham, 1971). In general this criterion has been previously determined by establishing a norm at which 50% or more of the children tested were successful in completing the item. A criterion-referenced test focuses on specific skills and concepts, and allows intratest comparison to measure individual growth in the areas tested. At the point when a child attains a predetermined level of proficiency it is assumed that he has mastered the specific concept and that he is ready to go on to the next, or a more difficult concept. The most significant difference between norm- and criterion-referenced tests is in the use made of the test results. Criterion-referenced tests lend themselves to curriculum building and pre- and post-testing.

Comparison of receptive and expressive language: semantic systems   One of the most widely used tests of language comprehension is the Peabody Picture Vocabulary Test (Dunn, 1965). This fairly brief test requires a child to choose the correct one of four pictures to identify the word named by the examiner. The test was first published in 1959 and revised in 1970. Despite the recent revision, the standardization group still includes only white children from the Nashville, Tennessee area. The test was designed to indicate "verbal intelligence" including an IQ score. Another test that may be used to measure vocabulary comprehension is the Ammons Full Range Picture Vocabulary Test (Ammons and Ammons, 1962). This test also requires the subject to point to the one of four pictures that best illustrates the word said by the examiner. The standardization group consisted of 458 individuals. The test yields a mental age and a percentile score.

The Auditory Reception subtest from the ITPA (Kirk, McCarthy, and Kirk, 1968) also measures knowledge of noun/verb vocabulary. In this subtest no pictures are involved, which makes it particularly valuable for use with children who might have difficulty in responding to picture material. The subject is required to give a "yes" or "no" response to the examiner's three-word questions, for example, "Do dogs fly?", "Do beverages quench?".

The above tests measure content words consisting of nouns, adjectives, and verbs. A recent test, the Vocabulary Comprehension Scale (Bangs, 1975), was designed to measure the comprehension of words of position, size, quality, and quantity only. Unlike the other tests, this vocabulary scale uses objects that may be manipulated. The vocabulary contains many function words (prepositions, pronouns, etc.). Because the total number of function words are limited, this vocabulary does not continue to increase. Once all the pronouns are mastered, for example, there are no more to learn. The Vocabulary Comprehension Scale is a criterion-referenced as well as norm-referenced test.

Expressive vocabulary is measured in most of the norm-referenced tests of ability previously discussed. The Bayley Scale of Infant Development (Bayley, 1969), the Birth to Three Developmental Scale (Bangs, in preparation), and the picture naming of Stanford-Binet may be used to evaluate specific vocabulary of children under 4 years of age.

The occurrence of a child's first words and the subsequent adding of words have been so well documented that an examiner should always attempt to ascertain from a parent the approximate number of words a rather silent child is capable of saying. A normal child of 12–18 months uses three or more words meaningfully, and by 24 months has acquired twenty or more meaningful words (Gesell et al., 1940; McCarthy, 1954; Darley and Winitz, 1961; McNeill, 1970). Comparison of a child's actual vocabulary with expected vocabulary size can provide valuable clinical insights for both examiner and parent.

During the 1970s increased attention has been paid to the semantic implications of vocabulary development. Bloom pointed out the sequential development of vocabulary. Her analysis of the negative form "no" from its initial use indicating nonexistence to rejection and finally denial (Bloom, 1970) illustrates this development. Eve Clark (1973a, b) deepened the examiner's insight into vocabulary development by illustrating how the child first identifies an object or action based upon critical perceptual features. A child may call any animal with four legs or running movements a "doggy" and only much later begin to use the appropriate term. Relational words are also frequently "overextended." Words such as "more, less; big, little; tall, short" constitutes pairs of marked versus unmarked words. The unmarked words, such as "tall," may be used nominally (The man is 6 feet tall) and developmentally precedes the other item. The concept of markedness is discussed more fully by Clark (1973a, b).

One linguistic test that compares receptive and expressive language development is the REEL Scale (Bzoch and League, 1971/8). This is an interview scale that evaluates a child's expressive and receptive language skills based upon the parent's or caregiver's responses to the examiner's questions. The scale yields a language age. The standardization group consisted primarily of children of members of the University of Florida staff, which may limit the test's applicability. The Birth to Three Developmental Scale also allows for specific comparison of receptive as opposed to expressive language skills (Bangs, in preparation). In general, however, the examiner must compare scores from separate tests being especially alert to measure comprehension in any child whose expressive language is deficient.

Comparison of receptive and expressive language: morphosyntactic systems The linguistic research resulting from insights provided by the theories of generative grammar focused heavily on syntax in the late 1960s and early 1970s. Before then, an examiner had to rely exclusively on clinical insight to evaluate a child's syntax; now, however, a number of tests are available to assist in this process. The Grammatic Closure subtest from the ITPA (Kirk, McCarthy, and Kirk, 1968) requires children to provide various morphologic markers (*Here is a foot. Here are two* ____. *The thief is stealing the jewels. These are the jewels that he* ____). This test measures expressive use of these forms; and it is assumed that most children who use a form expressively also comprehend the form. For children who do not use the form expressively, or whose speech is so defective that the examiner cannot understand their responses, there are other tests that measure only comprehension of morphosyntactic structures.

The Test for Auditory Comprehension of Language (TACL) (Carrow, 1973) measures the comprehension of various morphosyntactic structures by having the child point to the correct one of three stimulus pictures to identify the utterance of the examiner. Utterances range from a single word *painter* to a complete sentence, *The girl is not swimming*. The test yields percentile scores and has been standardized on Anglo, Mexican American, and black children. A Spanish edition is also available, as is a 25-item Screening Test for Auditory Comprehension of Language (STACL) (Carrow, 1973).

Assessment of Children's Language Comprehension (Foster, Gidden, and Stark, 1973) also assesses a subject's ability to process auditory information. This test requires a child to point to the correct picture to illustrate the examiner's utterance. The number of pictures per stimulus page varies from four to five. Items measured range from two elements (*dirty box*) to four elements (*happy little girl jumping*). The score is expressed in percent correct. Another measure of a child's comprehension of syntactic structures is the Morphosyntax Comprehension Scale (Lynch, in preparation). This scale uses the manipulation of objects to measure whether a child distinguishes six different types of morphosyntactic structures. Items such as *Which car is getting gas? Which car will get gas?* must be identified by the child from an actual scene. This test is both norm- and criterion-referenced.

To assist in determining a child's expressive use of grammatical forms, the Carrow Elicited Language Inventory (Carrow, 1974b) was developed. This test requires the subject to imitate the examiner. Utterances range from two words (*Cats jump*) to such a complex sentence as *If it rains, we won't go to the beach.* Responses are recorded on audio tape and analyzed later to derive an error score and deviation from the mean.

The Northwestern Syntax Screening (Lee, 1970) provides a measure of both receptive and expressive syntactic ability. On the receptive portion the subject is required to identify the correct one of four pictures described by the examiner in such words as *The car hits the train.* On the expressive portion there are two pictures that the examiner first describes. Then the subject is asked to describe one of the two pictures, such as *The cat is under the desk.* This test yields a percentile score and norms have been established to identify children with linguistic problems.

In addition to the standard tests there are other guidelines that may assist an examiner to evaluate a child's syntactic system. Bloom (1973) has looked at the constraints that determine when a child is ready to progress from single words to syntactic combinations of words. She challenges the oversimplification expressed by the belief that a child at the one-word stage actually is attempting to express an entire sentence by the use of that word.

Once children begin to combine words, usually by their 2nd year, the stages of linguistic growth may be divided according to the mean length of the utterance. This measure, not chronologic age, is commonly used to group children in order to study their language development. Roger Brown (Brown, 1973) divided initial language development into five stages according to mean length of utterance (MLU).

Rules for calculating mean length of utterance and determining upper boundaries are given by Brown (1973).

Stage	MLU	Upper boundary
I	1.75	5
II	2.25	7
III	2.75	9
IV	3.50	11
V	4.00	13

Crystal et al. (1976) pointed out an important problem with mean length of utterance, namely that this measure becomes less sensitive as an individual gets older and sentences become more complex. MLU can contribute only minimal information about linguistic complexity when utterances exceed five words per utterance. An utterance such as *The boy and girl have fed the fish and dog* is less complex than *The boy who owned the fish fed the dog*, although both contain 10 morphemes. Despite its drawbacks, however, calculation of mean length of utterance provides important linguistic information, and a linguistic assessment of a child producing short utterances is not complete without an estimate of mean length of utterance.

Probably the most rigorous linguistic studies have been devoted to the age and order of development of certain English morphemes (see Table 2). Some of those that have been most frequently studied have age ranges established. Examiner's awareness of these morphologic constructions and their median age of acquisition provide outside validation to results of the various standard tests as well as analysis of the language sample.

What function does the language serve? Bloom (1970) has suggested that in small children speech serves the following functions: 1) to give comments, 2) to give reports, 3) to give directions, and 4) to ask questions. The Russian neuropsychologists Vygotsky and Luria have discussed the directive function of language. It is essentially through language that an adult regulates the behavior of children. It is the child's internalization of language by which he eventually learns to control his own behavior.

Language also assists in establishing a child's self-image. A child's

Table 2. Median age of acquisition of certain morphologic constructions

Construction	Median age	Studies
Present progressive	2.4	Brown, 1973 Menyuk, 1963, 1969 deVilliers and deVilliers, 1973
Prepositions *in, on*	2.4	Menyuk, 1963, 1969 Brown, 1973 deVilliers and deVilliers, 1973
Plural nouns, regular	2.6	Menyuk, 1963, 1969 Brown, 1973 deVilliers and deVilliers, 1973
Personal pronouns	2.7	Menyuk, 1963, 1969
Articles *a, the*	3.0	Brown, 1973 Menyuk, 1963, 1969 deVilliers and deVilliers, 1973
Past regular	3.0	Brown, 1973 Menyuk, 1963, 1969 deVilliers and deVilliers, 1973
Past irregular	3.3	Menyuk, 1963, 1969 Brown, 1973 deVilliers and deVillicrs, 1973

Chapman, 1971.

feeling of differentiation from his mother is fostered by learning that his own name is different from everyone else's. Children reflect their awareness of this by questioning adults about whether their name will be changed when they grow up and their role in life changes (Rees, 1973). Evaluation of the functions served by a child's speech should be part of the linguistic analysis. The child's ability to sustain a series of utterances in conversational exchange is an essential linguistic skill that some linguistically disordered children may lack. Prutting estimated that by age 3 the normal child could sustain a series of 18–20 utterances (Prutting and Rees, 1977).

Language sample   This is one of the most traditional ways of studying language. The quality of the information derived from a language sample is related to the manner in which it is collected, the size of the sample, and the sophistication of the method of analysis.

The setting in which the language sample is obtained should be carefully controlled. A play or other "nontest" room is recommended for this purpose. A young child may need to be accompanied by a parent, friend, or sibling who has brought a favorite toy or snack from home. Activities that seem natural to the child should be planned.

The size of the language sample is of crucial importance. In her Developmental Sentence Analysis, Laura Lee (1974) used 50 utterances obtained by having the child verbalize while playing with toys, telling a story, and finally retelling a story, such as "The Three Bears." Menyuk in her 1964 study used under 100 utterances per child whereas Bloom (1970) used 1,500 utterances. Bloom recorded a child interacting with a parent, while in her studies Menyuk used language samples from three different situations, child with adult, child with child, and child at home. Despite all of these precautions it is not uncommon to read serious criticism of researchers for inadequate sampling. It has been suggested that a larger language sample is needed from a disordered child than from a normal child in order to analyze the language most accurately. The examiner must keep in mind the distinction between analyzing language to identify a disorder and analyzing language for the purpose of writing a grammar or hypothesizing rules about how children develop their first language. The latter usually requires a much larger sample.

One rigorous method of analysis of language samples is that developed by Laura Lee. In the 1971 discussion (Lee and Canter, 1971) it is stated that "a structure is not given a score unless all required syntactic and morphological rules have been observed." This rigor does not allow for the obvious incompleteness of spoken language. The text on Developmental Sentence Analysis (1974) still penalizes the child who may consistently omit articles, for example, yet otherwise uses rather sophisticated structure. The scoring system focuses heavily on verbs. Because of its rigor it provides much valuable information usable for planning therapy as well as for diagnostic purposes. Percentile scores are generated after scoring.

Another method of language sample analysis is presented by Crystal, Fletcher, and Garman (1976). They provide a system (LARSP: Language Assessment, Remediation, and Screening Procedure) for analyzing samples obtained during sessions of standard 30-min length. It is left to each clinician to present any stimuli that obtain verbalization. The LARSP yields a measure of the grammatical complexity of a child's sentences.

Even if formal systems of analysis are not employed, the language sample provides valuable information. The language sample provides ideal data for calculating the mean length of utterance. It also indicates the verbal productivity of the child. Morehead and Ingram (1973) found that the normal children in their study produced a mean of 175.5 utterances, whereas the linguistically disordered children produced a mean of 148.7 utterances when other factors were controlled. This study objectifies what parents, teachers, and examiners have long observed, namely, that linguistically disordered children tend to be less verbal than normal children. Such a verbal productivity rating has the potential of measuring test-retest improvement.

The language sample also gives information about the frequency of occurrence of certain utterance types in a child's language. One characteristic of the linguistically disordered child seems to be that he may use a form once or in only one context without generalizing it to other contexts. Analysis of a language sample may indicate whether the form occurred only once or routinely.

The language sample must be tape-recorded, or video taped, but to insure accurate transcription the recording must be supplemented by written notes. A suggested form for making hand-written notes is included in Appendix A.

Use of Extratest Data

In the administration of any objective test, there is a rate of expected error. This expected or standard error varies with different test instruments from ± 5–15 points. Test manuals typically report the standard error on specific instruments. This error is related to differences in examiner instructions, child's response and level of effort, test conditions, etc. Error in excess of the standard error might be controlled by administering the entire battery of tests several times within the same week, but such retesting is not feasible in a diagnostic situation. How can an examiner control for error? One method of control lies in the careful use of extratest data. This extratest data includes: 1) case history with the chief complaint, developmental information, and medical history plus the parent's description of the child's behavior; 2) examiner's subjective impressions of the child's behavior; and 3) report from other professionals. Extratest data should be used to confirm or deny the hypothesis the examiner has made based upon the information obtained during differential assessment and linguistic assessment.

Case history   "Chief complaint" is a term commonly used to refer to the reason for referral. The chief complaint tends to be the unifying factor among children with linguistic disorders. The majority of them, regardless of etiology or eventual diagnosis, are referred because of failure to learn to speak at the expected age.

The validity of the parental chief complaint is too often overlooked. A recent survey among parents of deaf children (Malkin, Freeman, and Hastings, 1976) shows that 75% of cases of deafness were first discovered by parents. Less than 10% were first identified by a physician. In the majority of the cases there was a 12-month delay between the time the parents first voiced their concern to a professional and the time when a diagnosis was finally made. The parent's chief complaint can be used as a point of reference for evaluating test results and for conducting the summary conference following the testing.

Case histories routinely contain questions about the child's development. Many parents will have difficulty recalling the exact ages at which a child attained developmental milestones. This often suggests that the behavior occurred at the age the parents expected and so little notice was taken of it. If a parent seems unable to provide developmental information, the examiner can assist them by asking them to recall some significant day, like the child's first Christmas or second birthday, and then describe what the child was doing at that time.

A significant aspect of the history is the parent's description of the child's behavior. Much information can be obtained by simply asking the parent to describe what the child most enjoys doing and how he spends his time at home, including any behavior that is a problem to the parents. This description of the child's behavior at home should be compared to the examiner's impression of the child's behavior during testing. If there are significant discrepancies the parent should be allowed to demonstrate the behavior being questioned.

The prudent examiner who looks at the case history for the first time will ask, "Would I expect the child described here to have any problems at all? If so, what type of problem appears likely?"

The examiner's subjective impressions The most obvious appraisal the examiner can make is of the child's overall appearance. Does the child's height and weight seem normal for his chronologic age? Next, the examiner should carefully observe the child's face. Is there any indication of hypoplasia or lack of development of the nose, maxilla, or mandible? Are there abnormalities of the lips and their movement? Are the eyes of expected size and position on the face? Do they focus and move normally? Is there ptosis or an epicanthal fold? Is the head of normal size or is it abnormal as in hydrocephaly or microcephaly? Examiners need to be familiar with manuals of congenital and genetic abnormality (Gorlin, 1976; Mysak, 1976) so that they recognize such stigmata and are alerted to their diagnostic implications.

The examiner has the entire period of the assessment to observe the child's behavior. These observations supplement the objective scores obtained and should answer the following questions:

1. How does the child relate to people? Is he warm, cooperative or aloof and manipulative of adults? How does the child attempt to secure what he wants? Does he use speech, gesture, or a tantrum?
2. How does child respond to test materials and situations? Is the child interested in the test materials and will he play imaginatively with any of them?
3. Is the child able to regulate his behavior appropriately for his age or is he very impulsive and overactive, flitting from one thing to another so quickly that no task is ever completed?
4. Does the child show any sign of learning during the testing situation?
5. What hand does the child use during testing? Does the child seem appropriately coordinated when handling test materials?

Reports from other professionals Reports of previous evaluations, summaries of medical examinations and academic progress reports are routinely requested. The sophisticated examiner uses these reports to support or refute his prior diagnostic impressions. Any impression that does not agree with a previous report should be questioned, although the examiner must guard against being unduly influenced by these previous reports. There is a natural tendency to try to replicate the test results reported by a highly respected colleague and to refute the results reported by a less respected professional.

Although the effectiveness of the concept of "at risk" registries has been disputed (Rogers, 1971) and the difficulties of specifying uniform rules are apparent, many hospitals attempt to maintain a closer watch on infants who meet their own criteria of being at risk. Examiners should be aware of the factors of high risk and look for them on medical reports. Meier (1973) has reviewed these factors in some detail. Children at risk are those who were delivered abnormally, who were fifth or later-born, or whose condition caused concern after birth. A high incidence of problems has been observed in children with low birth weight, and it has been determined that there is a relationship between severity of handicaps and low birth weight (Meier, 1973).

CRITERIA FOR FORMING DIAGNOSTIC IMPRESSIONS

The data collected from the objective procedures and from the extra-test sources must be interpreted to form the diagnostic impressions. It is the process of interpretation that puts the greatest demands upon the examiner's qualifications. Most serious students master the science of objective testing; many fewer students perfect the art of diagnostic interpretation.

As a guide to the examiner, this section presents differential assessment profiles that are characteristic of the normal child, the child with specific linguistic disorder, and the child with linguistic disorder secondary to hearing impairment, mental retardation, and emotional disturbance. The pattern of learning strengths and weaknesses determines the child's primary diagnostic classification. The points marked on the profile are based upon objective test scores calculated according to standard procedures for each test. A child who falls more than 6 months below expected performance for his chronologic age can be presumed to exhibit a problem in that area of development. The extent of the problem can be further clarified by analysis of language sample and various extratest data.

The Normal Child

Most children from middle class families are pleased by the opportunity to show the examiner all they have learned and often urge the examiner to teach them answers to questions they do not know. Their development follows the schedules of normal motor, cognitive, linguistic, and personal/social growth that constitute the literature of normal child development (Gesell et al., 1940; Jersild, 1960; Mussen, 1970). A predictable number of normal children are referred for testing. Their profiles are characteristic.

A child with the following profile might have been referred because he was forced to compete, either at home or at school, with children of superior ability. Some families and some schools contain few, if any, children of "average" intelligence. Such a child might have been enrolled in an academic program as one of the youngest children in the class and not be ready for formal school work.

Some normal children generate a more defective-appearing profile. The bilingual child, considered elsewhere in this volume, is one

Differential Assessment Profile — Normal Child

Language skills				Memory/attention		Nonverbal skills		
Oral language		Gesture language					Visual	
Compre-hension	Expres-sion	Compre-hension	Expres-sion	Auditory	Visual	Problem solve	Visual motor skills	Gross motor

such child. Current research emphasizes the "problems" children of poverty display, particularly the poor black child (Williams, 1970). Other studies of developmental norms indicate that black children in America may attain motor skills more quickly than do white children (Bayley, 1970), and studies of black children in Africa show that they attain the physical milestones of crawling, standing, and walking from 2–3 months in advance of white American children (LeVine, 1970). Bayley's studies (1970) suggest that the superiority in black children is maintained up to 12 months with other studies of black Africans suggesting that developmental superiority is maintained up to age 3 (LeVine, 1970). In America it seems to be a fact that poor children as a group receive lower scores on standard IQ tests than middle class children. Cross-cultural studies show that cognitive functioning (Piaget Tasks) is similar in a variety of cultures (Ginsberg, 1972). The examiner must be alert to the possibility that the objective test penalized certain children because of their cultural or socioeconomic background.

The Child with Specific Linguistic Disorder

This diagnostic designation does not appear in national surveys of educational problems. Generally it is included under the controversial class of handicaps called specific learning disabilities. A distinction is made between specific learning disability and minimal brain dysfunction, the latter being the medical designation (Myklebust, 1968). The prevalence of this problem is indicated by the estimate of the 35th International Council of Education (Department of Health, Education and Welfare, 1975a) which indicates that 10% of the public school children in the United States are exceptional because of learning disability.

The child with a specific linguistic disorder has failed to comprehend or speak his native language appropriately for his chronologic age. Like other disorders, linguistic disorders occur on a continuum. A characteristic profile of a child with linguistic disorder follows.

Differential Assessment Profile — Linguistically Disordered Child

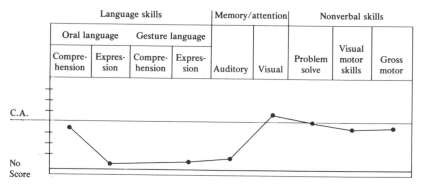

This child's most apparent deficits occur in auditory/verbal tasks. Because the most serious diagnostic confusion is with the hearing-impaired child, no diagnostic impressions can be made without complete and reliable audiologic testing. Behavioral differences also exist, however. The linguistically disordered child is sensitive to environmental sound and often is easily distracted by sound from an adjoining room or the hallway. The linguistically disordered child may give associate responses (*hot* for *stove, Hello* for *phone*). Behaviors such as these are not as characteristic of the hearing-impaired.

The linguistically disordered child demonstrates a predictable deficit in auditory memory with repetition of linguistic material (such as sentences) usually less adequate than repetition of nonlinguistic material. Tests for auditory perception, if administered, are usually defective. Rees (1973) and Liberman et al. (1967) suggest that auditory perception is a linguistic function and any linguistic impairment may be expected to affect auditory perception. This is not to imply that the linguistic disorder is caused by the perceptual problem, but rather that the two problems coincide.

Finally, on the profile the linguistically disordered child demonstrates fairly normal abilities in the nonverbal area of learning. This distinguishes such a child from one who is mentally retarded or emotionally disturbed.

The linguistic assessment of the linguistically disordered child yields information that can be analyzed in view of the rather extensive research that has been done exploring the differences between "language delay" and "language disorder." Both Menyuk (1964) and Lee (1966) feel that "language delay" is a misnomer. They find that linguistically disordered children use deviant forms. Lee, who emphasizes the verb system, feels that linguistically disordered children have great difficulty in learning verbs and they are particularly likely to omit the copula and auxiliary verbs. Errors with the auxiliary *be* are often found in disordered language (Lee and Canter, 1971), as are incorrect pronoun forms. Lee (1966) states that the linguistically disordered child produces atypical utterances such as *think no guess it*, and *got no guess*.

Linguistically disordered children also seem to deviate from the normal in the number of questions they ask. The often reported period of frequent questioning in normal children is not observed in disordered children. It was the conclusion of Menyuk and Lee that linguistically disordered children are not merely following the natural rate more slowly but are failing in certain key linguistic processes.

A study by Leonard (1972) analyzes the frequency of occurrence of certain structures in normal and linguistically disordered children. Normal 2 year olds used subject-verb utterances for 23% of their total utterances, whereas the linguistically disordered children used them only 4% of the time. Linguistically disordered 5 year olds used single word utterances and two-word utterances with the participle *-ing* (eat*ing* or sitt*ing* down) 22% of the time, whereas such structures were not heard at all among the normal children. Menyuk (1964) found that noun phrases and verb phrases were frequently omitted by linguistically disordered children.

Within the past several years other researchers have taken a second look at the conclusions of Menyuk and Lee regarding the nature of linguistic disorder. Johnston and Schery (Morehead and Morehead, 1976) studied 287 children with language disorders between the ages of 3 and 16 years. Among the measures they used were mean length of utterance and order of acquisition of the 14 morphemes studied by Brown. Brown's work (1973), supported by the study of deVilliers and deVilliers (1973), indicated that in normal children the order of progression of acquisition proved to be relatively stable across children, with the exact order being determined by the grammatical complexity of the form. Johnston and Schery (1976) calculated the mean length of utterance and the order of acquisition of these same 14 morphemes. Their results indicated remarkable similarities in the acquisition of these 14 morphemes. They also found a relationship between MLU and acquisition of morphological forms. Their study included a 6-month retest following language training, at which time a significant increase in MLU was found. Their conclusion was that linguistically disordered children take an abnormally long time to acquire language but that they learn the same forms in the same order as normal children. What differed was their developmental time table. By considering language disorders as a variant of normal language development Bloom and Lahey (in press) provide an integrated framework around which language disorders can be identified and goals for rehabilitation determined.

Extratest data obtained on the linguistically disordered child indicates that such a child achieves motor milestones within the limits of normal; however, he may be described as "awkward" or "clumsy." Although such children give the impression that they wish to cooperate with testing, their behavior may be more difficult to control, the incidence of tantrums is higher, and they may have difficulty in maintaining the necessary attention required in order to complete tasks.

Nonverbal language systems may be impaired in these children. They sometimes use gesture; but the system is primitive, especially when compared to that of the hearing-impaired child. They are not particularly responsive to visual or tactile cues, as a hearing-impaired child often is. Some are less sensitive to strangers and may accompany the examiner with little apparent awareness that he is a stranger. Parents may report difficulty in teaching the linguistically disordered child the kind of social customs or manners that the normal child "picks up" without teaching.

The Hearing-Impaired Child

The definition, incidence, and methods of testing for hearing impairment are discussed in detail elsewhere in this volume. Hearing impairment is a continuum, but significant hearing impairment, or lesser hearing impairment combined with other problems, results in

Differential Assessment Profile — Hearing-impaired Child

Language skills				Memory/attention		Nonverbal skills		
Oral language		Gesture language					Visual motor skills	Gross motor
Compre-hension	Expres-sion	Compre-hension	Expres-sion	Auditory	Visual	Problem solve		

predictable linguistic disorders. The most obvious linguistic symptom is moderate or severe delay in the development of comprehension and expression of oral language.

The profile of the hearing-impaired child is highly characteristic. Such a child may have little or no oral language, or else his expressive language may exceed his ability to comprehend. Hearing-impaired children babble like normal children until the age of 6 or 7 months, and may even use the vowel-consonant combination *a-mah* (interpreted by the parents to be *momma*) at approximately 1 year of age (Northern and Downs, 1974). A few hearing-impaired children have learned to say phrases, to name pictures, etc., and may score on these expressive test items. However, when a verbal exchange such as question and answer is expected, they are unable to perform.

Extratest data reveal that the motoric development of the hearing-impaired child follows normal developmental patterns, although self-help tends to be somewhat delayed. It has been noted that deaf children laugh aloud less than the normal child; but their smiling is not affected (Myklebust, 1954).

In the test situation the hearing-impaired child may seem over-active because of his need to explore the test environment. However, he plays with toys with interest and imagination. Such a child is sensitive to visual and tactile stimuli. Attempts to communicate with gesture are often observed, and some hearing-impaired children have developed sophisticated gesture systems. This child's attention and level of cooperation may seem less than adequate because of the examiner's difficulty in conveying the test instructions. Usually the child's attention improves on the nonverbal tests.

The Mentally Retarded Child

Mental retardation represents a continuum and its definition is extremely complex. Robinson and Robinson (1965) relate these difficulties to the problems in defining intelligence. They feel three characteristics are essential in defining mental retardation. These are impairment in the capacity to learn, inadequate knowledge acquired, and inability to adjust or adapt to the total environment. They further describe a mentally retarded child as one who falls at least one standard deviation below the mean of the general population (Robinson and Robinson, 1970). The incidence of mental retardation is said to be 3% of the general population (Bensberg and Sigelman, 1976).

Differential Assessment Profile — Mentally Retarded Child

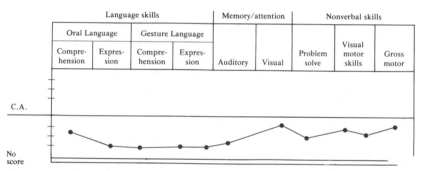

The profile of the mentally retarded child is characterized by the relatively uniform depression of test scores across the spectrum of achievement. The more severe the retardation the more depressed are all areas of functioning. Although language development may lag behind other performance there is minimal discrepancy between language and nonverbal skills. No areas of performance are appropriate for chronologic age. Because the development of the mentally retarded child occurs on an organismic basis it is expected that motor milestones will also be delayed. Myklebust (1954) found that the mean age for sitting was 10.3 months and for walking was 21.1 months.

The more severely involved retarded children tend to be mute; but others develop language. Karlin and Strazzula (1952) estimated that those with IQs below 30 said their first word between 3½ and 4½ years whereas those with IQs of 50–70 used their first word at about 3 years of age. Lenneberg (1967) indicates that passing of motor milestones best predicts the age of language acquisition. A study by Newfield and Schlanger (1968) indicates that retarded children seem to learn morphology in a manner comparable to normal children. The order of development was identical to the normals but the pace of the retarded was slower suggesting the differences are quantitative, not qualitative.

In other areas of behavior the mentally retarded child tends to perform characteristically for his mental age. Such a child of 4 or over may play happily with pull toys, dump trucks, etc., which would interest a much younger child. The mentally retarded child responds to sound as a younger child would. He is no more attentive to visual stimuli than any child of his mental age. Gesture, if used at all, tends to be rather primitive. His ability to relate to others is also characteristic of mental age. As the mentally retarded child becomes older and has more experience with failure, he may become increasingly fearful of new situations and be especially reluctant to respond.

The Emotionally Disturbed Child

Like other problems discussed, emotional disturbance is not a single disease but rather a group of related problems that are displayed on a continuum of severity. They range from mild behavior disorders that can be characterized into classes (Anthony, 1970) to more severe disorders. These classes include functional problems such as food fads, enuresis, nightmares, sleepwalking, head banging, and tics; affective problems such as unusual fears, apprehensions, panic, and separation anxieties; tension habits such as nail biting, thumbsucking and unexplained sadness, grief, or euphoria; and social behaviors such as excessively aggressive acts, destructive acts, withdrawal, negative behavior, controlling or clinging behaviors and masturbation. It is obvious that many children display one or even several of these problems without exhibiting any significant disorder, and there is no evidence that children with these behavioral problems are more likely to have linguistic disorders than any other child.

The more serious of the emotional disturbances have as one of their most significant symptoms inappropriate or lack of verbal behavior. These disorders are usually considered under the term "childhood psychosis" (Goldfarb, 1970). Childhood psychosis is not a single disorder but a group of related problems. Two of the most carefully described disorders are childhood schizophrenia (Bender, 1947, 1956) and infant autism (Kanner, 1942). Kanner feels that in autism there is withdrawal of the child from the very beginning of life with the first symptoms being apparent during the first 3 months. The etiologies are diverse and still not well specified.

The outstanding feature of the profile of the emotionally disturbed child is a lack of objective test scores. This profile reflects his inability to perform except for isolated items such as motor ability, which can be scored on the basis of examiner's observation. A possible exception is some nonverbal task that might have caught the attention of the child and that he did spontaneously with no interaction with the examiner. Such children will sometimes complete puzzles or block tasks that are left out in view or which the examiner is "playing with" in the child's view.

Differential Assessment Profile — Emotionally Disturbed Child

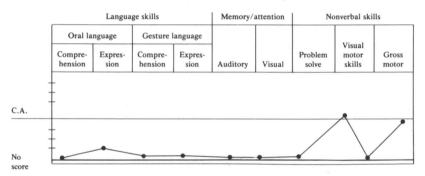

The generation of a profile reflecting "No scores" illustrates that lack of performance can yield valuable diagnostic information. Children who are difficult to test are often sent home with the recommendation to return in 6–12 months. Such a recommendation is unfounded. No child is too young to be tested when an overall behavioral approach is used; consequently nothing is gained by refusing to see a child until he is older. On the contrary, inability to cooperate suggests a serious problem and a recommendation to return in 6 months results in losing irreplaceable months of training during the primary language-learning period.

A recent publication on autism edited by Ritvo et al. (1976) describes autism as a "physical disease of the brain" whose victims share a neuropathophysiologic process that interferes with developmental rate resulting in disturbances of motility, language, and personality development. The onset is apparent before 3 years of age with children varying from totally mute to those whose speech is characterized by echolalia, usually accompanied by misuse or reversal of pronouns. This volume on autism contains a protocol for behavioral evaluation that lends itself to prescriptive teaching of the autistic child.

It also provides an excellent review of current research on the etiology and remediation of this problem (Ritvo et al., 1976).

Proposed levels for classifying the communication of these children (Ruttenberg and Wolf, 1967) give an indication of what the examiner may expect to observe in the case history and during the assessment of an emotionally disturbed child. The following is adapted from the author's guidelines:

1. No communication
   a. totally unaware
   b. primitive affect-undirected
   c. subtle signs of directed affect
2. Nonverbal communication
   a. occasional approach to a person
   b. regularly expressed awareness of another person
   c. a definite approach, some mutuality emerges
3. Verbal communication
   a. may be echolalic
   b. may have elaborate animal noises or sound effects
   c. may have pronoun reversals, may refuse to acknowledge pronouns
   d. may have perseverative remarks or taboo words
   e. may occasionally use well structured, sophisticated utterances.

The extratest data obtained on the emotionally disturbed child are characteristic. Kanner (1942) indicates that the autistic child develops motorically like the normal child, whereas the schizophrenic child is less adept motorically but generally within the range of normal. They seem to be healthy, robust, and physically attractive children. Both groups tend to reject activities that they are very capable of doing, such as dressing or feeding themselves. Autistic children display atypical motoric behaviors, such as hand-flapping in 70% of the cases studied by Ritvo et al. (1976).

The outstanding characteristic of these children is their aloneness. They seem to be unaware of the essential living character of people around them and unaware of their own personal identity and body. They seem to be nonhearing, nonsmiling, and tend to "look through" people. In general they are described as maintaining a tyrannical control over their environment and become panicky and desperate if any change occurs. At these times it is difficult to comfort them and several testing sessions may be needed before the child is willing to display any but screaming, panic behavior. Their aggression is indiscriminate and often self-directed. They will rock, whirl or bang their heads for long periods and may do severe damage to themselves in cases such as head banging if not forcibly restrained (Goldfarb, 1970).

REPORTING RESULTS

Test results are always recorded in written form and may also be reported verbally. All reports are communication and involve, as language always does, a speaker (usually the examiner) and a listener or reader (usually another professional or a parent). The style of the report should be concise and intelligible to the reader. A summary of the tests used to observe behaviors and the results of those tests including a profile need to be included.

Reports of the examiner's subjective impressions should be precise and avoid "cute expressions." For example, the examiner should specify that the child spent 40 min of the 60-min test session running about the test room rather than commenting that the child "climbed the walls." The examiner must guard against the tendency to gossip in the report. Some information revealed in the case history and the conference has no direct bearing on the problem. The fact that the mother has been married five times before marrying the child's father may be interesting but probably does not contribute to a linguistic problem. A concise summary of some of the rules for good report writing appears in Pannbacher (1975) and in Knepflar (1976).

Legally the examiner must have a signed release of information for each report sent. Ultimately it is the parents who control information about their own child.

Results of a differential assessment may be stated as follows.

"This child displays no linguistic disorder. According to our test scores both verbal and nonverbal skills are within the range of normal. Comprehension and expression of oral language are entirely adequate for a child of this age"; or

"This child exhibits a significant linguistic disorder, characterized by the following deviations from normal language patterns..."; or

"This linguistic disorder seems associated with response patterns that are seen in children who have been diagnosed as being...hearing impaired...mentally retarded...emotionally disturbed. This impression of linguistic disorder as secondary to the above condition is substantiated by the accompanying report from the audiologist, clinical psychologist, physician, etc."

If such reports from allied professionals are not available, then the first recommendation would be that appropriate diagnostic testing be immediately scheduled and final diagnostic impressions be deferred until all testing was complete.

Regardless of the impression derived from the differential assessment, the results of the linguistic analysis should be presented. Differences between comprehension and expression in terms of vocabulary and morphosyntactic systems should be described. Differences between oral language and gesture, if significant, can be included. An estimate of vocabulary size, including content versus function words and estimated mean length of utterance, and finally some estimate of overall verbal productivity is required for any child who exhibits a restricted linguistic system. Naturally, the intelligibility of the speech will be specified (the phonologic aspects of language are not discussed in this chapter). Finally, the function of the child's language should be described. When age norms are available, the examiner should provide these to clarify further the linguistic developmental age of the child.

After testing, a conference is usually scheduled with the parents. This conference should be an exchange of information, not a monologue by the examiner. Because few examiners have the benefit of formal course work in interviewing or conferencing, periodic review of interview techniques is appropriate. Sullivan (1954) provides considerable insight into this process. Further discussion of the topic plus references are included in the texts by Johnson, Darley, and Spriesterbach (1952), Doll (1953), and King and Berger (1971). In addition, an examiner can sharpen his own skills by tape recording conference sessions and reviewing the tapes several days later. Simple analysis of the percentage of time the examiner spoke as opposed to the time the parent spoke provides insight into the dynamics of the conference. An even more valuable check to conference efficiency is routine follow-up of parents to see what they feel the diagnostic impressions and recommendations were. The final proof of the effectiveness of the conferences is whether the parents followed the examiner's recommendations.

There are few studies on conference effectiveness. One study of patient understanding of physicians' presurgical conferences (JAMA, 1976) indicates the significant difference between what a professional actually said and how the patient perceived what was said. In an effort to communicate more effectively with the parents, and also to protect the examiner, a Parent Conference Form (Appendix B) may be used.

A copy of this form is given to the parents for their records. It also provides a format for the conference by requiring a mutually understood statement of the parent's chief concern and primary questions as well as a summary of test results and the examiner's recommendations.

CONCLUSION

The challenge of testing young children lies in the fleetness of their responses and the changeability of their moods. The marvel of testing the young child lies in the speed with which he changes from a mute, helpless infant to an independent preschooler, who by age 4 has already learned the structure and thousands of words of his native language. The child with a linguistic disorder is still primarily a child and only secondarily one with a problem. Such a child still has the wonderous growth potential common to all children. That potential is the hope that keeps the professional seeking more sophisticated methods of diagnosis and more developmentally sound systems of remediation.

REFERENCES

Abrahamsen, A. A. 1977. Child Language: An Interdisciplinary Guide to Theory and Research. University Park Press, Baltimore.

Administrative Guide and Handbook for Special Education. 1973. Texas Education Agency Bulletin 711.

Ammons, R. B. and Ammons, H. S. 1962. Ammons Full Range Picture Vocabulary Test, Psychological Test Specialists, Missoula, Montana.

Anthony, E. J. 1970. Behavior disorders of childhood. In: P. H. Mussen (ed.), Carmichael's Manual of Child Psychology, Vol. 2, pp. 667–764. John Wiley & Sons Inc., New York.

Arthur, G. 1949. The Arthur Adaptation of the Leiter International Performance Scale. J. Clin. Psychol. 5:1–5.

Bangs, J. L. 1947. A comprehensive historical survey of concepts regarding congenital language disability. Unpublished dissertation, University of Iowa.

Bangs, T. E. 1968. Language and Learning Disorders of the Pre-Academic Child. Appleton-Century-Crofts, Inc. New York.

Bangs, T. E. 1975. Vocabulary Comprehension Scale: Pronouns and Words of Position, Quality, Quantity and Size. Learning Concepts, Inc., Austin, Texas.

Bangs, T. E. Birth to Three: Assessment, Program Planning and Curriculum. In preparation.

Bar-Adon, A. and Leopold, W. (eds.). 1971. Child Language: A Book of Readings. Prentice-Hall Inc., Englewood Cliffs, New Jersey.

Bayley, N. 1969. Manual for the Bayley Scales of Infant Development. The Psychological Corporation, New York.

Bayley, N. 1970. Development of mental abilities. In: P. Mussen (ed.), Carmichael's Manual of Child Psychology, Vol. 1, pp. 1163-1209. John Wiley & Sons Inc., New York.

Becky, R. E. 1942. A study of certain factors related to retardation of speech. J. Speech Hear. Disord. 7:223-250.

Bender, L. 1947. Child schizophrenia: Clinical study of one hundred schizophrenic children. Am. J. Orthopsychiatr. 17:40-56.

Bender, L. 1956. Schizophrenia in childhood: Its recognition, description and treatment. Am. J. Orthopsychiatr. 26:499-506.

Bensberg, G. J. and Sigelman, C. K. 1976. Definitions and prevalence. In: L. L. Lloyd (ed.), Communication Assessment and Intervention Strategies. pp. 33-72. University Park Press, Baltimore.

Berko, J. 1958. The child's learning of English morphology. Word 14:150-177.

Bloom, L. 1970. Language Development: Form and Function in Emerging Grammars. The MIT Press, Cambridge, Massachusetts.

Bloom, L. 1973. One Word at a Time. Mouton & Co., The Hague.

Bloom, L. and M. Lahey. Language Development and Language Disorders. John Wiley & Sons Inc., New York. In press.

Bodenman, P. S. 1976. Some Aspects of Education in the United States. Paper presented to incoming educators from abroad. Washington, D.C.

Bowerman, M. F. 1974. Learning the structure of causative verbs: A study in the relationship of cognitive, semantic and syntactic development. Pap. Rep. Child. Lang. Dev. 8:142-178.

Bricker, W. A. 1972. A systematic approach to language training. In: R. L. Schiefelbusch (ed.), Language of the Mentally Retarded, pp. 74-92. University Park Press, Baltimore.

Bricker, W. A. and Bricker, D. D. 1970. A program of language training for the severely handicapped child. Except. Child. 37:101-110.

Brown, R. 1958. Words and Things. pp. 194-228. The Free Press of Glencoe, New York.

Brown, R. 1973. A First Language: The Early Stages, pp. 54-56. Harvard University Press, Cambridge.

Buros, O. K. (ed.). 1972. The Seventh Mental Measurement Yearbook. Vol. 1. The Gryphon Press, Highland Park, N.J.

Bzoch, K. R. and League, R. 1971/8. Assessing Language Skills in Infancy. University Park Press, Baltimore.

Carrow, E. 1973. Test for Auditory Comprehension of Language. Learning Concepts, Inc., Austin, Texas.

Carrow, E. 1974a. A test using elicited imitations in assessing grammatical structure in children, J. Speech Hear. Disord. 39:437-499.

Carrow, E. 1974b. Carrow Elicited Language Inventory. Learning Concepts, Inc., Austin, Texas.

Cattell, P. 1960. The Measurement of Intelligence in Infants and Young Children. The Psychological Corporation, New York.

Chapman, S. K. 1971. The age and order of acquisition of selected morphological constructions produced by children age 2 to 4 years of age, pp. 43-44. Unpublished dissertation, University of South Carolina.

Chomsky, N. 1957. Syntactic Structures. Mouton & Co., The Hague.

Clark, E. V. 1973a. What's in a word? On the child's acquisition of semantics in his first language. In: Timothy E. Moore (ed.), pp. 65–110. Cognitive Development and the Acquisition of Language.

Clark, E. V. 1973b. How children describe time and order. In: C. A. Ferguson and D. I. Slobin (eds.), Studies of Child Language Development, pp. 585–606. Holt, Rinehart, and Winston, Inc., New York.

Crystal, D., Fletcher, P., and Garman, M. 1976. The Grammatical Analysis of Language Disability: A Procedure for Assessment and Remediation, American Elsevier Publishing Co., Inc., New York.

Darley, F. and Winitz, H. 1961. Age of first word, review of research, J. Speech Hear. Disord. 26:272–290.

Darley, F. L. 1964. Diagnosis and Appraisal of Communication Disorders. Prentice-Hall Inc., Englewood Cliffs, New Jersey.

deVilliers, J. G. and deVilliers, P. A. 1973. A cross-sectional study of the development of grammatical morphemes in child speech. J. Psycholinguist. Res. 2:267–278.

Department of Health, Education and Welfare. 1975. Progress of education in the United States of America: 1972–73 and 1973–74. In: Report for the Thirty-Fifth International Conference on Education. Publication No. (OE) 76-19104. p. 11. United States Government Printing Office. Washington, D.C.

Doll, E. A. 1953. Measurement of Social Competence. American Guidance Service, Inc., Circle Pines, Minnesota.

Dunn, L. M. 1965. Peabody Picture Vocabulary Test. p. 34. American Guidance Service, Inc. Circle Pines, Minnesota.

Ewing, A. W. G. 1930. Aphasia in Children. Oxford University Press, New York.

Foster, R., Gidden, J. J., and Stark, J. 1972. Assessment of Children's Language Comprehension. Consulting Psychologists Press, Inc. Palo Alto.

Gesell, A., Halverson, M. Thompson, H., Ilg, F. L., Castner, M., Ames, L. B., and Amatruda, S. 1940. The First Five Years of Life. Harper and Brothers, New York.

Ginsberg, H. 1972. The Myth of the Deprived Child. Prentice-Hall Inc., Englewood Cliffs, New Jersey.

Goldfarb, W. 1970. Childhood psychosis. In: P. H. Mussen (ed.), Carmichael's Manual of Child Psychology. Vol. 2. pp. 765–830. John Wiley & Sons Inc., New York.

Goldstein, K. 1948. Language and Language Disabilities. Grune & Stratton, Inc., New York.

Gorlin, J. 1976. Syndromes of the Head and Neck. McGraw-Hill Book Company. New York.

Greenfield, P. M. and Smith, J. 1976. The Structure of Communication in Early Language Development. Academic Press, New York.

Hayes, J. R. 1970. Cognition and the Development of Language. John Wiley & Sons Inc., New York.

Head, H. 1926. Aphasia and Kindred Disorders, Vols. 1 and 2. Cambridge University Press, Cambridge, Great Britain.

Hiskey, M. S. 1966. Hiskey-Nebraska Test of Learning Aptitude. Union College Press, Lincoln, Nebraska.

Houston, S. H. 1969. A sociolinguistic consideration of the Black English of children in Northern Florida. Language 45:599–607.

Jackson, H. 1871. Singing by speechless (aphasic) children. Lancet 2:430–431.

Jakobson, R. 1968. Child Language, Aphasia, and Phonological Universals. Mouton & Co., The Hague.

JAMA. March 1976, Memories Can Fade After Surgery. 235 (10):993.

Jersild, A. T. 1960. Child Psychology. Prentice-Hall Inc., Englewood Cliffs, New Jersey.

Johnson, D. J. and Myklebust, H. R. 1967. Learning Disabilities: Educational Principles and Practices. Grune & Stratton, Inc., New York.

Johnson, W., Darley, F. L., and Spriesterbach, D. C. 1952. Diagnostic Methods in Speech Pathology. Harper & Row, Publishers, New York.

Johnston, J. R. and Schery, T. K. 1976. The use of grammatical morphemes by children with communication disorders. In: D. M. Morehead and A. E. Morehead (eds.), Normal and Deficient Child Language, pp. 239–258. University Park Press, Baltimore.

Kanner, L. 1942. Autistic disturbance of affective contact. Nerv. Child. 2:217–250.

Karlin, I. W. and Strazzula, M. 1952. Speech and language problems of mentally deficient children. J. Speech Hear. Disord. 7:286–294.

King, R. R. and Berger, K. W. 1971. Diagnostic Assessment and Counseling Techniques for Speech Pathologists and Audiologists. Stanwix House, Inc., Pittsburgh.

Kirk, S. A., McCarthy, J. J., and Kirk, W. D. 1968. Examiner's Manual Illinois Test of Psycholinguistic Abilities, p. 23. Western Psychological Services, Los Angeles.

Knepflar, K. J. Report Writing in the Field of Communication Disorders. The Interstate Printers & Publishers, Inc., Danville, Illinois.

Labov, W. 1971. The logic of Nonstandard English. In: F. Williams (ed.), Language and Poverty: Perspectives on a Theme. p. 170. Markham Publishing Company, Chicago.

Lee, L. L. 1966. Developmental sentence types: A method for comparing normal and deviant syntactic development. J. Speech Hear. Disord. 31:311–30.

Lee, L. L. 1970. A screening test for syntax development. J. Speech Hear. Disord. 35:103–112.

Lee, L. L. 1971. Northwestern Syntax Screening Test. Northwestern University Press, Evanston, Illinois.

Lee, L. L. 1974. Developmental Sentence Analysis. Northwestern University Press, Evanston, Illinois.

Lee, L. L. and Canter, S. M. 1971. Developmental sentence scoring: A clinical procedure for estimating syntactic development in children's spontaneous speech. J. Speech Hear. Disord. 36:315–340.

Leiter, R. G. 1969. Examiner's Manual for the Leiter International Performance Scale. Stoelting Company, Chicago.

Lenneberg, E. H. 1967. Biological Foundations of Language. John Wiley & Sons Inc., New York.

Leonard, L. B. 1972. What is deviant language? J. Speech Hear. Disord. 37:427–446.

Leopold, W. 1973. Patterning in children's language learning. In: A. Bar-Adon and W. Leopold (eds.), Child Language: A Book of Readings. Prentice-Hall Inc., Englewood Cliffs, New Jersey.

LeVine, R. 1970. Cross-cultural study in child psychology. In: P. H. Mussen (ed.), Carmichael's Manual of Child Psychology, Vol. 2, p. 574. John Wiley & Sons Inc., New York.

Lewis, M. M. 1936. Infant Speech: A Study of the Beginnings of Language. Harcourt Brace &World, Inc., New York.

Liberman, A. M., Cooper, F. S., Shankweiler, D. P., and Studdert-Kennedy, M. 1967. Perception of speech code. Psychol. Rev. 74:431–461.

Lynch, J. and Bricker, W. A. 1972. Linguistic theory and operant procedures: Toward an integrated approach to language training for the mentally retarded. Ment. Retard. 10:12–17.

Lynch, J. Morphosyntax Comprehension Scale. In preparation.

Malkin, S. F., Freeman, R. D., and Hasting, J. O. 1976. Audiol. Hear. Educ. 2:21–29.

McCarthy, D. 1954. Language development in children. In: L. Carmichael (ed.), Manual of Child Psychology. pp. 492–630. John Wiley & Sons Inc., New York.

McGinnis, M. 1963. Aphasic children: Identification and education by the association method. Alexander Graham Bell Association for the Deaf, Washington, D.C.

McNeill, D. 1970. The development of language. In: P. Mussen (ed.), Carmichael's Manual of Child Psychology. pp. 1061–1161. John Wiley & Sons Inc., New York.

Meier, J. 1973. Screening and Assessment of Young Children at Developmental Risk. DHEW Publication No. (05) 13–90. p. 48. Washington, D.C.

Menyuk, P. 1963. A preliminary evaluation of grammatical capacity of children. J. Verb. Learn. Verb. Behav. 2:429–439.

Menyuk, P. 1964. Comparison of grammar of children with functionally deviant and normal speech. J. Speech Hear. Res. 7:109–121.

Menyuk, P. 1969. Sentences Children Use. The MIT Press, Cambridge, Massachusetts.

Menyuk, P. 1972. Relationships among components of the grammar in language disorders. J. Speech Hear. Res. 15:395–406.

Menyuk, P. 1976. A problem of language disorder: Length versus structure. In: D. M. Morehead and A. E. Morehead (eds.), Normal and Deficient Child Language. pp. 259–279. University Park Press, Baltimore.

Moerk, E. L. 1977. Pragmatic and Semantic Aspects of Early Language Development. University Park Press, Baltimore.

Moore, T. E. (ed.). 1973. Cognitive Development and the Acquisition of Language. Academic Press, New York.

Morehead, D. M. and Ingram, D. 1973. The development of base syntax in normal and linguistically deviant children. J. Speech Hear. Res. 16:330–352.

Morehead, D. M. and Morehead, A. E. 1976. Normal and deficient child language. University Park Press, Baltimore.

Mussen, P. H. (ed.). 1970. Carmichael's Manual of Child Psychology, Vols. 1 and 2. John Wiley & Sons Inc., New York.

Myklebust, H. R. 1954. Auditory Disorders in Children. Grune & Stratton, Inc., New York.

Myklebust, H. R. (ed.). 1968. Progress in Learning Disabilities. Vol. 1. Grune & Stratton, Inc., New York.

Myklebust, H. R. (ed.). 1971. Progress in Learning Disabilities. Vol. II. Grune & Stratton, Inc., New York.

Mysak, E. D. 1976. Pathologies of Speech Systems. The Williams & Wilkins Company, Baltimore.

Nance, L. S. 1946. Differential diagnosis of aphasia in children. J. Speech Disord. 2:219–223.

Newfield, M. U. and Schlanger, B. B. 1968. The acquisition of English morphology by normal and educable mentally retarded children. J. Speech Hear. Res. 11:693–706.

Northern, J. and Downs, M. P. 1974. Hearing in Children. The Williams & Wilkins Company, Baltimore.

Orton, S. 1937. Reading, Writing and Speech Problems in Children. W. W. Norton & Company Inc., New York.

Pannbacher, M. 1975. Diagnostic report writing. J. Speech Hear. Disord. 40:367–379.

Penfield, W. and Roberts, L. 1959. Speech and Brain Mechanisms. Princeton University Press, Princeton, New Jersey.

Piaget, J. 1923. Le Langage et la pensée chez l'enfant. Delachaux et Niestlé, Paris. Translated by Marjorie Gabain. 1955. The Language and Thought of the Child. The World Publishing Company, Cleveland.

Popham, W. J. (ed.). 1971. Criterion-Referenced Measurement. Educational Technology Publications, Inc., Englewood Cliffs, New Jersey.

Prutting, C. A. and Rees, N. 1977. Pragmatics of Language: Applications to the Assessment and Remediation of Communication Behaviors. Short course presented at the American Speech and Hearing Association.

Public Law 94-142. 1976. Education for all Handicapped Children Act.

Rees, N. S. 1973. The view from Procrustes bed: Auditory processing factors in language disorders. J. Speech Hear. Disord. 38:304–315.

Ritvo, E. R., Freeman, B. J., Ornitz, E. M., Tanguay, P. E. (eds.). 1976. Autism: Diagnosis, Current Research and Management. pp. 5, 12. Spectrum Publications, Inc., New York.

Robinson, H. B. and Robinson, N. M. 1965. The Mentally Retarded Child: A Psychological Approach. McGraw-Hill Book Company, New York.

Robinson, H. B. and Robinson, N. 1970, Mental retardation. In: Paul Mussen (ed.), Carmichael's Manual of Child Psychology, pp. 615–666. John Wiley & Sons Inc., New York.

Rogers, M. G. 1971. The early recognition of handicapping disorders in childhood. Dev. Med. Child Neurol. 13:88–101.

Ruttenberg, B. G. and Wolf, E. G. 1967. Evaluating the communication of the autistic child. J. Speech Hear. Disord. 32:314–324.

Siegel, G. M. and Broen, P. A. 1976. Language assessment. In: L. L. Lloyd (ed.), Definitions and Prevalence in Communication Assessment and Intervention Strategies, pp. 33–72. University Park Press, Baltimore.

Strauss, A. A. and Kephart, N. C. 1955. Psychopathology and Education of the Brain-Injured Child. Grune & Stratton, Inc., New York.

Strauss, A. A. and Lehtinen, L. E. 1947. Psychopathology and Education of the Brain-Injured Child, p. 4. Grune & Stratton, Inc., New York.

Sullivan, H. S. 1954. The Psychiatric Interview. W. W. Norton & Company Inc., New York.

Terman, L. M. and Merrill, M. A. 1937. Measuring Intelligence. Riverside Press, Cambridge, Massachusetts.

Terman, L. M. and Merrill, M. A. 1960. Stanford-Binet Intelligence Scale. Houghton Mifflin Company, Boston.

Terman, L. M. and Merrill, M. A. 1972. Stanford-Binet Intelligence Scale, pp. 75–78. Houghton Mifflin Company, Boston.

Terman, L. M. and Merrill, M. A. 1973. Stanford-Binet Intelligence Scale. Manual for the Third Revision Form L-M. Houghton Mifflin Company, Boston.

Texas Education Agency Bulletin 711. 1973. Texas Education Agency, Austin.

Travis, L. E. 1931. Speech Pathology. Appleton-Century-Crofts, New York.

Vaisse, M. D. 1866. Des sourds-muets et de certains cas d'aphasie congenitale. Bull. Soc. Anthropol. 1 (2):146–150.

Van Riper, C. 1947. Speech Correction. 2nd Ed. Prentice-Hall Inc., Englewood Cliffs, N.J.

Wechsler, D. 1967. Manual for the Wechsler Preschool and Primary Scale of Intelligence. The Psychological Corporation, New York.

Wechsler, D. 1974. Wechsler Intelligence Scale for Children—Revised. The Psychological Corporation, New York.

Weiner, P. S. 1972. The language-related behavior of dysphasic children. In: R. L. Schiefelbusch (ed.), Language of the Mentally Retarded, pp. 192–193. University Park Press, Baltimore.

West, R. L., Kennedy, L., and Carr, A. 1947. The Rehabilitation of Speech Revised Edition. Harper & Brothers, New York.

Wilbur, H. B. 1867. Aphasia. Am. J. Insanity 24:1–28.

Wilde, W. R. 1853. Practical Observations on Aural Surgery and the Nature and Treatment of Diseases of the Ear. Blanchard and Lea, Philadelphia.

Williams, E. 1970. Language and Poverty: Perspectives on a Theme. Markham Publishing Company, Chicago.

Williams, R. L. 1972. The BITCH test (Black Intelligence Test of Cultural Homogeneity). Black Studies Program. Washington University, St. Louis.

APPENDIX A

Language Sample

Key to symbols

Name _____Date _____	· · · = lapse of time in speech
Birthdate_____C.A._____	⋮ = lapse of time: child active
Examiner_____Test time____	— — = unintelligible or "un-heard" words
	/ = end of utterance: falling inflection
Total number of words _____	
Number of utterances_____	? = question: rising inflection
Mean length of utterance _____	

Setting for language sample
Persons present:

Speech event:	Utterances
(Note child's gestures, actions, etc., which contribute to understanding utterances.)	

APPENDIX B

Child's name _____Case number _____
Staff member(s)_____Date_____
Reason for testing: _____
Parent's questions: _____
Test results

Differential Assessment Profile

	Language Skills				Memory/attention		Nonverbal skills		
	Oral language		Gesture language						
	Compre-hension	Expres-sion	Compre-hension	Expres-sion	Auditory	Visual	Problem solve	Visual motor skills	Gross motor
C.A.									
No score									

Language level

Recommendations

This information has been discussed with me and I have received a copy of this report.

_____
(Signed: Parent or Guardian)

Evaluation of Linguistic Disorders in Adults

Harvey Halpern

CONTENTS

Although noting the maze of terminology in the field of aphasia Professor Halpern skillfully guides the reader through definitions of the more significant terms in clinical use. In describing the evaluation of linguistic disorders in adults, the chapter begins with a brief history of test development starting with Henry Head's first test (Head, 1926) and includes a description of over a dozen of the most commonly used tests published since then. The focus of the chapter is on the responsibility of the speech pathologist to provide differential diagnosis for adults who have some type of communication problem secondary to brain damage. Professor Halpern notes that seven language categories (Halpern, Darley, and Brown, 1973) separate the aphasic from the patient with generalized intellectual impairment. Guidelines (Johns and Darley, 1970) that distinguish apraxia of speech from expressive aphasia and that separate the irrelevant speech of the patient with confused language from the auditory aphasic are specified. Criteria for identifying and classifying dysarthria are also detailed. The discussion on assessment includes prognostic factors and presents research data showing the influence of bilingualism on aphasia rehabilitation.   —Eds.

Quite often the speech pathologist is called upon to aid in the differential diagnosis of the brain-injured patient. His evaluation can help decide whether a patient has aphasia, generalized intellectual impairment, apraxia of speech, confused language, dysarthria, or any combination of these disorders. This information can be very useful, for it helps to determine whether speech treatment is recommended or not and to determine which kind of treatment is applicable. For example, treatment for the aphasic patient involves language training, whereas training for the patient with apraxia of speech might involve a phonetic or motoric approach.

Another advantage is that proper evaluation of the speech and language of a patient can offer the neurologist another diagnostic sign in determining whether a lesion(s) is of focal or diffuse origin. For example, confused language or generalized intellectual impairment is thought to be consistent with diffuse lesions, whereas aphasia and apraxia of speech are generally associated with focal lesions (Mayo Clinic, 1964, pp. 257-258). On the other hand, it is most likely that an attending physician will have made the referral and information such as onset and type of lesion, accompanying paralysis, visual and hearing problems, and course of treatment can be gleaned from him.

Although the literature is somewhat sparse, the difficulties involved in differentiating the five groups have been noted (Mayo Clinic, 1964, pp. 257-258; Darley, 1964, pp. 36-40; Stengel, 1964, p. 289; Zangwill, 1964, p. 297; Halpern, Darley and Brown, 1973). Each of the five groups will be discussed separately in detail.

APHASIA

Aphasia can be defined as a multimodality language disturbance caused by brain injury. It is a linguistic deficit that causes the individual to have difficulty in the comprehension or formulation of language symbols. Aphasia is not generalized intellectual impairment, apraxia of speech, confused language, or dysarthria, although components of any combination of those disorders may accompany aphasic disturbance (Halpern, 1972).

Although there is much confusion over the terminology and nomenclature in aphasia, a few definitions seem warranted to start any discussion of aphasic disturbance. Difficulty in the comprehension of spoken language symbols is generally known as auditory aphasia. Here the individual might have greater difficulty in understanding 1) abstract words as opposed to concrete; 2) longer words than short; 3) infrequently used words as compared with frequent; 4) certain parts of speech; 5) words that sound alike; 6) closely associated words; and 7) complex sentences. There can be a reduced auditory retention span and a general slowness of comprehension. Alexia is the term used when an individual has an impairment in the comprehension of written symbols (reading). Many of the same disturbances that apply to the auditory aphasic can be observed in alexia, except that here the difficulty is in comprehension through the visual modality.

Difficulty in the formulation of spoken language symbols can be called oral expressive aphasia. This problem may manifest itself as a reduced vocabulary, telegraphic speech, jargon, agrammatisms, reduced fluency, excessive fluency, circumlocutions, neologisms, paraphasias, phonemic changes, and word-finding difficulties.

An impairment in the formulation of written language symbols is called agraphia. Acalculia is a disturbance in handling numerical symbols either through comprehension in listening or reading, or formulation in speaking or writing.

As was stated in the definition, aphasia is caused by brain injury. It is most likely of focal origin. A major cause of aphasia in middle and old age is cerebrovascular accident. Cerebrovascular accidents consist of thromboses, embolisms, aneurysms, hemorrhages, and ischemias. A cerebral thrombosis is an occlusion of an artery to the brain by a clot. A cerebral embolus is a clot formed elsewhere and finally lodging in the brain. An aneurysm is a swelling or ballooning of a cranial artery. A cerebral hemorrhage is the rupture of a blood vessel with subsequent bleeding into the brain. Ischemia is deficient circulation in the brain. All cerebrovascular accidents have one thing in common, they deprive the brain of oxygen, thus causing brain damage.

Trauma to the brain is another major cause of aphasia. Gunshot wounds, automobile accidents, and falls are most likely involved in physical trauma to the brain. Brain tumors, both malignant and nonmalignant, are associated with causing aphasia. Quite often the extirpation of a brain tumor will cause aphasia. Abscesses, infectious diseases, and degenerative diseases of the brain can also result in aphasia.

Before presenting further characterization of aphasia, a review of aphasia testing is presented to indicate the evolvement of the tools available for making a differential diagnosis of the language-impaired adult.

Testing of Brain-Injured Adults

During the 1800s, the assessment and diagnosis of aphasia were limited strictly to clinical observations. After a while, short qualitative tests were performed to determine the kind and degree of aphasia. For example, the examiner would ask the patient to indicate by fingers how many weeks he spent in the hospital. At the turn of the century, the Proust-Lichtheim Test (Baker, 1954) investigated inner speech by having the patient hold up as many fingers as there were syllables in the word he could not pronounce.

Head (1926) devised a systematic evaluation of reading, writing, speaking, and auditory comprehension. Head, who was a disciple of Hughlings Jackson, based his test on the patient's symbolic formulation and expression. Both Jackson and Head stressed the psychologic components that exist in aphasic patients. Head's test included object naming, color naming, easy reading sections, clock tests, and following directions of a numerical and spatial nature. The sophistication of Head's tests provided the background for many of the procedures used today.

The utilization of mental and educational achievement tests for evaluating the aphasic was accomplished by Weisenberg and McBride (1935). Their test included items that assessed all the language modalities and items assessing nonlanguage modalities such as formboards, picture completion, drawing, and copying. The Weisenberg and McBride study gave three important advances in testing methodology. First, it was the first study to use a normal control group. Second, they compared performances of aphasic subjects with those of nonaphasic brain-damaged subjects. Third, they used standardized measurements for evaluation.

Chesher (1937) created a test to evaluate aphasic patients where the central features were the common objects: key, pencil, hammer, button, scissors, and comb. Subjects were directed to name objects, read aloud printed names, write names, point, repeat, copy names, and spell names of the common objects.

The Goldstein-Scheerer Tests of Abstract and Concrete Behavior (1941) were introduced at the beginning of World War II. They were derived from Goldstein's concept that the aphasic patient suffers from impairment of the abstract attitude. The test consisted of the following.

1. Stick Test: The patient has to copy stick figures while looking and then has to reproduce the sticks from memory after looking for a certain interval.
2. Cube Test: The patient has to reproduce with blocks a colored design printed on a card.
3. Color Sorting Test: The patient has to sort woolen skeins of vary-

ing hues and shades into groups according to different color concepts.
4. Color Form Sorting Test: The patient has to sort triangles, squares, and circles in different colors into color and form groups.
5. Object Sorting Test: The patient has to sort a set of objects into groups according to material, form, and colors.

Shortly after World War II, the Halstead-Wepman Aphasia Screening Test (1949) was developed. The test was designed to provide a rapid self-contained evaluation of aphasic language behavior.

In still a different approach, Taylor (1953) described a scale called The Functional Communication Profile. The Profile attempts to measure the functional dimensions of language performance not accounted for in clinical testing. It consists of a list of 48 communication behaviors considered common language functions of everyday life. Ratings of each behavior are made on an 8-point scale on the basis of informal interaction with the patient in a conversational situation. For example, the speaking section of the test records whether the patient can do the following: greetings, his own name, nouns, verbs, noun-verb combinations, phrases, directions, speaking on the phone, short complete sentences, and long sentences.

Eisenson's Examining for Aphasia Manual (1954) gave us a tool that uses the Weisenberg and McBride classification system and evaluates patients along predominantly receptive or predominantly expressive lines. Although the Eisenson Manual is quite subjective in its scoring and interpretation, its portability and screening portions make it still a very widely used and popular tool.

Recently, a number of tests have been devised to put scoring procedures on a more quantitative basis. Instead of simply scoring responses as correct or incorrect, attempts have been made to scale, categorize, and quantify the different types of aphasic responses.

The Language Modalities Test for Aphasia (Wepman and Jones, 1961) consists of film strips as the visual stimuli and the voice of the examiner as the auditory stimuli. The Language Modalities Test for Aphasia (LMTA) includes a 6-point scale for scoring oral and graphic responses. The 6-point scale is as follows. 1) Correct responses, 2) phonemic errors, 3) grammatical and syntactical errors, 4) semantic errors, 5) jargon errors, 6) no response, admission of inability to respond, or any automatic phrase. After examination, patients can be placed in one or more of the author's five classification categories of aphasia. These classification categories are: syntactic where the syntax or grammar is disturbed; semantic where the substantive language is disturbed; pragmatic where there is a lack of meaningful speech or no context can be found; jargon where speech is unintelligible; and global where little or no speech is available.

As an added feature to the LMTA, Wepman (1958) suggested a correction and recovery scale as a prognostic indicator of the patient's language ability. The scale ranges from level 1 through level 8. At level 1 the patient fails to recognize errors made in any modality, cannot recognize errors when they are pointed out, and therefore cannot correct errors. At level 8 the patient recognizes errors made in both speech and writing and corrects them easily without assistance.

Wepman and his associates used the LMTA in a series of subsequent studies. Jones and Wepman (1961) performed a factor analysis of 168 aphasic subjects and said the analysis clearly demonstrated the existence of several dimensions that underlie test performance of aphasic patients. This argues against the hypothesis that language disturbance after brain damage may be viewed as a unitary, general disorder. Spiegel, Jones, and Wepman (1965) classified 50 aphasic subjects into six groups on the basis of differences of their spontaneous speech. Their findings provided evidence that it is possible to predict, from the performance of aphasic patients on the LMTA, some general features of their spontaneous speech.

The Minnesota Test for Differential Diagnosis of Aphasia (MTDDA) developed by Schuell (1965) contains an in-depth evaluation of five major areas. Subtests in five areas measure disturbances in: a) auditory abilities with nine subtests, b) visual and reading abilities with nine subtests; c) speech and language abilities with 15 subtests; d) visuomotor and writing abilities with 10 subtests, and e) numerical relations and arithmetic processes with four subtests. Items in each subtest tend to go from simple to complex. A 6-point clinical rating scale ranging from no impairment to total impairment is used for evaluating the auditory, speech, reading, and writing areas. Patients are then classified according to Schuell's system.

A number of investigations and theoretical positions have led to the development of MTDDA and they include Brown and Schuell (1950); Schuell (1953); Schuell (1954); Schuell and Jenkins (1959); and Schuell, Jenkins, and Jiminez-Pabon (1964, Chapter 6). Schuell, Jenkins, and Carroll (1962) performed a factor analysis of 155 aphasic patients on 69 tests comprising 679 items of the MTDDA, and their findings indicated that there is a dimension of general language deficit in aphasia that is not modality specific. The authors feel there is no support for the hypothesis of a sensorimotor, a receptive-expressive, or an input-output dichotomy in aphasia. A short examination for aphasia by Schwell (1957) is available and consists of those tests from the MTDDA judged to have the highest diagnostic and prognostic value. Schwell (1966) describes a diagnostic and severity scale to help in the reliability of the Short Test of the MTDDA.

A slightly different approach to examining the aphasic patient is the Token Test by DeRenzi and Vignolo (1962; McNeil and Prescott, 1978). This test uses 20 tokens of varying shapes, sizes, and colors. Patients are asked to arrange the tokens according to simple and then progressively more complex instructions. Orgass and Poeck (1966) tested 66 subjects without brain damage, 49 subjects brain-damaged without aphasia, and 26 aphasic subjects with the Token Test. They found the discriminating power of the test remarkably high and felt the test could be suitable for selecting patients regardless of type of aphasia. Swisher and Sarno (1969) administered the Token Test to English-speaking left brain-damaged aphasics, right brain-damaged nonaphasics, and nonbrain-damaged control patients who were matched across groups for age and educational level. They found that all patients had increasing difficulty as the parts progressed, that the left brain-damaged aphasic patient made the greatest number of errors on all parts of the test, and no relationship was demonstrated between age and Token Test scores. Finally, Spellacy and Spreen (1969) constructed a shortened 16-item version with adequate discriminating power and reliability. They suggested that the short version of the Token Test is approximately as useful as the original.

The Sklar Aphasia Scale (Sklar, 1966) consists of auditory and visual decoding sections and oral and graphic encoding sections. Scoring is based on impairment where the higher the impairment the greater the score. A percentage of impairment profile is drawn with the categories: no impairment, mild, moderate, severe, and global.

The Porch Index of Communicative Ability (PICA) provides items for examining the auditory, visual, verbal, and graphic modalities (Porch, 1967). In addition, there is a gestural battery where subjects are required to respond nonverbally to instructions. Patient responses are scored on a 16-point scale that indicates the accuracy, completeness, facility, promptness, and responsiveness of the patient's reaction. The scale ranges from 1, indicating no response and no awareness of the item, to 16, indicating a complex response with spontaneous, accurate, and fluent elaboration about the test item.

The Neurosensory Center Comprehensive Examination for Aphasia (Spreen and Benton, 1969) consists of 20 tests of language performance and four control tests of visual and tactile function. The 20 language tests assess understanding and production of language, retention of verbal material, reading, and writing. The four control tests are designed to detect the presence of visual or tactile deficits that might affect performance on the language items and are given to a patient whenever his performance on certain tests (visual or tactile naming, reading) is subnormal. A distinctive feature of this examination is the provision for constructing a profile of directly comparable percentile scores, corrected for age and educational level, for any patient.

The Boston Diagnostic Aphasia Test (Goodglass and Kaplan, 1972) systematically evaluates conversational and expository speech, auditory comprehension, oral expression, understanding written language, and writing. It also provides for an aphasia severity rating scale and a rating scale profile of speech characteristics based on melodic line, phrase length, articulatory agility, grammatical form, paraphasia in running speech, word finding, and auditory comprehension.

In summation, it is evident that the assessment and diagnosis of aphasic patients has gone from a simple clinical observation procedure to the relatively sophisticated, systematic, quantitative testing methods of today. Scoring procedures and diagnostic nomenclature will vary depending upon the test used for evaluation. Test items related to discovering the symptoms of a generalized intellectual impairment, apraxia of speech, confused language, and dysarthria are discussed later in this paper. Those items can be added to any of the aphasia tests reviewed in order to make a differential diagnosis.

Characterization of Aphasia

Before deciding on who would make a good candidate for therapy, there are a number of prognostic indicators that might give some insight into the selection. Although the prognostic factors cited are gleaned from the literature in aphasia, many of these indicators might be applicable to patients with a generalized intellectual impairment, apraxia of speech, confused language, or dysarthria.

Eisenson (1949), Wepman (1953), Vignolo (1964), Darley (1972), and Emerick and Hatten (1974, pp. 249–251) have outlined the following prognostic indicators: 1) The younger the patient, the better the prognosis. 2) The sooner the patient enters therapy from the time of onset of aphasia, the better the prognosis. 3) The less extensive neurologic damage, the better the prognosis. 4) Trauma as a cause of aphasia seems to warrant a better prognosis than cerebrovascular accident. 5) If the aphasic patient has the will to improve and accept his limitations, the prognosis is better. 6) If the family of the aphasic patient has the proper attitude and provides encouragement to the patient, the prognosis is better. 7) The milder the language impairment at the initial evaluation, the better the prognosis.

As stated earlier in this paper, Wepman (1958) suggests an eight-level scale based on self-correction as a prognostic indicator of the patient's language ability.

Smith (1971), in a study involving 78 aphasic patients, analyzed some of the prognostic indicators mentioned above. He found that the severity of comprehension defects generally reflects the severity of overall language impairment. Keenan and Brassell (1974) in their study of 39 aphasic patients also analyzed a number of prognostic factors and found that initial listening performance, initial talking performance, motor speech impairment (accompanying apraxia or dysarthria), and speech stimulability (measures taken and success at correcting speech responses) showed a definite relationship with the patient's eventual speech performance levels. Although there are always exceptions, the prognostic factors listed above might provide insight and guidelines for recommending treatment as well as help in guiding and counseling the family. If in doubt about whether to recommend therapy or not my suggestion would be to recommend it. You can always release a patient from therapy if you find it is not beneficial, and nothing has been lost. Finally, even if a complete evaluation cannot be made during the initial diagnostic session, for whatever reason, I would recommend therapy anyway. This would provide time for an ongoing and complete diagnosis in addition to the benefits of therapy.

Related to prognosis, recovery, and treatment for the aphasic patient is the concept of bilingualism. Osgood and Miron (1963, p. 36) discuss three general hypotheses about loss and recovery of language in bilinguals: 1) Ribot's rule that the earliest language learned will be the last to be lost (and the easiest to recover); 2) Pitre's rule that the language most practiced before injury will be most resistant and recovered most readily (most automatized); 3) Minkowski's rule that the language most strongly supported by emotional or affective factors (prestige, language used by spouse, language of childhood, etc.) will be best.

Osgood and Miron (1963, p. 36; pp. 135–137), De Reuck and

O'Connor (1964, pp. 116–120), and Millikan and Darley (1967, p. 190) cite several studies such as the work done by Lambert and Fillenbaum, and no consensus can be reached regarding the influence of bilingualism in the recovery from aphasia. Charlton (1964) reviewed previous hypotheses concerning aphasia in bilingual and polyglot patients and a consecutive series of 10 unselected cases. Preferential loss of one language over another is shown to be the exception rather than the rule in such cases, and it was concluded that where such "monoglot" aphasia does occur, it is most likely not caused by organic factors alone, but to psychological reactions of various types to the organic impairment of an important faculty.

The work done with bilingual subjects may give insight when working with such aphasic patients. I agree with the findings that show that aphasic language disturbance strikes all languages in the bilingual patient without any preference of one language over the other. Too often, we are misled by the surface types of answers given by the aphasic patient in his non-English language. The lack of multilingual tests for aphasia and the scarcity of bilingual speech pathologists often force the examiner to ask simple questions. These simple questions in turn elicit simple correct responses. If the patient were treated with the proper materials, it is most likely that his non-English language would be as affected as his English language.

In a recent study by Halpern, Darley, and Brown (1973, p. 164) four groups of 10 patients each, with each group having a different neurogenic disorder of communication (aphasia; generalized intellectual impairment; apraxia of speech; and confused language), were tested for impairment in 10 language categories. "Each had been given a standard neurologic examination and a language examination which was an adaptation of Schuell's (1957) short examination for aphasia. From the verbatim recorded responses to the latter, each subject had been assigned a diagnosis of one of the four disorder categories (from Halpern, et al. 1973, pp. 162–173).

On an analysis of the speech and language data, the group with aphasia showed impairment in all 10 language categories tested—moderate in six of them and mild in four. Even the mild impairments, however, tended toward the moderate range; and the overall rating (mean 31) was in that range. Relevance and writing words to dictation were least impaired, and adequacy (semantic) and auditory retention span were most impaired.

These findings seem to corroborate the opinion that aphasia affects all language functions, but some more than others (Darley, 1964, p. 40; Schuell et al., 1964, p. 156; and Smith, 1971). It is noteworthy that auditory retention span was particularly impaired in aphasia but less so in the other disorders. Schuell et al. (1964) demonstrated the prominence of this disability in their study of aphasic patients. It appears to be a fundamental component of aphasia.

Fluency was reduced in the aphasic group because as a rule these patients did not have an easy flow of words for full replies to the stimulus. Our measure of fluency is different from that of Howes (1964, pp. 61–68), who studied the total words produced in ad libitum speech by aphasic patients and considered all words produced, regardless of appropriateness. Howes found a range of 12 to 220 words per minute in aphasia, whereas 100 to 175 words per minute is normal. Simple observation confirms that many aphasic patients have a distinctly sparse output of words whereas others have many words. (from Halpern et al., 1973, pp. 162–173)

The neurologic data showed that the aphasia group was of variable onset (seven were rapid with less than 10 days and three were slow) and variable duration (six with less than 3 months and four with more than 3 months) and was associated in nine cases with infarcts (5) or tumors (4) in predominantly posterior locations (on EEG, six showed posterior focus and two showed anterior focus on delta or dysrhythmia).

Summing up, we can say aphasia is a linguistic disturbance that can be characterized by difficulties in reception or expression. Language may be affected through the modalities unevenly, that is, some may be better than others. The aphasic patient wants to communicate. When he cannot, he will usually show signs of frustration. Semantic and syntactic errors are quite typical of aphasic responses. Although language structure may be in error, thought and content usually are relevant to the situation. Aphasics' responses typically are not bizarre.

GENERALIZED INTELLECTUAL IMPAIRMENT

A "generalized intellectual impairment (GII) implies a general lowering of intellectual functions." Performance on language tasks and nonmental tasks are about the same and lowered. The patient usually exhibits an "across the board" depression of mental faculties, personality changes, emotional lability, dull and bland behavior, and memory loss (Darley, 1964, p. 39; Mayo Clinic, 1964, pp. 238–239; Halpern et al., 1973). This disorder can resemble a mild aphasia.

Etiology of GII is attributed mostly to cortical degeneration (senile or presenile dementia) that would bring about diffuse lesions. Sometimes trauma and tumor are causes.

Critchley (1970, pp. 349–351) has stated that:

in dementia language impairment essentially entails a poverty due to inaccessibility of those different vocabularies which ordinarily we can utilize and which are called the speaking vocabulary, the writing vocabulary, and the reading vocabulary. These terms refer respectively to the stock of words which we are in the habit of employing in conversation; to the larger one we draw on in written compositions; and to that even greater depository which also includes terms we recognize but rarely venture to use. With advancing mental inelasticity and memory-loss ... the words utilized by the demented patients become severely restricted in conversation and to a somewhat lesser extent in letter writing.

The difficulty in word finding differs however from the anomia of aphasics. The demented patient does not necessarily show any hesitancy in putting a name to an object presented to him....

Semantic

errors in naming do not occur; nor yet neologisms, substitutions ... or portmanteau (brunch, smog) words. Neither does the patient seek to by-pass the elusive term by means of elaborate circumlocutions, as is common with aphasics. But on the other hand the demented patient finds it difficult to reel off the names of flowers, animals, vegetables,

unless the real object is before him. He lapses into a sort of concrete attitude.

Critchley further noted that:

a patient with early dementia (GII) may preserve a facade of normalcy for quite a long time, by resorting to small talk. As time goes by, his repertoire of things to say becomes more limited and more stereotyped ... "more laced with cliches and set phrases..." Later the subject remains taciturn unless directly addressed. This social seclusion ... does not embarrass or perturb the patient.

Perseveration, which might be indicative of an "ideational rigidity," is also present in written and spoken language.

Stengel (1964) and Zangwill (1964) have also indicated that in a question and answer session the GII patient may be able to answer ordinary simple questions that are concrete. But if a question is asked of a more abstract nature, the patient may be unable to answer. Typically he is not distressed and exhibits dull and bland behavior toward the situation.

From a medical viewpoint, Brosin (1967, p. 709) sums up a generalized intellectual impairment as a disorder "caused by irreversible, permanent, diffuse destruction of brain cells." It is "usually chronic and progressive, leading to dementia over a period of months to years."

In testing for generalized intellectual impairment, questions relating to time and place orientation and simple general information can be used along with the tests used in aphasia evaluation. If necessary, one can substitute one modality for another in an effort to elicit an answer. Even when using the different modalities, the patient may miss many of the following easy questions.

Examples of orientation questions are: 1) What day is it? 2) What month? 3) What is today's date? 4) What year? 5) Where are you now? 6) What city? 7) What state? 8) Why are you here?

General information questions are as follows: 1) When do we celebrate Christmas? 2) What is the capitol of the United States? 3) Who is the president of the United States? 4) Who discovered America? When? 5) How many states are there in the United States? 6)Who was the first president of the United States? 7) Who was president during the Civil War? 8) Who invented Mickey Mouse and Donald Duck? 9) What country is immediately north of the United States? 10) Who was Helen Keller?

The psychologic tests used for assessing brain damage have been reviewed by Benton (1967). These tests include the standard IQ tests; reasoning and problem solving tests; memory and orientation tests; tests of perception; and attention, concentration, and motor ability tests.

The language findings of the Halpern, Darley, and Brown (1973, pp. 169–170) study showed that:

> the group with general intellectual impairment manifested deficiency of seven language categories. The overall rating (mean 22) was in the middle of the mild range. Three categories stood out as moderately impaired (adequacy or semantic, reading comprehension, arithmetic), and a fourth (auditory comprehension) was nearly in that range. Syntax (at 11%) was almost unimpaired, and three (relevance, writing words to dictation, fluency, at 9 and 10%) were just within the range of no impairment.

> That this group suffers from a general reduction of language capability, as has been proposed earlier (Mayo Clinic, 1964, pp. 238–239), is confirmed by the finding of some impairment of most language functions and most of the greater disability on the same ones (adequacy, arithmetic) that were generally most difficult also for the other groups in the study.

> Since reading comprehension is one of the more complex language functions and is learned after the other language functions are available for a foundation (Staats, 1968, p. 218), one would expect the group with general intellectual impairment to have more difficulty with reading comprehension than with auditory comprehension, as they did. The reversal of this pattern by the aphasic group is surprising. Possibly the marked de-

ficiency in auditory retention span affected their overall auditory comprehension, for memory and recall are very much a part of comprehension.

The neurologic findings revealed that the general intellectual impairment group was of slow onset (one was rapid with less than 10 days and nine were slow with more than 10 days) and long duration (one with less than 3 months and nine with more than 3 months), associated with predominantly diffuse lesions (six showed generalized or bilateral dysrhythmia, suggesting projected rhythms from deep structures), and caused by degeneration (eight degenerations, one trauma, one tumor).

In summation, the generalized intellectual impairment patient can resemble a case of mild aphasia. Whereas the aphasic has an uneven disturbance of all the modalities, the GII patient has an even impairment affecting all modalities. This even disturbance is in the mild category and can be described as a "skimming off the top." These patients have a bland, benign, noncaring attitude and are generally not frustrated when they miss easy questions. Not only does GII affect all the modalities but it can cut across into memory, judgment, thinking, and abstracting abilities. Emotional lability, at times, can cause the patient to go from a benign attitude to a highly irascible state. Generally, their responses are relevant to the situation.

APRAXIA OF SPEECH

Apraxia of speech is an articulation disorder that results from impairment, due to brain damage, of the capacity to order the positioning of speech musculature and the sequencing of muscle movements for volitional production of phonemes and sequences of phonemes; but it is not accompanied by significant weakness, slowness, or incoordination of these same muscles in reflex and automatic acts (Darley, 1964, p. 36; Johns and Darley, 1970).

This disorder can resemble a good deal of the oral expressive language behavior of the aphasic patient. For example, the phonemic groping of the apraxic patient can resemble the word finding difficulty of the aphasic patient. The etiology for apraxia of speech is generally the same as for aphasia.

The studies cited below offer some guidelines in diagnosing apraxia of speech. One or more of the following error patterns would lead to such a diagnosis: 1) Numerous phonemic errors, including substitutions, omissions, additions, repetitions, and distortions, with a predominance of substitutions (La Pointe, 1969; Johns and Darley, 1970; Trost, 1970) in the absence of significant weakness, slowness, or incoordination of the speech musculature. 2) Phonemic error inconsistency (Darley, 1969); substitution of a variety of phonemes and phoneme clusters for correct phonemes; and inconsistently correct phoneme production, including islands of error-free fluency especially during a period of automatic-reactive speech (Shankweiler and Harris, 1966; La Pointe, 1969; Johns and Darley, 1970). 3) Difficulty with initiation of speech; effortful speech production during purposive-volitional speech, characterized by hesitant, groping movements of the articulators before and during speech production and numerous retrials at correct word production (Darley, 1969; La Pointe, 1969). 4) An increasing number of phonemic errors with increasing word length (Johns and Darley, 1970; Deal and Darley, 1972). 5) A marked discrepancy between speech perception and speech production; perception may be good, but production poor (Johns and Darley, 1970).

The idea that a separate term, apraxia of speech, be used instead of terms that need redescription seems quite evident when one looks at the literature. Some of the following studies use terms such as articulatory dyspraxia, cortical dysarthria, phonemic-articulatory disorders, and verbal apraxia, which in all probability actually describe the condition called apraxia of speech.

Critchley (1952) stated that many aphasic patients show disorders of articulate speech that are both varied and variable in their character. Dysarthria and dysphasia, although often occurring in combination, are actually separate phenomena. Articulatory dyspraxia is also an independent entity, although it may coexist with aphasia and contribute to defects of articulation. Bay (1964) reported on a study of 80 unselected aphasic patients and found a well defined and frequent group of speech disorders marked by a distinct apraxia of the articulatory muscles and impaired tongue movements in the glossogram test. Bay says he is describing what other people have referred to as motor aphasia, but what he calls "cortical dysarthria." His main point is that it is a motor disorder independent of language, and we must distinguish this motor disorder from the linguistic disorders called aphasia.

DeRenzi, Piezcuro, and Vignolo (1966) tested 105 aphasic patients and found a high correlation between the severity of oral apraxia and the severity of phonemic-articulatory disorders. Oral apraxia and Broca's aphasia were a common combination. Oral apraxia was present in about one-third of conduction aphasics and usually absent in Wernicke's aphasia. Oral apraxia was not considered to be a part of a general praxic disturbance.

Johns and Darley (1970) studied 10 apraxic and 10 dysarthric subjects and found that these patients typically display marked discrepancy between good perception of stimuli and poor oral production of the same stimuli. Specific phonemes do not differentiate dysarthric and apraxic patients, but types of errors and their consistency do. Dysarthric patients predominantly showed distortions and substitutions (frequently simplification) whereas apraxic patients showed predominantly unrelated substitutions, repetitions, and additions. Errors of dysarthrics were found to be highly consistent, errors of apraxics highly inconsistent. The mode of stimulus presentation affects performance: auditory-visual is better than auditory or visual alone. Few errors are simplification, suggesting inappropriateness of the term "phonetic disintegration."

In a follow-up study that used the same 10 apraxic of speech subjects as Johns and Darley (1970), Aten, Johns, and Darley (1971) found that apraxia of speech patients as a group made significantly more auditory perceptual errors than normal subjects, but varied considerably in their level of performance. The achievements of some patients were within the range established by the control subjects; that of others was unequivocally inferior. The major deficit in the apraxic group seemed to be impairment of ability to retain the second and third syllable consonant elements in three-word sequences.

Deal and Darley (1972) studied 12 subjects with apraxia of speech and minimal aphasic involvement in four experimental conditions: the effect of instructions, the effect of three different experimentally imposed response-delay intervals on a word-repetition task, the effect of noise, and the effect of visual monitoring. Also studied in one or more of these conditions were the loci of errors in oral reading, the apraxic subjects' ability to predict and to recognize their errors, and the nature of the errors made. Under the conditions in which they were studied, instructions, response-delay intervals, noise, and visual monitoring had no significant influence on phonemic accuracy. Subjects with apraxia of speech had significantly more difficulty with three-syllable words than with one-syllable words. They made more errors on words weighted high (Brown's word-weighting method) than on words weighted low. Word length and grammatical class seemed to be important characteristics influencing increases in errors. The ability of apraxic subjects to predict errors seems to be an individual characteristic. The ability to recognize errors seems to be a group characteristic. Subjects consistently made substitution, repetition, addition, and omission errors. The results support the contention that apraxia of speech is a motor-programming disorder.

Rosenbek, Wertz, and Darley (1973) tested 30 patients with apraxia of speech, 10 patients with aphasia and no apraxia of speech, and 30 normal subjects. They employed three oral sensory-perceptual measurements: oral form identification, two-point discrimination and mandibular kinesthesia. The apraxia of speech group was significantly inferior to the aphasic and normal groups on all three oral sensory-perceptual tests. The normal and aphasic groups did not differ significantly from each other. Apraxia of speech and oral sensory-perceptual deficit were related in that the more severe the apraxia of speech, the more profound the oral sensory-perceptual deficit. Not all patients with apraxia of speech demonstrated impaired oral sensation and perception; however, higher cortical sensory dysfunction frequently accompanied apraxia of speech.

Deal (1974) had five patients with apraxia of speech read a simple 100-word paragraph five times in succession. Results indicated that as a group the subjects made consistent word errors and demonstrated a significant adaptation effect.

Martin (1974) objects to the term "apraxia of speech" on the grounds that it implies that the phonologic impairment is motoric, and therefore separate and distinct from other language systems. The term "aphasic phonologic impairment" is suggested so as to permit investigation of the disorder without diagnostic prejudice.

Recently, La Pointe and Johns (1975) studied the phonemic abilities of 13 apraxic of speech subjects. The patterns of error obtained from articulatory confusion matrices of these subjects revealed the following. 1) Consonants were more susceptible to error than were vowels, as were consonant clusters when compared to single consonants. 2) Affricatives and fricatives were significantly more susceptible to error than all others, as were palatal and dental phonemes. 3) When substitution errors were tabulated as either anticipatory (prepositioning), reiterative (postpositioning), or metathesis, anticipatory errors outnumbered reiterative errors by a ratio of 6 to 1. 4) Feature analysis of substitution errors revealed that 38% were defective in two or more features and these productions bore little resemblance to the target sound. 5) No significant differences were found among error percentages for initial, medial, and final positions; and in voiced and unvoiced phonemes.

In testing for apraxia of speech, procedures such as the following can be used to supplement the tests used in aphasia evaluation. Look for the symptoms described previously and ask the patient to do the following: 1) prolong *ah*; 2) prolong *ee*; 3) prolong *oo*; 4) repeat *puh* rapidly; 5) repeat *tuh* rapidly; 6) repeat *kuh* rapidly; 7) repeat *puh-*

tuh-kuh rapidly; 8) repeat *snowman*; 9) repeat *gingerbread*; 10) repeat *impossibility*.

Responses can be scored as accurate and immediate and that will be considered the best; accurate but delayed or acceptable overall pattern with defective amplitude, accuracy, force, or speed will be considered second in order; and partial, perseverative, irrelevent, or nil will be considered the worst scoring.

The Halpern, Darley, and Brown (1973, p. 170) language findings showed that:

> the group with apraxia of speech revealed mild impairment in seven categories, but normal ability with respect to three. The overall rating (mean 14) fell in the lower portion of the mild range. The finding of only mild impairment of overall language function supports the belief that apraxia of speech is mostly a disorder of the programming of motor functions (Darley, 1964, p. 36; Johns and Darley, 1970). Except for arithmetic, only the oral expression of ideas (adequacy or semantic, fluency, and syntax) was more than slightly impaired.

> The prominence of impairment of fluency is the characteristic that distinguishes the apraxia of speech group from the other three groups. Most of their errors in fluency were pausing and hesitating. The groping for articulatory placement and their repeated efforts to produce the right word correctly seem to be the causes of the lack of fluency.

The neurologic findings revealed that the apraxia of speech group tended to be of sudden onset (10 were rapid with less than 10 days) but variable duration (six with less than 3 months and four with more than 3 months) and was associated with anterior infarcts (nine infarcts and one trauma but data insufficient in EEG).

Summing up, apraxia of speech can be described as a motor speech problem in which ability to volitionally sequence motor movements for speech is impaired. Apraxia of speech is not a linguistic disturbance, but rather a programming or transmissive problem. Theoretically, a pure apraxia of speech patient would not have difficulty in any modality except oral expression. Typically, apraxic patients are highly inconsistent in their errors. They may have difficulty starting speech. They will have the most difficulty when asked to say something upon confrontation or command. When in error, apraxics typically recognize the error and show frustration in their efforts to correct themselves. At times, they have the ability to give a correct production after a number of faulty attempts. Their reactions are relevant to the situation and they do not exhibit bizarre responses.

CONFUSED LANGUAGE

Confused language is a part of a condition where:

> the patient's responsiveness to his environment is impaired to a mild degree. Psychological responses are slower, restricted in scope and less adaptive. The behavior indicates that the patient is less able to recognize and understand the environment than in the normal state. Clearness of thinking and accuracy of remembering are impaired.

The patient usually manifests a disorientation of time and place, confabulation, and inability to follow directions, and unawareness of the inappropriateness of his responses (Darley, 1964, pp. 38–39; Mayo Clinic, 1964, p. 234; and Halpern et al., 1973). The bizarre, irrelevant responses typical of this disorder can easily resemble the responses of the aphasic patient who has a marked difficulty in comprehending spoken language. This type of aphasic patient will emit jargon or paraphasic responses much like that in the language of confusion.

The language of confusion can be caused by head injury, subarachnoid hemorrhage, rapidly increasing intracranial pressure, drug intoxication, withdrawal symptoms, acute infections, tumors, uremia, hepatic failure, and other types of metabolic disorders. The lesions are diffuse or disseminated.

Geschwind (1967, pp. 107–109) describes the syndrome of nonaphasic misnaming that

> typically occurs in disorders which diffusely involve the nervous system, especially when the disturbance comes on fairly rapidly. Characteristically the errors tend to "propogate." Thus the patient being asked where he is may say "In a bus," and may then say that the examining physician is the driver, that those around him are the passengers and that the bed he is in is used by the driver for resting. It is usually obvious once a sequence of questions is asked that ordinary aphasic misnaming is readily ruled out. Thus in aphasic misnaming there is no tendency to "propogation" although perserveration, i.e. repetition of the same incorrect word, occurs frequently.

> The "connected" or "propogated" character of the errors may show up particularly in relation to the hospital and the patient's illness. He may call the hospital a "hotel," the doctors "bell boys," the nurses "chambermaids," and will not accept correction.

> One feature which often characterizes non-aphasic misnaming is that spontaneous speech is usually (but not invariably) normal despite gross errors in naming. In aphasia, errors in confrontation naming are almost always accompanied by a disturbance in spontaneous speech in which

word-finding pauses, empty phrases, semantic or adequacy errors and circumlocutions appear.

Stengel (1964) has stated that people in confusional states, when called upon to name objects, do not respond in the same way as aphasics. Aphasics say, " I know what it is, but I can't find the word." Confused patients boldly and sometimes recklessly improvise and produce words on the spur of the moment. These words may show effects of perseveration, slang, and other associations. They may contain references to certain aspects of the correct concept. The words produced may show a creative inventiveness. Occasionally they embody references to the patient's personal problems. The patients show no awareness of error and when told to think again they insist that they are right. These nonaphasic misnaming responses are invariably associated with a more general change in behavior, whereby perception and motivation are altered. The disturbance of motivation is particularly obvious in relation to the task of naming and definition. These patients do not seem to care whether they obtain an accurate correspondence between the object and its generally accepted verbal representation. They disregard the function of language as a code of behavior and of communication.

Weinstein et al. (1966) compared 18 jargon aphasics with 26 standard aphasics.

> Jargon consisted of phonetic distortions, of mispronounced words, of neologisms, of standard English words put together in meaningless sequence and of sentences seemingly irrelevant to the subject under discussion. (p. 169)

Jargon subjects had bilateral brain involvement and showed confabulation, particularly about the onset of the illness or the reason for coming to the hospital; disorientation for place and time; unawareness of errors; did not show any catastrophic response;

> ... and in the course of clinical improvement, the jargon was replaced by confabulations, and forms of idiomatic speech such as cliches, puns and malapropisms. The greater the frequency of such verbalizations, the less was the degree of anxiety and overt concern. (p. 187)

It seems that jargon aphasia and nonaphasic misnaming resemble some aspects of confused language.

In a recent study by Chedru and Geschwind (1972), 24 patients with metabolic or toxic disorders of rapid onset, and without focal brain lesion, were selected as "confused" on the basis of an alteration of attention. They were given a short neuropsychologic examination, their performances being compared to those of 10 controls and to their own after recovering from confusion.

The following disorders were observed: a) disturbances of mood and behavior, disorientation, unconcern toward illness; b) mild word-finding difficulties, tendency toward verbal paraphasias in repetition and reading test, slowing of verbal fluency, marked dysgraphia; c) mild spatial disturbances (right-left recognition; test of Head), constructional apraxia, disturbances in finger recognition and in calculation, memory defect. Most of the disorders disappeared completely after clearing up of the acute confusional state.

Aspects of confused language can resemble certain elements of schizophrenic language. Critchley (1970, pp. 354–355), Stengel (1964), and others have compared the language of schizophrenia with aphasic language. They agree that despite certain similarities, the situation is basically nothing like that associated with language impairment in aphasia. The patient with aphasia fails in his verbal communication because of an inaccessibility, if not complete loss, of verbal symbols in thought. In schizophrenia the thinking processes themselves are disturbed, but the verbal symbols are intact.

The aphasic is an anxious person who may be very aware of his problem (except for the severely involved auditory aphasic who can show little or no awareness); he strives and strains to achieve mutual communication, showing a good deal of frustration when he fails. The schizophrenic, by contrast, may be aloof, negativistic, or non-caring about his problem.

Aspects of confused language can also resemble the language that comes as a result of right hemisphere lesions. Weinstein (1964) compared the errors in naming objects made by 20 patients with left hemisphere and 20 with right hemisphere lesions. Only right-handed patients were used.

In the 20 cases with left brain lesions, errors were made on 56% of the items presented. These errors were primarily of the syntactic or semantic (adequacy) type and involved no special predilection for the illness-connected items. The same number of patients with right brain lesions averaged only 3.5 errors on the 40 items. Here the majority (63%) of the errors fell into the hospital and illness-connected group.

The patients with left brain lesions did poorly in calculation, in interpreting idioms, in spelling, in giving rhymes, synonyms, and antonyms. The 20 patients in the left brain damage group made an average of 10 errors out of 13 idioms, being unable to transpose such expressions as *caught flat footed, hot under the collar,* as if they could not use the same element in more than one pattern. Yet, with one exception, these patients could name the hospital and their doctor, and only three made errors in month, year, and time of day. With the exception of one man, who could not name the hospital, all expressed awareness of their disabilities and did not confabulate.

On the other hand, patients with lesions of the minor hemisphere, who made two or more naming errors, showed more loss of relatedness to the environment. All were disoriented for place or date, expressed in misnaming or mislocating the hospital, condensing the distance between home and hospital or giving an erroneous month or year. Fourteen patients confabulated about their illness. Compared to the left brain lesion subjects, they did well in calculation, idioms, spelling, rhymes, synonyms, and antonyms. Although similar types of errors exist, the chief difference between the confused language patient and the right-brain damaged group described is the amount and spread of error.

From a medical point of view, Brosin (1967, p. 709) sums up confusion as a disorder caused by reversible, temporary, diffuse disturbance in brain function. It is usually brief but may be prolonged up to 1 month or longer. It may end in health and cure, death, or chronic disease.

In testing for confused language, the same procedures can be used as described in testing for a generalized intellectual impairment. You can add this to any aphasia battery.

Darley (1964, pp. 38–39) sums up testing for confused language with the following: 1) Is the patient oriented in space and time? Confused patients are frequently disoriented. 2) How well does the patient stay in contact with the examiner? The confused patient may unpredictably wander away from the conversation and engage in a colloquy upon some irrelevant subject. The confused patient may respond well to specific questions and discrete tasks but will "wander away" when given more freedom in response, as when he is asked open-ended questions or when he is required to explain proverbs or the functions of objects. 3) How aware is the patient of the inappropriateness of his responses? The confused patient tends to show clearly that he thinks he is "making sense" even when his responses are inadequate and irrelevant. 4) How well structured are the patient's responses? The confused patient may demonstrate normal sentence structure, whereas the content of the sentences is inappropriate.

The psychological tests used for assessing brain damage have been reviewed by Benton (1967). As stated before, these tests include the standard IQ tests; reasoning and problem solving tests; memory and orientation tests; tests of perception; and attention, concentration, and motor ability tests. In addition, Chedru and Geschwind (1972) offer some scoring criteria for evaluating the confused patient.

The language findings of the Halpern, Darley, and Brown (1973, pp. 170–171) study showed that:

> the group with confused language showed impairment of all the 10 categories measured. The overall rating (mean 28) fell near the upper border of the mild range, and four of the group scores were in the moderate range.

> The finding of overall impairment of language function seems consistent with the idea that confusion produces a disorientation with regard to language as well as time and place (Mayo Clinic, 1964, p. 234; Darley, 1964, pp. 38–39; Stengel, 1964, p. 289; Zangwill, 1964, p. 297). Since language reception and production require accuracy of interpretation and response, it is not surprising that this group showed a significant degree of overall language impairment. Although, it was the category least affected overall, relevance had fourth rank among the group with confused language and seemed to differentiate that disorder clearly from the rest. Patients with confused language gave bizarre responses to various stimuli, indicating that clearness of thinking and accuracy of remembering were impaired. They seemed unaware of the irrelevance of their responses and made no attempt at correction. This finding corroborates clinical impressions (Mayo Clinic, 1964, pp. 38–39, 234; Darley, 1964, pp. 38–39; Stengel, 1964, p. 289; Zangwill, 1964, p. 297).

> Writing words to dictation ranked third in the confused language group but much lower in other groups. The variety of the functions comprised in writing words after hearing them spoken and the concentration required may have been generally too much for the patients with confused language. This group also showed the most impairment in reading comprehension, which might interfere with their writing. Most of the errors made by this group were misspellings, but some were bizarre responses apparently unrelated to the stimulus.

> The finding that the patients with confused language failed more often to comprehend what they read than what they heard may be attributable to their inability to keep their attention on silent stimuli as closely as on the auditory stimuli, which were presented more actively by the examiner.

The neurologic findings revealed that the confused language group was of sudden onset (eight were rapid with less than 10 days and two were slow) and short duration (10 with less than 3 months), seven patients were associated with disseminated (multiple focal lesions or focal and diffuse) and three had diffuse lesions. EEG revealed a predominance of complex generalized or bilateral dysrhythmia mixed with generalized or focal delta patterns, suggesting rhythm from deep structures mixed with destructive lesions of hemispheres. Confused language was caused by trauma as often as by all other causes combined (five trauma, three hemorrhage or hematoma, one infection, and one tumor).

In summation, patients with confused language exhibit bizarre responses, irrelevant answers, confabulation, and propagation. They demonstrate disorientation to time and space. Many times, their language structure is proper, but thought and content are improper. They are not communicating with their listener and show no insight or awareness of their inappropriate responses. Because of their irrelevant responses, they can at times resemble the auditory aphasic. However, the auditory aphasic will do much better through the other modalities, whereas the confused language patient will be consistently bizarre or irrelevant, regardless of modality.

DYSARTHRIA

Many times a condition known as dysarthria can appear alone or accompany the speech and language disorders described previously. Peacher (1950), Grewel (1957), and others have offered concepts concerning dysarthria. Darley, Aronson, and Brown (1969a, p. 246) stated that:

> dysarthria is a collective name for a group of speech disorders resulting from disturbances in muscular control over the speech mechanism due to damage of the central or peripheral nervous system. It designates problems in oral communication due to paralysis, weakness, or incoordination of the speech musculature. It differentiates such problems from disorders of higher centers related to the faulty programming of movements and sequences of movements (apraxia of speech) and to the inefficient processing of linguistic units (aphasia).

They delineated six types of dysarthria with its neurologic and speech characteristics.

The first type is described as flaccid dysarthria and is generally found in the neurologic disorder called bulbar palsy.

> All patients in this group displayed evidence of a lower motor neuron lesion implicating motor units of the cranial nerves involved in speech (V, VII, IX, X, XII). (p. 250)

In addition to imprecise consonants, the outstanding characteristic of flaccid dysarthria is hypernasality.

The second type is described as spastic dysarthria and is generally found in the neurologic disorder called pseudobulbar palsy. The patients constituting the pseudobulbar group presented upper motor neuron disorder, presumed to involve combined damage to the pyramidal system and to a portion of the extrapyramidal system, because these arise from the same motor cortex areas.

Etiology may be multiple strokes, brain injury sustained in accidents, cerebral palsy of infancy, extensive brain tumors, encephalitis, multiple sclerosis, or progressive degeneration of the brain. In addition to imprecise consonants, the outstanding characteristics of spastic dysarthria is the harsh and strain-strangled voice.

The third type is described as a mixed dysarthria and is generally found in the neurologic disorder called amyotrophic lateral sclerosis.

> In amyotrophic lateral sclerosis there is progressive degeneration of both upper and lower motor neurons. One would expect the patients with this disease to have both bulbar (flaccid dysarthria) and pseudobulbar (spastic dysarthria) characteristics, truly a "mixed dysarthria." (pp. 253–254)

In addition to imprecise consonants, the outstanding characteristic of mixed dysarthria is the severe nature of hypernasality, breathy voice, and slow rate.

The fourth type is described as hypokinetic dysarthria and is generally found in the neurologic disorder called parkinsonism. In addition to imprecise consonants, the outstanding characteristics of hypokinetic dysarthria are severe monopitch and monoloudness, and reduced stress.

The fifth type is described as hyperkinetic dysarthria and is generally found in the neurologic disorders called dystonia and chorea. In addition to imprecise consonants, the outstanding characteristics of hyperkinetic dysarthria are the excess loudness variation (dystonia) and the interruptions of all speech processes because of continuous muscular movement (chorea).

> Common causes of all these movement disorders are encephalitis, degeneration of nerve cells due to aging or arteriosclerotic changes, repeated small injuries of the head, birth injuries and congenital diseases, exposure to certain toxins, and certain tranquilizing drugs. (p. 257).

The sixth type is described as ataxic dysarthria and is generally found in neurologic cerebellar disorders.

> When the causative lesion—whether tumor, progressive degeneration, trauma, multiple sclerosis, toxicity from alcoholic excess, strokes, or congenital conditions—involves both sides of the cerebellum and ataxia

of both upper extremities is observed, ataxic speech is generally noted as well. (p. 256)

In addition to imprecise consonants, the outstanding characteristics of ataxic dysarthria are the irregular articulatory breakdown and the excess and equal stress.

Relatively speaking, many a diagnostician has found dysarthric symptoms easily discernible from the language of aphasia, a generalized intellectual impairment, and confusion. Usually the difficulty comes in differentiating dysarthric from apraxic of speech symptoms. To help in differentiating the two syndromes, Johns and Darley (1970) studied 10 apraxic and 10 dysarthric subjects and found that dysarthric subjects erred more by distortion and substitution (generally simplification); whereas the apraxic subjects erred more by substitution and repetition; their substitutions being often unrelated and frequently additive (such as substitution of a consonant cluster for a consonant singleton). They found dysarthric errors were highly consistent, apraxic of speech errors highly variable.

To make a systematic evaluation of dysarthria one must sample several types of speech and voice production. Darley, Aronson, and Brown (1968) suggest that a sample of contextual speech can be elicited by having the patient tell about a picture representing a situation, or having the patient read a standard paragraph of simple prose containing all the consonants and vowels of English as well as some consonant clusters.

In additional testing for dysarthria, the following procedures can be used along with the tests used in aphasia evaluation. Look for the symptoms described under each type of dysarthria and ask the patient to: 1) prolong *ah, ee, oo,* as long, clearly and steadily as possible; 2) repeat *puh* as rapidly as possible (bilabial sound); repeat *tuh* as rapidly as possible (lingua-alveolar sound); repeat *kuh* as rapidly as possible (lingua-velar sound).

These procedures are the same as used in testing for apraxia of speech except one should note the outstanding characteristics of hypernasality (flaccid dysarthria); harsh, strain-strangled voice (spastic dysarthria); severe hypernasality, breathy voice, and slow rate (mixed dysarthria); severe monopitch, monoloudness, and reduced stress (hypokinetic dysarthria); excessive loudness variations and the interruption of all speech processes (hyperkinetic dysarthria); and irregular articulatory breakdown and excess and equal stress (ataxic dysarthria).

Oral perception factors might provide additional diagnostic clues.

Creech, Wertz, and Rosenbek (1973) studied 20 normal adults and 20 adults who demonstrated dysarthria. They compared the subjects on three measurements of oral sensation and perception. Results indicated that the dysarthric subjects displayed significant oral sensory and perceptual deficit on all three measures. Teixeira, Defran, and Nichols (1974) investigated patterns of errors made by three groups of neurologically impaired subjects with expressive disorders of speech: aphasia, apraxia, and dysarthria. Results suggest sensory-perceptual deficit in apraxics and, to a lesser degree, in dysarthrics and aphasics.

Recently, Kent and Netsell (1975) performed cineradiographic and spectrographic analysis to study the speech production of a subject who presented the classic neurologic signs of cerebellar lesion and who had speech characteristics similar to those that have been reported for ataxic dysarthria. Special attention was paid to the deviant perceptual dimensions that have been described for ataxic speech. Examination of the cineradiographic and spectrographic records revealed conspicuous abnormalities in speaking rate, stress patterns, articulatory placements for both vowels and consonants, velocities of articulatory movements, and fundamental frequency contours. In general, the physiologic and acoustic observations of ataxic dysarthria were compatible with the existing perceptual description of this condition.

Summing up, dysarthria can be viewed as a motoric problem that can involve paralysis of the speech mechanism. It is not on a linguistic level as aphasia nor a programming or transmissive level as apraxia of speech. These patients are consistent in their errors, usually have little difficulty in starting speech, and are not affected by speech being automatic or volitional. Typically, they do not have the ability to give a correct production after a number of faulty attempts. They are generally frustrated when in error, their syntactic and semantic qualities are typically intact; their responses are relevant to the situation; and their thinking, memory, and abstracting abilities are usually not impaired. Dysarthria is a motor problem that can affect articulation, voice, breathing, and prosody.

REFERENCES

Aten, J., Johns, D., and Darley, F. 1971. Auditory perception of sequenced words in apraxia of speech. J. Speech Hear. Res. 14:131–143.

Baker, E. E. 1954. An historical development of etiological concepts concerning aphasic speech and their influence upon aphasic speech rehabilitation. Unpublished Ph.D. thesis, New York University.

Bay, E. 1964. Principles of classification and their influence on our concepts of aphasia. In: A. V. S. de Reuck and M. O'Connor (eds.), Disorders of Language. Churchill Ltd., London.

Benton, A. 1967. Psychological tests for brain damage. In: A. Friedman and H. Kaplan (eds.), Comprehensive Textbook of Psychiatry, pp. 530–538. The Williams & Wilkins Company, Baltimore.

Brosin, H. 1967. Acute and chronic brain syndromes. In: A. Friedman and H. Kaplan (eds.), Comprehensive Textbook of Psychiatry, pp. 708–711. The Williams & Wilkins Company, Baltimore.

Brown, J. R., and Schuell, H. E. 1950. A preliminary report of a diagnostic test for aphasia. J. Speech Hear. Disord. 15:21–28.

Charlton, M. 1964. Aphasia in bilingual and polyglot patients—a neurological and psychological study. J. Speech Hear. Disord. 29:307–311.

Chedru, F., and Geschwind, N. 1972. Higher cortical functions in confusional states. Cortex 8:397–409.

Chesher, E. C. 1937. Aphasia: technique of clinical examinations. Bull. Neurol. Inst. N. Y. 6:134–144.

Creech, R., Wertz, R., and Rosenbek, J. 1973. Oral sensation and perception in dysarthric adults. Percept. Motor Skills 37:167–172.

Critchley, M. 1952. Articulatory defects in aphasia. J. Laryngol. Otol. 66:1–17.

Critchley, M. 1970. Aphasiology and other aspects of language. Edward Arnold Publishers Ltd., London.

Darley, F. L. 1964. Diagnosis and appraisal of communicative disorders. Prentice-Hall Inc., Englewood Cliffs, New Jersey.

Darley, F. L. 1969. Nomenclature of expressive speech disturbance resulting from lesions of Broca's area: 108 years of proliferation and confusion. Presented at the Academy of Aphasia, September 1969, Boston.

Darley, F. L. 1972. The efficacy of language rehabilitation in aphasia. J. Speech Hear. Disord. 37:3–21.

Darley, F. L., Aronson, A., and Brown, J. 1968. Motor speech signs in neurologic disease. Med. Clin. North Am. 52:835–844.

Darley, F. L., Aronson, A., and Brown, J. 1969a. Differential diagnostic patterns of dysarthria. J. Speech Hear. Res. 12:246–269.

Darley, F. L., Aronson, A., and Brown, J. 1969b. Clusters of deviant speech dimensions in the dysarthrias. J. Speech Hear. Res. 12:462–496.

Deal, J. 1974. Consistency and adaptation in apraxia of speech. J. Commun. Disord. 7:135–140.

Deal, J., and Darley, F. L. 1972. The influence of linguistic and situational variables on phonemic accuracy in apraxia of speech. J. Speech Hear. Res. 15:639–653.

DeRenzi, E., Piezcuro, A., and Vignolo, L. A. 1966. Oral apraxia and aphasia. Cortex 2:50–73.

DeRenzi, E., and Vignolo, L. A. 1962. The Token test: a sensitive test to detect receptive disturbances in aphasia. Brain 85:665–678.

DeReuck, A., and O'Connor, M. (eds.). 1964. Disorders of language. Little, Brown & Co. Inc., Boston.

Eisenson, J. 1949. Prognostic factors related to language rehabilitation in aphasic patients. J. Speech Hear. Disord. 14:262–264.

Eisenson, J. 1954. Examining for aphasia. The Psychological Corporation, New York.

Emerick, L., and Hatten, J. 1974. Diagnosis and evaluation in speech pathology. Prentice-Hall Inc., Englewood Cliffs, New Jersey.

Geschwind, N. 1967. The variety of naming errors. Cortex 3:97–112.

Goldstein, K., and Scheerer, M. 1941. Abstract and concrete behavior tests. Psychol. Monogr. 53:329.

Goodglass, H., and Kaplan, E. 1972. The assessment of aphasia and related disorders. Lea & Febiger, Philadelphia.

Grewel, F. 1957. Classification of dysarthrias. Acta Psychiatr. Scand., 32:325–337.

Halpern, H. 1972. Adult Aphasia. The Bobbs-Merrill Co., Inc., Indianapolis.

Halpern, H., Darley, F. L., and Brown, J. 1973. Differential language and neurologic characteristics in neurologic involvement. J. Speech Hear. Disord. 38:162–173.

Halstead, W., and Wepman, J. 1949. The Halstead-Wepman aphasia screening test. J. Speech Hear. Disord. 14:9–15.

Head, H. 1926. Aphasia and kindred disorders of speech. Vol. 1. Cambridge University Press, London.

Howes, D. 1964. Application of the word frequency concept to aphasia. In: A. V. S. DeReuck and M. O'Connor (eds.), Disorders of Language. Churchill Ltd., London.

Johns, D. and Darley, F. L. 1970. Phonemic variability in apraxia of speech. J. Speech Hear. Res. 13:556–583.

Jones, L., and Wepman, J. M. 1961. Dimensions of language performance in aphasia. J. Speech and Hear. Res. 4:220-232.

Keenan, J., and Brassell, E. 1974. A study of factors related to prognosis for individual aphasic patients. J. Speech Hear. Disord. 39:257–269.

Kent, R., and Netsell, R. 1975. A case study of an ataxic dysarthric: Cineradiographic and spectrographic observations. J. Speech Hear. Disord. 40:115–133.

La Pointe, L. 1969. An investigation of isolated oral movements, oral motor sequencing abilities, and articulation of brain-injured adults. Doctoral dissertation, University of Colorado.

La Pointe, L., and Johns, D. 1975. Some phonemic characteristics in apraxia of speech. J. Commun. Disord. 8:259–269.

Martin, A. D. 1974. Some objections to the term apraxia of speech. J. Speech Hear. Disord. 39:53–64.

Mayo Clinic Sections of Neurology and Section of Physiology. 1964. Clinical examinations in neurology. W. B. Saunders Company, Philadelphia.

McNeil, M., and Prescott, T. 1978. Revised Token Test. University Park Press, Baltimore.

Millikan, C., and Darley, F. L. (eds.). 1967. Brain mechanisms underlying speech and language. Grune & Stratton, Inc., New York.

Orgass, B., and Poeck, K. 1966. Clinical validation of a new test for aphasia. Cortex 2:222–243.

Osgood, C., and Miron, M. (eds.). 1963. Approaches to the study of aphasia. University of Illinois Press, Urbana.

Peacher, W. 1950. The etiology and differential diagnosis of dysarthria. J. Speech Hear. Disord. 15:252–265.

Porch, B. 1967. The Porch index of communicative ability. Consulting Psychological Press, Palo Alto.

Rosenbek, J., Wertz, R., and Darley, F. L. 1973. Oral sensation and perception in apraxia of speech and aphasia. J. Speech Hear. Res. 16:22–36.

Schuell, H. 1953. Aphasic difficulties understanding spoken language. Neurology 3:176–184.

Schuell, H. 1954. Clinical observations on aphasia. Neurology 4:179–189.

Schuell, H. 1957. A short examination for aphasia. Neurology 7:625–634.

Schuell, H. 1965. The Minnesota test for differential diagnosis of aphasia. University of Minnesota Press, Minneapolis.

Schuell, H. 1966. A re-evaluation of the short examination for aphasia. J. Speech Hear. Disord. 31:137–147.

Schuell, H., and Jenkins, J. 1959. The nature of language deficit in aphasia. Psychol. Rev. 66:45–67.

Schuell, H., Jenkins, J. J., and Carroll, J. B. 1962. A factor analysis of the Minnesota test for differential diagnosis of aphasia. J. Speech Hear. Res. 5:349–369.

Schuell, H., Jenkins, J. J., and Jimenez-Pabon, E. 1964. Aphasia in adults. Hoeber Medical Division, Harper & Row, Publishers, New York.

Shankweiler, D., and Harris, K. 1966. An experimental approach to the problem of articulation in aphasia. Cortex 2:277–292.

Sklar, M. 1966. Sklar Aphasia Scale: Protocol Booklet. Western Psychological Services, Beverly Hills.

Smith, A. 1971. Objective indices of severity of chronic aphasia in stroke patients. J. Speech Hear. Disord. 36:167–207.

Spellacy, F., and Spreen, O. 1969. A short form of the token test. Cortex 5:390–397.

Spiegel, D. K., Jones, L. V., and Wepman, J. M. 1965. Test responses as predictors of free-speech characteristics in aphasic patients. J. Speech Hear. Res. 8:349–362.

Spreen, O., and Benton, A. 1969. Neurosensory center comprehensive examination for aphasia. Neuropsychology Laboratory, University of Victoria, Victoria, Canada.

Staats, A. W. 1968. Learning, Language, and Cognition: Theory, Research, and Methods for the Study of Human Behavior and its Development. Holt, Rinehart and Winston, Inc., New York.

Stengel, E. 1964. Speech disorders and mental disorders. In: A. V. S. DeReuck and M. O'Connor (eds.), Disorders of Language. Churchill Ltd., London.

Swisher, L. P., and Sarno, M. T. 1969. Token test scores of three matched patient groups: left-brain damaged with aphasia; right brain-damaged without aphasia; non brain-damaged. Cortex 5:264–273.

Taylor, M. 1953. Functional communication profile. Department of Physical Medicine and Rehabilitation, New York University Medical Center.

Teixeira, L., Defran, R., and Nichols, A. 1974. Oral stereognostic differences between apraxics, dysarthrics, aphasics and normals. J. Commun. Disord. 7:213–225.

Trost, J. 1970. Patterns of articulatory deficits in patients with Broca's aphasia. Doctoral dissertation, Northwestern University.

Vignolo, L. 1964. Evolution of aphasia and language rehabilitation: a retrospective exploratory study. Cortex 1:344–367.

Weinstein, E. A. 1964. Affections of speech with lesions in the non-dominant hemisphere. In: D. Rioch and E. A. Weinstein (eds.), Disorders of communication. The Williams & Wilkins Company, Baltimore.

Weinstein, E. A., Lyerly, O. G., Cole, M., and Ozer, M. N. 1966. Meaning in jargon aphasia. Cortex 2:165–187.

Weisenberg, T., and McBride, K. 1935. Aphasia. The Commonwealth Fund, New York.

Wepman, J. 1953. A conceptual model for the processes involved in recovery from aphasia. J. Speech Hear. Disord. 18:4–13.

Wepman, J. 1958. The relationship between self-correction and recovery from aphasia. J. Speech Hear. Disord. 23:302–305.

Wepman, J., and Jones, L. V. 1961. Studies in aphasia: an approach to testing. Manual of administration and scoring for the language modalities test for aphasia. Education Industry Service, Chicago.

Zangwill, O. 1964. Intelligence in aphasia. In: A. V. S. DeReuck and M. O'Connor (eds.), Disorders of Language. Churchill Ltd., London.

SPEECH

Introduction

Sadanand Singh

Generally, the procedure for diagnosing speech problems needs to adhere to a series of steps followed in a regular, orderly, and definite fashion. If these orderly steps are a direct result of clinical research designed to test a given diagnostic procedure, then they become the part of a credible diagnostic battery. It must be added, however, that the experimentally tested steps may be subject to controversy because of conflicting results of different studies involved in testing the same hypothesis. Such conflicting results increase the clinician's awareness of the various ramifications of a diagnostic issue and put the burden on the clinicians for making "correct" judgment in their adoption of a given diagnostic procedure.

A growing number of speech pathologists recognize their responsibility to incorporate experimentally verified diagnostic procedures of speech. This has inspired contemporary speech scientists to be involved in the testing hypotheses of clinical consequences. The outcomes of these studies are increasingly becoming the foundation of diagnosis today. Diagnostic procedures based on one clinician's intuition is appropriately losing ground. It is not fully convincing to know only that a given procedure is worthwhile because "it works." We must also ask why something works. In other words, what are the theoretical and historical foundations of a given diagnostic procedure? Do such foundations also have a strong data base? How do the theoretical, historical, and experimental bases yield a powerful diagnostic procedure? For example, distinctive feature theory (Singh, 1976; Baltaxe, 1978; and Blache, 1978) has been the basis for outlining phonologic acquisition of normal (Weiner and Bernthal, 1976) and deviant speech (Singh and Hayden, 1978) as well as for determining a very explicit phonologic status of children with speech problems (Compton, 1975, 1976; McReynolds and Engmann, 1975; Singh and Hayden, 1978).

The objective of the chapters within this section is to highlight the impact of clinical research on diagnostic procedures in speech. Two chapters are devoted to articulation disorders: one to provide a present day diagnostic procedure on foundation of a historical perspective (Dr. Michel) and the other to concentrate exclusively on the role distinctive features play in the diagnosis of articulation problems (Drs. Weiner and Bernthal). The chapter on stuttering (Dr. Hood) is designed to elucidate the impact of different theoretical, experimental, and methodologic stances on this controversial topic. The chapter on voice (Dr. Fox) is a global overview of the topic. This is an important topic because it has relevance to so many speech problems of both children and adults.

Although in each of the four chapters presented in this section effort has been made to include the state of the art today, none of these four chapters reflects all prevalent views. For example, there are various approaches in applying distinctive feature principles to diagnosing articulation problems. There is simple feature substitution count approach (McReynolds and Engmann, 1975), there is a "feature gram" profile approach (Singh and Hayden, 1978), and then there is the phonologic rule approach (Compton, 1975, 1976). Each of these three approaches is based on the principle that the phonemes are processed by features and consequently the phoneme errors ought to be analyzed by features. It is clear, however, that these three levels represent three degrees of sophistication in the analysis of articulation errors. The level of writing phonologic rules at each stage of examination is time consuming and probably would not stand the cost/benefit analyses. However, it is necessary for the clinicians engaged in the diagnosis and treatment of articulation disorders to be versed with each of these three levels of analyses and exercise their option to evoke any of these levels of analyses as deemed necessary.

This section does not include all speech topics. Topics such as cerebral palsy, dysarthria, and connected discourse problems have not been independently covered. Some discussions of these topics are included in the chapters in this section and also in chapters under "Language" and "Hearing."

REFERENCES

Baltaxe, C. M. 1978. Foundations of Distinctive Feature Theory. University Park Press, Baltimore.

Blache, S. 1978. The Acquisition of Distinctive Features. University Park Press, Baltimore.

Compton, A. J. 1975. Generative studies of children's phonological disorders: A strategy of therapy. In: S. Singh, (ed.), Measurement Procedures in Speech, Hearing, and Language, pp. 55–90. University Park Press, Baltimore.

Compton, A. J. 1976. Generative studies of children's phonological disorders: Clinical ramifications. In: D. M. Morehead and A. E. Morehead (eds.), Normal and Deficient Child Language, pp. 61–98. University Park Press, Baltimore.

McReynolds, L. V., and Engmann, D. L. 1975. Distinctive Feature Analysis of Misarticulations. University Park Press, Baltimore.

Singh, S. (ed.). 1976. Distinctive Features: Theory and Validation. University Park Press, Baltimore.

Singh, S., and Hayden, M. E. 1978. Distinctive Features Analysis of Articulation Tests. Manuscript in preparation.

Weiner, F. F., and Bernthal, J. 1976. In: S. Singh (ed.), Distinctive Features: Theory and Validation, pp. 178–204. University Park Press, Baltimore.

Evaluation of Articulatory Disorders: Traditional Approach

Lorraine I. Michel

CONTENTS

In this chapter Professor Michel presents a traditional philosophical approach to articulation disorders that includes rather specific recommendations for administering the articulation test. History serves as the foundation for present practice and Professor Michel presents a succinct historical review of the evaluation of articulation disorders. She has divided these highlights in terms of decades, e.g., 1910–1920. Some of these historical concepts may be considered theoretically sound and feasible, even today. For example, Swift (1918) considered articulation as "phonetic defects." "Consonants slightly off standard" were considered by him to be a mild disorder, correctable by drill, whereas lisping and omissions were referred to as "real" defects. Swift recommended an order of sound selection for phonetic training starting with sounds formed at the front of the mouth, then mid, and finally back. Needless to say, this strategy has been confirmed for phonologic acquisition and articulatory substitution patterns in current literature (Singh and Frank, 1972). This chapter also presents an analytical section on definitions, including a much needed discussion of the scope of articulation disorders. Professor Michel explicitly presents methods of constructing an articulation profile and correlates the profile with different generic test types. After the profile acquisition, different analysis techniques are discussed. These two sections serve as building blocks for forming competent diagnosis, recommendation, and prognosis.   —Eds.

In the following chapter, a systematic approach to articulation testing is presented, which incorporates the contributions of many authorities in the area of articulation. This approach is intended to serve as a model, providing methods of categorizing and administering articulation tests, and providing methods of evaluating test results. The reader may supply the specific names of the articulation tests. Articulation tests that are available today may not be available tomorrow, and tomorrow will bring a new test, which the reader should be able to evaluate, place in this model, and selectively use for maximum effectiveness. It is not the intention of the author to indicate that the philosophy and methods as presented constitute the only approach to articulation evaluation, or even the best approach to articulation evaluation. This approach is one of several alternatives available to the examiner.

HISTORICAL PERSPECTIVE

During the many years that the topic of evaluation of articulation disorders has appeared in the literature (in actuality or by implication), numerous changes have taken place, not only in terminology but also in the scope of evaluation procedures. The following historical perspective highlights the evaluation procedures over the years, and is not meant to be a complete historical investigation. This review is directed toward four areas specific to the evaluation procedure: 1) definition of the term articulation disorder; 2) methods and instruments used for acquiring an articulation profile; 3) formulation of conclusions (a diagnosis) from the analysis of the articulation profile; and 4) formulation of recommendations concerning the articulation profile. The review, in 10-year periods, cites changes that occurred during that period.

1910–1920

During these years there was an attempt at defining terms, there was interest in determining etiology, and general remediation procedures and techniques were suggested. Certainly none of these areas was thoroughly described by today's standards. Little, if anything, was mentioned about methods of acquiring the articulation profile (a delineation of the misarticulations), nor about the analysis of the profile beyond the mandatory determination of etiology.

For example, Scripture (1912) discussed three categories of "lisping" that would be considered pertinent to articulation: 1) negligent lisping; 2) neurotic lisping; and 3) organic lisping. The individual who exhibited "negligent lisping" was one who did not realize he was misarticulating. This disorder was attributable to "mental carelessness." A description of the disorder included sound substitutions, and alluded to the distortions of sounds. The use of "tongue gymnastics," and the concepts of phonetic placement instruction, auditory and visual models, and drill were the recommended methods of therapy. If the disorder was not corrected, either through a lack of therapy or a failure of the therapy program, "neurotic lisping" resulted. This second category was caused by emotional disturbance, fright, or anxiety, and frequently was accompanied by stuttering. In "organic lisping," the individual misarticulated sounds because of oral mechanism defects such as "feeble lips," tongue defects, and obstruction of the nasal passages. The author felt that no special treatment could correct this latter condition, but for colds he recommended a laxative, and cleansing the nasal passages with antiseptic sprays.

Swift (1918) referred to articulation disorders as "phonetic defects." "Consonants slightly off standard" were considered by him to be a mild disorder, correctable by drill, whereas lisping and omissions were referred to as "real" defects, which were likely to become permanent. Recommended methods of therapy included imitation of a model and, as a last resort, phonetic placement, which Swift considered to be very uninteresting to children. He also recommended an order of sound selection starting with sounds formed at the front of the mouth (/m/, /p/, /b/, then further back (/n/, /t/, /d/), then

/s/, /l/, and /r/ or /η/, /k/, and /g/, after which he felt that the sound selection did not matter.

1920-1930

During the 1920s, in an attempt toward greater specification in the four areas of evaluation, it can be noted that: 1) the disorder was defined with examples; 2) testing procedures were described in some detail, and the use of a standardized test was recommended; 3) analysis of the test results for patterns was suggested; determining the etiology was still mandatory; 4) recommendations for remediation continued to be general in nature.

Borden and Busse (1925) expressed their concern about the need for greater accuracy in diagnostic procedures. Using examples for clarification, they defined the disorder in terms of "omissions," "insertions" (i.e., additions), "replacement" (i.e., substitution), and "inversion" (as in lantren for lantern) (p. 127), and stated that there were three aspects important to the diagnostic process. The first aspect was concerned with the acquisition of the articulation profile. The examiner needed to hear all of the errors. In order to accomplish this, the client was to read sentences that emphasized specific phonemes, and the examiner was to check all sounds incorrectly produced. The client was then to reread the incorrect sentences, or read selected word lists, in order for the examiner to confirm his initial judgment, and to "note the exact acoustic character of each defect" (p. 137) (interpreted as meaning to describe exactly how the sound was misarticulated). The examiner was cautioned that errors could be inconsistent, that is, the client "may omit a given sound unit or replace it by another, *only in certain acoustic contexts*" (p. 138). The second aspect of diagnosis was to determine whether any pattern or grouping of defects could be noted. Possibilities mentioned were patterns concerning voicing, consistent use of one manner of articulation for another, or consistent misuse of place of articulation. The third aspect of diagnosis was to classify the disorder by etiology. An oral mechanism examination provided information regarding structural adequacy, and client history provided information regarding foreign dialect, language spoken in the home, "speech provincialism" (i.e., dialect), "speech carelessness" (i.e., attitude toward speech), "speech infantilism," and "functional nervous disturbance." All of the above etiologies were defined at length.

Stinchfield (1928) stated that a standardized speech test was essential to an accurate diagnosis. The Blanton-Stinchfield Speech

Measurements test, devised in 1926, was recommended. Part one was concerned with judgment of, among other characteristics, the general area of enunciation. Part two consisted of an articulation test comprised of words with all the phonemes in all positions, and common consonant blends. Data were collected by the author using children and college-age female adults in order to have a means of comparison. The "Speech Hygiene Program," to be followed by all with speech disorders, included recommendations such as getting at least 9 hours of sleep nightly, going to sleep immediately with pleasant thoughts, assuring oneself that he knows he can make all the sounds of the English language, eating plenty of fruits and vegetables, and exercising for 2 hours daily.

1930–1940

In the 1930s 1) a common definition of "articulation disorder" generally was being used; 2) the evaluation process was described in detail; 3) determining an etiology, although important, was not mandatory; 4) analysis of the articulation profile was becoming even more complex; 5) the use of a standardized format for recording and analyzing test results was recommended.

Travis (1931) included in the text *Speech Pathology* an entire chapter concerned with general examination methods. Specific to articulation, he noted that the speech examination was to be based on "unemotional propositional speech" through the use of standardized tests where pictures were presented whose labels contained all the consonants in all positions. Articulation was also to be analyzed while the client was reading, reciting something from memory, and imitating. Speech sound discrimination was to be analyzed. The clinician was to have a "trained ear" in order to adequately judge the articulatory abilities of the client. The relative frequency of speech sounds in children's speech was included.

Van Riper's *Speech Correction: Principles and Methods* (1939) brought into focus the concepts and techniques basic to the diagnosis of articulation defects. He included information on normal articulation development, which the clinician was to use as a basis for comparison with the disorder being analyzed. He noted that systematic methods must be used when analyzing articulation and he detailed these methods. The clinician was to note what errors occurred in spontaneous speech through labeling pictures and answering questions, the responses from which used all consonants in all appropriate positions (initial, medial, final). The clinician was to note what errors occurred when the client imitated the clinician's model of words or nonsense syllables (stimulability). The clinician was to analyze articulation during reading and casual conversation. Finally, the clinician was to accurately imitate the misarticulated sound, pair it with the correctly articulated sound, and ask the client to select the correct production (sound discrimination). Actual test presentation was to vary according to the needs of the client, and was to occur after rapport had been established with the client. An ample supply of a variety of pictures cut from magazines was mandatory for the clinician (the use of published standardized tests was not mandatory). The results of the articulation tests were to be recorded in an "Articulation Test Report." Here the clinician was to indicate the nature of the error (omission, substitution, distortion, addition), describe the production if the sound was distorted, indicate the position of the error (initial, medial, or final), indicate any words in which the error sound was articulated correctly, and analyze the error sounds regarding manner of articulation (such as nasality), frequency of articulation, visibility of articulation, developmental order, and voicing. A sample form was included for the clinician to follow. Van Riper cautioned that determining the cause of the articulation disorder was frequently of little use because the cause sometimes no longer existed when the diagnosis occurred and remediation program was initiated. If possible, etiologic factors were to be removed, and the clinician help the client to adjust to speaking situations.

There was not a heavy emphasis on the evaluation of articulation disorders in journals such as the *Journal of Speech Disorders*, although there was mention of the need for special materials to be used for diagnosing articulation errors (Stinchfield-Hawk, 1939) and an article concerning dysarthria (Robbins, 1940).

1940–1950

In the 1940s we find 1) an emphasis on the effects of maturation on articulation (Roe and Milisen, 1942); 2) that articulation test responses be spontaneous and the clinician be cautious not to say anything that would allow the client to correctly imitate the target phoneme; and 3) texts (Anderson, 1942; Kennedy, Carr, and Backus, 1947) that carefully described phonetic placement for each phoneme, provided suggestions of phonetic placement for misarticulated phonemes, and provided remediation approaches for each phoneme. The existence of regional variations was stressed, as was careless articulation (e.g., /dIpθaŋ/ for /dIfθaŋ/) (Anderson, 1942). In some texts the etiology of the articulation defect was given prime emphasis in the body of the text, while evaluation procedures were relegated to the appendix (Kennedy et al., 1947). Included in these appendices were suggestions of tests to administer; a description of methods of test presentation was lacking. Analysis of articulation defects continued to be concerned with etiology as a primary factor. Analysis of the articulation profile emphasized patterns of voicing, manner of articulation, acoustic frequency, loudness of the phoneme, visibility, place of articulation, amount of intraoral air pressure required, and whether the phoneme was a vowel, semivowel, consonant, etc. An attempt was made to relate all of these patterns to some etiology.

1950–1960

The *Diagnostic Manual in Speech Correction* by Johnson, Darley, and Spriestersbach (1952) included 1) procedures to follow for obtaining an articulation profile; 2) information concerning normative articulatory development; and 3) factors related to speech development. Other texts were available that were concerned with the description of articulation disorders, possible etiologic factors, and remediation procedures (for example, Berry and Eisenson, 1956). Templin's *Certain Language Skills in Children* (1957) contained a comprehensive analysis of normal articulation development from ages 3–8, presented test instruments for evaluating articulation and sound discrimination, and provided a detailed procedure for administering these tests.

1960–Present

In the 1960s and early 1970s texts concerned only with diagnostic procedures were more prevalent, and each, in varying degree, was concerned with the evaluation of articulation disorders (Johnson et al., 1963; Darley, 1965; Emerick and Hatten, 1974). In addition, the emergence of distinctive feature analysis and behavior modification principles greatly influenced the analysis of the articulation profile, and the formulation of recommendations concerning therapy. Tongue thrust as a possible etiologic factor, programmed articulation therapies, the acceptance of minority dialect as a difference in articulation rather than a disorder of articulation, more stringent standards in test development, a greater number of published articulation tests, and even accountability (specification of results expected from therapy) have influenced the evaluation process.

The reader can note that many changes have occurred in the

area of evaluation of articulation disorders during this span of years. The boundaries and terminology of the area have become more consistent. The use of systematic evaluative procedures has increased from being nonexistent to being mandatory. Test instruments have become increasingly more sophisticated. The body of knowledge concerned with normal articulatory development and production and used as a basis for comparison with the disordered articulatory development and production continues to grow. There is a multidimensional interpretation of the articulation profile, with conclusions being reached not only in regard to etiology, but also in developmental and distinctive feature patterns. Data available on remediation procedures are being used to allow for more meaningful recommendations. The evaluative procedures are not static, but continue to change as new research reported in journals and texts refines and updates our thinking. The clinician must be alert for this new information and must be ready to alter procedures as new and better ideas are made available. We must strive for greater precision in the definition of terms, in the acquisition and analysis of the articulation profile, and in the formulation of recommendations.

DEFINITION

Articulation, one of several areas included in the term speech, is the speaker's verbal production of the sounds (phonemes) of his language by the use of the articulators, or parts of the oral mechanism, that may interrupt or modify the voiced or voiceless air stream. In normal articulation development, not all the phonemes of the language are mastered with equal precision at the same age. It is not unusual to hear a 2-year-old child say some sounds incorrectly (misarticulate): /aɪ hæ maɪ bɪŋkəˀz ɪn maɪ bɑkˌɪts/ (I have my fingers in my pockets.). Such misarticulation is not classified as disordered because of the age of the child.

Regional or dialect variations are also not included in the area of articulation disorders. The speech pathologist must recognize the standard articulation patterns for a specific region, and be especially alert if he moves to a new region, or if a potential client has just recently moved to the community. Such sentences as /mə kɑr hɛz nou pɑr/ (my car has no power), /tʃɛk jɜ ɔl/ (check your oil), and /aɪ pɑkt maɪ kɑ/ (I parked my car) are each common in a certain area of the country. Professional associates who have lived in the region for a while are a valuable source of information regarding regional articulation patterns to the newcomer. If a colleague is unavailable, the speech pathologist would do well to critically listen to the articulation of everyone encountered in the new town (grocer, gas station attendant, children, teacher, sales clerk, etc.) and determine the articulation pattern appropriate to that area. (See also Thomas, 1947.)

Language disorders also are not included in the realm of articulation disorders. In some instances errors in articulation are, on closer examination, disorders of language patterns at the morphologic level. For example, the examiner may note that the /s/ or /z/ phoneme is omitted in the final position of words such as *cats* or *dogs*, but is included in the final position in such words as *bus* or *nose*. Or the client's internalized rule for plurality may result in an omission of /s/ or /z/ in the final position of any singular noun (i.e., one *bu*, two *bus*; one *gla* and two *glass*). Error in the use of morphologic markers for past tense or the comparative, as well as the plural and others, results in articulation which appears disordered. When the examiner notices such articulation patterns, and determines that in other linguistic environments the phonemes are articulated correctly (3rd person singular *asks* and *goes*,for example), it is concluded that an articulation disorder is not present, but rather that the language patterns of the client should be evaluated more extensively.

An articulation disorder exists when a phoneme (vowel or consonant) is incorrectly produced so that it sounds different from the sound expected from that individual. The specific incorrect sound production can be categorized as one of the following:

1. Omission: the target phoneme is not articulated, it is omitted.

Example	Phoneme omitted
ay-cake—/eɪ/ instead of /keɪk/	/k/
bush-brush—/bʌʃ/ instead of /brʌʃ/	/r/
un-sun—/ʌn/ instead of /sʌn/	/s/

2. Substitution: the target phoneme is replaced by another recognizable phoneme.

Example	Substitution
tate-cake—/teɪt/ instead of /keɪk/	t/k
bwush-brush—/bwʌʃ/ instead of /brʌʃ/	w/r
thun-sun—/θʌn/ instead of /sʌn/	θ/s

3. Distortion: the phoneme is replaced by a production that is slightly to severely off the target, or by a sound not found in that language.

Examples

Make a whistle accompanying the /s/.
Make the air flow for the /s/ through the sides of the mouth. The re-
resulting sound is somewhere between the /s/ and the /ʃ/, and is a
distorted /s/.
Make the /tʃ/ sound with the blade of the tongue rather than the
tongue tip. The resulting sound is a distorted /tʃ/.

4. Addition: an extra phoneme is inscrtcd into the word. Some additions are common to specific regions of the country (idear for idea) and some additions have a high frequency of occurrence (athuhlete for athlete). The additions that are clinically note-worthy are those unique to the client being examined.

Examples	Additions
schlool-school—/sklul/ instead of /skul/	/l/
kritten-kitten—/krɪtn/ instead of /kɪtn/	/r/
singging-singing—/sɪŋgɪ ŋ/ instead of /sɪŋɪŋ/	/g/

When studying clients who only have articulation disorders, any com-bination of omissions, substitutions, and distortions can occur in the preschool age group. School-age children through age 8 tend toward a greater number of substitutions and distortions, with omissions much less frequent in occurrence. In adulthood, articulation disorders tend mainly to be distortions of phonemes, with some substitutions occurring. Additions are the least frequent type of misarticulation in any age population.

The severity of the articulation disorder or, stated in another way, the intelligibility of the speaker, depends upon five factors. 1) The number of phonemes misarticulated: the individual who misarticulates only one phoneme will be much more readily understood than the individual who misarticulates 5 phonemes, 10 phonemes, 20 pho-nemes, etc. 2) The frequency that each phoneme is misarticulated: the individual who misarticulates /r/ only in /r/ blends will be more easily understood than that person who always misarticulates the phoneme. 3) The consistency of the error: the individual who some-times substitutes /θ/ for /s/, sometimes /f/ for /s/, and sometimes omits the phoneme is more unintelligible to the listener because no pattern of articulation can be readily determined. 4) The frequency of occurrence of the phoneme in the spoken language: the phoneme /ʒ/ as in *azure* occurs much less frequently than the phoneme /s/ as in *sun*. Misarticulating the /ʒ/ will not cause as noticeable a disorder as misarticulating the /s/. 5) The uniqueness of the misarticulation: a /θ/ for /s/ substitution or a /w/ for /r/ substitution is relatively common and may even go unnoticed by some people. A /b/ for /s/ substitution will affect intelligibility of articulation to a much greater extent because it is unusual. A distortion that is slightly off target, such as a "weak" /r/ or /l/, will probably go unnoticed, whereas an omitted or severely distorted /r/ or /l/ will affect intelligibility to a much greater extent. The labeling of an articulation disorder as mild, or moderate, or severe (or mild-moderate, etc.) is a judgment made by the speech pathologist and generally relates to an estimate of intelligibility of speech. Sometimes an intelligibility rating will be stated rather than a rating of severity of disorder (for example "75% intelligibility in conversational speech").

Articulation disorders can be further classified based on the etiology or cause (regardless of whether or not an etiology is specifically determined). Articulation disorders can be developmental or acquired, organic or functional. Developmental articulation disorders occur when the client has never consistently articulated the phoneme correctly, when he is beyond the age where the misarticulation would be considered within normal limits for articulation development, and when there is no known organic etiology. Developmental articulation disorders are not age specific but they occur more frequently in children than adults. The adult who exhibits a developmental disorder either never had therapy to correct the disorder, or the therapy was limited in its success. In an acquired articulation disorder, the client's previously correct articulation patterns are incorrect because of organic trauma (such as a cerebral vascular accident (stroke)), or a degenerative disorder (such as multiple sclerosis), or even something as common as a loss of teeth (either primary teeth, with the child waiting for the new teeth to erupt, or permanent teeth, with the client needing to adjust to dentures, an empty space, or whatever). Acquired articulation disorders are also not age specific, though they are more common to the adult population.

An organic speech disorder is one where a specific and known organic difference exists that directly relates to and causes the articulation disorder. For example, a lingual frenum that is too short, paralyzed lips or velum, or brain damage can cause an articulation disorder. A functional speech disorder tends to include all other suspected etiologies such as inadequate learning, lack of stimulation, lack of motivation, etc. Again, neither the organic nor the functional articulation disorder is age specific.

The use of the above classification systems implies that an etiology has been determined. This author feels strongly that, if the speech pathologist is sure of the etiology (that is, there exists a definite cause-effect relationship), the etiology should be explicitly stated; for example, "This articulation disorder is attributable to severe hearing loss," or "...is attributable to imitation of the parent." If the speech pathologist does not know the cause, stating that the client's disorder is functional, or developmental, means relatively little beyond the label itself. Although it is recognized that the need to determine an etiology follows the medical model (where there is the catch-all term "idiopathic" meaning of unknown cause and peculiar to the individual) and although it is recognized that there are situations where a label is mandatory, the speech pathologist would do well, if at all possible, to use his time determining what the client can articulate, and how to most efficiently remediate what he cannot articulate, rather than be concerned with perfunctory labels.

ACQUIRING THE ARTICULATION PROFILE

Once the speech pathologist has defined what he is analyzing, he needs to consider how to analyze it and how often to analyze it. To consider that evaluation of articulation can occur in a single test session implies that the examiner can determine all there is to know about the client's articulation profile during that brief time. This is not the case. Although the examiner obtains a great deal of information during the initial evaluation, by no means does he have a complete picture. The client is in a strange place, is interacting with a stranger (in spite of establishing rapport), and has undetermined levels of anxiety and motivation. All these factors, and many more, are available to influence the client's level of articulatory performance that day. Consequently, the evaluation of articulatory proficiency must be considered an ongoing process. The emphasis here will be on procedures to follow for the initial evaluation. However, the reader must keep in mind that if a disorder in articulation is present the examiner/clinician must continually probe the articulation proficiency in order to maintain an up-to-date profile. When considering the initial articulation evaluation, there are several prerequisite competencies (both academic and performance based) that must be met by the examiner before actually administering a test.

Prerequisite Competencies

Sound discrimination ability   The examiner must be skilled at hearing differences in phoneme production. If, for example, the examiner cannot hear that the final /r/ is omitted, or cannot distinguish between a slightly distorted and correct production of a phoneme, or cannot hear an f/θ substitution or a dentalized from an alveolar /t/, then the examiner will not be scoring the articulation test accurately, and any interpretation of the results will be invalid. The examiner should know how reliable a listener he is. He should check his reliability as often as possible. This reliability check can be accomplished in any of several ways. He can check his listening skills as compared with standardized test responses (Irwin and Nickles, 1970). Or the examiner and a professional colleague can independently score an ongoing articulation test. Or both examiners can independently score a tape recording (high quality video or audio) of an articulation test. Each response score is checked against the other (a point-to-point check) and scored as agreed (+) or disagreed (−). The number of agreed response scores is counted, and a percentage is calculated. For example:

Test response	Examiner A	Examiner B	Agreement
1. *pig*[a]	correct	b/p	−
2. pu*pp*y	correct	correct	+
3. cu*p*	omission	omission	+
4. e*gg*s	correct	correct	+
			3/4 = 75%

[a]stimuli (from Henja, 1963)

If there are 80 responses to the articulation test, and the examiners agree on 76, the inter reliability (or percentage of agreement) is 95%. The examiners should have at least a 90% reliability score, but it is more important to be knowledgeable of your reliability as a judge of articulation. If possible, the examiners should listen again to the responses upon which they disagreed, either by replaying the tape or requesting the client to repeat his response, and agreeing on a score. During a live repetition, the client may change his response. Each new response must be scored as a separate entity.

The examiner should also periodically check his intrareliability, that is, how consistently the same response was judged. An audio or video tape is needed here. The examiner scores the test, waits for several days, and rescores the same test by replaying the tape. Response scores from the test are checked against the response scores from the replay, and the number of agreed response scores are counted.

For example:

Test Response	Articulation Test	Replay	Agreement
1. saw [a]	θ/s	θ/s	+
2. pencil	θ/s	θ/s	+
3. house	θ/s	D	−
69. swing	−	−	+
			¾ = 75%

[a]stimuli (From Pendergast, Dickey, Selmar, and Soder, 1965)

High intrareliability is not only necessary in the evaluation process, but is also very important when judging the progress made in therapy. If the examiner determines that his reliability for scoring articulation tests is poor, he should enroll in a refresher course in articulation, or at least enlist the help of a colleague to rebuild listening skills.

Knowledge of types of articulation tests Another important competency is knowledgeability concerning the wide variety of articulation tests that have been published. Historically it was advocated that each clinician develop his own articulation test from pictures cut from magazines, children's dictionaries, and picture books. This is an interesting exercise in finding large, clear, and age-appropriate pictures for all the phonemes to be tested in all positions, and should not be discounted as a learning experience for understanding the difficulties of stimulus selection in test development. However, the use of published tests with which other professionals are familiar is encouraged. The home-made test should be used only when no response is elicited using the standardized test. When using published tests, the examiner must be aware that 1) published articulation tests differ in concept and design; 2) published articulation tests differ in advantages and limitations; 3) newly published articulation tests should be studied regarding their construction and standardization procedures. An articulation test is selected for use based on several factors: 1) the examiner's purpose (screening or complete diagnosis); 2) the age of the client; 3) the expected attention span and general performance of the client; and 4) the ease of test administration as judged by the examiner.

Screening tests Screening tests at the word level are abbreviated articulation tests that analyze the production of only a limited number of phonemes, and perhaps blends, not necessarily in all testable positions. Screening tests either include only those sounds that developmentally should be articulated correctly by the specific age, or include the most difficult phonemes to articulate. Some complete diagnostic evaluation articulation tests have screening tests inherent in their design by stimulus selection (see, for example, the Templin-Darley *Tests of Articulation*, 1969; Fisher-Logemann *Test of Articulation Competence*, 1971). These screening tests tend to include the later developing phonemes. Articulation screening tests can also be found as a part of a language evaluation test (see, for example, Zimmerman, Steiner, and Evatt, *The Pre-school Language Scale*, 1969). The *Predictive Screening Test of Articulation* (Van Riper and Ericson, 1975) is designed to indicate which clients are most likely to require therapy, and which are most likely to self-correct their misarticulations. (See also Barrett and Welsh, 1975, for further discussion.) Screening tests may also be brief paragraphs (such as "My Grandfather," Van Riper, 1939, 1963; "The Rainbow Passage," Fairbanks, 1960) that contain all of the phonemes to be tested in at least one position. Use of such tests implies that the client has the ability to read so the examiner does not question whether the client has difficulty initiating articulatory movement. (This concept holds true for any articulation test that requires the client to read.)

Because screening tests are relatively easy to administer (that is, responses can be scored "right" or "wrong"), there is a tendency to assume that anyone can administer such a test. Training for administering a screening test is necessary, although not generally lengthy. The speech pathologist must determine the adequacy of the sound discrimination abilities of the person who is administering the screening test, and the speech pathologist must ensure that a consistent scoring system is used. In this case, the examiner must understand that the "diagnosis" made is either a) normal articulation or b) needs further evaluation.

Diagnostic tests   Diagnostic tests include all of the phonemes of American English (consonants, vowels, and diphthongs) and a large sampling of double and triple consonant blends, in all possible positions (initial, medial, final).

Word Tests: Some of the tests are designed to present one stimulus picture for each target phoneme (see, for example, Templin and Darley, 1969). Other tests are designed to evaluate several phonemes per stimulus, such as: *house*—/h/ and /s/ (see, for example, Goldman and Fristoe, 1969). If the examiner is new to testing procedures or if the examiner's reliability in determining phoneme accuracy is less than good, this latter type of articulation test is not recommended because the examiner must concentrate on the accuracy of production of more than one target phoneme. However, this type of test saves time.

Sentence Tests: Tests in which the client reads sentences containing the target phoneme(s) in several words (all possible positions) are available for the beginning reader and for the more advanced reader. (See, for example, Fairbanks, 1960, or Fisher and Logemann, 1971). The examiner is required to concentrate only on the target phoneme(s) for each sentence. The more experienced examiner will note all misarticulations found in each sentence and thereby be able to judge frequency and consistency of error from a larger verbal sample.

Repeat the Story Tests: In this type of test, a story with picture stimuli is read to the client. The examiner, when reading, emphasizes key words that contain the target phonemes. The client then repeats the story, using the pictures as a cue for the story sequence. The target phonemes are thus incorporated into the client's verbalization of the story (See Goldman and Fristoe, 1969).

Object Tests: The author is aware of no standardized object articulation test. However, the examiner may decide to use objects if other tests fail to elicit a response, and if the client is apt to respond favorably to objects. Object tests tend not to test all phonemes in all testable positions because of the difficulty of finding appropriate, easily recognizable objects.

Deep Tests: This type of test examines phonemes in many phonetic environments (see, for example, McDonald's *A Deep Test of Articulation*, 1964; Elbert, Shelton, and Arndt, 1967). Although other tests analyze the production of a phoneme in its relation to a few other sounds, deep tests help to determine in which of many phonetic environments the target phoneme is articulated correctly, and in which it is misarticulated.

High Intraoral Pressure Test: When the examiner questions velopharyngeal competence, an articulation test that emphasizes only those phonemes that require high intraoral pressure is recommended (see, for example, the *Iowa Pressure Articulation Test*, Templin-Darley *Tests of Articulation*, 1969). This type of test does not examine the production of all phonemes; such is not its purpose.

Systematic scoring system   Before initiating the actual test procedures, a clear and dependable note-taking system for scoring the articulation test should be devised. The examiner who writes "d" for "distorted," and later interprets this symbol as a substitution, (d/ –) has lost valuable information because of an unsystematic scoring system. Although each of us is sure he will remember the meaning of all his notations, the passage of even a small amount of time will affect memory, and notations that are not analyzed until perhaps much later that day or the next can easily be meaningless if they are not part of a consistently used and dependable system. Some tests will suggest the system to be used. Most tests do publish accompanying scoring sheets, which, at minimum, include the stimulus items in the order to be presented. The author recommends the following:

1. If using a published score form, score the target phoneme in the place provided, so there is no doubt concerning your judgment of the target phoneme. If the response is completely correct, do not write anything, even a check mark. Hastily written check marks can resemble dashes or phonemes such as /v, r, ʃ/. Writing nothing saves time, and means that no error has occurred.

2. If the client has made a substitution for the target phoneme, a slash (/) is written between the produced phoneme and the target phoneme (e.g., b/p or θ/s). Print IPA symbols as clearly as possible. Write a capital "D" when a distortion occurs. Write a dash (—) for omission rather than a capital "O" because a hastily written capital "O" can resemble a capital "D" (and vice versa).

3. In the area for comments regarding the target phoneme, or on a separate piece of paper matched numerically regarding stimuli, describe the distorted sound. Also note whether the response was imitated or spontaneous.

4. If other phonemes within the word were misarticulated, and you are scoring them, note these errors in a separate area. For example:

Number	Picture	Response	Comments	Margin
1.	valentine	b/v		w/l; m/n (MF); k/t
2.	stove	b/v	imitated response	s = D (lateralized); k/t
3.	rabbit	D	tongue not elevated	
4.	car	—		

1. The target phoneme was the initial /v/, which was substituted with a /b/; the client also substituted /w/ for /l/, /m/ for /n/ in both the medial and final positions, and substituted /k/ for /t/.

2. The target phoneme was the final /v/, which was substituted with a /b/. The client also distorted the /s/ by lateralizing the air flow, and substituted /k/ for /t/. The response was imitated (examiner modeled).
3. The target phoneme was initial /r/, which was distorted because of a lack of tongue elevation. The remainder of the word was articulated correctly.
4. The target phoneme was the final /r/, which was omitted. The remainder of the word was articulated correctly.

The importance of a clear, dependable, and consistent system of notation cannot be overstressed. Such a system is of paramount importance to the accuracy of the entire evaluation.

Oral mechanism evaluation The fourth necessary competency is the ability to administer and interpret an oral mechanism evaluation. All too frequently the examiner, with head turned at an awkward angle, steals a brief glance into an opening mouth, and then declares that the oral mechanism is adequate in form and function for speech purposes. Because the ability to articulate depends in part upon the presence of and correct function of the articulators, it is mandatory that the examiner systematically evaluate the oral mechanism. This author feels that an oral mechanism evaluation should occur even if the examiner is administering only an articulation screening test.

The details of a complete oral mechanism examination are beyond the purview of this chapter; however, the following procedural recommendations are offered:

1. Place the client at a comfortable level for you. Perhaps a child will have to sit on the table top or desk; or perhaps the examiner will need to stand when examining the mouth of an adult, or kneel on the floor when examining the child.
2. Study the oral mechanism front to back. That is, start at the lips, and proceed to study each articulator in turn toward the velum and pharyngeal wall. It is a waste of time to ask the client to open his mouth in order to look at the hard palate, then look at lip movement, then again request an open mouth to look at the teeth, then study tongue-to-lip movement, and then again request an open mouth to study velar action.
3. Use a high intensity flashlight, and some tool, such as a tongue blade, to aid you in viewing the oral mechanism. There is generally little difficulty in administering an oral mechanism evalu-

ation to a child if the child has had the opportunity to flash the light in the examiner's mouth, and hold a tongue blade. The author has frequently seen a child inspecting his mother's mouth, demonstrating that unusual game the examiner had done earlier! The examiner should use the tongue blade gently but firmly, so as not to hurt the client but yet to indicate confidence in his own ability to handle a tongue blade. If the child will not tolerate a tongue blade, a lollipop can function as a substitute.

4. The judgment of size of each part of the oral mechanism becomes meaningful only as that part relates to the whole oral cavity.

5. Although diadochokinetic rates have been determined for /pʌ/, /tʌ/, /kʌ/, and /pʌtʌkʌ/, the examiner should not feel lost if the child cannot remember the /pʌtʌkʌ/ sequence. Rapid repetition of *pattycake* (or *buttercup*) will also allow the examiner to analyze the coordination of rapid tongue and lip movements.

6. If a deviation from the normal is noted, the examiner should carefully evaluate whether and how this deviation affects articulation. Frequently, compensatory articulatory movements will result in an acoustically (and perhaps visually) correct sound. The individual with an immobile upper lip may well articulate the /p/, /b/, and /m/ using the lower lip and upper teeth. The resulting sounds look different but may sound accurate in context.

Further discussion relative to the interpretation of the oral mechanism evaluation occurs later. The author refers the reader to Travis' *Handbook of Speech Pathology and Audiology* (1971) for normative information regarding the oral mechanism.

Background information   The final prerequisite for an articulation evaluation is to have obtained any available background information from the client, or parent (or social worker, etc.) to aid in the interpretation of test results and in the formulation of the recommendations. A description of the complete case history form and interviewing techniques are outside the purview of this chapter. Consequently, we will discuss here only those questions pertinent to the articulation evaluation. The following questions do not pertain to every age group. The clinician should select or revise the questions to be client-specific.

Description of the problem   The reader should note use of the term "problem" here. The examiner has not yet evaluated the articulation to determine the existence of a "disorder," but because the client is present for an examination, there does exist a "problem."

Conversely, an individual could have a disorder but not recognize it as a problem.

The examiner should ask the client/parent to describe the problem as thoroughly as possible. This description should include under what circumstances the level of performance changes, whether there have been any attempts to remediate the problem, whether anyone has mentioned the problem (i.e., whether it is readily apparent to others), and how the client and others react to the problem.

Developmental history   The examiner needs to know the age at which the major developmental milestones were attained (sitting, walking, etc.) in order to evaluate motoric development. The client/parent should describe the speech development.

Medical and health history   The parent/client should describe any accident, injury, or surgery to the mouth area, and any significant medical history that may have affected articulation. (Although a broken arm can indeed be a traumatic experience, the examiner must pursue this medical area further to find a direct cause-effect relationship). High fevers, extended hospitalization, or any severe illness wherein the client's efforts were concentrated on life support areas rather than articulation development or articulation maintenance should be described. Present health status, and any medications needed should be discussed. The examiner should have permission to obtain information from other pertinent sources (such as physicians or dentists).

Family history   The examiner should ask if there is anyone among the client's immediate family or other relatives who exhibit similar speech patterns. The family's reaction to the speech patterns should be noted.

Educational history   The examiner should inquire whether the speech problem has influenced schooling in any way. A description of how the client functions in school is useful.

Society history   The examiner needs to know if the speech problem has influenced social adjustment, or peer interaction. What is peer reaction to the speech problem? Peers, neighbors, or other acquaintances who exhibit similar speech patterns should be listed.

In some situations, no background information is available. This is, of course, especially true in large scale articulation screening programs where all school children are tested. It is also sometimes true if the client is referred to the clinic, and brought to the clinic by someone other than the parent or an individual acquainted with the client's history. Grandparents, school teachers and nurses, social workers, pre-school aides, etc., may lack the specific background information you request. Sometimes even the mother or father may not remember details of previous years. As mentioned earlier, although historical information provides a basis for etiology and attitudinal information provides a basis for prognosis, it is the articulation performance of that day upon which the examiner makes judgments concerning whether it is disordered, whether therapy is recommended, and what therapeutic approach (program) to recommend.

Testing Procedures

Published tests frequently include procedures for administering the test in the examiner's manual. These recommended procedures should be followed in order to compare the results with any norms accompanying the test. Many instances arise where a deviation from the recommended test administration procedures is necessary. Although the tests results cannot then technically be compared with the data published with it, the examiner can still interpret the results, keeping in mind the circumstances in which the results were obtained.

When eliciting a response, the clinician should aim for a spontaneous response, be it the label of a picture, reading a sentence, or completing an intraverbal lead. If the client does not know the name of the picture, etc., the clinician should note that the response was not spontaneous, and delayed repetition should be used. Playing 20 questions with the client in an attempt to elicit a spontaneous response is time consuming, and all too frequently fruitless. Witness the following exchange:

Clinician: "What's this?"
Client: "I don't know."
Clinician: "Oh, your Daddy has one of them."
Client: Silence
Clinician: "He uses it to cut wood."
Client: "An axe."
Clinician: "No, he has to move his arm like this (motion)."
Client: "I don't know."
Clinician: "It has sharp teeth and a wooden handle."

The reader can quickly see the amount of time wasted in this exchange. In eliciting a delayed imitation response, the clinician models the target word, and then says something brief such as, "Say it." or "Tell me." The last verbalization heard by the client is not the target word, or, ideally, does not contain the target phoneme, and so the imitation factor is reduced.

Clinician: "What's this?"
Client: "I don't know."
Clinician: "Saw. Tell me that."
Client: "Saw."

In addition, when eliciting a response, the clinician should judge the first response made by the client; he should not have the client frequently repeat the response, which may change as attention is brought to it. This concept refers back to the good listening skills of the clinician.

Administering the screening test An articulation screening test should be used when the examiner needs to see many clients within a short period of time, the group has unknown presenting problems, and the examiner needs to determine only whether the articulation is normal or questionable. Such groups as school children, college students, nursery schools, and nursing home residents are frequently screened for articulation disorders. The test is brief, and, if accurately constructed, should not overlook anyone with an existing disorder. That is, screening tests tend to over-refer (false positives) rather than under-refer.

It is difficult to judge the time required to complete an articulation screening test. College students reading a short paragraph may complete the screening in 5 minutes; preschoolers trying to spontaneously identify the picture stimuli may take 15 minutes.

The purpose is to be brief, however. The typical procedure is as follows:

1. Social conversation, which puts the client at ease and allows the examiner to judge general articulation performance in spontaneous conversational speech.
2. Read the paragraph, or label the words, etc. (see earlier description of screening tests).
3. Oral mechanism examination.
4. Any articulation error noted (dependent upon test norms) results in a referral for a complete articulation evaluation.

From the screening test, no recommendations are made beyond the referral for a complete articulation evaluation. No description is made of the disorder (nor is a definite statement made that the articulation is indeed disordered).

Diagnostic test procedures   Diagnostic test procedures are used to determine whether or not a disorder exists, to describe the disorder, and to make recommendations concerning a course of action for the disorder. Because the client's age and some background information should have been available to the examiner, an appropriate articulation test should have been selected before initiation of the evaluation. Back-up tests should also be available in case the expected age, performance level, or attention span of the client is erroneous. The procedures are as follows:

1.   Conversation: that period of time, frequently referred to as "establishing rapport," should be audio recorded for later articulation transcription. In addition, the examiner should note, in writing, any phonemes that are misarticulated, and the environment in which they are found (position, and phoneme preceding and following). At least 2 minutes of conversation from the client are needed (excluding the examiner's conversation).

2.   Test administration: the examiner may select more than one test to administer. For example, perhaps he wants to see how the adult responds to a sentence articulation test (read), as well as a spontaneous word articulation test. Or, the examiner may administer the spontaneous word articulation test, and then a portion of a deep test to further analyze the misarticulated phonemes. Or, the examiner may administer a spontaneous word articulation test, and a target word in sentence test. Or, noting that phonemes requiring high intraoral pressure are misarticulated, or that there is a hypernasal quality, the clinician may elect to administer an articulation test evaluating velopharyngeal competence.

3.   Stimulability: after the examiner has determined which phonemes are misarticulated, he then determines whether or not the client is able to correct the error with minimal attention and training on the phoneme. Some published tests include a stimulability test (see Goldman and Fristoe, 1969). In essence, the examiner is to determine whether the client, with an accurate model to imitate, can articulate the phoneme correctly and, if so, at what complexity level. The examiner models the phoneme in isolation, nonsense syllables (NSS), at the word level, or at the short phrase level. Some clients articulate the phoneme correctly in NSS but not in isolation or words, some in isolation but not in NSS or words, some in the medial but not in the initial or final positions, or any other combination of events. The examiner can select

any vowel environment for the stimuli. However, if possible, the examiner should select phoneme environments where he has noted correct and also incorrect productions in order to determine consistency of error. The examiner can also use visual cues, phonetic placement cues, and descriptive cues along with the auditory model. If all these attempts fail to elicit a correct production at any complexity level (isolation to short phrase), and in any position (initial, medial, final), then that phoneme would be categorized as one not easily mastered. Because the examiner is attempting to see how rapidly the client learns to articulate the sound correctly, this information would be valuable in determining which phoneme(s) to select initially for the remediation program.

4. Sound discrimination: research studies to date do not agree on the role the client's sound discrimination ability plays in his articulation disorder. Is it because the sound is not discriminated correctly that it is misarticulated? Or is it because the sound is misarticulated that it is not discriminated correctly? Does sound discrimination training affect the articulatory production of the target phoneme? Or does production training affect the discrimination of that phoneme? (See Williams and McReynolds, 1975; McReynolds, Kohn, and Williams, 1975). Some speech pathologists do analyze the client's sound discrimination ability. They note whether the client is able to discriminate between the correctly articulated phoneme and another phoneme (as in a substitution), between a distorted and a correctly articulated phoneme, and between the presence and absence of the phoneme (as in an omission). The examiner should look for new information pertaining to sound discrimination, which will help to determine the importance of this analysis in the evaluation process.

ANALYSIS OF THE ARTICULATION PROFILE

After administering the tests for evaluating the client's articulation proficiency, the examiner should have the following information: articulation errors made in conversational speech, errors made on the standard articulation test(s), errors made on the deep test, the client's response to stimulability tests on the error phonemes, and form and function of the oral mechanism. Perhaps the examiner will have client history (see earlier discussion of situations in which this may not be the case), and perhaps the examiner will have elected to study sound discrimination of the error phonemes. The error phonemes should then be analyzed by the examiner in the following ways. (Distinctive feature analysis is discussed at length in the next chapter.)

Pattern Analysis

The phonemes that have been misarticulated should be charted to determine whether any pattern of misarticulation can be noted. In the most basic pattern analysis, the misarticulated phonemes are charted by position in the word (initial, medial, final) and type of misarticulation (substitution, distortion, omission, addition). (See Figure 1.) Observable patterns occur when the misarticulated phonemes are only in the initial (or medial or final) position, or if the client only omits (or substitutes) phonemes, or any combinations thereof (omits in the final position and distorts in the medial position). Consistency of the misarticulations can also be noted. That is, in the initial position does the client sometimes substitute and sometimes distort the target phoneme? Or, does the client substitute the target phoneme with more than one phoneme? Distortions should be analyzed for any consistent articulatory behavior.

A different charting system can be used to analyze the misarticulations by place of articulation (as bilabial, lingua-alveolar, lingua-velar, etc.), manner of articulation (how the sound is formed), and voicing (with or without voice) (see Figure 2.) Observable patterns occur when the misarticulated phonemes are of one type, be it attributable to place (all lip-involved phonemes), manner (all plosives, for example), or voicing (for example, all voiceless). A combination of the two charts, or combining the data from the charts, offers the examiner a great deal of information concerning the characteristics of the misarticulated phonemes (see Figure 3). Information obtained

TYPE	OMISSION	SUBSTITUTION	DISTORTION	ADDITION
INITIAL				
MEDIAL				
FINAL				

POSITION

Figure 1.   Charting consonant misarticulations by position and type of misarticulation.

PLACE	VOICE	MANNER				
		PLOSIVE	FRICATIVE	AFFRICATE	NASAL	GLIDE
BILABIAL	+					
	−					
LABIO-DENTAL	+					
	−					
LINGUA-DENTAL	+					
	−					
LINGUA ALVEOLAR	+					
	−					
PLATAL	+					
	−					
LINGUA-VELAR	+					
	−					
GLOTTAL	+					
	−					

Figure 2.   Charting consonant misarticulations by place, manner, and voicing.

from the oral mechanism evaluation should be combined with the test results in determining cause-effect relationships between oral mechanism function and misarticulation. Information available from the client history should also be combined with test results for etiologic purposes.

The examiner should also analyze the misarticulated phonemes concerning acoustic frequency. That is, are the misarticulated phonemes all high frequency sounds, which may possibly indicate hearing loss? And, the examiner should view the misarticulated sounds regarding amount of intraoral breath pressure required. That, com-

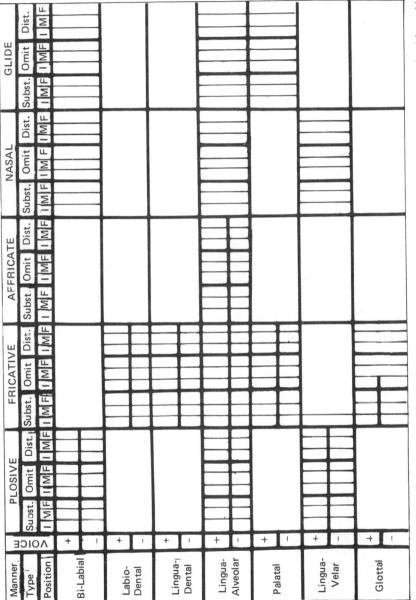

Figure 3.   Charting the consonant misarticulations by type, place, manner, voicing, and position. (*Wh* has been omitted from this chart.)

bined with hypernasality, may suggest a submucous cleft or inadequate velopharyngeal function. Perhaps the examiner had noted this tendency during the testing procedures, and administered further tests analyzing intraoral pressure.

The abovementioned charts (Figures 1, 2, and 3) should be used as visual aids when verbally reporting the results to the parent/client (see p. 455).

Developmental Analysis

The clinician should analyze the misarticulated phonemes with regard to the age at which the phonemes should be articulated correctly based on normal developmental data. Obviously such analysis is not necessary if the client is well over the age of 8. Age 8 is the point when, developmentally, all phonemes (in any environment including triple blends) should be articulated correctly. The most comprehensive information concerning normal articulation development is by Templin (1957). She studied the articulatory development of 480 children aged 3–8. The normative data that resulted for 25 phonemes (studied in the initial, medial, and final positions) indicate the age at which at least 75% of the subjects articulated each phoneme correctly. Prather, Hedrick, and Kern (1975) studied the normal articulatory development of youngsters aged 2–4 years. Also using a 75% criterion, they found earlier age levels than Templin found for 20 of the 25 phonemes (studied in the initial and final positions). Seventy-five percent of their subjects had not achieved correct production of the remaining five phonemes by age 4. The developmental sequence of the phonemes was similar in the two studies. Rather than study only the upper age limits of correct phoneme production, Sander (1972), incorporating the data of Templin and others, studied the average age or customary production of 24 phonemes. His description, then, indicated the ages where 50–90% of the subjects correctly produced each of the phonemes. In addition to these sources of information on articulation development, some articulation tests indicate age limits by which clients should be articulating each of the tested phonemes (see, for example, Henja, 1963, or Fisher and Logemann, 1971).

Regardless of which system is used, the misarticulated phonemes should be charted developmentally by age level, with the client's chronologic age clearly specified on the chart. The example offered here is adapted from Templin's data (see Figure 4). Again, the chart is a very useful visual aid when discussing the articulation test results with the parent. The developmental norms on the chart you use should be revised as often as new data are made available.

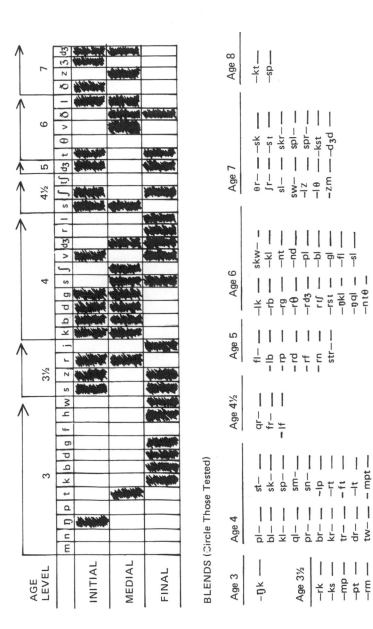

Figure 4. Charting consonant articulations according to developmental norms. (Adapted from Templin, 1957.)

Stimulability Analysis

Results of the stimulability test are to be analyzed according to the complexity level(s) at which a correct response occurred (see Figure 5). The error phonemes are listed. In the complexity level columns, the phonemic environments tested are listed and the accuracy of the responses noted. Comments should be entered on the form regarding the type of stimulation presented (such as the use of visual stimulation, auditory stimulation, phonetic placement cues, or combinations thereof). The examiner can then note at a glance which phonemes responded readily to stimulation, and at what complexity level. Rapid learning of an error phoneme is important information that is used when formulating recommendations regarding therapy programs.

Severity Analysis

As noted earlier (see p. 426), the examiner must also judge the severity of the articulation disorder, or how it affects the intelligibility of the speaker. This judgment is derived from the conversational speech sample as well as from the number, frequency, and consistency of the misarticulated phonemes.

Vocabulary Analysis

Although vocabulary is beyond the realm of the analysis of articulation, the number of picture stimuli presented that the client could not spontaneously label should be noted. Generally, published articulation tests have selected picture stimuli that are easily recognizable. The client who cannot spontaneously label the pictures, but rather responds only imitatively, should be further evaluated for a possible language deficit.

Diagnosis

After the examiner has put all of the information together in a systematic fashion, he must determine whether an articulation disorder exists, and, if so, describe it using the information obtained in the analysis. Possible diagnoses include 1) normal articulation, 2) delayed articulation, and 3) deviant articulation

Normal articulation   The articulation of the client is normal if the examiner concludes that the individual is using dialect or regional variations, or consistent misuse of morphological markers (see pp. 424–425). The articulation is also within normal limits if the client is within developmental norms. That is, all of the misarticulated pho-

COMPLEXITY LEVEL / POSITION	ISOLATION	TYPE OF STIM.	NONSENSE SYLLABLES	TYPE OF STIM.	WORD	TYPE OF STIM.	PHRASE	TYPE OF STIM.
ERROR PHONEMES s^I	correct	Phonetic placement	æ-correct, i-correct, u-correct, ε-incorrect → Mirror	Phonetic placement and Mirror	sun, Sally }incorrect, sip	Auditory model		
s^M			æ }correct, i, u }incorrect, ε	Phonetic placement and mirror	incorrect	Auditory model		
s^F			æ, i, u, ε }incorrect		incorrect	Auditory model		

Figure 5. Charting the results of the stimulability test. Example for phoneme /s/ is given for all positions (initial, medial, and final).

nemes are phonemes that are expected to be accurately articulated at a later age. The client who is age 4 and misarticulates the $/\theta/$ is within normal limits developmentally, according to the Templin data.

The diagnosis that the articulation is within normal limits also occurs when the misarticulation is so slight that it does not draw attention to itself, the client is not aware or concerned about it, and it probably will not affect any future goals. This articulation performance technically is deviant, but has a very low severity rating. It is sometimes difficult to judge whether the slight misarticulation will affect any future goals of the client, and the examiner should discuss this issue with the client in detail before formulating recommendations. For example, is it significant that a school teacher has a slightly lateralized /s/? Many education training institutions do not have any articulation competency levels for their majors. Is correct articulation necessary for public speaking endeavors? Many advertisers on television employ people who misarticulate, perhaps as an attention getting device, perhaps because the misarticulation is not considered by them to be significant, or perhaps because they are unaware that the articulation is actually incorrect. For the remainder of this chapter, this type of articulation is considered disordered. However, the reader should recognize the technical point involved.

Delayed articulation   The articulation of the client is considered to be delayed if it is following normal developmental patterns, but at a slower rate. The 5-year-old client who correctly articulates all phonemes through the age 4 level and thereafter misarticulates the phonemes is considered to have delayed articulation. Those clients who exhibit "baby talk" or infantile articulation patterns usually have delayed articulation. Frequently, a language disorder is also present.

Deviant articulation   Any other error pattern such as the misarticulation of all fricatives, or all voiceless phonemes, or no determinable pattern without further analysis is indicative of the existence of deviant articulation.

Populations with Higher Incidence of Articulation Disorder

Very frequently the speech pathologist is among the first of the professionals analyzing a problem in which communication (in this case, an articulation disorder) is one of several or many symptoms. Communication plays such a significant role that a lack of its development, or its degeneration, is quickly noted. Other symptoms may take longer to be recognized or can more easily be ignored. Thus the examiner should be aware of disorders that include misarticulation as a frequent or common symptom. Texts are available that describe in detail the articulation patterns characteristic of these various populations. Only a brief comment is provided here. It must be stressed that characteristic patterns are discussed, without reference to the wide range of individual differences.

Mental retardation   One possible etiology for delayed or deviant articulation is mental retardation. Within this population, language disorders are also common. It is, of course, up to the examiner to determine which of the two disorders more significantly affects the client's communication and therefore warrants more immediate and intensive attention. The client who has a pronoun substitution (me/I, etc.) and who misarticulates 15 different phonemes needs a concentrated articulation program, with work on language. The client who has a vocabulary of 25 words needs intensive language therapy, and articulation therapy only after there is enough language to determine an articulation profile.

Cleft palate and palatal disorders   The client with a cleft palate or with velopharyngeal incompetence will have difficulty channeling the air flow through the mouth, and phonemes that require high intraoral pressure (the plosives, fricatives, and affricates) are misarticulated. The plosives are frequently substituted by a glottal stop; the fricatives and affricates may be very weak or distorted. The vowel quality (hypernasal) is readily apparent (see Travis, 1971).

Congenital hearing loss   The child's oral communication development can be directly related to the amount and nature of the hearing loss: the greater the hearing loss, the greater the communication deficit. Thus the child with a profound hearing loss will not only have delayed articulation, but delayed language as well. The child with a mild to moderate loss may only have deviant articulation, which will then be dependent on the characteristics of the loss. Frequently, phonemes with high acoustic frequency will be distorted or omitted (/s/, /z/, /f/, /θ/, etc.), the client will have a tendency to misarticulate the phonemes that are not highly visible (the velar plosives, for example), and self monitoring of articulation and discrimination will be affected.

Acquired hearing loss   The older child or adult, after acquiring a hearing loss, may experience a deterioration in the preciseness of articulation performance, dependent upon the amount and characteristics of the hearing loss. The client with a high frequency loss will show signs of high frequency phoneme distortion, and may have difficulty incorporating these phonemes into newly acquired vocabulary.

Brain damage   The classification system devised by Darley, Aronson, and Brown (1975) delineates six types of dysarthrias: spastic, ataxic, hypokinetic, hyperkinetic, flaccid, and mixed. These differ according to the site of the brain lesion, and can also be classified according to the causal disease (such as Parkinson's disease, myasthenia gravis, multiple sclerosis, etc.). Regardless of the classification, articulation performance is affected because of a loss of strength, loss of range of movement, and a loss of ability to coordinate the articulators. Plosives and fricatives are weak or omitted, vowels are imprecise, medial and final consonants pose greater problems than initial consonants, and there is a progressive deterioration of articulation as the length of the verbal utterance increases. The misarticulations are relatively consistent in nature. Specific muscle weakness will determine which phonemes are more likely to be affected (i.e., bilabials, or the phonemes requiring tongue tip elevation, etc.). Velar paralysis or paresis can occur, which results in hypernasality; prosody, respiration, and phonation are also affected.

The apraxic individual does not exhibit weakness or incoordination when automatically (or reflexively) using the articulators. There is no apparent impairment of muscle function. However, when purposively speaking, if indeed the client attempts volitional speech, errors in articulation are inconsistent in nature. Substitutions, additions, and repetitions occur as opposed to omissions or distortions. A phoneme may be articulated correctly once, and then substituted by another phoneme far removed (by distinctive feature) from the target phoneme. In children, developmental apraxia manifested by a severe articulation disorder must be differentiated from the functional articulation disorder.

For both apraxia and dysarthria, a thorough oral mechanism evaluation is essential for the role it plays in differential diagnosis. The reader is referred to Darley et al. (1975) for further information on the evaluation of dysarthria and apraxia.

ARTICULATION PROFILE INFERENCES
Recommendations

After the examiner has concluded whether or not a disorder exists, and the type and severity of the disorder, he must decide whether any recommendations should be made, and if so, what the recommendations should be. The great variations in clients and their individual circumstances must be kept in mind when formulating recommendations. This section will review the most frequently occurring recommendations. The examiner coordinates the unique circumstances of the client and the conclusions reached from the testing in order to determine the appropriate recommendations for the specific client. The four most common recommendations are: 1) normal articulation—no recommendations; 2) re-evaluate the articulation—no therapy recommended; 3) articulation disorder—no therapy recommended; and 4) articulation disorder—therapy recommended.

Normal articulation—no recommendations   If the client's articulation is well within normal limits for his age, or if no phonemes are misarticulated by the individual older than age 8, the client has normal articulation, and no remediation (therapy) program is necessary. However, this recommendation should not preclude the examiner from discussing 1) articulation stimulation procedures to the parent; 2) situations that may occur in the near future to the client that may affect articulation; and 3) any steps that should be taken to make the articulation even more intelligible.

Re-evaluate articulation—no therapy recommended   In some instances, a delay in articulation may be accompanied by information in the client's history that indicated an unusual reason for the delay, with a probable normal learning profile thereafter. Or perhaps an incident had recently occurred and the client had not had time for the articulation performance to stabilize. Under these circumstances, a re-evaluation of the articulation within 6 months (to 1 year) should be recommended. This particular recommendation is frequent when the client is very young (age 3, for example), has numerous misarticulations, and is unintelligible, but responds to stimulability testing, is proficient in other motoric skills, and has no language deficit. A well defined articulation stimulation program presented by the parents to the child may offer sufficient impetus to the child to develop his articulation skills more rapidly. If the recommendation for a re-evaluation is made, the articulation profiles of the evaluation and re-evaluation should be compared at the time of the re-evaluation. If no progress is noted in self-correction of the misarticulated phonemes, a remediation program may then be recommended because, in spite of the excellent response to stimulability testing and the good articulation stimulation, the child is unable to make the correcting adjustments without more concrete assistance.

Articulation disorder—no therapy recommended As mentioned in a previous section, articulation disorders do occur that are so very mild that they can, for all purposes, be considered "within normal limits." The well-trained ear of the examiner should discriminate even the most mild of misarticulations. However, the examiner must be a realist when deciding whether or not to recommend a remediation program, and whether or not to tell the client that his articulation is indeed disordered. In some instances, thinking that one's articulation is disordered (for example, because of an inconsistent and slightly distorted /3/) may be much more devastating than the misarticulation is worth. Although the client should be aware of the misarticulation, he also should be realistic about its importance. The frank conversation as described, concerning the relative importance of the misarticulation and the goals of the individual (both immediate and long term), should offer the examiner sufficient information to decide whether or not to recommend a remediation program. For adults, in many instances, the prognosis is poor for generalizing (carrying over) the corrected phoneme to conversation, and so therapy is not recommended.

Articulation disorder—therapy recommended In most instances where the examiner concludes that there is an articulation disorder, therapy is recommended. Then, the examiner recommends 1) the frequency of therapy sessions; 2) the type or program of therapy to follow; 3) the starting point of that program. (In some clinics, the speech clinician who offers the remediation program is not the same person who conducted the initial evaluation, and the speech clinician decides on the above three items. In other settings, the examiner may also conduct the remediation program for that client.)

Frequency of therapy sessions Although scheduling according to individual needs is the ideal, there are many circumstances that prevent the ideal from occurring. School settings with itinerant clinicians do not lend themselves easily to an irregular schedule for any one client. Clinicians who service several nursing homes generally find it is not feasible to make a special trip to meet the need of one client who is also serviced on a regular routine.

Young children generally are scheduled for half-hour sessions because that is an appropriate time length for their attention span. Older children and adults generally are scheduled for 45–60 minutes.

A client may be seen as frequently as twice daily, to as infrequently as once every 2 weeks. The scheduling of sessions should meet the needs of the client while at the same time be feasible for the clinician.

There is yet another factor to consider in determining scheduling: the client himself, or the parent of the client. Sometimes the travel distance is too great for frequent, short sessions. The reader can add the many other reasons that might be mentioned for determining schedules.

Type or program of therapy to follow   The examiner may recommend that the client follow a specific therapy program. Certain articulation profiles lend themselves to a specific program, some clinicians prefer to use one type of program over another, or certain theoretic approaches may be advocated. For example, there are those who feel that a youngster who has many misarticulations would benefit from a multiarticulation approach where all the phonemes are trained simultaneously. There are those who advocate the use of published training programs that are phoneme specific (see Mowrer, Baker and Schutz, 1970; Shriberg, 1975). Or the deviant articulation pattern may lend itself to a distinctive feature remediation approach rather than working on an individual error phoneme. Or the clinician may choose to work on the phoneme that responded most readily to stimulability testing, is developmentally supposed to be articulated correctly, or is readily visible.

Regardless of which approach is selected for the remediation program, the use of ongoing evaluation is mandatory. The clinician must frequently administer probe tests to determine whether correction of the target phoneme (or feature) has occurred, and whether there is generalization of training to other more complex environments, or to other phonemes. As mentioned previously, the clinician must know the amount of progress being made, and must maintain a recent articulation profile.

Starting point of therapy program   Because the examiner has judged the client's response to stimulability testing, obtained information from deep testing, and determined the accuracy level in various environments, he can determine in phoneme specific therapy approaches at which level to begin training. The client may articulate the phoneme accurately in isolation and nonsense syllables, but inaccurately at the word level, etc. The client should not be placed into a step of the program that is too difficult and there is little opportunity for success. Likewise, the learning process is slowed if the training is concentrating on a step that already can be accurately performed.

Entrance into a distinctive feature program is discussed in the next chapter.

Prognosis

The prognosis is a statement that estimates the extent of progress that can be expected based upon the available information. A prognostic statement should include the goal toward which the judgment is being made. For example:

A. This client has a good prognosis. . .
B. The prognosis for correct articulation patterns in conversational speech is good. . .

Statement A is much too general; it does not give the reader the specific information needed concerning the prognosis. Statement B provides that information. Although a client may have a good prognosis for correcting the error phonemes in single words, that same client may have a very poor prognosis for incorporating the corrected phonemes into conversation.

In addition to clearly defining the goal to which the prognosis is related, the examiner should also include the information upon which the prognostic statement is based. The factors that 1) are known to exist and 2) concern the client are the most meaningful: the client's age, extent of disorder, organic involvement, attention span, learning ability, motivation, and health, for example. Thus the prognosis might read as follows:

C. Based on his age (76), extent of hearing loss, and disinterest in his speech, the prognosis for the correct production of the /s/ phoneme in conversation is poor. . .
D. Based on his age (4½), the number of misarticulated phonemes (5), his response to stimulability tests on the error phonemes, his good attention span, and that the phonemes are inconsistently articulated correctly, the prognosis for the self-correction of the error phonemes is excellent. . .

Any statement initiated by "if": "if the client enters a preschool program," or "if the parent cooperates with a home program," or "if the client increases his attention span" is tenuous as a basis for a prognosis. These factors may well contribute to a successful change in articulation, but are subordinate to client-centered factors. A parent could take a rock to speech therapy, never miss a session, work diligently on a home program, and the prognosis for the rock for learning to articulate remains poor.

The third part of the prognosis indicates whether or not speech therapy is vital to the prognosis. Is it assumed that therapy is necessary, or will the goal be attained without therapy? Thus, example C above would include "...with therapy," and example D would include "...without therapy," to make the prognosis complete.

Presentation of Conclusions and Recommendations

The examiner should be prepared to present the conclusions and recommendations to the parent or client, who deserves more information than 1) that an articulation disorder does (or does not) exist; 2) that the client articulates many sounds including the /s/ wrong; and 3) that a therapy program would be "good." At the conference, if the parent (or client) had not already been told the agenda of the evaluation, he should be so told. The conversation would be similar to the following: "During the examination, I (examiner) administered several types of tests to analyze your (child's) ability to say the different sounds (or "articulation" if you have already defined it), examined your (child's) mouth to see if there was any part of the mouth that could not function correctly for speech..." Then the conclusions that have been reached should be explained, using the visual aids the examiner prepared in reaching those conclusions. If a developmental profile had been prepared, show it with the client's age clearly indicated (see Figure 4). If the misarticulated phonemes have been charted to determine deviant patterns, show these patterns to the parent/client. Discuss stimulability test results, and that the client responded to these phonemes but not to other phonemes. The examiner should not race through the conclusions and recommendations, and then, as an after thought, inquire whether the parent has any questions. Techniques for presenting information in the most meaningful manner should be used.

The parent or client may well ask how long therapy will be necessary to correct the disorder. This question is one for which a data base is beginning to be gathered. At the present time there is no existing standard that can be followed that equates a description of the articulation disorder with the time required for correction. At best, now, the clinician can cite, from experience, the length of time required to correct similar cases, or can cite the factors that helped determine the prognosis.

REFERENCES

Anderson, V. A., 1942. Training the Speaking Voice, p. 266. Oxford University Press, New York.

Barrett, M., and Welsh, J. W. 1975. Predictive articulation screening. Lang. Speech Hear. Serv. Schools 6:91–95.

Berry, M., and Eisenson, J. 1956. Speech Disorders: Principles and Practices of Therapy. Appleton-Century-Crofts, New York.

Borden, R. C., and Busse, A. C. 1925. Speech Correction, pp. 127, 128, 137, 138, 150, 152–154. F. S. Crofts and Company.

Darley, F. L. 1965. Diagnosis and Appraisal of Communication Disorders. Prentice-Hall Inc., Englewood Cliffs, New Jersey.

Darley, F. L., Aronson, A. E., and Brown, J. R. 1975. Motor Speech Disorders. W. B. Saunders Company, Philadelphia.

Elbert, M., Shelton, R. L., and Arndt, W. B. 1967. A task for evaluation of articulation change: 1. Development of methodology. J. Speech Hear. Res. 10:281–288.

Emerick, L., and Hatten, J. 1974. Diagnosis and Evaluation in Speech Pathology. Prentice-Hall Inc., Englewood Cliffs, New Jersey.

Fairbanks, G. 1960. Voice and Articulation Drillbook. 2nd Ed. Harper & Row, Publishers, New York.

Fisher, J., and Logemann, J. A. 1971. The Fisher-Logemann Test of Articulation Competence. Houghton Mifflin Company, Boston.

Goldman, R., and Fristoe, M. 1969. Test of Articulation. American Guidance Service, Inc., Circle Pines, Minnesota.

Henja, R. F. 1963. Developmental Articulation Test. Speech Materials. Ann Arbor, Michigan.

Irwin, R. B., and Aleki Nickles. 1970. Articulation: Evaluation. Ohio State University Department of Photography. Reference in: The use of audiovisual films in supervised observation. Asha 12:363–367.

Johnson, W. F., Darley, F, and Spriestersbach, D. 1952. Diagnostic Manual in Speech Correction. Harper & Brothers, New York.

Johnson, W., Darley, F., and Spriestersbach, D. 1963. Diagnostic Methods in Speech Pathology. Harper & Row, Publishers, New York.

Kennedy, L., Carr, A., and Backus, O. 1947. The Rehabilitation of Speech. (Revised Ed.). Harper & Brothers, New York.

McDonald, E. 1964. A Deep Test of Articulation. Stanwix House, Inc., Pittsburgh.

McReynolds, L., Kohn, J., and Williams, G. C. 1975. Articulatory defective children's discrimination of their production errors. J. Speech Hear. Disord. 40:327–338.

Mowrer, D. E., Baker, R. L., and Schutz, R. E. 1970. Modification of the Frontal List Programmed Articulation Control Kit. Educational Psychological Research Association, Palos Verdes Estates, California.

Pendergast, K., Dickey, S., Selmar, J., and Soder, A. 1965. Photo Articulation Test. The King Company Publishers, Chicago.

Prather, E. M., Hedrick, D. L., and Kern, C. A. 1975. Articulation development in children aged two to four years. J. Speech Hear. Disord. 40:179–191.

Robbins, S. D. 1940. Dysarthria and its treatment. J. Speech Disord. 5:113–120.

Roe, V., and Milisen, R. 1942. The effect of maturation upon defective articulation in elementary grades. J. Speech Disord. 7:37–50.

Sander, E. K. 1972. When are speech sounds learned? J. Speech Hear. Disord. 37:55–63.

Scripture, E. W. 1912. Stuttering and Lisping, pp. 123, 160, 162, 173. The Macmillan Company, New York.

Shriberg, L. 1975. A response evocation program for /3/. J. Speech Hear. Disord. 40:92–114.

Singh, S., and Frank. D. C. 1972. A distinctive feature analysis of the consonantal substitution pattern. Lang. Speech 15(3):209–218.

Stinchfield, S. M. 1928. Speech Pathologist with Methods in Speech Correction, pp. 73–98. Expression Company, Boston.

Stinchfield-Hawk, S. 1939. The year 1938 in speech correction. J. Speech Disord. 4:87–95.

Swift, W. B. 1918. Speech Defects in School Children and How To Treat Them. Houghton Mifflin Company, New York.

Templin, M. 1957. Certain Language Skills in Children. University of Minnesota Press, Minneapolis.

Templin, M., and Darley, F. 1969. The Templin-Darley Tests of Articulation. (2nd Ed.). Bureau of Educational Research and Service. Division of Extension and University Services. The University of Iowa, Iowa City.

Thomas, C. K. 1947. Phonetics of American English. The Ronald Press Company, New York.

Travis, L. E. 1931. Speech Pathology, p. 206. D. Appleton and Company, New York.

Travis, L. E. (ed.). 1971. Handbook of Speech Pathology and Audiology. Appleton-Century-Crofts, New York.

Van Riper, C. 1939. Speech Correction: Principles and Methods, pp. 156–182. Prentice-Hall Inc., New York.

Van Riper, C. 1963. Speech Correction Principles and Methods, p. 484. (4th Ed.). Prentice-Hall Inc., Englewood Cliffs, New Jersey.

Van Riper, C., and Ericson, R. 1975. Predictive Screening Test of Articulation. Western Michigan University Press, Kalamazoo, Michigan.

Williams, G. C., and McReynolds, L. 1975. The relationship between discrimination and articulation training in children with misarticulations. J. Speech Hear. Res. 18:401–412.

Zimmerman, I. E., Steiner, V. G., and Evatt, R. L. 1969. Preschool Language Scale. Charles E. Merrill Publishing Company, Columbus, Ohio.

Articulation Feature Assessment

Frederick F. Weiner and John Bernthal

CONTENTS

The need for evaluation of articulation disorders in light of the currently available phonological theories has made necessary the consideration of distinctive features in testing, diagnosis, and treatment of articulation disorders. Professors Weiner and Bernthal present the underlying assumptions and criticisms of traditional articulation testing. These assumptions are that: a) there exists a heirarchy of severity depending upon the type of articulation errors in which the description of errors are merely substitution, distortion, and omission (SDO) of phonemes; b) the greater the number of SDO errors the more severe the problem; and c) SDO are mutually exclusive diagnostic categories. This approach is tied closely to the intelligibility of speech rather than to an in-depth analysis of the speakers' knowledge of the underlying rules that generate a given set of responses. In this chapter a concise discussion of distinctive feature components of the generative theory and a correlation of distinctive

459

features with the speech output are presented. Articulation clinicians may have to be concerned with both the speakers' intuitive knowledge of a rule (distinctive feature as an underlying phonologic abstraction) as well as the speakers' ability to manifest the rule (phonetic feature) in the speech output. Having developed a foundation for the distinctive feature approach, drawing support from theoretical (Chomsky and Halle, 1968) and experimental (Singh, 1976) domains, Professors Weiner and Bernthal present a step-by-step method of evaluating misarticulation in ongoing speech based on distinctive features.   —Eds.

A NEED FOR CHANGE

There are at least two possible approaches to the assessment of a child's speech sound productions. In one approach, the child's speech is viewed as a unique and independent language system without reference to an idealized adult standard. The child's language system is treated as an unknown and the various sound productions are examined to determine how they function in his language system. The alternate approach is to view the child's speech relative to an adult standard. The child's sound system is viewed as an impoverished or underdeveloped version. The assessment task for the speech clinician is to note differences between the standard phonological system and the child's speech sound output.

The comparison of the child's sound productions to an adult standard has been the most widely used of the two approaches. This approach provides the speech clinician with structure, is easy to interpret, and is the least time consuming of the two. The alternate approach of describing the child's unique sound system relies on the resourcefulness of the examiner's insights and provides no standard for comparing children.

Evaluation of misarticulations by comparing them to a target phonological system is a relatively new application of linguistic principles. The general and growing acceptance of these procedures results from a dissatisfaction with the method of classifying speech sound errors as substitutions, distortions, and omissions (SDO). Many speech clinicians find the SDO procedure of assessment imprecise and lacking in therapeutic information. To understand the criticism of SDO scoring, it is important to discuss some of the assumptions behind this scoring procedure.

One major assumption of the SDO scoring system is that there is a hierarchy of severity depending upon the type of articulation error. Usually, omissions are considered the most severe error, substitutions next, and distortions the least severe. Thus children with a predominance of omission-type disorders are considered to have more severe articulation disorders, which are more resistent to modification.

A second assumption of SDO scoring of misarticulations is that the more errors a child demonstrates, the more severe is his problem. Norms have been established to compare the overall number of errors of a particular child to expected performances of the normal child.

A third assumption is that articulatory errors can be categorized as substitutions, distortions, or omissions. That is, each of these categories is mutually exclusive and all sound errors fall within these categories.

These are three major operating assumptions underlying SDO scoring. These assumptions are rarely verbalized and many speech pathologists who use SDO scoring would probably disagree with one or more of them. A case in point would be the assigning of a severity hierarchy for substitutions, distortions, and omissions. Templin (1957), in her investigation of the acquisition of speech sounds, found that omissions were the most frequent type of error in young children's speech, followed by substitutions and then distortions. Based on Templin's investigation some speech clinicians have assumed that children with speech sound omissions have more severe articulation disorders than children who do not omit speech sounds. In terms of intelligibility, this hierarchy for type of misarticulation seems to be truc (Jordon, 1960). However, if the severity criterion is "prognosis for behavioral change," then the hierarchy does not hold true (Turton, 1973; Winitz, 1969). The problems in this case is one of semantics. Severity judgments based on SDO scoring only relate to intelligibility. There is no proven relationship between intelligibility and prognosis for behavioral change. Thus, SDO scoring falls short as a prognostic indicator.

A second assumption of SDO scoring is that the absolute number of SDO errors is also thought to be an index of severity. There is little provision for determining the similarity between sound productions and the target. Thus, an /f/ for /θ/ substitution contributes as much to the numerical index of a child as /ʔ/ for /θ/ substitution. It is generally assumed that f/θ is more typical than ʔ/θ. Yet, the two errors are assumed to be equal, at least in the reporting of the results. Following this reasoning, the status of two children's articulation may look quite similar based on a numerical index, although one child may have less typical errors and require a completely different remediation strategy than the other child. In reality, most clinicians recognize that the nature of the actual error may be important in determining a remediation strategy. Yet, the results obtained via SDO scoring do not support this notion.

A third assumption of SDO scoring relates to the requirement that speech clinicians categorize misarticulations as substitutions, distortions, or omissions. A problem arises however, when looking for consistent definitions of these terms. If pressed, the speech clinician would probably describe a substitution as the replacement of a target sound by another sound that is outside the phoneme boundary of the target sound; a distortion as the replacement of the target sound by a phonetically similar sound not recognizable as any other phoneme; and an omission as the absence of the target sound. In reality, the differentiation of speech sounds into such discrete categories is artificial. Most likely, the only difference between substitutions and distortions is that a distortion is replaced by an uncommon English sound whereas a substitution is replaced by a common sound (Winitz, 1975). To illustrate the point: a native Spanish examiner might label a bilabial fricative that replaced /b/ as a β/b substitution, whereas a native English speaker may label the same production as a distorted /b/. This example shows that distortions often reflect the examiner's inability to accurately describe or perceive aberrant speech productions. As the examiner's repertoire of symbols expands and his ability to detect small differences between various speech sounds increases so do the number of uncommon substitutions he recognizes.

Likewise, the category of omission is a potential source of confusion. The traditional definitions of omissions are vague, inconsistent, and frequently do not reflect linguistic reality. Van Riper and Irwin (1958) suggested that some sound omissions are unvoiced oral or lingual postures, glottal stops, or short exhalations. In support of Van Riper and Irwin's contention, Bernthal and Weiner (1977) reported a spectrographic examination of sound omissions in which stop gaps or pauses and glides were present when the target sounds were perceived to have been omitted. Based on these results one might infer that the substitution or replacement of the target sound by a glide transition or a pause could be scored as a substitution.

It seems unreasonable to make judgments about severity or prognosis on the basis of SDO scoring. Before doing so there should be better agreement as to what constitutes these categories, or the presentation of evidence that these categories exist at all.

There are some other disadvantages to SDO scoring in addition to the difficulty in scoring misarticulations as substitutions, distortions, and omissions. First, such a scoring system does not provide information as to patterns of articulation errors. Rather, errors are counted and the absolute number is compared to a standard, based on normal articulation development. All errors are treated independently and there is usually no provision for determining whether errors are similar to each other on the basis of phonetic characteristics. Second, no provisions are made to determine the phonetic similarity or dissimilarity of the actual production to the target production. When errors are classified as distortions, the clinician is uncertain as to the degree of distortion. The clinician does not know whether the actual production and the target are produced with similar voicing manner or place. The SDO scoring system does not provide information for the selection of treatment sounds based on the above phonetic characteristics. Instead, the sound selected for instruction is usually based on developmental norms.

Because of the inadequacies of SDO scoring, many speech clinicians have sought alternative procedures for assessing articulation performance. Determination of error patterns seems to be the prerequisite for alternative assessment procedures. It is generally agreed that patterns of errors can provide information as to the starting point for articulation management and insight into possible instruction strategies.

TRADITIONAL METHODS
FOR DESCRIBING PATTERNS OF ARTICULATION ERRORS

The identification of patterns of articulation errors is not a new concept. Van Riper and Irwin (1958) used the modifying adjectives lateral, occluded, interdental, nasal, etc., to describe how error sounds are produced. They suggested that if the same modifying descriptions apply to several articulation errors, the clinician should consider beginning the treatment sequence with instruction for elimination of characteristics in error in several speech sounds.

Cruttenden (1972) presented a procedure in which spontaneous speech samples were examined for errors in manner, place, and voicing. In this procedure, the child's consonant sounds are systematically compared with each target consonant. To illustrate the procedure, Cruttenden transcribed a 200-word spontaneous sample of a 5-year-old boy with an articulation disorder. Table 1 is a listing of the results of the transcription. Table 1 compares the child's sounds on the right (with the number of each occurrence indicated) with the

Table 1. Transcription results of child's spontaneous speech sample[a]

Manner	Type	Labial	Dental	Alveolar	Palatal	Velar	Glottal
Plosives (inc.)	Fortis	p p^2		t t^2s^2	tʃ	k s^1k^{11}	.
	Lenis	b p^1b^8		d d^9k^1	dʒ $\theta^1t^1s^1$	g g^{13}	
Affricates							
Fricatives	Fortis	f f^2s^1	θ	s $s^5t^2s^1$	ʃ s^3		h s^{121}
	Lenis	v	ð ð^{1}d^7	z	ʒ		
Nasals		m m^9w^1		n n^{12}		ŋ	
Lateral				l $\theta^1j^1l^3$			
Approximant		w w^4m^2		r v^7w^2	j j^{14}		

From Cruttenden, 1972. Reprinted by permission.

[a] Illustrating target productions and the child's actual productions with the number of occurrences of each production indicated.

target phonemes on the left. From this data, the child's ability to preserve manner, place, and voicing during the production of consonants was evaluated. Table 2 is a matrix to illustrate the procedure for evaluating manner of articulation. Similar matrices are used to evaluate place and voicing. According to the matrix, 43 plosive sounds were attempted. The child produced a plosive for a fricative 38 times and a fricative for a plosive 5 times. Had the child produced every consonant correctly, there would only have been entries along the diagonal. Thus entries outside the diagonal represent errors. For this child, it can be concluded that the major error in his speech is attributable to an unestablished contrast between plosives and fricatives. By viewing the matrix, this pattern of errors is made readily apparent.

PHONOLOGY AND DISTINCTIVE FEATURES

To achieve more precision in the description of misarticulations, speech clinicians have begun to apply phonological principles to the assessment of children with delayed speech development. It has been shown that the phonology of these children is far from being random. Although the speech samples seem impoverished, much of the apparent randomness is quite regular (Oller, 1973). There are numerous processes of simplification in terms of the adult system, yet the manner of simplification in many instances is a highly complex and systematic process.

One method of determining the complexity of these processes is to describe speech output in rule form and evaluate the rules for similarity. The object of this procedure is to find sounds that are similar to each other on the basis of certain characteristics. The specific

Table 2. Matrix to illustrate procedure for evaluating manner of articulation [a]

	Plosive	Fricative	Nasal	Lateral	Approximant
Plosive	38	5			
Fricative	10	15			
Nasal			21		1
Lateral				3	1
Approximant			2		32

From Cruttenden, 1972. Reprinted by permission.
[a] The left margin lists manners of target sounds and manner labels above represent manners of actual production.

characteristics are usually subunits of the sounds and are referred to as distinctive features.

Complex objects or events have subunits or recognizable properties. In fact, objects or events are apt to be uniquely identifiable only by virtue of a bundle of properties. Not all the properties, however, are important for recognition of the object. The perceiver selects certain of these properties and they become meaningful to him for purposes of differentiating the object from similar objects. These properties or features make the object distinctive to the perceiver and are thus the distinctive features. To see how the concept of distinctive features is important in recognition of objects, consider the following situation reported by Gibson (1969).

> A psychologist arrives at an animal behavior station which has available for experimentation a large herd of goats. He is not familiar with goats. He plans his experiment and selects his subjects from a card file giving each animal's age, history, and so on. Now he must find his animals in the herd. They are tagged, but examining tiny ear tags of sixty animals is a lengthy process, so he must learn to recognize the animals by more obvious characteristics. After all, the goats appear to be able to distinguish one another. The goats, at first, look to him almost identical except for one or two characteristics, such as large or small, which are by themselves quite inadequate. But after a few months' acquaintance, he can spot his goat in the herd at a moment's notice and even from a fair distance. Furthermore, it is not only this goat which he has learned to recognize. He can enroll a new subject and find him, now, without a three-month or even a three-day warm-up. He has learned the distinctive features of goats and can recognize a new pattern of features with very little practice. (Eleanor J. Gibson, Principles of Perceptual Learning and Development © 1969, p. 82. Reprinted by permission of Prentice-Hall Inc., Englewood Cliffs, New Jersey.)

The distinctive features of speech are usually articulatory descriptions or acoustic consequences that serve to contrast one phoneme with others. For example, /p/ is contrasted with /b/ on the basis of vocal fold vibration or voice, and /p/ is contrasted from /t/ on the basis of place of articulation in the oral cavity.

The choice of what determines whether a feature is a distinctive feature is based on linguists' experience of languages and phonemic structures. But there is another objective criteria. The distinctive features of a sound must provide a unique pattern for each phoneme so that the minimal distinction between any two phonemes is one distinctive feature. However, a pair of phonemes may differ by a number of features.

Most distinctive features systems presented to date have a plus and minus value that defines bipolar qualities of the same property. A unique bundle for each phoneme can be represented in feature charts such as the one in Table 3. This is a chart of the distinctive features proposed by Chomsky and Halle (1968). By comparing the patterns of pluses and minuses for the features the uniqueness of any phoneme can be demonstrated. However, it should be noted that the chart is merely a listing of the minimal number of distinctions between phonemes. Thus, the feature bundle for each phoneme does not include all of the phonetic elements necessary to produce the sound, rather it is a phonemic representation. This is an important point to make because distinctive features have been erroneously assumed to represent articulatory events (Walsh, 1974; Parker, 1976).

The most widely used distinctive feature systems stem from either phonemic or generative theory. Phonemic theory assumes a direct correspondence between distinctive features and the speech signal. Distinctive features are considered to carry discriminating information capable of distinguishing between phonemes of a language. Features are present on an abstract phonemic level and a phonetic level. The phonetic level is considered to be roughly equivalent to the speech signal and has physiologic correlates. Although the assumptions of phonemic theory have been questioned (Parker, 1976), the tenants of phonemic theory are widely adhered to by speech pathologists.

In generative theory there is no one-to-one correspondence between distinctive features and speech signals. The aim of generative theory is to capture what the speaker knows about his language. It is assumed for instance, that speakers know that certain base morphemes have various manifestations. An example is seen in the word "electricity," which is generated from the word "electric" by the application of a phonological rule. Thus, the /s/ in electricity is a derivative of the /k/ in electric. The goal of generative theory is to describe such instances as two different phonetic representations derived from a single form. This level of description is considered to be phonetic. On this level, descriptions are made of changes in phonetic forms. There is no provision as there is in phonemic theory to describe the physiologic correlates of production.

Regardless of whether the feature system comes from generative or phonemic theory, features have been used as a vehicle for describing articulatory patterns. The description is achieved by showing the similarity of the behavior of groups of sounds that share a common

Table 3. Chomsky and Halle (1968) feature system

Consonant specification [a]

Feature	p	b	t	d	tʃ	dʒ	k	g	f	v	θ	ð	s	z	ʃ	w[b]	r	l	j[b]	h	m	n
Vocalic	0	0	0	0	0	0	0	0	0	0	0	0	0	0	0	0	1	1	0	0	0	0
Consonantal	1	1	1	1	1	1	1	1	1	1	1	1	1	1	1	0	1	1	0	0	1	1
High	0	0	0	0	1	1	1	1	0	0	0	0	0	0	1	1	0	0	1	0	0	0
Back	0	0	0	0	0	0	1	1	0	0	0	0	0	0	0	1	0	0	0	0	0	0
Low	0	0	0	0	0	0	0	0	0	0	0	0	0	0	0	0	0	0	0	1	0	0
Anterior	1	1	1	1	0	0	0	0	1	1	1	1	1	1	0	0	0	1	0	0	1	1
Coronal	0	0	1	1	1	1	0	0	0	0	1	1	1	1	1	0	1	1	0	0	0	1
Voice	0	1	0	1	0	1	0	1	0	1	0	1	0	1	0	1	1	1	1	0	1	1
Continuant	0	0	0	0	0	0	0	0	1	1	1	1	1	1	1	(1)	1	1	(1)	1	0	0
Nasal	0	0	0	0	0	0	0	0	0	0	0	0	0	0	0	(0)	0	0	(0)	0	1	1
Strident	0	0	0	0	1	1	0	0	1	1	0	0	1	1	1	(0)	0	0	(0)	0	0	0

[a] /ʒ/ and /η/ not included in this table. The feature specifications for these two phonemes can be easily extrapolated.
[b] Parenthesized values added.

feature or bundle of features. Thus, for example, a child who deletes /f, v, θ, ð, s, z, ʃ, and ʒ/ in the word final position can be said to delete + consonantal, + continuant sounds in the word final position. The specification of + consonantal, + continuant serves as a short hand for /f, v, θ, ð, s, z, ʃ, and ʒ/. The notational conventions employed in phonology, however, are not to be regarded as abbrevatory tricks for saving space when writing rules. They are intended to capture relevant aspects of phonological processes.

APPLICATION OF PHONOLOGICAL RULES TO MISARTICULATION

There are various published reports of applications of phonological rules to misarticulations. Three representative procedures were published by Haas (1963), Compton (1970), and Oller (1973).

Haas (1963) presented one of the first phonological analyses of a child's misarticulations. He considered the child's delayed language to be an idolect. He used the techniques of comparative linguistics to describe the child's phonological system. His subject used only seven consonants. One sample finding was that /t/ seemed to correspond to English phonemes /b, d, t, g, k/. Haas suggested that the child would have to distinguish the /t/ phoneme from /b, d, k, g/. He postulated that therapy should not emphasize training of articulatory positioning but rather a matter of deciding what phoneme contrasts a child demonstrates and bringing these contrasts in line with those of the adult language.

Compton (1970) demonstrated that a child's actual sound production was guided by underlying principles or phonological rules that translated the "standard" sounds into other phonetic forms. Sound errors of the form:

$$tʃ \rightarrow s \text{ obligatory}$$
$$dʒ \rightarrow d \text{ obligatory}$$
$$ʃ \rightarrow s \text{ optional}$$
$$s \rightarrow k \text{ optional}$$
$$d \rightarrow g \text{ optional}$$
$$k \rightarrow k \text{ optional}$$
$$t \rightarrow k \text{ optional}$$
$$p \rightarrow p \text{ optional}$$

were the result of the following phonological rules:

1. $\begin{bmatrix} \text{Place}_5 \\ \text{Voice} \pm \end{bmatrix} \rightarrow \begin{bmatrix} \text{Place}_4 \\ \text{Voice } \alpha \\ \text{Nasal} - \end{bmatrix}$ Obligatory

2.
$$\begin{bmatrix} \text{Place}_4 \\ \text{Voice} \pm \\ \text{Nasal} - \end{bmatrix} \rightarrow \begin{bmatrix} \text{Place}_6 \\ \text{Voice} + \\ \text{Nasal} - \end{bmatrix} \quad \text{Obligatory}$$

3.
$$\begin{bmatrix} \text{Stop} + \\ \text{Voice} - \end{bmatrix} \rightarrow \begin{bmatrix} \text{Stop} + \\ \text{Voice} - \\ \text{Aspiration} - \end{bmatrix} \quad \text{Optional}$$

Rule 1 states that both voiced and voiceless consonants belonging to palatal class are to be replaced by non-nasal consonants of the alveolar class. Rule 2 states that voiced and voiceless, non-nasal consonants of the alveolar class are sometimes replaced by non-nasal consonants of the velar class. Rule 3 states that voiceless stop consonants are sometimes unaspirated. According to Compton (1970) these rules or generalizations of observed articulatory errors provide for an economy of description. Only three rules are needed to explain eight errors. Furthermore, Compton postulates that an economy in therapy may be achieved. The therapist would only have to work on one rule to improve production of several sounds.

Oller (1973) used generative notational conventions to describe abnormal speech production. He found more regularity in abnormal speech than would be found using conventional analysis procedures. Using formal generative notational conventions, Oller was not only able to observe the kind of generalizations reported by Compton (1970) but was also able to describe speech production in specific phonetic environments. An example of Oller's descriptive procedures can be seen in a cluster simplification rule used by one of his subjects. The rule was derived from the following phonetic notation.

$$s \rightarrow \phi / - \begin{Bmatrix} p \\ t \\ k \\ w \end{Bmatrix}$$

$$1 \rightarrow \phi / \begin{Bmatrix} f \\ s \\ p \\ b \\ k \end{Bmatrix} - \text{Optional}$$

$$r \rightarrow \phi / \left\{ \begin{array}{c} \left\{ \begin{array}{c} p \\ b \\ t \\ a \\ k \end{array} \right\} - \text{Optional} \\ \\ - \left\{ \begin{array}{c} p \\ t \\ m \\ s \end{array} \right\} \end{array} \right\}$$

This notation is interpreted as: 1. /s/ drops out before /p, t, k, w/; 2. /l/ drops out after /f, s, p, b, k/; 3. /r/ drops out before /p, t, m, s, t, ʃ/ and after /p, b, t, d, k/. This phonemic explanation is at the cost of 19 rules. Oller (1973) uses feature notation to describe the same speech behaviors but at a cost of two rules. The feature notation, cluster simplification rules are rewritten accordingly as follows:

$$\left[\begin{array}{c} + \text{Consonantal} \\ + \text{Continuant} \\ - \text{Nasal} \end{array} \right] \rightarrow \phi / \left\{ \begin{array}{c} [-\text{Vocalic}] - \text{Optional} \\ \\ - [-\text{Vocalic}] \end{array} \right\}$$

These two rules state that consonantal, continuant, and non-nasals drop out before and after –vocalic phonemes.

APPLICATION OF DISTINCTIVE
FEATURES TO MISARTICULATION

Other researchers have been less interested in the general phonological rules than in the uses and misuses of actual distinctive features. Four representative examples of published procedures for distinctive feature assessment include reports by McReynolds and Huston (1971), Pollack and Rees (1972), Walsh (1974), and Carins and Carins (1971).

McReynolds and Huston (1971) evaluated the articulation of 10 children. The Deep Test of Articulation (McDonald, 1964) was used to test 28 phonemes in 46 contexts each. Figure 1 represents the results of the proportion of substitutions errors on each of the 28 sounds by one child tested. Sixteen phonemes were lacking almost completely from the child's articulatory repertoire.

Each substitution error was then analyzed using the Chomsky and Halle (1968) distinctive feature system. The features selected were: vocalic, consonantal, rounded, tense, nasal, continuant, voice,

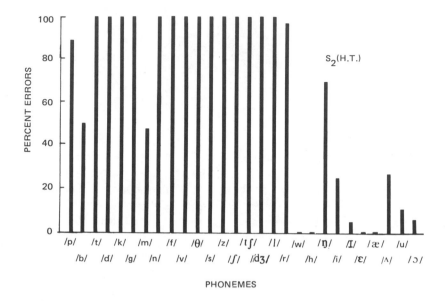

Figure 1.   Results of the proportion of child 2's substitution errors on each of 28 sounds reported by McReynolds and Huston (1971). A distinctive feature analysis of children's misarticulations. (Reprinted by permission.)

strident, coronal, high, low, back, and anterior. The analysis procedure consisted of comparing the idealized feature complex of the target phoneme with the idealized feature complex of the phoneme that replaced the target phoneme, and scoring all differences as errors.

This analysis of the sound errors for the above child revealed that the feature errors for all 28 sounds were seen in only seven features as exemplified in Figure 2. Furthermore, there were 16 sounds in error more than 80% of the time whereas there were only two features in error more than 80% of the time. McReynolds and Huston suggested on the basis of these results that a greater economy in treatment time may be achieved by teaching features rather than individual sounds.

Pollack and Rees (1972) presented a procedure that used Halle's (1964) system of distinctive features to analyze the speech of children. The distinctive features of voice, nasal, continuant, strident, grave, diffuse, vocalic, and consonantal were examined at three intervals during clinical management procedures to note changes in a child's phonologic system. Pollack and Rees are strong advocates for the

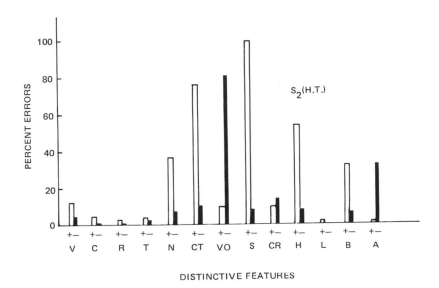

Figure 2. Analysis of child 2's substitution errors by distinctive features as reported by mcReynolds and Huston (1971). A distinctive feature analysis of children's misarticulations. (Reprinted by permission.)

application of distinctive features in the analysis and treatment of children with articulation disorders. They state that "...the distinctive feature concept may be applied constructively at every stage of clinical management of a child with an articulatory disorder."

Although the scoring of distinctive feature errors was similar to that reported by McReynolds and Huston (1971), the interpretations made by Pollack and Rees were somewhat different. They hypothesized that the prognosis for articulatory change may be inferred from a tabulation of the number of feature differences between the target sound and the error sound. They reasoned that the more differences between target sound and error sound the more severe the error. For example, h/s, t/s, and θ/s can be rank ordered on the basis of prognosis of articulatory change by comparing the number of feature differences between target and actual productions. There are four feature differences between /h/ and /s/, two feature differences between /t/ and /s/; and one feature difference between /θ/ and /s/. Thus, h/s is the most severe error and θ/s is the least severe error based on the above hypothesis.

Walsh (1974) described a phonetic system based on language-specific articulation features. His intent was to provide a system of assessment that would aid in the description of aberrant speech. He presented a classificatory system of features based on speech production. The system contains seven major class features. The following is Walsh's description of these features:

Segmental Feature

> *Segment.* The segmental feature specifies that a phoneme is present or absent in a given environment. Thus—*segment* indicates that a phoneme has been omitted.

Vocal Tract Configuration Features

> *Open.* A relatively unobstructed oral tract is characteristic of true vowels.

> *Stopped.* Fully occluded stop consonants and affricates, but not fricatives and sonorant sounds, are positively marked by this feature.

> *Constricted.* Constricted sounds include fricatives, glides, nasals, and liquids, in the production of which the degree of openness in the vocal tract exceeds that of the stop consonants and is less than that of vowels.

Consonant Placement Features: Lower

> *Lower Lip.* This feature normally pertains to bilabial and labiodental phonemes /p/, /b/, /m/, /w/, /f/, /v/.

> *Tongue Tip.* The tip of the tongue is the lower articulator, either contextually or habitually, of certain varieties of /t/, /d/, /s/, /z/, /θ/, /ð/, /l/, /r/, /n/, /tʃ/, and /dʒ/.

> *Tongue Blade.* This feature is the normal lower articulator for /ʃ/ and /ʒ/, also for certain retracted varieties of consonants normally produced with the tongue tip.

> *Tongue Dorsum.* The dorsum serves as the lower articulator for /k/, /g/, and extremely retracted varieties of /r/.

Consonant Placement Features: Upper

> *Upper Lip.* The upper lip is the normal articulator for /p/, /b/, /m/, and /w/. It is sometimes substituted for the upper teeth in misarticulated labiodental fricatives.

> *Upper Teeth.* This feature applies in normal speech only to /θ/ and /ð/, but serves as the upper articulator for certain consonants usually articulated at the tooth ridge.

> *Tooth Ridge.* The tooth ridge is the characteristic upper articulator for /t/, /d/, /s/, /z/, /l/, /n/, and the extended varieties of /j/, /r/, /ʃ/, /ʒ/, /tʃ/, and /dʒ/.

> *Prepalate.* The forward edge of the hard palate is the place of articu-

lation for the retracted varieties of /r/, /ʃ/, /ʒ/, /tʃ/, and /dʒ/, and for extremely forward articulations of velar stops.

Velum. The normal locus of articulation for /k/ and /g/.

Tongue Positions for Vowels

The monophthongs of American English are best described by reference to the positions of the tongue body in relation to its "neutral" position just before speaking. The tongue features along the vertical axis are high, mid, and low, and along the horizontal axis, front, central, and back. For the description of normative vowels one need not use all of these oppositions. The monophthongal vowels, for instance, may be specified as follows:

	/I/	/ɛ/	/æ/	/e/	/a/	/ʊ/	/c/
Front	+	+	+	−	−	−	−
Back	−	−	−	−	−	+	+
High	+	−	−	−	−	+	−
Low	−	−	+	−	+	−	+

Diphthongs should logically be described bisegmentally according to the terminals of the transition.

Release Features

In most distinctive feature systems, release features are neglected in favor of major class features and placement features. However, for several English phonemes the manner of release constitutes the actual distinctive marker. Among the distinctive release features for English are retroflex, lateral, nasal, frication, and abrupt. No distinctive release feature is provided for glides, since misarticulations resulting in glides usually are the consequence of the nonapplication of a typical release feature, often accompanied by or resulting from a shift in articulation.

Supplementary Features

Features that supplement oral configuration, placement, and release features may be distinctive or redundant. Typical supplementary articulation features are voice, aspiration, length, fortis, and lip rounding. (Walsh, 1974, pp. 40–41, reprinted by permission)

Walsh demonstrated the application of his feature system in the description of j/l substitution.

	/l/	/j/
lower articulation:	+ tongue tip	+ tongue blade
	− tongue blade	− tongue blade
upper articulation:	+ tooth ridge	− tooth ridge
	− prepalate	+ prepalate
release feature:	+ lateral	− lateral

This substitution error is seen as retraction of the articulators possibly rendering a lateral release impossible.

One additional application of distinctive features is seen in the concept of markedness (Cairns and Cairns, 1971). The use of distinctive features allows the linguist to group sounds into natural classes. For example, the natural class of all voice sounds is (+)voice. However, phonologists expect that the phonemes of a given natural class will all evidence similar phonological behavior. That is, a phonological rule will apply to all the phonemes that are members of a natural class. For example, if a child was devoicing he should do so for all or most (+)voice segments. However, most clinicians know from experience that if a child devoices, he will not necessarily devoice /m, n, ŋ, l, w, r, j/. These sounds are quite different from /b, d, g, v, ð, z, ʒ, dʒ/. The former are sonorants and the latter are obstruents. Phonologically, voiced obstruents behave as a class and participate in phonological processes that are different from these sonorants. Consequently, a system was needed to allow the voiced obstruents and voiced sonorants to be separated into two different natural classes. The solution was found in markedness theory.

On the basis of markedness theory, the production of voicing in obstruents involves more articulatory complexity than does the production of voicing in sonorants. The rationale for this assumption is described in Cairns and Cairns (1971). Because of the articulatory complexity, voicing becomes marked in obstruents. Similarly, all other features are assigned a marked (M) or unmarked (U) value. Table 4 is a listing of the M/U values for the Chomsky and Halle (1968) feature system (Cairns and Cairns, 1971).

There are two major assumptions of markedness theory that bear discussing. First, the ease of production of a specified feature varies across phonemes. Markedness theory provides support for this notion and a logical explanation for these production differences. Second, markedness theory promises to provide information about ease of sound production. Proponents of markedness hypothesized that the more marked features within a phoneme, the more difficult the phoneme should be to produce. Unfortunately, little has been done experimentally to validate the application of markedness to distinctive feature analysis of sound errors. McReynolds, Engmann, and Dimmit (1974) found limited support for these assumptions on the basis of analyses of articulatory defective children. Weiner and Bernthal (1976) found conflicting support for markedness theory in an investigation of normal feature acquisition in children.

OUR SYSTEM OF DISTINCTIVE FEATURE ASSESSMENT

The application of distinctive features to the assessment of children

Table 4. A listing of the marked and unmarked values for the Chomsky and Halle Feature System

Feature	Phonemes																					
	z	s	ð	θ	d	t	v	f	b	p	tʃ	dʒ	ʃ	g	k	w	h	y	l	r	m	n
Vocalic	U	U	U	U	U	U	U	U	U	U	U	U	U	U	U	M	M	M	M	M	U	U
Anterior	U	U	U	U	U	U	U	U	U	U	M	M	M	M	M	U	U	U	U	U	U	U
Coronal	U	U	M	M	U	U	U	U	M	M	M	M	M	U	U	U	U	M	U	U	M	U
Continuant	M	M	M	M	U	U	M	M	U	U	M	U	U	U	U	U	M	U	U	U	U	U
Strident	U	U	M	M	U	U	M	M	U	U	U	U	U	U	U	U	U	U	U	U	U	U
Voiced	M	U	M	U	M	U	M	U	M	U	U	M	U	M	U	U	U	U	U	U	U	U
Lateral	U	U	U	U	U	U	U	U	U	U	U	U	U	U	U	U	U	U	M	U	U	U
Nasal	U	U	U	U	U	U	U	U	U	U	U	U	U	U	U	U	U	U	U	U	M	M
Complexity	2	1	4	3	1	0	3	2	2	1	3	3	2	2	1	1	2	2	2	1	2	1

with articulation disorders should appeal to the speech pathologist for at least three reasons. Distinctive feature analyses procedures provide 1) subphonemic assessment, 2) an organization of the assessment information, and 3) a description of the patterns of errors. A major criticism of previously reported distinctive feature assessment procedures has been the use of phonemic features to describe phonetic events. Unlike the phonemic and generative feature systems, our system is totally phonetic. The features are entirely related to articulatory characteristics of speech sound production, and not intended to differentiate speech sounds from each other. Most English phonemes could be differentiated on the basis of these articulatory features. However a distinctly different combination of features for each sound was not a necessary requirement in the selection of this feature system. Rather the features selected were intended to 1) represent the essential articulatory characteristics of all English sounds and 2) provide a means for describing aberrant speech productions. The features and their corresponding articulatory correlates are listed in Table 5. Table 5 is by no means intended to be an exhaustive list. However, through clinical experiences we have found that most speech sound errors can be adequately described by these articulatory features.

Testing Sequence

There are two levels of testing administered to each child identified as having an articulation problem. The first level is designed to screen children's speech for patterns of feature errors. On this level, each of 21 sounds is elicited once in the prevocalic position and once in the postvocalic position. Children whose pre- or postvocalic errors are more than or equal to a criterion level on either the plus or minus aspect of any one feature are administered a second level test. This test is a 20-item deep test for each plus and minus specification found to meet or exceed the error criterion.

Obtaining a Speech Sample

One of the questions in articulation assessment is what constitutes an adequate and representative speech sample. Spontaneous speech samples are obviously more representative of a child's conversational speech than a sample of single word utterances elicited via picture stimuli. Nevertheless, utterances elicited using pictures are obtained much faster and allow for phonetic content to be controlled. For

Table 5. Twelve features and their articulatory descriptions

Feature	Articulatory description
Anterior	Made with primary constriction at or forward of the alveolar ridge.
Apical	Made with the tip of the tongue.
Dorsal	Made with the tongue body raised from the neutral position.
Glottal	Made with the tongue body lowered from the neutral position.
Retracted	Made with the tongue body retracted and slightly raised from the neutral position.
Nasal	Made with an abnormally large velopharyngeal valve opening.
Lateral	Made with a side channel for air flow created by lowering one or both sides of the tongue.
Continuant	Produced with the primary constriction in the vocal tract, not narrowed enough to completely constrict the air flow.
Voiced	Produced with vocal fold vibration.
Friction	Produced by forcing a continuous breathstream through a small or restricted opening.
Delayed release	Made by creating a narrow passageway so turbulence can be generated during the brief period immediately following release of the articulatory.
Distributed	Made with relatively long anterior to posterior constriction in the oral cavity.

these reasons we recommend that picture stimuli be used in this assessment procedure.

The production of speech sound errors is variable and frequently inconsistent. The production of speech sounds is influenced by such factors as phonetic context, rate of speech, and word position. Obviously, articulatory features are similarly variable. It is rare to find articulatory features that are consistently in error 100% of the time. Usually children have instances in which an articulatory feature is produced correctly. Many times the correctness of an articulatory feature is related to the manner of production of the target phoneme. In other words, in one child the (+)voice characteristic may be in error during the production of obstruents but correct during the production of sonorants. For this reason, three different profiles, each representing feature errors associated with three different classes of speech sounds should be obtained. One profile is obtained for friction-continuants, one for nonfriction continuants, and one for noncontinuants. We have found that many times a feature will be in error in only one of the three sound class profiles. Weiner and Bernthal (1976) report a similar finding in a study of feature acquisition in normal children.

Elicitation Procedure

The elicitation procedure involves instructing the child to name each picture presented. When stimuli do not evoke appropriate picture labels, the child should be instructed to imitate the examiner's production, but the response is not scored. After the presentation of two more stimulus items, the inappropriately named picture stimulus item should again be presented. In the event that he still does not label the picture appropriately the clinician should score the imitative response.

Stimuli

There are no standardized picture stimuli for use with this assessment procedure. Clinicians should choose items appropriate for the child being evaluated. Factors such as ability of the item to elicit the desired response and appropriateness of the vocabulary are important considerations in selecting stimuli. In some instances after the clinician becomes skilled in feature analysis, this assessment procedure could be performed using a spontaneous speech sample.

The first task of the examiner is to select pictures for Level I testing. Pictures that elicit CVC words are recommended because they are easy to score. Pictures from many of the standardized articulation tests are appropriate as Level I stimuli.

Level II stimuli should elicit a variety of sounds containing the feature that is being deep tested. For example, if (+)friction were being tested in the prevocalic position, pictures that elicit /f, v, θ, s, z, $\int$/ three times each and /ð twice could be used as the 20 stimulus items needed. It is also recommended that for this level pictures that elicit CVC words be used.

Scoring

Figure 3 shows the articulation feature assessment score sheet for first and second level testing. The top half of the score sheet consists of three scoring blocks to record feature errors during production of friction-continuants, noncontinuants, and nonfriction continuants. Each block has 12 major divisions headed by abbreviations for the 12 features. Beneath each abbreviation is the criterion number of errors needed to do Level II or deep testing for both the plus and minus

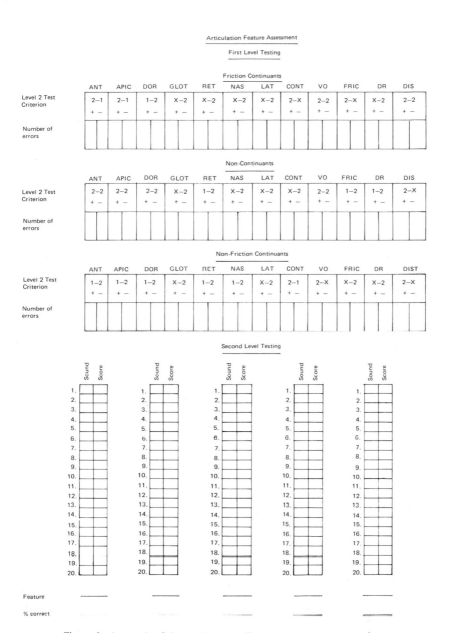

Figure 3. A sample of the Articulation Feature Assessment score sheet.

aspects of each of the 12 features. The blank section labeled *number of errors* is reserved to record plus and minus feature errors noted. Scoring is done as the child names each stimulus item. To aid in scoring, templates are used for each sound elicited in Level I testing. A sample template is presented in Figure 4. Above either the plus or minus specifications of each feature label in this figure is a *blackened square*. These squares correspond to the idealized feature specifications of each sound. To aid in construction of the templates, a listing of the idealized feature specifications of each sound is presented in Table 6. In actual practice, feature specifications represented by blackened squares on the templates serve as a list of "yes/no" questions about each of the 12 articulatory features. The checklist of questions corresponding to the blackened squares of the /f/ template is presented in Table 7. Each "no" answer to these questions should be scored as an error. For example, an answer of "no" to the first question (was the sound produced at or anterior to the alveolar ridge?) would indicate that the child's attempt to produce /f/ resulted in a sound whose primary constriction was posterior to the alveolar ridge. A "no" answer to the second question (was the sound produced without the tip of the tongue?) would indicate that the child's attempt to produce /f/ resulted in a sound in which the tip of the tongue was involved.

For ease in scoring, templates should be equal in size to the scoring blocks of the articulatory feature assessment scoring sheet. Before each sound is elicited, the template for that sound should be placed beneath the scoring block as pictured in Figure 5. The examiner then formulates his questions depending upon whether the plus or minus specifications of each features is blackened. For each "no" response a check mark is placed above the corresponding *blackened square* in the *number of errors* box. The prevocalic stimuli and postvocalic stimuli are scored on separate sheets. If, for either score sheet, the number of check marks equals or exceeds the "Level II test criterion" Level II testing should be done for the appropriate specification of that feature.

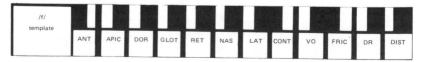

Figure 4. The template for scoring /f/ productions in Articulation Feature Assessment.

Table 6. Idealized feature specification of 21 consonants

Feature	\multicolumn{21}{c}{Sounds}

Feature	f	v	θ	ð	s	z	ʃ	p	b	t	d	k	g	tʃ	dʒ	m	n	w	r	l	j
Anterior	+	+	+	+	+	+	−	+	+	+	+	−	−	−	−	+	+	−	−	+	−
Apical	−	−	+	+	+	+	+	−	−	+	+	−	−	+	+	−	+	−	+	+	−
Dorsal	−	−	−	−	−	−	+	−	−	−	−	+	+	+	+	−	−	+	−	−	+
Glottal	−	−	−	−	−	−	−	−	−	−	−	−	−	−	−	−	−	−	−	−	−
Retracted	−	−	−	−	−	−	−	−	−	−	−	+	+	−	−	−	−	+	−	−	+
Nasal	−	−	−	−	−	−	−	−	−	−	−	−	−	−	−	+	+	−	−	−	−
Lateral	−	−	−	−	−	−	−	−	−	−	−	−	−	−	−	−	−	−	−	+	−
Continuant	+	+	+	+	+	+	+	−	−	−	−	−	−	−	−	−	−	+	+	+	+
Voiced	−	+	−	+	−	+	−	−	+	−	+	−	+	−	+	+	+	+	+	+	+
Fricative	+	+	+	+	+	+	+	−	−	−	−	−	−	+	+	−	−	−	−	−	−
Delayed release	−	−	−	−	−	−	−	−	−	−	−	−	−	+	+	−	−	−	−	−	−
Distributed	+	−	−	−	+	+	+	+	+	+	+	+	+	+	+	+	+	+	+	+	+

Table 7. Checklist of questions corresponding to the idealized feature specifications of /f/

Checklist of questions corresponding to the /f/ template

1. Was the target produced with primary constriction at or forward of the alveolar ridge?
2. Was the target produced without the tip of the tongue?
3. Was the target produced without raising the tongue body from the neutral position?
4. Was the target produced without lowering the tongue body from the neutral position?
5. Was the target produced without a retracted tongue body?
6. Was the target produced with the velopharyngeal valve in the closed mode?
7. Was the target produced without a side channel for air flow?
8. Was the target produced so that the primary constriction did not completely obstruct the air flow?
9. Was the target produced without vocal fold vibration?
10. Was the target produced by forcing a continuous breath stream through a small or restricted opening?
11. Was the target produced so that when the articulators were released there was not a brief period when a narrow passageway was formed and turbulence generated in the vocal tract?
12. Was the target produced with a relatively short anterior to posterior contruction in the oral cavity?

Scoring for Level II is much easier than for Level I. Level II scoring only requires the examiner to focus on one articulatory feature. Sounds to be elicited are selected and recorded in the *sound* column for each feature tested. As responses to stimuli are elicited, the examiner notes in the *score* column incorrect usages of the articulatory features being tested. For purposes of establishing a baseline to determine the success of treatment procedures, the Level II testing items could be randomized and presented again.

Interpretation

There are several approaches to the remediation of articulation errors when training focuses on features. Most of these approaches use either a paired comparison or multiple sound treatment model. In the paired comparison model, the clinician selects two sounds that differ by the feature in error. The client is then given instruction so that he is able to produce the two sounds. The assumption underlying this model is that following successful production of the sounds containing

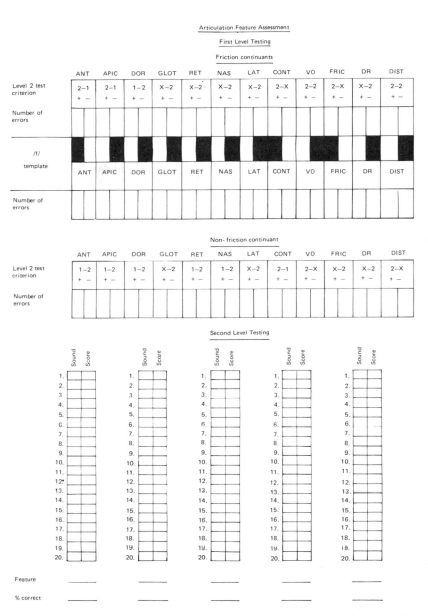

Figure 5. A sample of the Articulation Feature Assessment score sheet showing where to position templates during speech evaluations.

plus and minus aspects of the treatment feature generalization of the feature will occur to other sounds in which the feature was in error (McReynolds and Bennett, 1972).

In the multiple sound approach, several sounds are selected that contain the feature in error. Attention is focused on only that aspect of each sound affecting production of the target feature. Consequently, a child who substitutes stops for fricatives would be instructed to focus on the (+)friction characteristic in /f/, /v/, /θ/, /ð/, /s/, /z/, and /ʃ/. The (+)friction characteristic might, for purposes of instruction, be equated with the term "flow" and the client would be asked to make the above sounds flow (Weiner and Bankson, 1978). All productions resulting in correct use of (+)friction would be accepted regardless of whether the sound was actually produced correctly.

Irrespective of which therapy model the clinician chooses, he must first decide which feature to begin training. We have attempted to isolate several factors that the clinician should consider in the selection of a feature for training. This discussion of feature selection assumes that the Articulation Feature Assessment scoring procedure discussed earlier in this chapter will have been utilized to aid the clinician in identifying features which are in error. It should be cautioned, however, that these selection factors are based on a minimum of empirical evidence and need further investigation.

Feature Redundancy

Below is a matrix of the plus and minus specification of anterior and distributed for the sounds /f/, /v/, /θ/, /ð/, /s/, and /z/. As seen in the matrix, the plus and minus specifications are not independent. The values for (+)anterior can be predicted on the basis of (−)distributed. That is, (−)distributed sounds are always (+)anterior. In terms of teaching features, it would not be economical to teach a redundant feature like (+)anterior within /f/, /v/, /θ/, and /ð/ because (+)anterior would be produced correctly if (−)distributed was produced correctly.

	f	v	θ	ð	s	z
anterior	+	+	+	+	+	+
distributed	−	−	−	−	+	+

To provide a practical example of interpretation on the basis of redundancy, the results of Articulation Feature Assessment of a 6-year-old are presented in Figure 6. These results provide an illustration of (+)continuant as a redundant feature. A matrix of the specifications of continuant and friction for /f/, /v/, /θ/, /ð/, /s/, /z/, /ʃ/, /r/, /w/, /1/, and /j/ are presented below to show that the specifications of continuant and friction are not independent. The (+)friction sounds are alway (+)continuant and therefore redundant within the (+)friction sounds. Thus, when deciding whether to teach (+)continuant or (+)friction the decision should be to teach (+)friction.

	f	v	θ	ð	s	z	ʃ	r	w	l	j
continuant	+	+	+	+	+	+	+	+	+	+	+
friction	+	+	+	+	+	+	+	−	−	−	−

Similarily, a decision should be made about teaching production of (+)anterior and (+)apical because when (+)anterior is in error, (+)apical must also be in error. To help in the decision, a matrix of the specifications of anterior and apical is presented for the (+)friction sounds. According to this matrix for (+)friction sounds: 1) (−)apical sounds are always (+)anterior; 2) (−)anterior sounds are always (+)apical; 3) (+)anterior sounds are sometimes (−)apical and sometimes (+)apical; and 4) (+)apical sounds are sometimes (+)anterior and sometimes (−)anterior. Therefore, (+)apical cannot be predicted from (+)anterior or vice versa. The two features are independent and not redundant within (+)friction sounds. In fact, (+)apical differentiates /f/ and /v/ from /θ/ and /ð/, and (+)anterior differentiates /s/ and /z/ from /ʃ/ and /ʒ/.

	f	v	θ	ð	s	z	ʃ	3
anterior	+	+	+	+	+	+	−	−
apical	−	−	+	+	+	+	+	+
friction	+	+ ·	+	+	+	+	+	+

It is important to know that (+)apical and (+)anterior are sometimes related, especially when planning the treatment sequence. However, the clinician cannot use redundancy as a means of determining whether to begin teaching (+)apical or (+)anterior. That decision must be determined by other factors.

Number of Different Features in Error

If one considers the plus and minus aspects of each feature, there are 24 possible features that could be deep tested. For certain children,

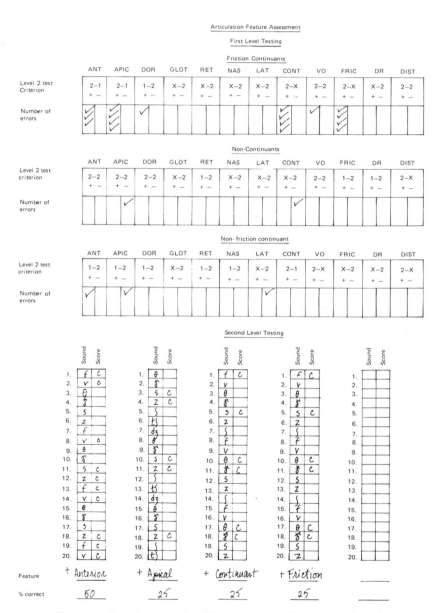

Figure 6.   Sample results of a child's Articulation Feature Assessment.

deep testing will only be necessary for few features, whereas other children will require deep testing on several features. We suggest that for the child with few features in error, the feature to be treated first should be one with the lowest percentage correct on Level II testing. Whereas, when a child requires deep testing for several features, the feature to be treated first should be one with a high percentage correct on Level II testing. Although data are not available to support our contention, the following illustration serves as an explanation for our rationale. Let us suppose that two children are administered Articulation Feature Assessment and child 1 scores one feature error while child 2 scores five feature errors. For child 1 each misarticulation is different from the target sound by one feature. Work on that feature will affect every misarticulation in the child's sound inventory. If child 1 had two features in error, 75% and 25%, it would make best sense to teach the feature that was 75% in error. Correction of this feature would naturally have the greatest effect on overall articulation.

For child 2 each misarticulation will be between one and five features different from the target sound. Training on one feature will have a lesser effect on overall articulation than for child 1. Because child 2's overall sound patterns will not change significantly regardless of which feature is trained, the clinician should work on the one that will best introduce the concept of features. It seems logical that a feature from this child's inventory of feature contrasts that is almost established should be the first feature selected. This choice should provide a feeling of success for the child while gradually introducing the concept of features.

Ease of Feature Instruction

It is our experience that certain features are easier for children to understand and learn than others. Again, we do not have data to support our notion except from clinical experience in which we attempt to teach feature concepts. For example, voicing and most manner features are easier for children to learn than are place features. One possible reason that we have had more difficulty in the instruction of place features is that several articulatory contacts many times occur within one place feature. In English, (+)anterior includes labial, labialdental, linguadental, and linguaalveolar or a total of four articulatory contacts under the heading of (+)anterior. In contrast, friction has only one parameter for each of its specifications (albeit there may be different degrees, but the degree of friction is not distinctive in

English). In short, we believe that voicing or features related to manner should be taught before features related to place.

Acoustic Contrast

Another factor that should be considered when selecting a feature for training is the acoustic contrast between the plus and minus aspects of a feature. An example of a maximum acoustic contrast can be seen in the features friction or nasal. The acoustic difference between the plus and minus aspects of these features is easily detected. The plus and minus aspects of the feature distributed do not provide a maximum acoustic contrast. For example, the (+)distributed sound /s/ is difficult to differentiate from the (−)distributed sound /θ/. Usually, features in which the plus and minus aspects are not acoustically distinctive are more difficult for children to learn. Interestingly, the features related to place of articulation do not provide maximum acoustic contrast. Most likely, the difficulty in teaching place features relates to both the lack of binary opposition seen in many place features and the lack of acoustic contrast.

Visibility

Another factor that may affect the ease with which a feature can be taught is the visibility of the articulatory movement associated with a particular feature. If the articulatory movements can be observed by the child in one feature but not observed in the second, in most instances the more visible feature will be easier for the clinician to teach. Visibility is useful in the instruction of some place features. For example, (+)apical is more visible than (+)retracted and therefore should be easier to teach. The usefulness of the visual cues as instructional aids is not a new concept to speech clinicians. Individuals employing traditional phoneme instruction have used this concept for years. Sounds like /p/, /b/, and /m/ are frequently referred to as easy sounds to teach; less visible sounds like /k/ and /g/ are considered more difficult.

Frequency of Usage

Frequency of usage is a prime consideration when selecting a feature to teach. Features such as (+)nasal, (+)delayed release, and (+)lateral occur in English less often than do features such as (+)anterior, (+)apical, and (+)voice. The clinician, when selecting a feature for training, must concern himself with the effect his training will have on overall articulation patterns. Correction of (+)lateral will only be beneficial in /l/ production and thus unacceptable in terms of efficiency.

Physiologic Constraints

The structural integrity of the speech mechanism should be assessed before deciding which feature to teach. Needless to say, it would be unwise to teach (−)nasal to a child with an unrepaired cleft palate or to teach (−)distributed to a child with missing teeth.

Integration of Feature Selection Factors

The above seven factors to consider when selecting a treatment feature were derived through clinical experience. Conclusions we have drawn on the basis of these factors are not invariable across subjects. Furthermore, there are no absolutes in deciding which feature to teach. For example (−)distributed has a minimal acoustic contrast but is highly visible. In the end, the clinician must take all the factors into account, weigh the results, and then make a clinical judgment as to which feature to begin training. Discussion of the above factors is intended only as an aid for the clinician in his selection of process.

To show the process a clinician might use to select a training feature the Articulation Feature Assessment results presented in Figure 6 will be evaluated:

1. Instruction should be initiated on (+)friction feature because: a) it is a manner feature, b) it is a contrast that is easy to perceive, and c) it has a high percentage of errors compared to other features in error.
2. The (+)continuant feature would not be taught because it is redundant. It will be corrected when (+)friction is taught.
3. After (+)friction, (+)apical or (+)anterior should be taught. Determining which of the two features to select first is a difficult decision. In this case we would recommend (+)apical because of the lower percentage of correct production. (+)apical is 25% correct whereas (+)anterior is 50% correct. Furthermore, correction of the (+)apical feature will result in concurrent correction of the (+)anterior feature in /θ/, /ð/, /s/, and /z/. Of the two features, (+)apical should be easier to teach than (+)anterior because (+)apical is binary and (+)anterior is not.

We have attempted to provide a method for evaluating misarticulations in ongoing speech. The evaluation procedure should help the clinician in making more precise descriptions of misarticulated speech.

For some clients this analysis procedure will provide useful information. For other children there may be as many feature errors as there are sound errors and the precision and economy of the system will have been lost. At this point, we do not claim that feature treatment and analysis will be useful for all children. Nevertheless, determining whether a speaker's sound system can be accounted for on the basis of a hand full of features may be reward enough for using Articulation Feature Assessment.

REFERENCES

Bernthal, J., and Weiner, F. 1977. A re-examination of the sound omission: Preliminary considerations. J. Childhood Com. Disord. 1:132–137.

Cairns, H., and Cairns, C. 1971. Linguistic Perspectives. In: F. Williams (ed.), Analysis of Production Errors in the Phonetic Performance of School-Age Standard Speaking Children, pp. 4–18. United States Department of Health, Education and Welfare.

Chomsky, N., and Halle, M. 1968. The Sound Pattern of English, pp. 170–180, 300–315. Harper & Row Publishers, New York.

Compton, A. J. 1970. Generative studies of children's phonological disorders. J. Speech Hear. Disord. 35:315–339.

Cruttenden, A. 1972. Phonological procedures for child language. Br. J. Disord. Commun. 7:30–37.

Gibson, E. J. 1969. Principles of Perceptual Learning and Development, Appleton-Century-Crofts, New York.

Haas, W. 1963. Phonological analysis of a case of dyslalia. J. Speech Hear. Disord. 28:239–246.

Halle, M. 1964. On the basis of phonology. In: J. A. Fodor and J. J. Katz (eds.), The Structure of Language: Readings in the Philosophy of Language, pp. 324–333. Prentice-Hall Inc., Englewood Cliffs, New Jersey.

Jordan, E. P. 1960. Articulation test measures and listener ratings of articulation defectiveness. J. Speech Hear. Res. 3:303–319.

McDonald, E. T. 1964. Articulation Testing and Treatment: A Sensory Motor Approach. Stanwix House, Pittsburgh.

McReynolds, L. V., and Bennett, S. 1972. Distinctive feature generalization in articulation training. J. Speech Hear. Disord. 37:462–470.

McReynolds, L. V., Engmann, D., and Dimmitt, K. 1974. Markedness theory and articulation errors. J. Speech Hear. Disord. 39:93–103.

McReynolds, L. V., and Huston, K. 1971. A distinctive feature analysis of children's misarticulations. J. Speech Hear. Disord. 36:155–166.

Oller, D. K. 1973. Regularities in abnormal child phonology. J. Speech Hear. Disord. 38:36–47.

Parker, F. 1976. Distinctive features in speech pathology: Phonology or phonemics? J. Speech Hear. Disord. 41:23–39.

Pollack, E., and Rees, N. S. 1972. Disorders of articulation: Some clinical applications of distinctive feature theory. J. Speech Hear. Disord. 37:451–461.

Singh, S. 1976. Distinctive Features: Theory and Validation. University Park Press, Baltimore.

Templin, M. 1957. Certain Language Skills in Children. University of Minnesota Institute for Child Welfare, Monogr. 26.

Turton, L. J. 1973. Diagnostic implications of articulation testing. In: W. D. Wolfe and D. J. Goulding (eds.), Articulation and Learning, p. 195-218. Charles C Thomas, Publisher, Springfield, Illinois.

Van Riper, C., and Irwin, J. V. 1958. Voice and Articulation. Prentice-Hall Inc., Englewood Cliffs, New Jersey.

Walsh, H. 1974. On certain practical inadequacies of distinctive feature systems. J. Speech Hear. Disord. 39:32-43.

Winitz, H. 1975. From Syllable to Conversation. University Park Press, Baltimore.

Weiner, F., and Bernthal, J. 1976. Acquisition of phonetic features in children two to six years old. In: S. Singh, Distinctive Features: Theory and Validation, pp. 178-204. University Park Press, Baltimore.

Weiner, F., and Bankson, N. 1978. Teaching features. Lang. Speech Hear. Serv. Schools 9:24-28.

Winitz, H. 1969. Articulatory Acquisition and Behavior. Appleton-Century-Crofts, New York.

Evaluation of Voice Disorders

Donna Russell Fox

CONTENTS

Definitions of the evaluative parameters of voice remain ambiguous, thus making it difficult to standardize strategies for screening and diagnosis. After presenting historical perspective, discussing the incidence of voice cases, and formulating diagnostic guidelines and screening methods, Professor Fox clearly outlines the factors for evaluation of voice problems. Special attention has been given to patient history, medical examination findings, and physical, acoustic, and psychologic parameters of voice. In addition, Professor Fox clearly defines the role of a voice pathologist: "The real role of the voice pathologist is to synthesize information from medical examination findings, patient history, and voice function evaluation in order to determine the ways in which physical, acoustic, psychologic, and historical factors interact to maintain the vocal dysfunction."

The foundation of a very informative deliberation in this chapter has been Professor Fox's years of clinical experience diagnosing and treating voice disorders. This chapter is organized with utmost practical consideration. Detailed protocols for the various prerequisites for voice evaluation have been outlined with case citations and examples. This is a broadly based chapter covering the continuum of voice problems from the transient hoarseness of the child to the more serious voice problem of the patient whose larynx has been removed because of cancer.   —Eds.

Whether performed by a speech pathologist, voice pathologist,[1] or a composite team of experts, the goal of evaluating voice dysfunction is to identify any problem that exists and suggest means of intervention. The speech pathologist involved in the evaluation of vocal disorders should have academic training in the areas of voice science, vocal function disorders and medical pathologies, as well as clinical experience with voice patients, qualifying him/her for a subspecialty in voice disorders. As a rule, a team approach is probably most effective in evaluating vocal dysfunction. This team generally includes a voice pathologist, an otolaryngologist with specific interest and training in voice dysfunction, and a clinical psychologist. In the case of a singer or other person whose profession necessitates voice usage, a vocal teacher interested in voice pathologies should also be included. In the case of a child, both the classroom teacher and the school's speech pathologist should join the team. The real role of the voice pathologist is to synthesize information from medical examination findings, patient history, and voice function evaluation in order to determine the ways in which physical, acoustic, psychologic, and historical factors interact to maintain the vocal dysfunction.

HISTORICAL PERSPECTIVE

The clinical techniques in the modern armamentarium have their roots in ancient philosophy. Galen, a second century physician, originated the concept that vocal exercise is important for health. He wrote that "deep breathing is the specific exercise of the thorax and lung; so is phonation and the use of the phonetic organs" (Finney, 1968 p. 423). Galen's book on health and medicine was translated into Latin in the early 1500s, and his idea of proper exercise as a means of preserving health was followed with varying degrees of advocacy during the 16th and 17th centuries. In these early writings,

---

[1]In this chapter, voice pathologist refers to a speech pathologist who has chosen to specialize in the diagnosis and treatment of voice disorders.

the voice was described as the center of the soul, and was thought to be in direct contact with the heart. Throughout most of history, voice problems have been investigated from an exclusively medical viewpoint. The medical advances that have been made provide a basis for the variety of approaches used today.

In the early 1740s, Antoine Verrein named the vocal cords and defined their function (Finney, 1968). Almost 100 years later, in 1855, Manuel Garcia stimulated the study of laryngeal disease by inventing the laryngeal mirror, although this technique of indirect laryngoscopy had earlier been devised independently by Babington in 1829. Laryngoscopy was introduced in America in 1858, was popular in this country by the turn of the century, and was thought to be a great advancement toward diagnosis and treatment of voice disorders. Thus, the use of laryngoscopy to examine the larynx became routine. Fetterolf (1909) urged physicians to be able to recognize signs of larynx malfunction, advising them to make an examination of the interior of the larynx whenever a voice change was persistent. The main causes of voice problems in the 19th and 20th centuries were tuberculosis, syphilis, cancer, and papilloma of the vocal cords.

The modifications developed over time have made both direct and indirect laryngoscopy usable and accessible. The discovery and use of cocaine in 1884 was of help as an anesthetic in examining the larynx. The suspension laryngoscope was introduced in 1913 by Killian and was considered to be a great improvement. Modern techniques of endoscopy were developed and described by Chevalier Jackson in the 1920s. His instruments and techniques form the basis of laryngoscopy as we know it today (Ransone, Holden, and Bull, 1973). Major improvements in the last decade include: 1) the modification of the self-retraining laryngoscope, which is held in place on the physician's head by an arrangement of bars and straps, leaving the hands free to examine and operate on the larynx; and 2) the application of micro-laryngoscopy, the use of a microscope in conjunction with the laryngoscope, which allows far more exact laryngeal examination and surgery. The most dramatic and well known case of voice pathology, that of the Crown Prince Frederick who was treated by the famous British physician Morrell MacKensie, might have had a different outcome if microlaryngoscopy had existed at that time. The Prince had carcinoma of the larynx, but because of conflicting diagnosis, surgery was not performed. The Prince, by then Kaiser, subsequently died, and Morrell MacKensie was disgraced for the remainder of his career.

The literature on testing, evaluation and diagnosis of voice problems spans recent history. The first color movies of the vocal cords were developed in 1930 (Russell and Tuttle, 1930). In 1936, a test for functional aphonia was developed (Asherson, 1936). This test required the patient to read aloud while both ears were simultaneously occupied by noise. Breiss published a new method for evaluating vocal dysfunction in 1957; his method consisted of four individual tests of muscle function, which enabled him to "classify voices very exactly as to type and character," and to "indicate which muscle pairs are functioning out of balance." The first to use pressure on the thyroid cartilage as a diagnostic test for mutational falsetto was Gutzman. Isshiki, Yanagihara, and Morimoto (1966) endeavored to establish a more accurate way of diagnosing hoarseness by measuring noise and harmonic components of the voice. Except for the abovementioned study, very little of the literature before 1970 dealt with clinical testing techniques or procedures for evaluating vocal dysfunction. More recent publications have specified procedures (Boone, 1971; Moore, 1971; Moncur and Brackett, 1974; Fox and Blechman, 1975).

In spite of the availability today of such instruments as the sonograph, spirometer, and ultra high speed cinematography, the principal instrument for clinically judging voice function and quality is still the clinician's ear. Speech pathologists today use many of the same techniques for evaluation as were used 20-40 years ago (Fairbanks, 1940), perhaps because very little data are available to support any specific clinical method of evaluation, or possibly because of the cost and inaccessibility of modern instrumentation. Henderson wrote an article in 1913 called "The Need of a Standard in Voice Production" in which he refers to the various standards used to judge the singing voice. His plea for a universal standard is still appropriate today for both the singing and speaking voice.

INCIDENCE

Because of the variability of methods in data collection and population selection, estimates of the occurence of vocal dysfunction vary from 1-10%. Van Riper (1964) estimated that 1-2% of school children have voice disorders. Gillespee and Cooper's 1973 data concurred; however, Senturia and Wilson (1968) estimated the figure to be as high as 6%. Shearer (1972) indicated that hoarseness may be the most common vocal disorder in children; and in addition, Baynes (1966) reported that 7% of all children he evaluated demonstrated chronic hoarseness. Silverman and Zimmer (1975) reported that of the 38 children in their sample, only 10 were seen by otolaryngologists for a follow-up to determine the presence of vocal pathology. Their results further demonstrate the difficulty in ascertaining the true incidence of vocal disorders. A study performed by Laguite (1972) indicated that between 5 and 10% of the adult population had some type of laryngeal or nasopharyngeal pathology that produced a deviant voice quality.

Further investigation into the area of incidence is needed. Many incidence figures are based on an individual clinician's categories. In some geographic areas, one clinician may receive an inordinate number of voice cases while another may have none; thus, conflicting percentages in caseloads appear. In our own clinic, the number of patients treated for vocal dysfunction as opposed to speech disorders such as stuttering, articulation, and various language disorders varies greatly from week to week. Physicians often treat voice disorders that result from inflammation and infection. Thus, these figures are difficult to statistically incorporate into current incidence data.

Significant differences in incidence also occur because of varying expertise in recognizing and labeling voice disorders (e.g., nasal resonance classified as a resonance problem, voice problem, speech problem or as "cleft palate speech"). Coupled with this is the fact that some medical diagnostic categories, such as vocal nodules and vocal polyps, are used interchangeably. Consequently, the clinical case review has not proven to be particularly reliable. The most that can be stated about the incidence of voice problems is that it varies in different populations and geographic areas and etiologies; and recent texts on voice do not address the problem of incidence (Murphy, 1964; Boone, 1971; Moore, 1971; Moncur and Brackett, 1974).

GUIDELINES FOR DIAGNOSIS

The voice pathologist needs to differentiate between a normal and an abnormal voice. If the voice is abnormal then the following distinctions must be made: 1) abnormalities caused by a transient condition (i.e., those that may result from excessive yelling at a football game and treated by vocal rest, or an inflamed, engorged vocal mechanism resulting from an infectious disease and treated by medication; 2) those attributable to habitual and learned conditions (chronic misuse and abuse, environmental stress); and 3) those caused by psychologic stresses or disturbances (aphonia, mutational falsetto). Some types of voice problems are really not treatable by the voice pathologist, but are of concern in the differential diagnosis of voice disorders. The truly defective voice—in which the behavior of the voice is judged to be abnormal in terms of pitch, loudness, timing, or quality—must be dealt with from both a diagnostic and a therapeutic point of view. In addition, the factors that are important for understanding etiology and past and present functioning must be delineated by the diagnostician in order to appropriately refer and intervene. The voice pathologist must decide which aspects of the voice are deviant to such a degree that the voice is judged defective. The clinician judges the voice of the patient, realizing that the communication behavior must be in accordance with age, sex, physiologic condition, psychosocial status, and perceptual acceptability to both listener and speaker.

When clinician judgment indicates that the patient has a defined voice disorder, and the severity of the disorder is designated, the clinician must decide which of the factors are remediable and which cannot be changed. Referral to a physician for medical management may be made. If the patient is already under medical care, the findings must be referred to his physician. The patient may be in need of psychologic investigation or remediation for attitude, interpersonal relationships, lifestyle management, etc; an appropriate referral should be made. If voice function is in need of management, the clinician must decide on the most appropriate method or technique of treatment, either through his own services or those of some other speech pathologist whose major interest is voice function.

If the patient is a professional voice user and is involved in singing, a voice teacher is an appropriate adjunct referral. When the voice patient is a professional speaker, the use of the speech teacher may be necessary if the speech pathologist is not trained in the art of public speaking. To ensure the best possible care, the efforts of all the team must be coordinated. Specific duties for treatment and management should be clearly defined.

The speech pathologist who cannot recognize the characteristics of serious pathology requiring medical intervention, should not take the responsibility of diagnosing and treating vocal dysfunction. Any patient experiencing voice symptoms for 2–4 weeks should be seen by an otolaryngologist. Stress should be placed on the need for a specialist in vocal disorders, because most general practitioners or specialists in other areas are not skilled in examining the larynx. Thus, each speech pathologist should know the availability and skills of the medical practitioners in his area. In some areas, a pediatrician or an allergist may be skilled in examining the larynges of children, and may prove to be the best source of contact.

The quality of hoarseness is always suspect, both in children and adults. Although the most frequent cause for persistent hoarseness in a child is the presence of nodules from vocal abuse, hoarseness may occasionally signal the presence of papilloma, which is not amenable to vocal treatment and may be life-threatening. Hoarseness in adults may result from vocal nodules, but can also signal carcinoma or other malignant or benign lesions. Infrequently, long abuse to cords may result in organic changes in the larynx that are considered "precancerous."

Persistent or variable resonance problems, on the other hand, usually signal organic pathology and should be treated within the limits of the structure. The speech pathologist's role in this instance may be more diagnostic than therapeutic; hence, evaluation of the structure as related to function is paramount. The two most commonly missed defects of palatal structure are the submucous cleft and the congenitally short palate. Careful examination of the palate by palpation, visual observation, and other available clinical and objective techniques should reduce the numbers of patients treated by speech intervention when the structure cannot support normal speech. In such cases, the structure may be assessed by the team effort of a plastic surgeon and a speech pathologist; however, the speech pathologist is primarily responsible for relating function to the speech product. Ocasionally, an otolaryngologist may assess palatal structure, but more often his responsibility lies in assessing the ear or laryngeal pathology. Here again, knowing the particular skills available in the community becomes part of the role of the speech pathologist involved in voice and resonance disorders.

VOCAL SCREENING

Need for Programs

Voice disorders are often missed because of the lack of organized screening. At present, no standard model for vocal screening exists. Perhaps the ear provides the only necessary screening criteria, but this assumes that the attention of the clinician is directed toward voice deviation. A pilot study of 68 clinicians was conduced by Hurtz (1976) to determine if speech and hearing therapists (legal name designated by the Texas Education Agency) in the San Antonio area public schools listened for voice abnormalities. These clinicians were asked to identify their basis for evaluating voice disorders. Their answers were as follows: three clinicians used Boone's *Voice Evaluation* (1971, pp. 77, 82–83); five, Johnson, Darley, and Spriesterbach's *Voice Profile* (1973); four, Fairbanks' *Voice Profile* (1940), and 14 used a self-made check list or some nonstandard technique.

Thirty-eight (over 50%) of the clinicians in these schools did not test for voice dysfunction. Their screening procedures were directed toward identification of articulation, stuttering, and language disorders, and did not include any attention to voice. Those who used a specific screening technique obtained the majority of their cases from those children who failed voice screenings. The years in which voice screening was most frequently administered were kindergarten and first and second grades. Thus, the number of children systematically screened for voice disorders is very small. These factors emphasize the need for some kind of defined screening procedure. In the study cited above, 46 responses to the question, "How do you obtain your voice cases?" indicated that the primary method of obtaining voice patients was through a referral procedure. The majority of the school speech clinicians felt that less than 10% of those holding administrative positions were capable of effective voice referral. This same group of clinicians judged themselves to be less qualified to recognize and work with voice disorders than any of the other communication disorders. These data seem to indicate a need for increased training in the identification and evaluation of voice disorders.

Method

Vocal screening, which ought to be part of any communication evaluation, should provide a quick means of testing function and a direction for further evaluation. A screening procedure should sift out what is not a problem and indicate what is a problem. Either formal or informal testing methods can be used. A determination of whether the patient's voice production is normal or abnormal may be all that is necessary for screening purposes. Many well trained and experienced clinicians can make this initial judgment after a few minutes of conversation, but this ability is usually the sum of many years of experience, practice, and familiarity with vocal dysfunction. A more formal pattern of testing may better enable the less experienced clinician to focus attention on actual voice production and identification of deviant factors. The following is a screening procedure that can be completed in about 5 minutes by a trained observer. (See appendix for recording form).

1. Is this voice production normal or abnormal? (quality) Obtain samples of spontaneous speech and listen to quality (harsh, hoarse, breathy, incorrect resonance), breathing pattern, and evidence of tension. Use any activity that can demonstrate the extremes of the pitch range, flexibility, and control.
2. Is pitch adequate? Have patient sing up and down a scale, count up and down in a step by step progression, or slide up and down the scale using phrases such as "How are you?" The point of this exercise is not to determine range in terms of a scale unit, but rather to decide where on the range vocal function is best. Optimum and habitual pitch should be the same.
3. Is loudness adequate? Listen to appropriateness of loudness in the testing situation. Ask patient to demonstrate loud voice and soft voice.
4. Can phonation be sustained adequately? Have patient say *ah* or *ee* and time length of phonation. Normal is 10 seconds for a child and 20 seconds for an adult.
5. Is breath support adequate and equal or inadequate and unequal for phonation time? Ask patient to sustain /s/ and then /z/. Time and compare. The normal time should be approximately the same for both, but each should be at least 10–20 sec in length. In cases of vocal pathology, phonation time may be decreased. The significance of these two measures lies in the comparison of the control of breath stream for unphonated and phonated sounds.

A word of caution: A monologue is the best way to obtain a spontaneous speech sample, but voice production can become monotonous. Therefore, it is best to get more than one sample. In addition, allow the patient several trials for each behavior request in order to get some indication of the best (and occasionally the worst) effort.

The screening process can be administered by any trained member of the voice evaluation team. If the patient fails the screening process, diagnostic testing usually follows. Vocal dysfunction may arise from: 1) vocal misuse or abuse, 2) structural abnormalities (acquired or congenital), 3) neurologic abnormalities (acquired or congenital), 4) endocrine and other systemic disorders, and 5) psychologic or environmental stress. No single area of expertise can assume the total responsibility for determining the etiology, type, and treatment of the vocal dysfunction. When dysfunction is evidenced, in-depth evaluation is necessary.

Because of the unique position of the speech pathologist, a voice patient may be identified initially through routine screening and may not have seen any other member of a voice evaluation team. In this case, proper background history, assessment of vocal status and function, and physical and psychologic status must be obtained by the speech pathologist. Referral for otolaryngologic assessment is essential if dangerous pathology is to be eliminated. This may be accomplished by an initial contact with a family physician or by direct referral. Referral policy depends on the rules of various employers. Some settings demand that a minimum of three names be given a patient for any specialty, others have available contracted specialty consultants.

The clinician in private practice makes direct referrals and chooses specialists in designated areas. Close cooperation among various specialists is essential for good case management, and knowledge of interprofessional protocol facilitates information exchange.

Background information and tests for hearing, language, and articulation are essential in providing the clinician with information about the past and present functioning of the patient. Once screening has been completed, proper referral or interdepartment assessment in specific areas provide the definitive information necessary for successful intervention. The school or the parents can best aid the speech pathologist in understanding a patient who is a child. For an adult, work history and past education provide clues to lifestyle and function.

INTERVIEWING

One of the best methods for collecting past history is from the patient himself. Clinicians are accustomed to asking the adult patient about the onset and development of this problem. This approach is also appropriate for children, although questions may have to be worded more simply. All too often the clinician may overlook the information available from the young child regarding his feelings about the voice problem and his attitudes toward his ability to function. This information may be important. The clinician may have difficulty separating fact from fiction, but interviewing and counseling even young children seems essential for progress in remediation. In the public school setting, parents are often unavailable to the speech pathologist; however, much pertinent information can be gained from school academic and health records, and from nurses' and teachers' comments, as well as from the child himself and his siblings. Thus, answers ordinarily provided by parents may be obtained from other sources.

The patient history should be seen as a picture of his past physical, social, and psychologic function. The questions necessary to complete that picture vary among clinicians (Murphy, 1964; Bonne, 1971; Moore, 1971; Fox and Blechman, 1975). The search for possible etiology includes the broad categories of congenital or acquired structural differences, environmental or psychic stress, and hyper- or hypofunction. Changes in vocal function are usually danger signals and are therefore considered important. A sensitive clinician will pursue areas of patient history that may be pertinent to that particular voice problem. He must be alert to what is normal or unusual for the particular patient in question and be able to assess inter-relationships of vocal function and available medical, physical, social, and psychologic data.

EVALUATION OF VOICE FUNCTION

Behavioral testing of the voice focuses on pitch, loudness, and quality. The performance of specific tasks can be judged against clinical and objective criteria for voluntary control, flexibility, and optimum function. Perkins (1971) defines optimal function aesthetically (ranging from normal acceptability to others up to the aesthetic excellence exemplified by the opera singer), acoustically (most efficient frequency range), and hygienically (least amount of effort). These definitions form a workable basis for the clinical evaluation of voice.

To evaluate the functioning of a voice, the voice pathologist should develop an organized routine. A patient's own evaluation of his vocal problems can provide a beginning reference. If the patient has been referred by another speech pathologist for consultation, investigation may focus on treatment possibilities; however, if the patient has been referred from an otolaryngologist, the primary need may be for differential diagnosis, with intervention a lesser consideration. If the patient has traveled a considerable distance for the evaluation and will return home afterward, or if he has come at the insistence of his otolaryngologist or employer, further intervention or follow-up may not be feasible. The patient's answer to the question, "What is your complaint?" should be recorded precisely. This can be a beginning point for counseling as well as a means of directing attention to a specific problem. The patient should not leave the office of the clinician feeling that his specific complaint has not been dealt with adequately. In other words, the clinician should not overlook the patient's questions while seeking answers to his own questions.

The first meeting with the patient generally provides an excellent opportunity to observe characteristics of manner and appearance. Personally greeting the patient in the waiting room is a good practice; it offers a chance to observe his individual approach, gait, manner, and the ease with which he presents himself. Shaking hands can give the clinician some indication of muscle tone and muscular coordination. Walking down the hall with the patient provides the opportunity to observe any difficulties in walking, such as unusual gait or posture, or an unusually brisk or slow pace.

To encourage conversational speech, the clinician may ask: "Did you receive the history form that we sent you in the mail?" This question not only gives the clinician useful information, but also puts the patient at ease. Mailing a case history form to the patient before the appointment is a good idea. It permits the patient to go through the questions in advance, and the clinician can note any unanswered questions or particularly ususual responses. Give the patient an opportunity to describe his concerns, how he first noticed the difficulty, and what he has done about the vocal problem. This verbal description can be compared with the history form. During the conversation, the clinician should pay close attention to language, vocal usage, and to the information the patient has given about the development of the voice problem. Unusual sitting postures, head or neck tension, body tension, rate and rhythm of speech, and unusual dysfluency or hesitancy should also be noted.

Tape recordings may begin at any point. Taping is done to determine base line behaviors and document improvement during consecutive sessions. The voice pathologist must decide how much to record and which specific behavior sample will be pertinent. Patient permission, either in written form or on the tape itself, is usually obtained before recording.

Evaluation procedures outlines in the book, *Clinical Management of Voice Disorders*, (Fox and Blechman, 1975), provide the clinician with a structured sheet for vocal testing. If certain areas listed on the evaluation sheet do not apply to a particular patient, those areas may be omitted. However, if the clinician does not work with voice disorders daily, the entire procedure should be used to structure the evaluation. In-depth analysis of vocal function must explore the covarying relationships that determine the specific dysfunction.

The primary distinction that a clinician must make is between the normal and the deviant. If the voice has an unpleasant sound, the clinician must decide whether or not that unpleasant quality indicates abnormality. This decision will depend on the perception of the listener and explains why training is the clinician's most elegant tool.

BEHAVIORAL ANALYSIS

Pitch

The pitch of the voice is an important indicator of vocal control and flexibility. Although there are many ways to evaluate pitch, only a few techniques will be mentioned. The normal voice should have a range of 1½-2 octaves. Having the patient sing up and down the scale or speak at designated pitches, along with observing intonation during conversation, allows the clinician to determine any abnormalities in ability to produce and use the total voice range. The clinician should note the effects of raising and lowering the pitch on both the quality and loudness of the voice. As an alternative to singing the scale, the clinician may have the patient pretend to walk up a flight of stairs, raising his voice with each step upward and continuing until his voice can go no higher. Whether or not to provide a model for imitation is left to the discretion of the individual clinician; however, if the patient is resistent, a model may be necessary. In this case, only a model of the desired behavior should be provided; do not give a tone on which to begin. If the singing is demonstrated, let a few moments elapse before having the patient begin. This assures that the patient will begin on a tone that is comfortable for him and near his habitual tone. Time should be allowed for the patient to practice and relax before recording the production. At times, because of tension and anxiety, the first tone that is produced is higher than the one that the patient would ordinarily use. Muscular tension in the vocal cords or in the entire vocal tract, has an effect on the quality, pitch, and loudness of the voice. Determine the normality of range usage, pitch discrimination, and ability to carry a tune. Notice differences between singing and speaking. Singing and speaking should be congruent with the total range available to the patient. Later, the clinician will decide how important the observations of pitch are with regard to total voice dysfunction.

In addition to these clinical techniques, a number of laboratory techniques are available for pitch determination. Sound spectrography, for example, analyzes the voice by relating acoustic energy to physiology, and charts the dimensions of sound (frequency, intensity, and time). Such instrumentation is available comercially, but is often not available to the practicing voice clinician; thus, the patient may need referral to other facilities where such instrumentation is available. Other less expensive means of pitch determination such as the PAD pitch meter and the B and K Beat Frequency Oscillator, are also available; they are discussed in Boone (1971, pp. 90-94). Generally, the range of vocal cord frequencies used in normal speech extends from about 60-360 Hz (over 2 octaves), but normal usage of any one person's range is about 1½ octaves. Fundamental pitch is about 125 Hz for the normal male and 200 Hz for the normal female.

The habitual pitch range usage and the ranges best suited to that larynges (optimum pitch) should be the same for maximum vocal hygiene. Clinicians need not have the ability to locate specific pitches on a musical scale for this judgment. The essential thing is to determine: a) whether or not the patient demonstrates adequate vocal range and flexibility, and b) if habitual pitch range usage falls within the ranges best suited to that particular laryngeal structure. Experimenting with different pitch levels may reveal that changing customary pitch brings improvement in quality, loudness, or pitch production. There is evidence to support the clinical impression that pitch use changes in males over age, (Hollien and Shipp, 1972) and probably in females as well (Van Gelder, 1974). Thus, pitch usage must be judged in terms of an individual's specific vocal structure, sex, and age.

The patient must remain relaxed in order for his performance to be a demonstration of his ability. Practice trials can serve to relax the patient, and the clinician should administer several trials and record the best one. Many adults are resistant to any kind of singing. They may make such comments as, "I can't sing," "I can't do this," or "My voice is no good for this." This usually indicates a feeling of discomfort. If a patient is reticent toward a portion of the testing, the clinician should move to other areas and return to the areas of difficulty later in the session. Another way to eliminate uneasiness is to test in a sound booth. The assurance that no one will hear him is comforting to the patient. Still another approach is to explain the rationale for a task. The patient will often become less resistant if he understands what the clinician is attempting to do.

Loudness

Loudness, the perceived characteristic of sound wave amplitude, seems to be the second most often heard complaint of the patient with vocal disorders. "I can't seem to talk very loud" or "my voice fades out after a little while" are typical comments. Rarely does a patient complain of being too loud, although with questioning he may admit that friends say he talks in a loud voice. Greater air flow past the vocal cords, and often increased tension, contribute to increased loudness. Thus, procedures for testing breathing economy, phonation time, and constriction are essential for a definitive description of loudness control, flexibility, and optimal function. Excessive loudness, accompanied by excessive tension, is probably the greatest culprit in voice disorders, resulting in nodules or other changes in vocal cord mass.

Evaluation by the clinician of the vocal use should answer the following questions about loudness. Is the voice too loud or too soft? Are there bursts of loudness that may interfere with the communication process? Can phonation be sustained over a 10-sec period? What is the degree of vocal constriction? The full procedure recommended for loudness testing has been previously outlined (Fox and Blechman, 1975), but several suggestions are further discussed here. Having the patient sustain a vocal tone for the maximum possible time indicates how well phonation can be sustained and controlled. The time phonation can be maintained may vary with loudness because loudness is controlled by air flow and vocal constriction. For a voice to be considered normal, voice production should be maintained 15–20 sec by adults and at least 10 sec by children. Increasing loudness may significantly decrease phonation time in the pathologic voice. Another technique to test loudness control and flexibility is to have the patient read aloud while wearing earphones. The noise input to the earphones is then elevated in order to observe any change in the patient's increase in vocal intensity. Does the patient increase loudness smoothly and efficiently (normal), or does phonation become impossible or uncontrollable (pathologic)? If during the evaluation the clinician observes evidence of vocal constriction, tension in the head and neck area, or general postural tension that seem to interfere with vocal control, the clinician may suggest that the patient change his posture and continue speaking. If resistance is encountered, have the patient stand across the room and call to you in a loud voice, or ask the patient to speak loudly to you from inside the sound booth while the microphone is switched on. With many voice disorders, patients may not be able to increase volume. When they attempt to increase loudness, little or no phonation is achieved. Vocal control may be present only when using a very soft voice produced with little or no tension. In such cases, the optimal function may not fall within the usual or normal range but is the best a particular structure can achieve without too high a price in terms of vocal tension and abuse.

Details of vocal use during a typical day and week of activities may provide information to use in selecting testing techniques for that patient. For example, a young male supervisor of an export company was referred for hoarse voice quality with the laryngeal findings of thickened cords and beginning vocal nodules. He was able to sustain phonation for only 7 sec. Nothing in his typical day's vocal activities indicated excessive use or abuse. However, when discussing a typical week's activities, he indicated that his responsibility in his army unit was to give commands for marching drills. When he demonstrated this activity, excessive loudness and tension, accompanied by hard glottal attack and raised pitch were evident.

In addition, the patient with a loudness disorder is always suspect for hearing problems. All cases of voice problems should be screened for hearing sensitivity. The loudness disorder patient is more likely to need in-depth audiologic assessment to fully ascertain the relationship between voice and hearing.

Laryngeal Quality

Quality is a difficult aspect of voice to evaluate although the literature abounds in descriptive terms and definitions for quality (Fairbanks, 1940; Perkins, 1971; Moncur and Bracket, 1974; Fox and Blechman; 1975). Pleasantness versus perceptually insulting unpleasantness serve as opposite poles for judgments of voice quality. Spectrography provides a means of physical measurement of voice. Clinically, quality may be viewed as a continuum ranging from harshness through hoarseness to breathiness. Harshness may result from close approximation of the vocal cords with a sharp sudden closure; breathiness results from slight approximation of the cords, which allows unphonated air to escape before, during, and after a vocal attempt. Hoarseness may lie somewhere between these two extremes.

Harshness is perceived as a tense, hard vocal attack accompanied by a sudden initiation of tone. This voice quality is often normally found in people when they are angry. Breathiness is the physical result of inadequate approximation of the cords and can be found normally in those affecting a sultry, sexy tone, or may accompany the normal speaker with stage fright. The tension and low pitch of the hoarse voice are produced by vocal cords that do not approximate properly as in normal attempts to lower pitch, but more often in cases of misuse or organic diseases such as carcinoma and inflammation of the cords from either abuse or infection. Hoarseness can be described relative to apparent tension, the duration of a sustained tone, pitch, and phonation control.

Experimentally, abnormal voice qualities are now being investigated by Murry, Singh, and Sargent (1977). They report at the outset that "hoarseness is a complex concept and probably not fully accountable on any one perceptual dimension. That is, a voice that is hoarse evokes different perceptual constructs from the listeners." A similar statement can be made regarding judgments of harshness and breathiness. Assuming inherent multidimensional perceptual attributes in the judgments of voice qualities these authors "determined the perceptual attributes of a group of non-normal voices." The results showed that the perceptual attributes of voice can be explained by acoustic, psychologic, and physiologic factors. "The significant correlate of breathiness was air flow, and nasality correlated significantly with both F_1 and F_2." The physical aspect correlating with a rating of hoarseness was the degree of noise present in the acoustic spectrum.

The initial interview will provide a voice sample for a general quality judgment but should probably not be the only measure. Some sounds have more affinity for certain types of voice quality and can be used as a means of testing quality in a systematic design: e.g., "Eddie raised the braves average," used for harsh attack, and "who took the folks to the coast" (Fairbanks, 1940) to demonstrate breathy quality. Variability of quality may be a significant factor in differential diagnosis and treatment. For example, if a patient has inconsistent breathiness, testing for specific conditions that increase or decrease this quality can support or refute the clinician's hypothesis regarding the likelihood of a successful intervention as well as point to possible etiologies.

Techniques for testing quality are discussed in various texts (Perkins, 1971; Moncur and Bracket, 1974; Fox and Blechman, 1975). Whatever the method, recording the patient using a standard reading or spoken passage with increased and decreased loudness and pitch changes usually indicates quality consistency. In addition, the ability of the patient himself to recognize quality changes should be assessed.

Resonance

A final vocal attribute to be observed is resonance. There is some question whether resonance should be considered a quality of the voice or a separate "speech" disorder, but for present purposes, it will be defined as an aspect of voice quality. Thus far, sound produced by the larynx has been the primary concern; however, resonance results from sound transmission above the larynx. Normal resonance is a laryngeal tone that has been modified through the pharyngeal and oral cavities (with the exception of the /m/, /n/, and /g/ sounds in English, which are directed through the nose). Resonance is usually categorized as oral, pharyngeal, or nasal. The interaction of tongue and palate is responsible for a variety of resonance differences. Too much or too little use of any of these resonating cavities is considered abnormal. Nasal resonance on non-nasal phonemes is considered unpleasant and unacceptable, although various regional dialects in this country accept differing amounts of nasality. The three major types of nasality are: hyper- (excessive nasal resonance), hypo- or denasality (insufficient nasal resonance), and cul-de-sac (directed through the nose, but not allowed to escape). A fourth type, assimilative nasality, occurs when vowels before and after nasal consonants are produced with excessive nasal resonance. The etiology may be either organic or nonorganic. Hypernasality can be characterized by a mild to excessive nasal resonance, with or without facial grimace and excessive nasal air flow. The denasal quality is produced by a blockage occurring at the posterior part of the nasal cavity or slightly above the palate; the sound is similar to that of a person suffering from a cold. Cul-de-sac resonance may be produced by a blockage in the anterior portion of the nose because of deviated septum, polypoid growth, injury to the anterior portion of the nose, or pinching the nares with the thumb and forefinger. Thus, even though the sound is emitted orally the nasal quality remains perceptible. Some techniques used to determine whether the resonance is nasal or non-nasal are: Ask the patient to sustain the sound of *ah* or *ee* and then open and close the nares by pinching to see if there are any differences in the sound. If there is an excessive nasal flow one will hear a cul-de-sac resonance on the *ah* or *ee* sound. To determine whether good nasal resonance is present, use the sound *mmm*. Ask the patient to hum a sound and close the nares with the thumb and fingers. The voice should stop if sound is being emitted through the nose because of vocal damping. However, if the *mmm* sound continues, this may indicate that the sound is being made by both nasal and oral resonance, and that complete bilabial contact is not being maintained. Thus, the patient is allowing the sound to escape through the lips while still maintaining a close acoustic approximation of the correct *mmm* sound (this can be observed in some allergic rhinitis patients). If *mmm* is produced but cannot be sustained for about 10 sec, nasal deviation or blockage may also be suspected.

STRUCTURAL EVALUATION

The structure examination may be performed before or after the vocal function testing. This author prefers that this procedure be the last examination. Begin by looking at the total configuration of the face. Look for asymmetry in the forehead, eyes, nose, and lips. Notice the face shape and any head deformities.

The muscles of the face can be tested by having the patient wrinkle the forehead and then frown. Then have patient protrude and retract the lips to determine whether they are symmetrical while moving. To note any deviation in strength or motion, ask the patient to open and close the mouth and protrude and retract the tongue. Also check lip protrusion and retraction for muscle strength, symmetry, and sensation. When scars are present, function or sensation may be diminished. Palatal function should be checked visually by having the patient tip his head back and say *ah* a number of times. Note the symmetry of the palate during movement and any evidence of scarring or abnormality of uvula, fauces, or tonsils. If the patient has a bifid uvula or if nasal resonance is evident, the clinician should palpate the palate and check for evidence of submucous clefting. Also, a check should be made for notching into the hard palate, midline indentation, or zone of light. Velopharyngeal valving may be observed by means of one or several of the following clinical techniques: a) Hunter oral manometer, b) Iowa Pressure Articulation Test of the Templin-Darley Articulation test (Morris, Spriestersbach, and Darley, 1961), c) holding a mirror under the nostrils and having the patient say the *s* or *z* sound or blow air out of the mouth to check the nasal air flow, d) use of a nasal olive to determine whether there is nasal air flow or non-nasal speech such as "Suzy sat by the seashore," e) tongue anchor (Fox and Johns, 1970), f) air paddle (a piece of paper cut into a paddle shape for gauging air flow through the nose versus the mouth (Bzoch, 1975).

Abnormal resonance, established through voice testing, can indicate a need for more sophisticated, objective methods of testing such as cineradiography, lateral skull x-rays, Taub oral panendoscope, or inspection of velopharyngeal function through the flexible nasopharyngoscope. Nevertheless, in any case in which structural intervention is being considered, some combination of these processes should be part of the general work-up.

The laryngeal examination that the voice pathologist performs is not in any sense medically diagnostic. However, for the speech pathologist involved in vocal therapy, assessment of laryngeal structure and function is essential. The best way to perform indirect laryngoscopy is to have the patient face the clinician and place a strong light over his right shoulder. Using a head mirror to direct the light onto the mirror, move the mirror straight back, touching the palate and lifting it slightly while tipping the mirror to look down onto the vocal cords. The general configuration of the larynx and appearance of the cords during phonation should be noted. Have the patient say *ah* or *e* while producing a high pitched tone. This extends the vocal cords and allows them to be seen in their entirety. Observe any abnormality in color or general appearance, and any growths on the cords. By becoming familiar with the laryngeal appearance of each patient, the clinician can judge whether the vocal therapy is producing any structural changes. Whether or not a speech pathologist may perform a laryngeal structure examination may be mandated by employment policy or state legal restriction. However, if the speech pathologist is to function as a voice specialist, the ability to perform laryngeal examinations is probably a necessary skill.

PSYCHOLOGIC FACTORS

The voice pathologist must have an awareness of the interaction between personality, life style, and vocal function. Voice problems resulting from emotional disturbance may take almost any form. Symptoms may mimic those associated with organic voice pathology, or there may be complete loss of voice (aphonia). Lay literature often refers to the voice as being an indicator of emotions, personality, and individuality. The results of Rice and Gaylin (1973) indicate that different vocal qualities are representative of personality styles that have a general relation to cross-sensory modality. Although some authors feel that symptoms of neurosis may be interpreted on the basis of vocal quality alone (Sharp, 1963; Moses, 1954), cultivating one's ear for voice quality is probably no substitute for cultivating an understanding of personality dynamics, human relationships, and the interaction between the individual and the group to which he belongs (Courtney, 1975).

Aronson (1973) divides the system of classification for functional disorders of phonation into three major headings: 1) vocal abuse, 2) environmental stress, and 3) self-image bound. These categories provide a framework from which to evaluate a specific vocal dysfunction. However, vocal abuse and environmental stress can cause pathologic changes of the larynx, which may have nothing to do with psychologic etiology, whereas self-image bound disturbances lend themselves best to the concept of psychogenic voice disorders. In this category may be found such examples as mutational falsetto, the childlike speech of adults, and exaggerated masculine or feminine speech (such as that found in the homosexual or in the transsexual). In order for the clinician to make a differential diagnosis with regard to suspected psychogenic voice disorders, the following guidelines are helpful. One should determine: 1) if the history indicates sudden onset concomitant with emotional stress, 2) if an observable laryngeal pathology other than that caused by misuse or abuse is present, 3) if other psychosomatic complaints of wide range are present, 4) if the voice symptoms are variable, and 5) if the patient's insight and verbal commitment to change are congruent with his ability to act positively regarding vocal change. Additional tools used in such cases may be hypnosis, projective tests, and objective psychometric testing and evaluation. The influence of psychic factors in certain voice disorders may be of an endocrine origin (Van Gelder, 1974). Therefore, data regarding endocrine function and blood composition may be essential for a correct diagnosis. The practicing clinician should become adept at choosing appropriate tests for unusual types of problems (i.e., individuals who have specific structural deviations or deficits such as cleft palate, cerebral palsy, or laryngectomy) as well as differentiating subtle psychogenic and environmental stresses.

ETIOLOGY

Structural changes of the larynx may be congenital or acquired. Examples of congenital changes are webbing, papilloma, and laryngofissure; acquired structural changes include nodules, polyps, edema, contact ulcers, hyperkeratosis, etc. (Boone, 1971). The interview, together with the physical examination of the larynx, should be sufficient to assess vocal structure. Ascertaining vocal function should enable one to draw inferences regarding the relationship between structure and function. Structural changes may be caused by genetic factors, disease processes, or hyper- or hypofunction as an interaction between the person and his internal or external environment. One internal environment that may alter laryngeal function and affect vocal usage adversely, through changes in general response and degree of activity, is the endocrine system. Disorders of the thyroid, parathyroid, adrenal, and gonad are most likely to affect the voice. When hormonal disorders are present, exogenic factors such as smoking, coughing, and other vocal abuse activities may compound the problem. Therefore, knowing how to read medical reports of both clinical and laboratory types is an essential skill for the speech pathologist responsible for intervention in vocal dysfunction. Awareness of the effects of systemic diseases such as anemia, viral infection, etc., can often save time and money for the patient who may otherwise spend hours of frustration attempting to modify vocal behavior that is not amenable to behavioral intervention.

Boone (1971) reports that many voice disorders are the result of faulty vocal cord approximation (hyper- or hypofunction of the larynx). Approximation of the cords can be interfered with by a variety of conditions, but the symptomatic correlates are excessive loudness and tension or, conversely, loss of loudness and tension (Moncur and Brackett, 1974). The extrinsic muscles of the larynx also contribute to total vocal function. They too may be hyper- or hypotensive, and thus change vocal product.

Unfortunately, vocal symptom alone is not sufficient to indicate etiology. The symptom most often reiterated in complaints of the patient and description of clinicians is hoarseness. Jackson, Coates, and Jackson (1929) enumerate more than 50 etiological factors for chronic hoarseness. Any symptoms that suggest interference or impairment of normal laryngeal function must be investigated from both organic and nonorganic standpoints, and the voice pathologist must decide whether or not his evaluation supports behavioral intervention to change vocal function.

The history obtained from the patient should include both known etiologic factors and suspected contributors to vocal dysfunction. An example may demonstrate this point: A 10-year-old boy was referred to a voice pathologist by an otolaryngologist with the report that the child had been hoarse for a period of 1 month. Although the vocal cords were slightly edematous, the quality was abnormally hoarse. The child's vocal function indicated hoarse quality with slight restriction of pitch range. No abnormal voice use or indications of misuse were discovered in the history; however, further inquiry by the voice pathologist into environmental changes brought out the fact that the boy's mother had recently redecorated his room, painted and acquired a new mattress. The voice pathologist asked the mother to check the content of the mattress, and it was found that an unusual amount of Sisal was listed in the fiber content. Because the mother could not bring herself to discard the new mattress, she moved it to her own bedroom and put the old mattress back in the boy's room. One week later, when they returned for follow-up, the boy's vocal symptoms had totally disappeared; however, the mother had become hoarse.

Although not in any way a medical diagnostician, the voice pathologist should be a synthesizer of factors that may possibly affect total vocal product. Another case may demonstrate the covariability of etiologic factors and the difficulty of sorting out and weighing elements contributing to the total vocal product. Recently, Karen, age 14, was referred by an otolaryngologist with the report of edematous, red vocal folds with accompanying hoarseness. The child was not seen by the voice pathologist until 1 week following the original diagnosis. In the meantime, Karen had attended a football game after which she was totally aphonic for a period of 1 day. This was sufficient motive to call for an appointment with a voice pathologist, who began an evaluation of the vocal product. This child had, at the time of the vocal examination, a hoarse voice quality, restricted pitch range, and reduced loudness level. In addition, the second laryngeal examination indicated edematous cords, pink to red color, and the presence of two small vocal nodules. The history revealed that the child was in a state of leukemia remission and was beginning to show signs of pubescence. Thus, the voice abnormality resulted from interrelationships of vocal abuse, systemic disease (leukemia), and endocrine changes, and presented a challenge for the voice pathologist in assessing and weighing each contributing factor.

SPECIAL PROBLEMS

Cleft Palate

The speech and language problems presented by individuals with cleft palate or other cranial-facial abnormalities are variable and complex. This population generally combines a voice (usually resonance) and an articulation disorder with language problems evidenced early in life (Fox, Lynch, and Brookshire, 1976). Many of these problems are related to the structure and function of the velopharyngeal mechanism and may be compounded by factors of hearing loss, language deficit, retardation, or neurologic dysfunction. Evaluation by the speech pathologist must take all these factors into consideration. However, no single method of assessment has proved totally satisfactory. The clinician must ultimately make decisions regarding presence and severity of speech, voice and language problems, and whether these are related to the physical condition or to learned behavior. Thus, a detailed structural evaluation is essential to determine physiologic limits, along with usual language and learning measures.

Voice evaluation for the patient with cleft palate is very similar to that previously outlined, but special emphasis is placed on techniques to gauge resonance and quality disturbance. Evaluation techniques can be divided into those that involve clinical judgments and those that are measures of physical attributes. Additional clinical measures, in conjunction with those already discussed in the evaluation of resonance, should be employed. The Iowa Pressure Test, taken from the Templin-Darley Test of Articulation, relates air pressure, consonant production, and velopharyngeal closure to one another. Nasal air flow can be checked with a mirror or air paddle under the nostrils. Unpleasant or recognizable nasal resonance on isolated phonemes, as found in running speech, can be rated in terms of severity and consistency. The quality of nasality is important for ascertaining whether the mechanism is able to support normal resonance, and if so, under what specific conditions. For example, can the patient sustain non-nasal resonance on *ah* or *ee*, and if so, for how many seconds? Does this resonance change with greater effort or conversational speech? Is excessive effort indicated by facial grimace? Maintenance of air pressure can be checked with the Hunter oral manometer and the modified tongue anchor.

In addition to resonance differences, vocal quality may deviate in other ways. For example, a hoarse or harsh quality may be present because of laryngeal pathology (vocal nodules, intubation granuloma, papilloma, etc.) The presence of a cleft palate does not preclude other problems, and the clinician must be alert to all possibilities. In our cleft palate clinic, the otolaryngologist routinely examines the patients' larynges by indirect laryngoscopy to determine the condition of the mechanism. An example of a rating scale for some of these attributes can be found in the references (Subtelney, Van Hattum, and Meyers, 1972).

Direct measures of physical attributes are used as complementary alternatives to assess structure and function. Lateral skull x-rays give a static picture of the relationship between the palate and pharynx; however, cinefluoroscopy allows the observation of speech structures in motion. Mesiolateral movement can be observed by viewing the base of the skull during cinefluoroscopy or by using a flexible laryngoscope or bronchoscope through the nose, maintaining it above the velopharyngeal port. This latter technique allows the direct observation of the movement and relationship of the parts of the entire mechanism. The use of such modern technology, including various air flow measurements and electromyography is described further in the literature (Bzoch, 1972). Differing methods are used in centers throughout the world, but probably none uses all of the available techniques routinely, particularly when cost is prohibitive.

The evaluation techniques employed are usually combinations of those available and familiar to the clinicians. These techniques may be used for evaluation both before and after surgical intervention. Normal resonance may be attained after surgery with no further intervention necessary. Data on these cases, however, is scarce and often dependent on what the listener views as being deviant speech. Lay persons as well as professionals other than speech pathologists often accept greater deviation in a cleft patient's voice production.

Cerebral Palsy

The evaluation and subsequent treatment of the language and speech problems of the cerebral palsy patient requires multivariant techniques to assess the many aspects of the problem. Usually there are few language or speech problems that are uniquely characteristic of the individual with cerebral palsy. Symptoms depend on which neural centers have been damaged and the extend of that damage. Various aspects of voice may be affected. Pitch may be too high or low, accompanied by marked monotony or uncontrollability. Rate may vary, and is most often slower than average. Phonation may be characterized by bursts of loudness rather than controlled loudness. Voice quality may be impaired because of vocal cord paralysis or inability to coordinate vocal muscles. Breathing often represents the most abnormal pattern and is accompanied by gasping and poor control. Attempts to speak may be deterred by faulty phrasing and rhythm, speaking on residual air, or inconsistent patterns of phonation. In this case, the diagnostic assessment may need to focus primarily on breathing, both for maintenance of life and phonation. In the child with cerebral palsy, the most frequent abnormalities of respiration that interfere with voice production are irregular cycling, rib flaring, and thoracic-abdominal opposition (reversed breathing). Because breath support provides the basis for vocal production, the smoothness and control of exhalation and inhalation must be assessed. Exhalation provides the air flow that is then modified by the larynx and resonance cavities. In vocalization, inhalation is rapid and exhalation is prolonged; in relaxed respiration, the cycles alternate equally. The clinician must assess breathing for adequacy, control, and timing (e.g., number of breaths per sec), and note differences between quiet respiration and speaking. As a child matures, breathing rate changes. A normal adult's rate ranges from 10-20 inspirations per min (Lencione, 1968). Sufficient air must be taken into lungs to support vocalization for at least 5 sec (preferably 10 sec), to support continuous speech (a measure of adequacy) and controlled exhalation. Phonation must be voluntarily controlled and coordinated. A clinician may compare production of the voiceless consonant with the voiced cognate for length of production and vocal onset.

Phonation in the cerebral palsied is affected by the type and control of respiration, by the varying degree of ability to control tension in the vocal folds, and by the rate of expelling the vocal air stream (Morley, 1972). The three common types of laryngeal involvement affecting the phonation of the cerebral palsied are: 1) adductor spasms, in which the vocal cords are held together and phonation is initiated with difficulty, 2) abductor spasms, which prevent approximation of the vocal folds or cause a pulling apart of the vocal folds during phonation, resulting in breathiness or aspirate vocal quality, and 3) varying tensions in laryngeal muscles, resulting in atypical and variable pitch, intensity, and quality. These parameters can be tested by using the previously mentioned techniques for vocal evaluation; special attention should be placed on the inter-relationships of the parameters. How well the patient can match or imitate pitch, loudness, and quality indicates the amount of voluntary control and subsequently affects the prognosis.

Laryngectomy

Evaluation of the laryngectomized patient may begin preoperatively and continue as an ongoing process. The examiner should ascertain the patient's understanding of the projected surgery and the role of the speech pathologist in providing postsurgical methods of communication. The artificial larynx may be demonstrated to the patient or a laryngectomized patient using esophageal speech can be present in order to reassure the patient that there will be several methods of communication available to him. Family counseling may also be used as part of the presurgical evaluation. After surgery, information should be obtained from the medical report. The voice clinician must be aware of the consequences of different types of surgery and their possible effect on the learning of esophageal speech or the use of the artificial larynx. Damage to the .nerve supply of the pharynx and tongue can contribute to difficulty with swallowing, chewing, and air intake. Examination of the oral anatomy is necessary if a thorough assessment of the laryngectomy is to be accomplished. The speech clinician must determine: 1) how well the patient can swallow, 2) whether the soft palate is intact and if the velopharyngeal closure is adequate, 3) whether tongue mobility is sufficient for compression of air and moving the air bolus back into the pharynx, 4) whether the lips, jaw, and teeth can be used adequately for articulation. Breathing should be coordinated with air intake into the esophagus and expulsion for pseudophonation, even though breath support is no longer necessary for phonation control, but is used only for smooth and quiet respiration.

In this disorder, perhaps more than any other, one of the most important factors to consider is that of emotional stability, with depression and motiviation the two primary factors to judge. Sensitivity to and awareness of emotional trauma are essential ingredients of any clinician's armamentarium.

If a patient already has some type of air-trapping mechanism and is able to use some esophageal speech, a 7-point descriptive scale (Wepman et al., 1953) may be used for assessment. The scale is useful both for self-evaluation and for clinical observation and evaluation. From basic sound production to speech proficiency, it provides a heirarchy of goals for patient achievement. A similar scale devised by Snidecor et al. (1968) designates nine levels of achievement for evaluative purposes. Either of these may serve as a means of collecting base line data and measuring progress. New quantifying measures are being refined that will help establish selection and termination criteria. The initial evaluation may be performed either immediately or after an interval of time subsequent to removal of the larynx, and prognosis for pseudovoice acquisition determined. In this latter case, further intervention may be necessary for better speech acquisition. Four specific skills of "good" esophageal speakers, as defined by Berlin and ZoBell (1963), provide an excellent basis for evaluating and predicting esophageal speech proficiency. Patients must have the ability to 1) phonate on demand, 2) shorten the latency period between injection and phonation, 3) sustain a vowel for an adequate duration and 4) increase the number of plosive syllables produced on one inflation. These skills form the basis of therapy as well as serving to measure improvement.

Glossectomy or Mandibulectomy

Most speech pathologists have worked with an individual who has had a laryngectomy, but only a few have been exposed to the type of training necessary to deal with the glossectomy or the mandibulectomy patient. Because of the recency of this surgical intervention and thus the past scarcity of such referrals to a speech pathologist, few techniques have been developed for evaluation and treatment. The most recent publication is by Skelly (1973) and much of the information regarding patient treatment and evaluation was gathered at the Veteran's Administration Hospital in St. Louis.

Because of the large number of cancer patients treated in other centers, more of these patients are now being seen by local communication specialists. Surgical procedures are generally directed toward partial removal of the mandible or tongue rather than total removal. Subsequently, the speech pathologist should make a judgment regarding the relationship between remaining structure and the effect on intelligibility of acquired resonance and articulation deficits. If the patient has not been seen presurgically, some type of nonverbal measurement of learning and problem solving, visual deficits and imperceptions, motor coordination, self-correction, and speed of processing are additional avenues for evaluation. All of these evaluative techniques are contained under the category of articulation and language rather than voice, because phonation is not usually interrupted by these surgical procedures. However, the integration of phonation patterns with new structure and the need for retraining in compensatory movement does mandate that particular attention be paid to timing, rhythm, resonance, and inflection patterns, which may be essential for treatment in this area.

PROGNOSIS

The final function of the clinician is to indicate the prognosis for the patient. This can be done with and without a treatment variable. For example, the prognosis for a patient with bilateral vocal nodules who has received no vocal treatment can be stated in both positive and negative frames as shown in the following examples: 1) the patient will probably continue to have vocal problems until the vocal nodules are either diminished by means of vocal therapy or excised surgically,

2) this patient would probably do well with vocal therapy and should proceed into a program of voice re-education, or 3) this patient does not indicate any interest in following through with vocal re-education and will probably continue to have difficulties with his voice.

What then are the guidelines that can be used for predicting patient progress? In an article, Wheelis (1969) examines how people can or cannot change and indicates that the cycle of change is suffering, insight, will, and action. In light of this theory, the clinician may want to estimate how able the patient is to change his vocal behavior. When the patient tries some indicated vocal change (saying a sentence very softly, with a higher pitch, or monitoring throat clearing for about 5 min), success or failure is an indication of the prognosis. The patient's ability to understand his problem and the necessity of treatment and his feelings about what should be done to alter the problem, versus what the clinician feels should be done, often provide important clues for predicting the outcome.

Whatever the case, the expectations of the patient and the clinician must be reconciled. Many patients will want to know how long the process will take and what the cost will be, and the diagnostician should be prepared to answer these questions in an ethical and meaningful way. Estimates of time in treatment are now becoming more commonplace, and the estimate seems to depend upon these criteria: 1) the ability of the patient to change, 2) the ability of the clinician to initiate and direct change, 3) the physiologic and psychologic state of the patient and 4) the presence of treatable high risk factors. These variables are inter-related, and the clinician must make judgments about each one individually as well as in relation to each other. The first factor is estimated during the initial interview by the information gained from the past history and the trial intervention. The second factor is usually the combination of the clinician's training, experience, and creativity. The third is the result of history and testing; the fourth involves the interaction of the patient and his environment. "High risk" factors in voice disorders include shouting, screaming, prolonged talking or singing, smoking, inhaling chemicals, and other activities that may result in vocal pathology. How much can be changed by the patient and how much he is willing to change will be factors in his prognosis. Some working environments are conducive to voice problems, but changing jobs is not always an acceptable solution. Compromise and reconciliation are usually the final outcome.

Regardless of how the patient describes the vocal dysfunction, structure and function must be analyzed and differentiated as explicitly as possible. In all instances, the evaluation must be followed by differential diagnosis and an outline for treatment. The more tools and techniques available to the clinician, the more variable the ways of approaching the patient. However, a well structured voice evaluation with a stable rationale can bring order to the observation and direction to the treatment of voice disorders.

REFERENCES

Aronson, A. E. 1973. Psychogenic Voice Disorders: An Interdisciplinary Approach to Detection, Diagnosis and Therapy (Audio Seminars in Speech Pathology). W. B. Saunders Company, Philadelphia.

Asherson, N. 1936. Test for functional aphonia and for detection of unilateral nerve deafness. J. Laryngol. Otol. 51:527–529.

Baynes, R. 1966. An incident study of chronic hoarseness among children. J. Speech Hear. Disord. 31:172–176.

Berlin, C. I., and ZoBell, D. H. 1963. Clinical measures of esophageal speech acquisition. J. Speech Hear. Disord. 28:389–392.

Berry, W. R. 1966. The use of the artificial larynx in laryngectomee rehabilitation: proceedings of a conference. p. 118. V.A. Hospital, Memphis, Tennessee.

Boone, D. R. 1971. The Voice and Voice Therapy. Prentice-Hall Inc., Englewood Cliffs, New Jersey.

Briess, F. B. 1957. Voice therapy. I. Identification of specific laryngeal muscle dysfunction by voice testing. Arch. Otolaryngol. 66:375–381.

Bryce, D. P. 1974. Differential Diagnosis and Treatment of Hoarseness. Charles C Thomas, Springfield, Illinois.

Bzoch, K. R. (ed.). 1972. Communication Disorders Related to Cleft Lip and Palate. Little, Brown and Company, Boston.

Bzoch, K. R. 1975. Demonstration of techniques for evaluation of speech. Presented at Texas Speech and Hearing Association, October, Galveston, Texas.

Castiglioni, A. 1947. A History of Medicine. Alfred A. Knopf, Inc., New York.

Cooper, M. 1974. Spectrographic analysis of fundamental frequency and hoarseness: Before and after vocal rehabilitation. J. Speech Hear. Disord. 39(3):286–297.

Courtney, B. 1975. Other voices, other rooms: Voice changes as manifestations of ego changes. Psychiatry 28(4):375–379.

Fabricant, N. D. 1973. Laryngeal involvement in systemic diseases. The Eye, Ear, Nose, and Throat Monthly. 42:56–57.

Fairbanks, G. 1940. Voice and Articulation Drillbook. 1st Ed. Harper & Brothers, New York.

Fetterolf, G. 1909. The symptomatology of tuberculosis of the larynx. Med. Rec. 75:143–145.

Finney, G. 1966. Medical theories of vocal exercise and health. Bull. Hist. Med. 40:395–406.

Finney, G. 1968. Vocal exercise in the sixteenth century related to theories of physiology and disease. Bull. Hist. Med. 42:422–449.

Fisher, H. B., and J. A. Logemann. 1970. Objective evaluation of therapy for vocal nodules: A case report. J. Speech Hear. Disord. 35:277–285.

Fox, D. R., and D. Johns. 1970. Predicting velopharyngeal closure with a modified tongue-anchor technique. J. Speech Hear. Disord. 35:248–251.

Fox, D. R., and Blechman, M. 1975. Clinical Management of Voice Disorders. Cliff Notes, Inc. Lincoln, Nebraska.

Fox, D. R., Lynch, J. I., and Brookshire, B. 1976. Development of cleft palate children between two and thirty-three months of age. Presented at the American Cleft Palate Association annual meeting, May 1976, San Francisco.

Gillespie, S. K. and Cooper, E. B. 1973. Prevalence of speech problems in junior and senior high schools. J. Speech Hear. Res. 16(4):739–743.

Henderson, W. V. 1913. The need of a standard in voice production. Laryngoscope. 23:1–4.

Hollien, H., and Shipp, T. 1972. Speaking fundamental frequency and chronologic age in males. J. Speech Hear. Res. 15(1):155–159.

Hurtz, K. 1976. Voice screening in the San Antonio area schools. Presented at the University of Houston Spring Seminar.

Isshiki, N., Yanagihara, N., and Morimoto, M. 1966. Approach to the objective diagnosis of hoarseness. Folia Phonia 39:393–401.

Jackson, C. Coates, G., and Jackson, C. 1929. Nose, Throat, and Ear and Their Diseases. W. B. Saunders Company, Philadelphia.

Johnson, W., Darley, F. L., and Spriestersbach, D. C. 1963. Diagnostic Methods in Speech Pathology. Harper & Brothers, New York.

Laguite, J. K. 1972. Adult voice screening. J. Speech Hear. Disord. 37(2):147–151.

Lencione, R. 1968. A rationale for speech and language evaluation in cerebral palsy. Br. J. Disord. Commun. 3:161–170.

Moncur, J. and Brackett, I. P. 1974. Modifying Vocal Behavior. Harper & Row, New York.

Moore, P. 1971. Organic Disorders of Voice. Prentice-Hall Inc., Englewood Cliffs, New Jersey.

Morley, M. 1972. The Development and Disorders of Speech in Childhood. pp. 239–245. The Williams & Wilkins Company, Baltimore.

Morris, H., Spriestersbach, D. C., and Darley, F. 1961. An articulation test for assessing competency for velopharyngeal closure. J. Speech Hear. Res. 4:48–55.

Moses, P. J. 1954. The Voice of Neurosis. Grune & Stratton, Inc., New York.

Murphy, A. 1964. Functional Voice Disorders. Prentice-Hall Inc., Englewood Cliffs, New Jersey.

Murry, T., Singh, S., and Sargent, M. 1977 Multidimensional classification of abnormal voice qualities. J. Acoust. Soc. Am. In press.

Perkins, W. H. 1971. Vocal function: assessment and therapy. In: L. E. Travis (ed.), Handbook of Speech Pathology and Audiology, pp. 505–534. Appleton-Century-Crofts, New York.

Ransone, J., Holden, H., and Bull, T. R. 1973. Recent Advances in Otolaryngology. Churchill & Livingston, London.

Rice, L., and Gaylin, N. 1973. Personality processes reflected in client vocal style and Rorschach performance. J. Consult. Clin. Psychol. 40(1):133–138.

Russell, G. O. 1931. Speech and Voice. The Macmillan Company, New York.

Russell, G. O. and Tuttle, C. H. 1930. Color movies of Vocal cord action—an aid in Diagnosis. Laryngoscope 40:549–552.

Senturia, B. H., and F. B. Wilson. 1968. Otorhinolaryngic findings in children with voice disorders. Ann. Otol. Rhino. Laryngol. 77:1028–1044.

Sharp, F. 1963. Judgments of psychosis from vocal clues. J. Speech Hear. Disord. 28:371–374.

Shearer, W. 1972. The diagnosis and treatment of voice disorders in school children. J. Speech Hear. Disord. 37:215–221.

Silverman, E. M., and Zimmer, C. H. 1975. Incidence of chronic hoarseness among school-age children. J. Speech Hear. Disord. 40(2):211–215.

Skelly, M. 1973. Glossectomy Speech Rehabilitation. Charles C Thomas, Publisher, Springfield, Illinois.

Snidecor, J. C. and others. 1968. Speech Rehabilitation of the Laryngectomized. pp. 183–193. 2nd Ed. Charles C Thomas, Publisher, Springfield, Illinois.

Subtelney, J. D., Van Hattum, R. J., and Meyers, B. B. 1972. Ratings and measures of cleft palate speech. Cleft Palate J. 9:18–27.

Van Gelder, L. 1974. Psychosomatic aspects of endocrine disorders of the voice. J. Commun. Disord. 7:257–262.

Van Riper, C. 1964. Speech Correction—Principles and Methods. Prentice-Hall Inc., Englewood Cliffs, New Jersey.

Wepman, J., MacGahan, J. A., Rickard, J. C., and Shelton, N. W. 1953. The objective measurement of progressive esophageal speech development. J. Speech Hear. Disord. 18:247–325.

Wheelis, A. 1969. How people change. Commentary. May: 56–65.

Wilson, F. B. 1973. The voice disordered child: A descriptive approach. Lang. Speech Hear. Service in Schools. Am. Speech Hear. Assoc., Washington, D.C. 1(4):14–22.

APPENDIX

Voice Screening Form

Patient's name _____

Age _____ Date _____

Rate the patient on the following form:

	Normal	Abnormal	Type
Quality	_____	_____	_____
Pitch	_____	_____	_____
Loudness	_____	_____	_____
Breathing	_____	_____	_____
Phonation time	_____	_____	_____
s/z Comparison	_____	_____	_____

Write in one of the following if the abnormal column has been checked.
Quality—harsh, hoarse, breathy, nasal, denasal, cul-de-sac
Pitch—high, low, breaks up or down
Loudness—loud, soft
Breathing—clavicular, other
Time—number of seconds sustained phonation on *a* or *i*
s/z—number of seconds for each then divide (should be 1.00)

Clinician _____

The Assessment of Fluency Disorders

Stephen B. Hood

CONTENTS

This chapter begins with Professor Hood's caution that stuttering remains the subject of continuing theoretical speculation. The clinician must be sensitive to the influence of the social context in evaluating stuttering. Speech samples obtained during a diagnostic session may not be representative of the "real world" of the stutterer. A list of 14 common speech pressures is provided, including samples of these pressures. Dr. Hood emphasizes that many questions still remain about the relationship of language and fluency. Traditionally respected diagnostic techniques such as adaptation and consistency are also questioned (Prins, 1968; Kroll and Hood, 1974). Measures of fluency based only on stuttered words per minute are said to be insufficient. Basic procedures for Dr. Hood's transcript analysis are explained and scoring is illustrated. In addition, 19 other selected methods of evaluation, all available commercially, are reviewed. The special problems of evaluating children are treated in some detail and adaptation of techniques such as the "Draw Your Family Test" are presented. Dr. Hood stresses that no clear distinction can be made between diagnosis and therapy. Finally, suggestions are made for successful interviewing and counseling of the stutterer and his family.   —Eds.

Diagnostic procedures for clinical disorders are intended to answer questions concerning the nature and etiology of the problem, the severity of the problem, prognosis, and appropriate remedial measures. With stuttering, as with most other speech disorders, our present state of knowledge and the methods and materials available for assessment do not provide complete and definitive answers for these questions.

The nature, including the etiology of stuttering, remains the subject of extensive theoretical speculation. Although research findings have helped clarify certain factors involved in the problem, many of the findings are in the nature of empirical observations, amenable to varied interpretations. For example, Wingate (1962a–c) reinterpreted much of the research data of Johnson and associates (1959) and arrived at conclusions quite different from those of the original researchers. Likewise, there is no agreement among workers in the field as to the relative importance of various factors that are usually considered in the determination of the severity of stuttering. "Behaviorists" emphasize the observable and measurable characteristics of stuttering, whereas "psychotherapeutically oriented" clinicians emphasize the attitudes, feelings, and emotions that are part of the problem of stuttering. There is also the question of severity, and whether it is assessed from the point of view of the speaker or the listener. In clinical practice it is not unusual to come across a person who evidences very few breaks in the flow of speech, yet who believes that he has a severe problem. There are others who "stutter" on nearly every other word, yet consider it as no more than a minor irritation. Severity has two dimensions, one as perceived by the speaker, and the other as perceived by the listener. Although neither can be ignored in the determination of severity, the relative importance of each dimension is often a matter of the clinician's bias.

The observable characteristics of stuttering have both auditory and visual components. Despite the fact that most research has been based on tape recorded samples of stuttered speech, ratings of severity change markedly when one, rather than both, factors are considered (Luper, 1959; Williams, Wark, and Minifie, 1963; Hood and Stigora, 1972). The clinician is faced with the problem of deciding how much importance should be attached to each of these components for the determination of severity. The answer, of course, is largely a matter of opinion.

Stuttering is highly variable in relation to the social context. It is not uncommon to find that during a diagnostic work-up a stutterer evidences very few fluency interruptions yet reports that it is all but impossible to talk at work. On the other hand there are those with whom a clinical interview is very difficult because the interruptions are numerous and of long duration, and yet who report that their problem is not nearly as severe in most other situations. Speech samples obtained during the diagnostic session may not be representative of the "real world." How are we to determine severity on the basis of a potentially biased sample? The stutterer himself and those around him cannot always be relied on to give a valid estimate of difficulty in various social situations. Apart from all other considerations, this factor alone may dishearten the prospective diagnostician in his attempt to determine the severity of stuttering. In order to arrive at an 'intuitive judgment" of stuttering severity, many clinicians rely on the self-reports of the stutterer or other persons in his immediate environment, coupled with observations during the diagnostic session.

There are no easy, established procedures to determine the severity of stuttering and each clinician will have to develop his own criteria. Within limits, one set of criteria may be as good as any other. Although there can at present be little pretension of objectivity and scientific rigor in the determination of severity of stuttering, it is hoped that this will change in the near future.

Prognosis in stuttering is as varied as the disorder itself. Conjectures as to the factors that supposedly influence prognosis abound. Many years ago, for example, Bryngelson (1938) listed several factors important to favorable therapeutic outcome. No single factor, or combination of factors, has yet been proved to influence prognosis. Indeed, an important confounding variable in the determination of prognostic variables, at least in children and adolescents, is the high rate of spontaneous recovery (Wingate, 1964; Shearer and Williams, 1965; Sheehan and Martyn, 1966). Paradoxically, speech therapy and spontaneous recovery are not highly correlated (Sheehan and

Martyn, 1969). Therefore, until research delineates those variables that significantly influence fluency improvement, with or without therapy, prognostication will remain an unreliable process.

It is against this rather pessimistic background that we now attempt to chart a course through the maze of fluency and fluency disorders. We agree with Van Riper (1971) that clinicians urgently need better measures of stuttering severity, that our basic assessment techniques and procedures are at best prescientific, and we share his hope that "someday we will have good measures of stuttering severity" (p. 235). Unfortunately, we do not yet have clear and unambiguous diagnostic tests or assessment inventories. We may be coming closer, but we have a long way to go because the problems involved in assessment are complex and controversial. If we are to better understand the relationships among the variables associated with fluency disorders, then we must be more molecular in our approach. We must look at the specific components involved in the frequency, duration, intensity, and type of disfluency. In addition, we must attend to those behaviors involved in the avoidance of fluency disruptions, because "stuttering" involves far more than the disruption of fluency. Stuttering may represent either a "behavior" or a "problem." When we speak of stuttering as a behavior, we refer to the overt speech acts that are observable, definable, and measurable both in terms of their quantity and type. These overt behaviors are probably developed, maintained, and modified through instrumental (operant) conditioning (Shames and Egolf, 1975; Ryan, 1974). When we speak of stuttering as a problem, we refer to the more covert features: emotions, attitudes, feelings, and self concept. These are probably learned, maintained and modified through respondent (classical) conditioning (Brutten and Shoemaker, 1967; Wolpe, 1969). Assessment is not an easy task.

It is essential that we have a reason for doing what we do. Too often we seek only the method and procedure without a proper appreciation for the underlying rationale. Williams states the issue as follows:

> I wish clinicians would place more stress on the asking of meaningful questions that can be answered by systematic observation... [Clinicians] spend relatively little time defining the questions to which they are attempting to seek answers. (1968, p. 53)

Indeed, a diagnostic evaluation for one particular client is similar to a research investigation based on one subject. Consider the following analogous components. The review of literature corresponds to the background and case history; the research methods and procedures are like the diagnostic evaluation; the results of research are like the results of the evaluation; the discussion of the research findings is like the clinical interpretation; the recommendations for further research relate to the implications for therapy. Although the analogy is far from perfect, the basic relationships are valid and stress the importance of being systematic. Clinicians often confess that they do not know what to do to help a given client. The underlying problem, more often than not, is that they do not understand the nature of the problem for that particular client. Research tends to focus on groups of subjects; assessment and treatment is specific to the individual. Therefore, the diagnostician must play the role of Sherlock Holmes and do a considerable amount of detective work. The asking of meaningful and answerable questions is an essential first step. In this chapter we attempt to present some of the basic and logical questions to be asked and answered. The answers to these questions help determine the basic starting points for therapy. For the reader who is appalled by the tremendous number of potential factors to be considered we can make no apology. All we can say is that they may be important contributors that predispose a person toward disruptions in fluency, precipitate specific instances of disfluency, or serve to maintain the problem in its chronic state. Therefore, many of the aspects considered will be those believed to influence fluency/disfluency for people in general; it will then be the clinician's task to systematically determine those variables that are operating for any one particular client, to assess their significance, and to plan for their remediation.

GENERAL CONSIDERATIONS

The essential purpose of assessing fluency disorders is to determine whether a clinically significant problem exists and to determine how and where to begin treatment. In order to do this, the clinician must have a firm understanding of the nature of stuttering. Within the past decade alone, extensive work has been published concerning this subject. The space available in this chapter does not permit a complete review of the various theories, experiments and approaches to clinical management that currently are available (Brutten and Shoemaker, 1967; Sheehan, 1970; Van Riper, 1971, 1973; Williams,

1971; Ryan, 1974; Bloodstein, 1975; Eisenson, 1975; Shames and Egolf, 1976). We will attempt to review some of the major principles involved in the nature of stuttering based on the assumption that it is against these principles that the diagnostician bases his assessment. As Van Riper (1971) has pointed out, it is unfortunate that we have no "Bureau of Standards" for the assessment of stuttering severity (p.221). Indeed, "severity" is largely a perceptual event that involves far more than just the overt disfluency behavior(s) emitted by a speaker (Giolas and Williams, 1958; Boehmler, 1958; Williams and Kent, 1958; Sander, 1965). The perceptual set of the listener is of crucial importance, as is the self-definition of the speaker. We shall attempt to summarize the basic nature of stuttering, highlight the major components involved in the concept of "severity," and urge the reader to become as familiar as possible with the current literature in stuttering.

Stuttering as a Behavior—Stuttering as a Problem

Johnson (1963) has suggested that there are three general meanings for the term "stuttering." He proposed that stuttering may represent the "name for something the speaker does," that it may represent "a name for a classification made by a listener," and that it may represent a "name for a problem." More recently, Van Riper (1971) indicated that stuttering may be used as a noun or verb and that stuttering may be thought of as a behavior, or as a disorder. Williams (1957) has cautioned that we use care in our terminology and strive to be descriptive, rather than animistic in our use of language. Different meanings are derived from such parental descriptions as: 1) Johnny stutters, 2) Johnny is a stutterer, 3) Johnny has a stuttering problem, 4) Johnny repeats parts of words a lot, 5) Johnny gets stuck a lot when he talks. The language we use to conceptualize the problems is important. Do we use the language of self-responsibility and view stuttering as something the person does, or do we see it as a magical something that the person has? We agree with Williams that both the stutterer's and clinician's points of view and beliefs about stuttering are important (1957, 1971, 1972).

It is appropriate to think of stuttering both in terms of the "behavior" involved and in terms of the "problem" involved. When we discuss stuttering[1] as a behavior, we refer to the audible and inaudible components that are overt, observable, measurable, and quantifiable. These include such specific types of disfluency as repetition, prolongation and fixation, as well as, associated degrees of tension, struggle, and avoidance behavior. For the young child who is "just beginning to stutter" the behavior and the situations where it is observed to occur are considered, because the child has not yet developed self-awareness of having a problem. The child emits the behavior; the parents, teachers, and clinicians perceive the potential problem. Therefore, we are concerned about the frequency and type of behavior emitted, and more importantly, the antecedents to its occurrence. It is later in the development of stuttering that the person internalizes the feeling that he has a problem and develops emotions of frustration, shame, embarrassment, guilt, and fear. We must differentiate the "problem" from the "behavior."

The Question of Severity

How mild is mild? How severe is severe? These are questions that have plagued clinicians for many years. When we consider the various aspects of severity we come to the conclusion that many components interact in ways that preclude a unitary score or measure. We must cope with the various overt features of disfluency in terms of their frequency, duration, and type. We must also account for the associated tension and struggle that is manifest in the stutterer's attempted escape from the moment of stuttering and for the avoidance behaviors that are manifested before a moment of fluency disruption in an attempt to prevent its occurrence. In addition, client attitudes, feelings, and emotions must be considered. The issue is further complicated by the fact that stuttering is highly intermittent and not totally consistent.

Age is also a factor, and stuttering is generally viewed as a developmental disorder. The easy and effortless repetitions and bobbles of the preschooler who is "just beginning to stutter" differ markedly from the tense, fragmented speech of the transitional stutterer who is frustrated by his stuttering and trying to learn how to escape from it. The advanced exteriorized stutterer may show disfluency in the extreme: moments of stuttering that are frequent, blocks that are of long duration, tense forms of escape behavior, and both subtle and obvious attempts at avoidance. Emotions also change. The beginning stutterer who is unaware of his disfluency differs markedly from the later developmental stages where awareness, frustration, shame, guilt, and fear are involved. Negative emotion exists in many degrees! Age does not always correlate highly with severity. We have worked with too many youngsters who would be considered "severe" and too many adults who would be considered "mild" to make such a statement. Nevertheless, we know that if our program for prevention is not successful, or if our therapy for retraining is ineffective, stuttering will tend to become worse.

Developmental Perspectives

Historically, the development of stuttering was thought to involve two basic phases: primary and secondary stuttering (Bluemel, 1935). Unsatisfied with this dichotomy, some writers chose to discuss stuttering in terms of the trichotomy of primary, transition, and secondary stuttering (Van Riper, 1954). During the 1960s there were attempts to look at stuttering as developing in four rather discrete steps (Bloodstein, 1960a, b; 1961; Van Riper, 1963; Luper and Mulder, 1964). During the present decade there has been a move away from this admittedly artificial model of stuttering development as evidenced by the recent criticisms of Van Riper (1971) and Brutten (1975). We agree that the four-stage model is lacking, and that there is overlap among the developmental stages. We further agree that many stutterers fail to fit clearly into any one particular stage of development. Nevertheless, we would encourage the reader not familiar with these approaches to take the time to study them, for within them are descriptions of the basic overt and covert features involved in the disorder of stuttering. Whether or not they represent discrete steps along a complex continuum is immaterial; what is important is that they give a basic, although static framework against which to begin to conceptualize the concept of severity. Further we would encourage the reader not familiar with the concepts of "interiorized" and "exteriorized" stuttering to review the work of Douglass (1954), Douglass and Quarrington (1952) and Freund (1966). There are many severe "interiorized" stutterers who show little or no outward manifestation. Their problem is severe; their behavioral manifestations are minimal.

Reciprocity Between Assessment and Treatment

It is our contention that there can be no clear distinction made between "diagnosis" and "therapy." A diagnostic evaluation should be therapeutic and therapy should involve continuous evaluation. All that can really be gained from the initial evaluation is a basic yardstick concerning where the person is at that point; a yardstick against which to measure changes that result as a function of therapeutic intervention. Indeed, the attitudes and behaviors evident at the beginning of therapy will change markedly over the course of treatment. We need ongoing reassessment. We know clinicians who fall at both ends of the continuum. Some clinicians do a minimal amount of testing. They wish only to have an index as to where the person should begin the therapy program (Mowrer, 1976). Others (Brutten, 1975) spend a great deal of time trying to determine what type of stutterer the person is so that a differential treatment program can be considered. Our own approach falls somewhere in between. Much information is to be gathered, but relatively little is actually obtained during the initial evaluation session. With respect to taking the case history and providing counseling to the parents of a child in the incipient stages of development, it is often many weeks before we feel that we have gathered sufficient information to make specific recommendations. With the adult, it is often many sessions before we can determine whether the actual stuttering behaviors and related emotions are of primary or secondary importance. We feel it is possible to err either by being too brief or too extensive in the time we allot to the formal diagnostic battery. We save much of the testing until later in the course of treatment; in fact, testing continues to occur throughout the course of treatment. We continually assess and reassess.

FACTORS TO BE CONSIDERED IN ASSESSMENT OF FLUENCY DISORDERS

Etiology

The question of etiology has been debated for many years and controversy has centered around three major areas of concern: that stuttering results from some organic/physiologic/neurologic difference; that stuttering is the outward symptom of a deeper neurosis; that stuttering is a learned behavior (see Van Riper, 1971; Bloodstein, 1975). As partial support for the organic position is the evidence of disfluency and stuttering among brain-damaged populations such as the aphasic or cerebral palsied. Evidence in support of the neurotic position is provided by the literature in psychology and psychiatry. Support for the learning theory approaches is based on the developmental changes that occur, both emotionally and behaviorally, as the disorder progresses and the fact that the behavior is modifiable by classical and operant conditioning procedures.

The question of etiology is potentially misleading because it refers to the study of "causes," and because it is generally impossible to isolate the exact point in time where a difference, disorder, or problem first began. Therefore, those factors that may be first order, second order, or third order, etc., often remain unknown. Furthermore, the fact that certain behaviors, emotions, or events are highly correlated is of little real help because correlation does not imply cause and effect relationships. Our approach to assessment is based on the assumption that we must attempt to determine various types of causes: predisposing, precipitating, and maintaining. Sometimes they are obvious; unfortunately, they are all too often well hidden. We take the position that there is much to be learned regarding the question of etiology and that essential research has yet to be completed. Theories must consider this issue, and eventually therapies must also. For the present time it seems best to consider the individual person as an entity unto himself. It is our contention that both diagnosis and treatment must be individualized for the one specific person under consideration (See Sheehan, 1958, p. 79; Beech and Fransella, 1968, pp. 31-32). Therefore, we look primarily at those factors that precipitate and maintain the problem and give relatively less attention to factors that may originally have predisposed the person toward a fluency problem at some point in the past. We are concerned about an individual, not a group, because members of groups show individual differences. There may well be a stuttering syndrome or syndromes, but at the present we do not have enough information to know (St. Onge, 1963; Andrews and Harris, 1964).

Precipitating and Maintaining Factors

Because there is nothing we can do to change the past, we typically concentrate on the present and plan for the future. We take the position that moments of fluency disruption are, at least in part, reactions to communicative pressure and stress. Underlying organic or emotional conditions may predispose one person to break down more easily than another, but it is the situations under which this happens that concerns us. We wish to know those factors that precipitate instances of fluency disruption in their sporadic form, and later serve to maintain them. Listed below are some of the variables that relate to communicative pressure and stress that demand our scrutiny. We attempt to determine their presence or absence in several ways: through information reported on the case history; through parent interviews; by means of our interactions with the child in both formal and informal settings; through observing the child as he interacts with his parents and siblings; and often through visits to the child's home or school. We view communicative stress as the single most important variable to be considered, and yet stress per se is not the only critical item. The way the child copes is also important, for it has been our observation that many children who are prone to fluency problems show a low degree of frustration tolerance and a high degree of sensitivity. What are some of the things to look for? Primarily, they involve the antecedents to moments of fluency disruption. What was happening just before the child emitted a disfluency? Who was the child talking with? What was the subject of the conversation? Listed below are some of the communicative pressures that tend to increase the frequency of disfluency. When we find them operating, we try to minimize them as much as possible. Van Riper (1972, pp. 293–294) lists six common pressures that tend to increase the likelihood of fluency disruption.

1. Inability to find or remember the appropriate words. "I'm thinking of-of-of-of-uh that fellow who-uh—of yes, Aaronson. That's his name." This is the adult form. In a child it might occur as: "Mummy, there's a birdy out there in the ... in the ... he's ... uh ... he ... he ... he wash his bottom in the dirt."
2. Inability to pronounce or doubt of ability to articulate. Adult form: "I can never say sus-stus-susiss-stuh-stuhstiss-oh, you know what I mean, figures, statistics." The child's form could be illustrated by: "Mummy, we saw two poss-poss-uh-possumusses at the zoo. Huh? Yes, two puh-pos-sums." Tongue twisters, unfamiliar sounds or words, too fast a rate of utterance, and articulation disorders can produce these sources of speech disfluency.
3. Fear of the unpleasant consequences of the communication. "Y-yes I-I-I uh I t-took the money." "W-wi-will y-you marry m-me?" "Duh-don't s-s-spank me, Mum-mummy." Some of the conflict may be due to uncertainty as to whether the content of the communication is acceptable or not. Contradicting, confessing, asking favors, refusing requests, shocking, tentative vulgarity, fear of exposing social inadequacy, fear of social penalty in school recitations or recitals.
4. The communication itself is unpleasant, in that it recreates an unpleasant experience. "I cu-cu-cut my f-f-finger. . . awful bi-big hole in it." "And then he said to me, 'you're f-f-fired.'" The narration of injuries, injustices, penalties often produces speech hesitancy.

5. Presence, threat, or fear of interruption. This is one of the most common of all the sources of speech hesitancy. Incomplete utterances are always frustrating, and the average speaker always tries to forestall or reject an approaching interruption. This he does by speeding up the rate, filling in the necessary pauses with repeated syllables or grunts or braying. This could be called "filibustering," since it is essentially a device to hold the floor. When speech becomes a battleground for competing egos, this desire for dominance may become tremendous.

6. Loss of the listener's attention. Communication involves both speaker and listener, and when the latter's attention wanders or is shifted to other concerns, a fundamental conflict occurs. ("Should I continue talking ... even though she isn't listening? If I do, she'll miss what I just said ... If I don't, I won't get it said. Probably never .... Shall I? ... Shan't I") The speaker often resolves this conflict by repeating or hesitating until the speech is very productive of speech hesitancy. "Mummy, I-I-I want a ... Mummy, I ... M ... Mumm ... Mummy, I ... I ... I want a cookie." Disturbing noises, the loss of the listener's eye contact, and many other similar disturbances can produce this type of fluency interrupter.

To the above list, we would add several others, realizing full well that there may be overlap.

7. Competition for talking time: Although the "rules of the game" suggest that one person should listen while the other talks, this is not always the case. We recently observed a dinner situation where a 4-year-old made 11 attempts to begin a sentence before anyone even began to listen.

8. Time pressure: When we have a lot to say and a short amount of time in which to say it, we typically feel time pressure. For the child who feels hurried to complete his message the pressure may be sufficient to cause fluency breakdowns. Nearing the completion of a lengthy long distance phone call, he author's son announced that "I wanna talk to granddaddy." His father's abrupt warning to hurry up resulted in "but-but-but I only have one-one-one more question to ask him."

9. Verbal showing off: Parents often have a tendency to brag about what their children can do. In addition, they often make their children perform for Aunt Jane and Uncle Rick. Comments such as "Show Mrs. Ames how you can count to 20" and "Show Mr.

Preston how you can spell Mississippi" are to be found in every family. The question is how often do they occur, when do they occur, and are they spoken as requests or as demands? We worked with the son of an English Professor who was determined that his 9-year-old would have the best vocabulary in the department. He did! And some of the words he stuttered upon included: indigenous, surperfluous and tumultuous. Therapy involved allowing the boy to use what the parents considered "baby talk," and in a short time the stuttering vanished.

10. Demand speech: We agree with Van Riper (1973) that demand speech is an extremely potential fluency disruptor. However, unlike verbal showing off, here the child is forced to answer demands, answer questions, account for what he has or has not done, and confess his wrongdoings. We believe that activities such as self-talk and parallel talk are conducive to speech and language development; however, by the time the child reaches age 3 or 4, many parents replace these forms with excessive and typically unnecessary demands that require extensive verbalization from the child.

11. Statements of demand and support: Sheehan has emphasized this important concept (1970). We listen carefully for whether the parents speak in a manner that is supportive or demanding. In addition to the actual semantics of the utterance we pay particular attention to the rate, intensity and loudness with which the statement is made. "Haven't you finished your milk yet" can be spoken as a sentence or question. This same idea can also be expressed as "Your milk is nearly gone, how about finishing it up."

12. Positive and negative statements: We listen carefully for the ways in which parents teach their children to do things. Is the child taught how to ride a bicycle, or how not to fall off? Is he encouraged to eat carefully, or not spill? Is the child praised for his successive approximations, or reprimanded for his "less bad" behaviors or performances? We find this particularly important in view of Williams' comments concerning the fact that many children with stuttering problems are afraid to make mistakes in the process of talking (1971). We feel this relates to the issues of perfectionism, hypersensitivity to mistakes, frustration over mistakes that have been made and the resultant positive/negative attitude that develops with respect to learning something new.

13. Listener reactions to disfluency: Listeners differ with respect to their ability to tolerate disfluency in the speech of others; some

are quick to react. The type of disfluency is of particular importance. Listeners are quicker to react negatively to part-word repetitions, audible prolongations, tense pauses, and disrhythmic phonations than they are to revisions, interjections, word and multiple word repetitions. We become particularly concerned about both the quantitative and qualitative ways in which listeners react to the child's disfluencies. We wish to know the types of speech breakdown that result in listener reactions and to the types of reaction that follow. Do the listeners call attention to the disfluency? Do they ask or demand that the child stop, start over, and say it again? Or, do they adjust their own listening pattern in order to be a better listener who is able to pay attention without interrupting, contradicting, or otherwise acting as an aversive stimulus for the child?

14. Talking when excited: Sporadic periods of excitement tend to elicit increased disfluency. The child who has just completed building a fantastic big fort with his new set of Tinker Toys may be excited to tell about it. So may the adult who has just been picked as a contestant on a television game show. Typically such situations are random and no cause for concern. It is when the child is constantly excited and on the go that we become suspect. Joey is a case in point: always on the move, seldom remaining with any activity more than several minutes, totally manipulative of the surrounding environment, behaviorally but not medically hyperactive, and disfluent on approximately 65% of the words spoken. We attempt to pinpoint those situations where this marked activity level is present and systematically work to change it. Typically, this helps the parents as well as the child.

Collecting Speech Samples

The collection of valid speech samples is more complicated than one might suspect. This is particularly true in light of the fact that disfluencies occur intermittently and vary from situation to situation. Stuttering varies in relation to many internal and external factors: audience size; the age of the listener(s); whether the person is engaged in monologue or dialogue; whether the person is speaking or reading; whether the person is speaking at home or school or in the therapy room; and, whether the person is in a good or bad mood. We cannot assume that any one speech sample is representative. Even under similar circumstances we must be cautious for we know of too many stutterers who make both "good" phone calls and "bad" ones.

We attempt to sample the person's speech behavior in a number of different speaking situations. In addition, we request reports from other persons in the environment (parents, teachers, peers, spouse, business associates, employer). In the case of children we often send the "Descriptions of Stuttering" checksheet (see Appendix B) to a number of different people and ask that they complete it. We sometimes find high levels of agreement among the respondents. This typically suggests that the person's speech behavior is relatively consistent across speech situations and that the listeners perceive the speech in a similar way. In other cases there is disagreement. Does this mean that the listeners have different standards for fluency? Does it mean that the child's speech differs depending upon the person to whom he is speaking? We follow up with further investigation.

Highly related to the topic of speech sampling is the recent work of Silverman (1971a, b, 1972, 1973, 1974a). She found that differences in the disfluency of nonstuttering preschoolers apparently depend upon the speaking situation: talking with playmates and adults at school, talking at home with the family, and talking with the clinician in an interview situation. She also found that it made a difference whether the child was engaging in egocentric or socialized speech and whether the child was attempting to exchange ideas with the listener. The clinician must sample broadly. In particular, speech samples should be obtained from those situations that have been identified as causing concern.

With preschool and young school-age children we should collect speech samples in situations such as: rote tasks such as counting or saying the alphabet, reciting a familiar verse, telling a story, talking with puppets, describing a picture, relating an event, engaging in conversation, arguing, asking permission, and under other circumstances that involve various degrees of communicative pressure and threat. With older children and adults we also obtain fluency samples during oral reading, telephoning, talking to groups, talking to authority figures, and other situations that the person has identified as difficult. Our goal is to sample a range of behaviors. We want the "easy" ones as well as the "hard" ones. Later, we can develop a more specific hierarchy of speech situations.

Speaking and Reading

Although most of the above listed speech samples involved spontaneous speech, we also want to determine the person's level of fluency during oral reading. We wish to emphasize, however, that the selection of the reading material is extremely important. In adults, both normal nonfluency and stuttering increase proportionally with increased information value of the reading passage (Schlesinger et al., 1965; Taylor, 1966; Kroll and Hood, 1976). In an attempt to determine whether this is the case with children, Perry (1975) asked 80 normal speaking children from grades 3, 4, 5, and 6 to read orally passages of various levels of difficulty. As expected, significantly more disfluency was emitted during the reading of the more difficult passages. What was of particular interest, however, was her finding that the so-called "stuttered disfluencies" of part-word repetition, tense pause, and disrhythmic phonation increased at a faster rate than did such disfluency types as revision, interjection, and word and phrase repition. Blood (1976) employed an identical procedure, but used 40 stuttering children from grades 3-6. His results showed that an increased level of reading material had an even more pronounced effect than was the case with the nonstuttering children used by Perry. Again, part-word repetitions, tense pauses, and disrhythmic phonations increased at a faster rate than did the other disfluency types. We took an informal poll of practicing clinicians at a recent Ohio Speech and Hearing Association Conference and were sorry to learn that many clinicians are indiscriminant with respect to the reading material they use for diagnostic and therapeutic purposes.

Adaptation and Consistency

We would be remiss if we did not briefly discuss the question of stuttering adaptation and consistency. Adaptation refers to the successive reduction in the frequency of disfluency and stuttering across repeated reading of the same material. Consistency refers to the fact that stutterings that persist in the later readings tend to be among the original words stuttered. Although these measures were traditionally believed to have prognostic value, such an interpretation has recently been shown to be erroneous (Prins, 1968). One apparent reason for this is the finding that stuttering does not "adapt" in successive trials of spontaneous speech (Kroll and Hood, 1974). Moreover, Kroll and Hood looked at the way in which the specific frequency of part-word repetitions, disrhythmic phonations, interjections, word repetitions, and tense pauses changed as a function of repeated reading and spontaneous speech trials. The specific types of disfluency showed different rates of adaptation both among themselves, and between the reading and spontaneous speech conditions. Currently, we do tend to use an adaptation measure in reading as part of our assessment battery, but we do so with caution. We use the results to observe relative relationships among the types of behaviors emitted and their rate of decrease because we believe this helps in the planning of therapy. We also look at relationships obtained during spontaneous speech. Sometimes the degree of consistency gives clues as to which of the disfluency types might be most resistant to extinction. Within the adaption task, therefore, we think that it is significant both when there is and is not a high degree of consistency. A more detailed review of the issues involved in adaptation and consistency, as well as their use in a specific behavioral assessment battery, is provided by Brutten (1975).

Language and Disfluency

At the present time the research data concerning potential relationships between language and disfluency are neither complete nor conclusive. Our purpose, therefore, will not be to review the literature involved, but merely to point out some of the variables that may be operating. One reason for this is that generalizations based on group data many not be appropriate to individual cases. Individual differences exist and we must be appropriately cautious.

We believe that linguistic ability and the frequency of disfluency are inversely related. That is, as the child gets older he uses more sophisticated forms of language; concurrently, the frequency of disfluency decreases. It may be more than coincidental that the peak period of "normal nonfluency" occurs during the period of rapid language acquisition. Although Davis (1940) concluded that linguistic ability was not an important factor in the frequency of children's repetitions, Muma (1973) found that his highly fluent subjects used more complex language than did his highly disfluent subjects. Muma interpreted his results as support for a non loci explanation of the relationship between disfluency and syntax and suggested that disfluencies are related more to the complexity of the syntactic encoding process than to specific types of grammatical forms. Yet, the variability of children's language behavior is as marked as the variability and intermittency of disfluency. This was pointed out long ago by McCarthy (1929) and more recently by Longhurst and Grubb (1974). Difficulties related to the effects of the stimulus materials designed to elicit the speech sample, as well as the person who obtains the sample, have been well documented (Minifie, Darley and Sherman, 1963; Cowan et al., 1967; Mintun, 1968; Lee, 1974). We believe it is wise for the clinician to evaluate the kinds of language the child uses in general conversation; we feel it is essential that the clinician determine the types of language behaviors the child uses during periods of increased disfluency and stuttering.

In an attempt to better understand potential relationships between disfluency and language, Haynes and Hood (1977) investigated the language and disfluency of 30 children at the discrete chronologic ages of 4, 6, and 8 years. They used the Developmental Sentence Scoring (DSS) technique (Lee, 1974) to measure language complexity, and determined the frequency of occurrence of interjections, part-word repetitions, phrase repetitions, revisions, incomplete phrases, tense pauses, and disrhythmic phonations. As expected, linguistic abilities increased, and disfluency decreased as the children's age increased. The predominant disfluency type also changed. Factor analysis of a correlation matrix composed of the fluency and language variables revealed high correlations within the language variables and within the fluency variables. However, there were no meaningful correlations between any of the language and disfluency variables. Even when the children were later subdivided into groups based on those who were "most" and those who were "least" disfluent, no differences in language ability were found. The most disfluent children averaged 9.5 disfluencies per 100 words spoken and had a mean DSS score of 10.9. The least disfluent children averaged 4.5 disfluencies per 100 words spoken and had a mean DSS score of 10.52.

Emrick (1970) attempted to determine language and disfluency relationships. Her subjects were all kindergarten and 1st grade children. Ten of the children were considered to have stuttering problems, 10 were considered to be highly disfluent nonstutterers and 10 were considered to be typical nonstuttering children. With respect to both the measures of disfluency employed and the measures of language employed, the typical nonstuttering group differed significantly from both the stuttering and highly disfluent nonstuttering groups. Seldom did the stuttering and highly disfluent nonstuttering groups differ. The finding that the nonstuttering group made significantly fewer grammatical errors suggests that some aspects of linguistic ability may indeed be operating.

We cite the above related research by Haynes and Hood (1977) and Emrick (1970) to stress the fact that there remains much to be learned about potential relationships between language and fluency. We also cite this to indicate, however indirectly, that many children who are beginning to stutter can benefit from a language-oriented approach to therapy in which direct emphasis is placed on verbal encoding skills that are commensurate with the child's ability to maintain fluency. Additional support for this position is provided by the finding that children are more disfluent when they model complex as opposed to simple sentences (Haynes, 1976). The contention that increased grammatical load is associated with increased disfluency suggests that clinicians attend not only to the disfluencies observed, but also to the language forms emitted.

THE ASSESSMENT OF FLUENCY DISORDERS

We now turn our attention to the actual assessment process and to various procedures that are helpful in better understanding both the behavior and problem of stuttering. Our observations and interpretations will ultimately be based upon our own direct observations and upon the information supplied by informants.

Direct Assessment of Stuttering Behavior in Children and Adults

We are concerned with the frequency, intensity, duration, and type of disfluency emitted. In order to make this assessment, speech samples are collected from those situations that have been identified as producing various degrees of communication difficulty (monolog, dialog, picture description, spontaneous speech, telephoning, participating in show and tell, etc.). Our measures of duration are timed either with a stop watch or sweep second hand (See Riley, 1972). Measures of intensity or struggle may be obtained in a manner similar to that described by Van Riper (1971, p. 225). These assessments are generally easy to accomplish and will not be elaborated.

We want to emphasize the importance of the frequency measures, and the assessment of the specific disfluency types. In so doing, we work from the assumption that verbal efficiency in terms of words and syllables spoken per minute is important, and that it is against the verbal output that frequency measures should be based (Hood, 1974a, b). Because speech rate is highly variable, we do not feel that measures of frequency based solely in terms of "stuttered" words per min (Ryan, 1974) are sufficiently sensitive.

We are concerned that many clinicians and researchers lump together numerous diverse and complex behaviors within the general construct of a "moment of stuttering." To make such an all inclusive grouping of behaviors, however, fails to distinguish among the multiplicity of behaviors present and prevents any systematic consideration of the relationships that exist among the various behaviors. What the stutterer does at any point in time is in part the behavioral consequence of what he has already done. The stuttering behaviors that we observe are the culmination of certain tensing, speeding, avoiding, postponing, holding back, struggling, or escaping behaviors that have already occurred. Stuttering behaviors are sequential, cumulative, and often simultaneous; one behavior becomes superimposed upon another, and that on still another, until a total behavioral complex emerges as the moment of stuttering. However, these moments of stuttering differ in their components.

The molecular analysis of the components within the moment of stuttering has been suggested by Webster (1965) as a means of minimizing the effect of one behavior masking out another behavior. The research of Prins and Lohr (1968) revealed similar findings. Hood (1969) found that within 2,908 moments of fluency disruption there were 4,395 specific types of disruption. Similarly, Zenner (1971) discovered that within 2,775 molar elements of stuttering there were a total of 4,804 molecular behaviors that could be determined. The "moment of stuttering" is a misleading term when used in a global or molar way (Brutten, 1975).

The moment of stuttering is a dynamic event that fails to conform to the criteria of static analysis. The moment is actually comprised of both antecedent and subsequent behaviors and behavioral intents. It is impossible to clearly demarcate the dividing points that separate the predisruption, disruption, and postdisruption periods. Furthermore, it is not always possible to clearly differentiate the actual talking or stuttering behavior from the evaluation of the intention for which a particular behavior was used. Yet, the clinician routinely makes these judgments in both diagnosis and therapy. At the behavioral level the clinician may be concerned with such behaviors as part-word repetitions, word repetitions, multiple word repetitions, audible or inaudible fixations of articulatory posture, tense pauses, disrhythmic phonations, and various combinations thereof. At an inferential level, however, the clinician's task becomes more complex. Inferential constructs such as starters, timers, postponements, avoidances, circumlocutions, and various combinations thereof are assumed to exist. For example, the clinician must distinguish between the behavioral description of a "pause," the inference that this pause served to "postpone" the initiation of an utterance because of the anticipation of stuttering, or the inference that the pause occurred because of uncertainty in linguistic encoding. Furthermore, within an actual moment of fluency disruption a distinction can be made between the behavioral description of a "multiple word repetition" and the inference that this behavior was intended to "start" or "restart" the utterance. Indeed, a given behavior may be used to avoid an anticipated moment of stuttering before it has occurred, or may be used to escape from a moment of stuttering while it is occurring. Regardless of the theoretical posture from which the clinician operates, it is essential that both behavioral and inferential assessments be made. We need a systematic means of adding precision to our judgments and we must differentiate definitional-behavioral levels of analysis from the inferred intent of the behavior.

Assessment of Overt Features

Stuttering therapy, broadly defined, is a process of behavior modification that can take orientation from any number of theoretical postures. Regardless of his theoretical approach to therapy, the clinician generally selects several target behaviors toward which to direct his clinician attention. All too frequently, however, the clinician defines only superficially these target behaviors and fails to define, observe, and measure the frequency of their occurrence in various communicative situations. A representative sample of behaviors and behavioral intentions is presented in Table 1. From this general list an analysis of the speech behaviors of a particular client can be made along the lines suggested in Table 2. Other behaviors and behavioral intents could and should be used depending upon the particular client under consideration. The proportionate relationships among behaviors are shown in Table 3. A comparison of reading, spontaneous speech, and picture description analyses at the beginning and end of therapy is shown in Table 4. The analysis presented in this paper is taken from tape-recorded samples; this is done because tape-recorded samples are easy to obtain and because video tape equipment is not routinely available to clinicians. Although research concerning the relative usefulness of video tape and tape-recorded samples is equivocal, our own clinical and experimental evidence suggests that video-taped samples are generally superior to tape-recorded samples. This is particularly true with the disfluency types that are inaudible or non-vocalized (Quarrington and Douglass, 1960; Van Riper, 1971; Hood and Stigora, 1972).

The basic procedure for transcript analysis is presented in Tables 2 and 3. Listed below are definitions of terms and the measurement ratios used.

1. Verbal Output: Verbal output is considered the number of meaningful words and syllables spoken per unit of time. Extraneous words related to the stuttering pattern are not counted. The efficiency of communication may be calculated in terms of words or syllables spoken per unit of time.

2. Number of Moments of Disruption: This is the traditional concept of the "moment of stuttering." Each molar disfluency complex is counted. The relative frequency of these molar units may be calculated in terms of the number of meaningful words or syllables spoken, or per unit of time.

3. Total Disfluency Types: This is the tabulation of each and every distinct disfluency type within any given moment of disruption. Often several specific disruption types occur within a moment of disruption. Specific disfluency types are grouped into the categories of audible-vocalized, audible-nonvocalized, inaudible-nonvocalized, and avoidance-escape. Other categories could and should be chosen depending on the stuttering patterns exhibited by a particular client.

4. Disruption Ratios: Many possible disruption ratios are possible. The following are seen as being of primary importance.
   a. Meaningful syllables spoken per minute
   b. Moments of fluency disruption per syllable
   c. Total number of disfluency types per number of moments of disruption.
   d. The relationship among specific disfluency types per syllable
      1) audible-vocalized disruptions per syllable
      2) audible-nonvocalized disruptions per syllable
      3) inaudible-nonvocalized disruptions per syllable
      4) avoidance-escape behaviors per syllable
   e. The relationship of specific disfluency types to the total disfluency types. This shows the proportion of all disruption types accounted for by each group.
      1) audible-vocalized disruption per total disruption types
      2) audible-nonvocalized disruption per total disruption types
      3) inaudible-nonvocalized disruption per total disruption types
      4) avoidance-escape behaviors per total disruption types

Several important advantages result from the use of this measurement procedure. The major factor is that of increased precision in the systematic description, classifications, and quantifications of behaviors and behavioral intents related to stuttering. It becomes possible to

Table 1. Schematic portrayal of emotions, behaviors, and behavioral intentions related to the moment of stuttering

Preonset	Fluency disruption	Postdisruption
[a]Anticipation	[c]Disfluency	[a]Guilt
[a]Expectancy	[c]Fluency failure	[a]Humiliation
[a]Fear	[c]Stuttering	[a]Relief
[a]Negative emotion		[a]Shame
[a]Apprehension	[c]Audible-vocalized	[a]Embarrassment
[a]Anxiety	part-word repetitions	[a]Withdrawal
(etc.)	word repetitions	[a]Anxiety
	multiple word repetitions	[a]Tension reduction
[b]Avoidance	sound prolongations	[a]Hostility
[b]Postponement	[c]Audible-nonvocalized	(etc.)
[b]Disguise	part-word repetitions	
[b]Antiexpectancy	sound prolongations	
[b]Timers	disrhythmic phonations	
[b]Starters	[c]Inaudible-nonvocalized	
[c]Pauses	silent fixations of articulatory	
[c]Interjections	posture (blocking)	
[c]Word substitutions	tense pauses	
[c]Circumlocutions	[c]Struggle-escape behaviors	
[c]Bodily movements	[c]Broken words and retrials	
(etc.)	[c]Broken words and word	
	substitutions	
	[c]Recoils	
	(etc.)	

(rate changes)   holding back   speeding and tensing   (rate changes)

Adapted from Hood, 1974a.
[a]Attitudes and emotions
[b]Behavioral intentions
[c]Behavioral descriptions

Table 2. Transcript analysis of 1-minute speech sample

d   HKIA   F   kd   d   da   h   IKI   HF a
And I come from Springville Ohio and the town's ah got about five thousand

       da   I   ad I   H   d
people and it's ah got a bowling alley and ah there's a building that makes,

     LdKIL   da   d   a   it
It's m...It's the world's largest caster maker and it's called ah Corbets. And

    JH   ld   d   a   dd
then there's a-well I got one brother and that's it. I live.....[a]

Analysis of specific disruption types within moments of stuttering:
Audible-vocalized disruptions

a. part-word repetitions _H1|||_   Total _8_

b. word repetitions _____   Total _0_

c. multiple word repetitions _____   Total _0_

d. sound prolongations _HT HT ////_   Total _14_

                                                    Total _22_

Audible-nonvocalized disruptions

e. part-word repetitions _____   Total _0_

f. sound prolongations _///_   Total _3_

                                                    Total _3_

Inaudible-nonvocalized disruptions

g. hard contacts _____   Total _0_

h. silent fixations _HT_   Total _5_

                                                    Total _5_

Avoidance-escape behaviors

i. vocalized pauses and starters _HT ///_ Total _8_

j. Silent pauses _/_   Total _/_

k. Broken words, word postures, and
    recoils _////_   Total _4_

l. substitutions and circumlocations _///_ Total _3_

                                                    Total _16_

Total of all disruption types ____46____

[a]Nonmeaningful words are crossed out. Italic portions of transcript represent molar moments of stuttering. Letters above italic words represent specific disfluency types from molecular analysis.

Table 3. Example of scoring procedure based on data presented in Table 2

Client	John Smith	Clinician	Sally Jones
Task	Spontaneous speech	Date	June 12, 1972

Frequency counts
1. Number of meaningful words spoken 49
2. Number of meaningful syllables spoken. 63
3. Time duration of speaking task. 60
4. Total number of moments of disruption. 28
5. Total number of all disruption types. 46
    a. Audible-vocalized disruptions. 22
    b. Audible-nonvocalized disruptions. 3
    c. Inaudible-nonvocalized disruptions. 5
    d. Avoidance-escape behaviors. 16

Ratios of stuttering behaviors
1. Words per min 49 ; Syllables per min 63 .
2. Total moments disruption per word $28/49 = 0.57$; per syllable $28/63 = 0.44$
3. Total disruption types per word $46/49 = 0.94$; per syllable $46/63 = 0.73$
4. Total disruption types per moment of disruption $46/28 = 1.64$
5. Specific disfluency types

		Per Syllable	Per Total Disruptions
a.	Audible-vocalized	$22/63 = 0.35$	$22/46 = 0.48$
b.	Audible-nonvocalized	$3/63 = 0.05$	$3/46 = 0.07$
c.	Inaudible-nonvocalized	$5/63 = 0.08$	$5/46 = 0.11$
d.	Avoidance-escape	$16/63 = 0.25$	$16/46 = 0.35$

determine the major disfluency types that interfere with communication and the sequence in which they occur. When appropriate, certain types of disfluency may be further divided: for example, a part-word repetition with the proper coarticulation pei - pei - peipɜ or improper coarticulation of the vowel pʌ - pʌ - peipɜ. This knowledge helps the clinician to develop clinical strategies for working with the person who stutters. Because of the improved measurement precision afforded by detailed transcript analysis, a yardstick is provided against which to measure behavioral changes that occur within the course of therapy and during follow-up evaluations. Indeed, for some of our clients we have found it instructive to perform a transcript analysis on a weekly or biweekly basis in order to monitor changes in stuttering behavior (see Table 4). In addition, when the plan of therapy involves helping the client identify and confront his talking or stuttering behaviors, both the client and clinician can discuss the speech samples and transcript analyses. Often this joint inves-

Table 4. Master summary sheet of form-type disfluency analysis

	June 12[a]			June 27		
	Reading	Spontaneous	Picture	Reading	Spontaneous	Picture
Words/minute	58	49	55	157	152	133
Syllables/minute	73	63	67	199	188	154
Total disruptions/word	0.47	0.57	0.42	0.01	0.05	0.05
Total disruptions/syllable	0.37	0.44	0.34	0.01	0.04	0.04
Total disruption types/word	0.67	0.04	0.64	0.01	0.05	0.05
Total disruption types/syllable	0.53	0.73	0.52	0.01	0.04	0.04
Total disruption types/total disruptions	1.43	1.64	1.52	1.00	1.14	1.00
Per syllable disruptions						
Audible-vocalized	0.29	0.35	0.36	0.01	0.02	0.03
Audible-nonvocalized	0.09	0.05	0.07	0.00	0.00	0.01
Inaudible-nonvocalized	0.06	0.08	0.01	0.00	0.01	0.00
Avoidance-escape	0.10	0.25	0.07	0.00	0.02	0.01
Per syllable disruptions						
Audible-vocalized	0.54	0.48	0.69	1.00	0.38	0.60
Audible-nonvocalized	0.16	0.07	0.14	0.00	0.00	0.20
Inaudible-nonvocalized	0.12	0.11	0.03	0.00	0.25	0.00
Avoidance-escape	0.18	0.35	0.14	0.00	0.38	0.20

[a]Data taken from Table 2.

tigation between client and clinician provides insight for both persons involved, and helps to differentiate the behavior from the intent for which the behavior was used.

We hasten to point out that several potential drawbacks to the above mentioned procedures exist. The major problems concern the time and clinical judgements involved in classifying certain behavioral intents. For example, there are times when it is difficult to determine whether the intention of a short pause was related to linguistic encoding behavior as opposed to avoidance and postponement related to stuttering and it is sometimes difficult to determine whether the intention of such behavior represented a short silent pause or a brief, silent fixation of articulation posture. Moreover, it is sometimes difficult to distinguish between avoidance and escape behaviors because of the temporal sequencing of these behaviors; indeed, some behaviors may be used for either purpose. It is wise to follow Van Riper's advice: "When doubt arises we try only to be consistent. We count all doubtful times or none of them" (1971, p. 229). Finally, it is important to distinguish constructs that are of an explanatory nature (starters, postponements, etc.) from behaviors that are descriptive (part-word repetitions, sound prolongations, etc.).

We have found this procedure to be effective in assessing the frequency and type of behaviors emitted (Hood, 1974). Again, however, we strongly urge that the specific disfluency types be modified in order to best represent the behaviors typically evidenced by a particular stutterer. Further, we recommend that the clinician compare the results obtained with the normative data currently available (Johnson, 1961a, b; Johnson et al., 1963; Silverman, 1974b). A brief summary of other assessment procedures is presented in Table 5.

Assessment of Stuttering as a Problem for Children

If it becomes apparent that a child is aware that something is "different" or "wrong" with his way of talking, we attempt to get to the nature of these concerns. In some cases they are vague and undifferentiated; in others, they are clear and specific. One way we do this is through the use of projective questioning (Hood, 1970). We find that children generally reveal a good deal of information about themselves, but we are extremely cautious with our interpretations. We use them only as leads for future follow-up; we are reluctant to draw strong conclusions until we have additional information.

Aspects of self concept It is essential that greater efforts be made to understand the total child and how he relates to the significant

Table 5. Selected methods for the assessment of stuttering

Author	Reference source	Brief description
Ammons and Johnson	The Iowa Scale of Attitudes Toward Stuttering (Johnson et al., 1963).	Designed to determine the person's tolerance or intolerance for stuttering. Composed of 45 statements about stutterers and stuttering and how people should/should not feel about them.
Brutten and Shoemaker	Behavior Checklist (Brutten and Shoemaker, 1974b).	Behavior checklist comprised of 97 specific behaviors considered to be adjustive responses used either to avoid stuttering before its occurrence or to escape from it during its occurrence. Different forms for children and adults.
Brutten and Shoemaker	Speech Situation Checklist (Brutten and Shoemaker, 1974a).	Determines stutterers emotional reactions and degree of speech interruption on a 1–5 scale for 51 different speaking situations. Different forms available for children and adults.
Brutten and Shoemaker	Southern Illinois Modification of the Fear Survey Schedule (Brutten and Shoemaker, 1974c).	Determines degrees of emotional arousal for states of general, rather than speech-specific, emotionality. Subjects rate the degree of perceived emotionality on a 5-point scale. Different forms for children and adults.
Cooper	Cooper Chronicity Prediction Checklist for School-aged Stutterers (Cooper, 1973).	Designed to determine which children might spontaneously recover from stuttering. Clinician indicates response to 27 questions of chronicity in terms of historic, attitudinal, and behavioral indicators.
Cooper	Personalized Fluency Control Therapy: An Integrated Behavior for Relationship Therapy for Stutterers (Cooper, 1976).	Presents many useful forms to aid the clinician in assessment: 1) Stuttering Attitudes Checklist, 2) Situation Avoidance Checklist, 3) Concomitant Stuttering Behavior Checklist, 4)

	Stuttering Frequency and Duration Estimate Record, 5) Parent Attitudes Toward Stuttering Checklist, 6) Client and Clinician Perception of Stuttering Severity Ratings, 7) Longitudinal Stuttering Assessment Summary Sheet, 8) Fluency Analysis Checklist, and 10) Client Readiness for Fluency Control Inventory.
Erickson	Assessing Communication Attitudes Among Stutterers (Erickson, 1969).	Presents a 39-item severity scale based on true-false statements differentiating stutterers from nonstutterers. Also presents 28 adjectives that differentiate self-descriptions of severe versus mild stutterers.
Griffith	Uses of the Sheehan Sentence Completion Test in Speech Therapy for Stutterers (Griffith, 1969).	Stutterer completes 80 ambiguous sentence stems related to feelings and attitudes toward self, aspects of speaking situations, interpersonal relationships, and levels of conflict. Griffith suggests scoring in terms of: feelings toward others, emotional states and attitudes, stuttering or speaking behavior, family relationships, and miscellaneous concepts.
Johnson	Iowa Scale for Rating Severity of Stuttering (Johnson, 1963).	Presents a 7-point scale for the rating of stuttering severity.
Lanyon	The Measurement of Stuttering Severity (Lanyon, 1967).	64 true-false statements relative to the stutterer's behaviors and attitudes are answered.
Luper and Mulder	Stuttering: Diagnostic and Evaluative Checklist (Luper and Mulder, 1964).	Presents an evaluation form for use in case history and parent interview.
Riley	A Stuttering Severity Instrument for Children and Adults (Riley, 1972).	Assessment of three parameters: frequency, duration, and physical concomitant behaviors. Ratings are made for each parameter. Results in global rating of severity.

—continued

Table 5—*continued*

Author	Reference source	Brief description
Ryan	Table III: Types of Disfluencies and Stuttered Words and Examples (Ryan, 1974).	Lists nine types of disfluency, five of which are believed to represent normal disfluency and four of which are believe to represent stuttered words.
Ryan	Pre-School/Primary Form of the Stuttering Interview (Ryan, 1974).	Allows assessment of stuttered words per minute in various speech tasks: automatic, echoic, reading, picture naming, speaking alone, speaking with puppet, monolog, giving commands, talking while gesturing, speech competition, saying difficult words, speaking rapidly, talking while drawing, answering questions, telephoning, conversing, and observations in a natural setting.
Shames and Egolf	Operant Conditioning and the Management of Stuttering (Table 3.1. Suggested Occasions and Tactics for Evaluating Stuttering.) (Shames and Egolf, 1976).	Suggests tactics to use in sampling speech behavior under the following conditions: variations in audience size, talking to various people, different situations, competition for talking time, differing lengths of utterance, various topics of conversation, states of emotional excitement, social and verbal interactions, linguistic units and functions, and time pressure.
Sheehan, Cortese, and Hadley	Guilt, Shame, and Tension in Projections of Stuttering (Sheehan et al., 1962).	Describes a projective technique based on the stutterer's drawings representative of his behavior just before, during, and after a

Shumak	A Speech Situation Rating Sheet for Stutterers (Shumak, 1955).

moment of stuttering. Suggests method of viewing stuttering in terms of tension, shame-humiliation, sadness-dejection, and guilt. Stutterers rank 40 speaking situations in terms of how frequently they would be in them, how severely they would stutter, emotional reactions toward the situation and extent to which they would try to avoid the situation.

Van Riper	Profile of Stuttering Severity (Van Riper, 1971).

Presents a 7-point rating scale for each of the following components: frequency, tension-struggle, duration, and postponement-avoidance.

Van Riper	Guidelines for Differentiating Normal and Abnormal Disfluency (Van Riper, 1971).

Within the nominal categories of syllable repetitions, prolongations, gaps, phonation, articulatory postures, reactions to stress, and evidence of awareness, 26 features that may differentiate stuttering from normal disfluency are presented.

Woolf	Perceptions of Stuttering Inventory (Woolf, 1967).

In response to 60 items, the stutterer indicates those that are currently indicative of his current attitudes or behaviors. Items are equally divided among struggle, avoidance, and expectancy.

people in his environment. To work solely with the overt communicative behaviors may eliminate from consideration certain associated variables critical to an optimum therapeutic outcome. The child lives as part of a family unit. As a member of the family he is assigned, or assumes, certain roles: big brother, daddy's little boy, family brat, baby-talker, stutter-box, and others. The child's perception of self within the family constellation and the perceptions of the child by his parents and siblings is often an important correlate to therapeutic success or failure. Is the child loved and respected, overprotected, merely tolerated, or totally left to himself? What is the relationship between the child's communicative and other behaviors? What is the child's degree of self-understanding? Are the child's perceptions congruent with those of other members of the family? Moreover, these same questions should be asked concerning the child's relationships with peers and teachers at school and with children in the neighborhood.

The Draw Your Family Test (Machover, 1951) has been suggested as one means of tapping the nature of family relationships and the child's perception of self within the family. The child is told to "Draw me a picture of your family; be sure to include yourself. After you have finished your drawing we can talk about the people who live at home with you." The child completes his drawing on a plain white sheet of paper, using a pencil that has an eraser. As the child draws, the clinician makes note of such things as the order in which the persons are drawn, the care taken in the drawing, the size relationships among people, which persons are next to each other, those members who seem to be most/least dominant, characteristics of orderliness, perfection, attention to detail, and the closeness among members. Does the family seem to be united or distant, happy or unhappy, friendly or unfriendly? From the drawing the clinician begins to generate hypotheses for further inquiry. The clinician may use the child's drawing as a springboard to gather additional information. The family picture may serve as a stimulus about which the child can generate a story. The child may be asked to tell a story about each of the people in the picture. The child can be asked to clarify, expand, or further explain the story or the relationships that he perceives to exist among the people involved. Specific questions may be asked such that both positive and negative valences are tapped. Representative questions might include some of the following:

Of all the people in your family, including yourself, which person would you most like to be? Why?

Of all the people in your family, including yourself, which person would you least like to be? Why?

Of all the people in your family, including yourself, which person would most like you to change the way you talk? Why?

Of all the people in your family, including yourself, which person would least like you to change your speech? Why?

Of all the people in your family, which other person do you most like to be with? Why?

Of all the people in your family, which other person do you least like to be with? Why?

What is the very best thing you can think of about each person in your family?

What is the very worst thing you can think of about each person in your family?

If you could change just one thing about each person in your family, what would you change? Why?

If each other person in your family could change just one thing about you, what would they change? Why?

If you overheard the other persons in your family talking about you behind your back, what kinds of things do you think they would be saying? Why?

If you overheard the other persons in your family talking about you behind your back, what kinds of things would you like them to be saying? Why?

The working hypotheses gathered from this procedure may be further explored in therapy. Moreover, a comparison of the perception of the child, as compared and contrasted to the perception of the parent(s) yields further hypotheses for consideration and use in parental or child counseling.

In addition, we sometimes develop our own incomplete sentence stems and ask the child to complete the message. "Now, Billy, let's have this boy make up some sentences. I'll begin the sentences and I want you to finish them. Ready, O.K. then, here we go." Examples of our sentence stems include the following: "My mommy likes to _____, but she doesn't like to _____." "My daddy (sister, brother, teacher, etc.) likes to _____, but he doesn't like to _____." "It's good to make people _____, but it's bad to make people _____." "The best thing about me is _____, but the worst thing about me is _____." A variation on the above themes is to ask the following three questions. "Suppose you heard your family talking about you when they didn't know you could hear them. What do you think they would be saying? What would you not like for them to be saying? What are the very best things they could be saying?"

Things to be changed We all have a real, as well as ideal, self-concept, and for all of us there is something we would like to change. We ask, "Suppose I were a magical person and could change three things about you. What would you like me to change?" Other variations include: "If you could change three things about (your mother, your father, your sister or brother, teacher, etc.) what would you change? If your (mother, father, sister, brother, teacher, etc.) could change three things about you, what do you think they would change?"

Before proceeding, let us stress that we never let this projective probing seem like a test. We space the questions across several sessions, and generally attempt to insert them as "fillers" within the other activities. We attempt to minimize potential defensiveness.

Aspects concerning the environment We want to know how the child relates to his environment. What are his perceptions about home, his playmates, the classroom? Many of these will be tapped by responses to other questions. When they are not, additional time is spent probing.

Aspects of speaking We ask the child to describe his way of talking and to tell us the good and bad things about the way he talks. We probe gently into his awareness of situations that he finds more or less difficult, and we ask him why he believes this to be the case. We try hard to differentiate what the child believes and what the child has been told by others that he should believe. Has the child identified persons, places, or situations as stressful? If so, what are they? We want to know if the child ever does "special things" to help him talk more easily, and if so, what they are. We ask if other people have reacted to his way of talking and if so, how.

Potential secondary gain and the problem of avoidance For some children who are aware of their problem, we need to determine factors related to secondary gain and avoidance. Is the child either forced into or excluded from activities? At the age of 6, Brian told us that he did not have to bring anything for Show and Tell "because I stutter and don't have to do that." If the child is beginning to use his speech as a tool for secondary gain or avoidance, we need to know this in order to plan for therapy.

The child's use of language We wholeheartedly agree with Williams (1957, 1971) that the child's use of language is of critical importance. Does the child feel that he "has a stutter" or does he believe that he behaves in certain ways that interfere with the process of talking?

Does the child view the problem as a mysterious "it" that happens, or does he feel it is something he does? In therapy, we attempt to use the language of self-responsibility (see Williams, 1971).

Parental perceptions of the child We spend much time determining how the parents perceive the child and how they would ideally like to perceive the child; that is, to what extent the child is meeting parental expectations. We are impressed by the fact that much communicative pressure results from situations in which the child is acting in ways that run counter to what the parents desire. This is even more true with older children and adolescents. Let us give one brief example and discuss means of tapping this important consideration.

When we first began working with Kelly, he was 11 years old. It was obvious that the parents did not condone many of his behaviors. When asked to describe him, the parent were emphatic: He is a slob—his room is always a mess; he is always late—he is never home for dinner on time; he is lazy—he never does anything to help. In addition to working with Kelly on his talking/stuttering behavior, we devised a behavior modification program in which he earned points for cleaning his room, being home on time, and helping around the home. We believe his improvement in therapy was related less to the direct speech work than to helping Kelly behave in ways that earned more parental acceptance and praise. We use concepts derived from use of the semantic differential to aid us in assessing parent-child relationships.

The semantic differential (Osgood et al., 1957) is a measuring instrument designed to assess variations in attitudes toward constructs. Typically, the differential consists of a series of interval scales separating bipolar adjectives. In recent years the semantic differential has been used as a research tool to evaluate differences in similar groups for different constructs (i.e., clinicians' rating of stutterers and nonstutterers) or different groups for similar constructs (i.e., speech clinicians' and lay peoples' rating of stutterers.) Our purpose is not to review the research that has been conducted using the semantic differential. Numerous sources are available for the interested reader (Hansen, 1964; Jakobovits, 1966; Fisher, 1968; Tracy, 1974; Woods and Williams, 1976). Our purpose is, however, to point out the potential use of adjective scales for the description of attitudes toward individual persons who stutter. This is particularly important since recent investigations have indicated that people generally hold negative stereotypes toward persons who stutter (Erickson, 1968; Yairi and

Williams, 1970; Woods and Williams, 1971; Erickson, 1968; Tracy, 1974; Woods and Williams, 1976). Based on the above research, it is likely that significant adults in the child's environment react, both overtly and covertly, in ways that might be tapped using adjective scales constructed in a manner similar to the format of the semantic differential. We list in Table 6 a procedure that we shall soon begin to use at our clinic (We have always used the concepts. We are now attempting to be more systematic). We make no pretense that it will be of great value, although it does seem to have high face validity. The attempt is to combine the Q-technique (Stephenson, 1953) with the semantic differential in order to determine the real and ideal attitudes of significant adults toward the stuttering child. Various significant adults can be asked to complete two adjective checklists: the first section asks that they describe the way they perceive the child now; the second asks that they describe how they would ideally like the child to be.

The concepts involved in the 20 adjectives are actually things that we have routinely dealt with during the parent interview and counseling sessions. Our purpose will now be to use this form as part of the pre-evaluation questionnaire. In addition, we shall have this form completed by a number of different significant adults who have contact with the child. The reason for this is severalfold: First, we will want to look for similarities and differences among the respondents. In cases of disagreement, we will then want to determine the source of difference. Is the child, in fact, "different" when he interacts with various people, or is the child actually "similar" but perceived differently? Second, we will want to use this to determine behavioral change that occurs over time. Finally, we plan to further develop and standardize this instrument for potential use as a diagnostic tool.

THE CASE HISTORY, INTERVIEWING, AND COUNSELING

Many volumes have been devoted to taking the case history, interviewing informants and providing counseling (Murphy and FitzSimons, 1960; Johnson et al., 1963; Emerick, 1966). These topics could involve several separate chapters. Consequently, we wish only to highlight some of the major considerations involved.

The Case History

We attempt to determine the developmental history by means of various pre-evaluation instruments and personal interviews. Let us

Table 6. Assessment of perceptions of general personality traits

Name of person making this evaluation _____ Date _____
Name of person being evaluated _____ Relationship of person making this evaluation to person being described (parent, teacher, grandparent, etc.) _____ .

Listed below are a number of adjectives commonly used to describe people. Please indicate the extent to which you agree or disagree that the person being described is similar or dissimilar to the adjective, by circling the appropriate letter. Register your answer according to the following scale.

A = Definitely Agree
a = Somewhat Agree
? = Undecided
d = Somewhat Disagree
D = Definitely Disagree

Complete your rating twice. For the adjectives listed at the left, describe the way the person is at the present time. For the adjectives listed to the right, indicate the way you would ideally like this person to be.

		What the person is now					What you would like the person to be in the future				
1.	Outgoing	A	a	?	d	D	A	a	?	d	D
2.	Talkative	A	a	?	d	D	A	a	?	d	D
3.	Cooperative	A	a	?	d	D	A	a	?	d	D
4.	Excitable	A	a	?	d	D	A	a	?	d	D
5.	Anxious	A	a	?	d	D	A	a	?	d	D
6.	Nervous	A	a	?	d	D	A	a	?	d	D
7.	Sensitive	A	a	?	d	D	A	a	?	d	D
8.	Pleasant	A	a	?	d	D	A	a	?	d	D
9.	Perfectionistic	A	a	?	d	D	A	a	?	d	D
10.	Secure	A	a	?	d	D	A	a	?	d	D
11.	Fearful	A	a	?	d	D	A	a	?	d	D
12.	Self-conscious	A	a	?	d	D	A	a	?	d	D
13.	Relaxed	A	a	?	d	D	A	a	?	d	D
14.	Confident	A	a	?	d	D	A	a	?	d	D
15.	Spontaneous	A	a	?	d	D	A	a	?	d	D
16.	Awkward	A	a	?	d	D	A	a	?	d	D
17.	Quiet	A	a	?	d	D	A	a	?	d	D
18.	Shy	A	a	?	d	D	A	a	?	d	D
19.	Timid	A	a	?	d	D	A	a	?	d	D
20.	Expressive	A	a	?	d	D	A	a	?	d	D
21.	Athletic	A	a	?	d	D	A	a	?	d	D
22.	Artistic	A	a	?	d	D	A	a	?	d	D
23.	Thoughtful	A	a	?	d	D	A	a	?	d	D
24.	Hard working	A	a	?	d	D	A	a	?	d	D
25.	Intelligent	A	a	?	d	D	A	a	?	d	D

stress at the outset that it is both with enthusiasm and skepticism that we make use of currently available instruments. We are enthusiastic because they provide us with general information of potential importance. We accept the information with reluctance, however, and are always careful to compare and contrast it with our own perceptions. Informants cannot be relied upon to have clear recollections of historical events, and to be valid in their interpretation of them. Moreover, our own judgments, perceptions, and interpretations are subject to error. Just as there is no clear distinction to be drawn between "assessment" and "treatment'" so too there is no way of knowing when the full history has been taken. We continue to gather background information throughout the course of treatment. Our major concern is with those aspects of psychosocial, emotional, intellectual, communicative, and "general" development that might serve as predisposing, precipitating, and maintaining agents. Our ultimate goal is to integrate the information received, determine those components that are relevant, and make decisions regarding appropriate methods for clinical intervention. Let us sketch below some of our general procedures, but before doing so, let us emphasize that we are flexible and make variations when appropriate.

Pre-evaluation information We typically ask that the following information be completed before scheduling the initial evaluation session. For children suspected of being in Stages I or II (Van Riper, 1963) the parents complete the children's form of the stuttering information sheet, the descriptions of stuttering checksheet and the release of information forms. We usually obtain additional information regarding the child's physical and academic status from the physician and classroom teacher. For persons suspected of being in Stages III or IV (Van Riper, 1963) we request completion of either the child or adult form of the stuttering information sheet, the Speech Situation Checklist (Brutten and Shoemaker, 1974a) and the Behavior Checklist (Brutten and Shoemaker, 1974b), as well as relevant academic and medical information. Although we often use the Sheehan Sentence Completion Test (Griffith, 1969), the Fear Survey Schedule (Brutten and Shoemaker, 1974c), the Iowa Scale of Attitude Toward Stuttering and the Stutterer's Self-Ratings of Reactions to Speech Situations (Johnson et al., 1963), we tend not to give these until after several sessions of diagnostic therapy have been completed.

The initial interviews We view the initial interviews as extremely important in the establishment of a positive working relationship. We use the time to clarify information provided on the pre-evaluation forms, to expand and clarify the issues involved, and generally to get a better appreciation for both the person and his behavior. To reiterate a point raised earlier, the clinician plays the role of Sherlock Holmes and does a lot of detective work. Rather than elaborate, let us again simply state that the clinician must have a firm understanding of the various theories of stuttering, the nature of stuttering as both a problem and behavior, and awareness of many approaches to treatment, for it is against this framework that the assessment is based. Our task will have several separate yet overlapping components: obtaining information, determining the significance of the information obtained, providing information, giving support and encouragement, and making direct suggestions.

It has been our observation that beginning clinicians are typically "overly nice and polite." They are concerned about the establishment of rapport, and as such, often only skirt the important issues. As one beginning graduate student said, "I guess my problem is that I'm just the easy going Marcus Welby type. I forget that he can be a real s.o.b. at times without losing a good relationship." Rapport means far more than just the fact that the client or parents like us; rather, it means that we are working systematically to alleviate a disorder. We are both gentle and firm, permissive and dogmatic, condoning and condemning. We are, in fact, behavior modifiers. We can be sensitive and helpful, honest and truthful; we must learn when to make a statement and when to refrain, when to come on strongly and when to back off, and when to honestly admit that we do not know. (See Emerick and Hood, 1974, for related philosophical considerations.)

We invite the client or parents to join us in our detective work, for the assessment and treatment of stuttering represents a team approach. As Van Riper has pointed out, we cannot assume motivation and there will most certainly be resistance to overcome (1973). In so doing, we reject the use of first and third person singular. Statements such as "*I* would like for you to tell *me* about ..." are commonly made. The implication is that "*I* want you to tell *me*, so that *I* can tell *you* what to do." This adversary relationship if often counterproductive. Both by word and tone, we stress the first person plural. "Why don't *we* talk a bit about Johnny so the jointly *we* can come to better understand him, and determine some things that might be helpful."

Counseling

With respect to therapy, our goals are to determine and subsequently minimize those factors that precipitate and maintain the disorder, to help the person to cope with situations that for some reason cannot be minimized, and to teach the person adaptive ways to modify his speaking behavior. Obviously, the specific procedures will depend upon the client's age, intelligence, perceptivity, motivation, and severity. We take the position that interviewing and counseling are closely related and not clearly separable. We now wish to briefly present a model for interviewing and counseling that has proved to be extremely helpful. It is based on Brutten and Shoemaker's Two-Factor theory of stuttering (1967). Brutten and Shoemaker view stuttering as a form of fluency failure that is the involuntary consequence of negative emotion. Stuttering is defined as part-word repetitions and prolongations; other behaviors are viewed as instrumental acts to avoid or escape stuttering. Brutten has taken the position that the antecedents to fluency failure/stuttering are at the crux of the problem, and has recommended deconditioning and counterconditioning procedures as bases for treatment. Brutten has argued that children are normally fluent, and are so during 950/1,000 words spoken. Johnson, on the other hand, argued that children are normally disfluent, and are so at the rate of 50/1,000 spoken (1961a). Whereas Brutten would tend to work to eliminate the negative antecedent conditions that elicit involuntary fluency failure, Johnson stressed the need to ensure that significant listeners not mislabel the otherwise normal nonfluency. We choose not to take sides in this debate because we feel that each issue has strong evidence in its favor. Rather, we wish to present a modification of the Brutten and Shoemaker model, and ask the reader to consider its application to both the interview and counseling aspects of treatment.

Table 7 presents the model we use in parent interviewing and counseling, adapted from Brutten and Shoemaker. The reader not familiar with this position is strongly encouraged to study chapters 1 and 2 of *The Modification of Stuttering* (1967). We do not use the model in a theoretical sense, and we avoid all reference to the underlying concepts of respondent and instrumental conditioning. Our purpose is to help the person visualize and conceptualize relationships. By drawing the model and explaining it in general, nonprofessional terms, we find ourselves better able to focus our attention on critical relationships and interactions. Often, this model helps people to determine positive, neutral and negative aspects of speaking situations, types of talking/stuttering behavior, as well as the adaptive and mal-

Table 7. A model for interviewing and counseling

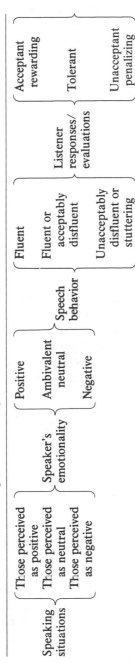

Speaking situations	Speaker's emotionality	Speech behavior	Listener responses/ evaluations
Those perceived as positive	Positive	Fluent	Acceptant rewarding
Those perceived as neutral	Ambivalent neutral	Fluent or acceptably disfluent	Tolerant
Those perceived as negative	Negative	Unacceptably disfluent or stuttering	Unacceptant penalizing

1. The clinician explains and discusses the following:
    "In situations perceived as positive, the speaker tends to respond with positive emotionality. His verbal output is fluent and listener responses are favorable. Situations perceived as negative result in negative emotionality, are usually accompanied by increased fluency disruptions and unfavorable listener reactions."

2. The clinician and interviewee explore potentially significant relationships.
    "Let's talk about Scott. Let's try to identify some of the favorable and unfavorable speaking situations he faces, how you think he feels about them, the various different ways he speaks, and the various types of reactions he receives from different listeners."

3. The clinician and informant explore means for changing harmful environmental influences.
    "Now that we have identified some of the negative factors, let's examine some possible ways to confront them and improve upon them. For example, you indicated that the dinner hour is particularly chaotic, with everyone trying to speak at the same time. What are some ways we might deal with this?"

4. The clinician and informant explore the significance of different types of speech behaviors.
    "We need to realize that different types of disfluency mean different things. There is an important distinction to be made between easy, effortless and infrequent repetitions of words and phrases, and revisions that are a part of the thought process and language formulation, as opposed to physical tension associated with sound and syllable repetitions, and when Scott 'freezes' on sounds. There are qualitatively different. Let's explore how the type of disfluency is related to the situation in which Scott is talking, and how listeners are apt to react to him."

adaptive aspects of how the speaker feels in a particular situation and how listeners react to the speech output. Although the model is far from perfect, it helps the clinician, client, and parents to sharpen their detective skills.

Based on the information we obtain through the pre-evaluation forms completed by the client or informants, and the information gathered during the initial interviews and during treatment, we attempt to determine the relationships between the situations the child enters, how he feels, how he talks, and how others react. Based on this, we attempt to minimize the negative and maximize the positive speaking situations, desensitize the person to negative feelings about the situation, and improve the reactions of listeners to the way the child is talking. With youngsters who manifest developmental nonfluencies we work directly with general language and communication skills, but not with the disfluency. With older children, we do work directly with the overt stuttering.

In Table 1 we listed numerous behaviors and attitudes related to stuttering. We attempt to relate these to the concepts presented in Table 7. Our task is to determine from the client or his family (or teacher, peers, etc.) the critical relationships that are involved. Examples of stressful speaking situations that might be associated with negative feelings can often be determined from the Speech Situation Checklist and Iowa Scales. Others might be determined through interviewing. Examples of talking that is considered better than average might include only occasional fluency disruptions in the form of phrase and word repetitions. Examples of talking that is considered worse than average might include disruptions in the form of tense pauses, disrhythmic phonations, and triple-unit part-word repetitions. Examples of good listener reactions might include people who are attentive and pay attention; bad reactions might include interruption, contradiction, and loss of listener attention.

In closing, let us make one final observation. We have found it extremely useful to conduct our interviewing and counseling from behind a one-way mirror. When the parent or parents watch their child working with a clinician, they tend to observe things relevant to the discussion at hand. They are often able to be more objective about their child and often perceive cause-effect relationships more clearly. Observation of a skilled clinician teaches more than a hurried 2-minute summary as parent and child leave the confines of a busy waiting room.

CONCLUDING THOUGHTS

Assessment is an ongoing process. People change, and so do behaviors and problems. The issues involved in diagnosis and assessment hinge upon the ability to compare and contrast who the person is, how the person feels, and how the person talks, to what the person was and what the person might ultimately become. Therefore, the clinician must ask and answer many significant questions. Of paramount importance is the ability of the clinician to perceive changes that occur during the process of therapy. Whatever "truths" result from the assessment process, they are at best tentative and subject to change.

> The therapy process doesn't really start with the clinician's decision to start therapy. So far as the child is concerned, the therapist's attitude, his special knowledge, his insights, and the way he reacts to the child's stuttering have an impact on the child and his frame of mind. Indeed, therapy has started during the diagnosis even though the first "therapy session" may not yet have been scheduled. (Luper and Mulder, 1964, p. 34)

ACKNOWLEDGMENTS

Appreciation is extended to present and past students who have contributed in so many ways to the assessment procedures discussed in this chapter, especially in developing the procedures used for determining the overt molecular analysis: Joseph Stigora, Robert Kroll, Michael Curran, Williams Haynes, Gordon Blood, Christine Perry, Kristen Kaylor, Cynthia Norbut, Karen Tracy, and Candice Hudson. Gratitude is extended to John Johnson, Marilynn Wentland, William Haynes, Michael Curran, and Gordon Blood for reading and critiquing portions of the manuscript. Very special appreciation is extended to Janet Watson, Gerri Nagy, and Marilyn Slatton for typing the various drafts of the manuscript.

REFERENCES

Ammons, R., and Johnson, W. 1944. The Iowa Scale of Attitudes Toward Stuttering. In: W. Johnson, F. Darley, and D. Spriestersbach, Diagnostic Methods in Speech Pathology. Harper & Row, Publishers, New York.
Andrews, G., and Harris, M. 1964. The Syndrome of Stuttering. Heinemann Ltd., London.
Beech, H., and Fransella, F. 1968. Research and Experiment in Stuttering. Pergamon Press, New York.

Blood, G. 1976. Comparison of the effect of difficulty of reading material on disfluencies in the oral reading of stuttering and nonstuttering children. Unpublished thesis, Bowling Green State University.

Bloodstein, O. 1960a. The development of stuttering: I. Changes in nine basic features. J. Speech Hear. Disord. 25:219–237.

Bloodstein, O. 1960b. The development of stuttering: II. Developmental phases. J. Speech Hear. Disord. 25:366–376.

Bloodstein, O. 1961. The development of stuttering: III. Theoretical and clinical implications. J. Speech Hear. Disord. 26:67–82.

Bloodstein, O. 1975. A Handbook on Stuttering. National Easter Seal Society for Crippled Children and Adults, Chicago.

Bluemel, C. 1935. Stammering and Allied Disorders. The Macmillan Company, New York.

Boehmler, R. 1958. Listener responses to non-fluencies. J. Speech Hear. Res. 1:132–141.

Brutten, G., and Shoemaker, D. 1967. The Modification of Stuttering. Prentice-Hall Inc., Englewood Cliffs, New Jersey.

Brutten, G., and Shoemaker, D. 1974a. Speech Situation Checklist. Southern Illinois University, Carbondale.

Brutten, G., and Shoemaker, D. 1974b. Behavior Checklist. Soutern Illinois University, Carbondale.

Brutten, G., and Shoemaker, D. 1974c. The Southern Illinois Modification of the Geer Fear Survey Schedule. Southern Illinois University, Carbondale.

Brutten, G. 1975. Stuttering: Topography, assessment, and behavioral change strategies. In: J. Eisenson (ed.), Stuttering: A Second Symposium, pp. 199–262. Harper & Row, Publishers, New York.

Bryngelson, B. 1938. Prognosis in stuttering. J. Speech Disord. 3:121–123.

Cooper, E. 1973. The development of a stuttering chronicity prediction checklist: a preliminary report. J. Speech Hear. Disord. 38:215–223.

Cooper, E. 1976. Personalized Fluency Control Therapy: An Integrated Behavior for Relationship Therapy for Stutterers. Learning Concepts, Inc., Austin, Texas.

Cowan, R., Weber, J., Hoddinott, B., and Klein, J. 1967. Mean length of spoken responses as a function of stimulus, experimenter and subject. Child Dev. 38:191–208.

Davis, D. 1940. The relation of repetitions in the speech of young children to certain measures of language maturity and situational factors. Parts 2 & 3. J. Speech Disord. 5:235–246.

Douglass, E. 1954. The development of stuttering and its diagnosis. Can. Med. Assoc. J. 71:366–371.

Douglass, E., and Quarrington, B. 1952. The differentiation of interiorized and exteriorized secondary stuttering. J. Speech Hear. Disord. 17:377–385.

Eisenson, J. (ed.). 1975. Stuttering: A Second Symposium. Harper & Row, Publishers, New York.

Emerick, L. 1966. The Parent Interview. The Interstate Printers & Publishers, Inc., Danville, Illinois.

Emerick, L., and Hatten, J. 1974. Diagnosis and Evaluation in Speech Pathology. Prentice-Hall Inc., Englewood Cliffs, New Jersey.

Emerick, L., and Hood, S. (eds.). 1974. The Client-Clinician Relationship: Essays in Interpersonal Sensitivity. Charles C Thomas, Publisher, Springfield, Illinois.

Emerick, C. 1970. Language performance of stuttering and nonstuttering children. Unpublished doctoral dissertation. The University of Iowa.

Erickson, R. 1969. Assessing communication attitudes among stutterers. J. Speech Hear. Res. 12:711–724.

Fisher, M. 1968. The anal-obsessive structure of the stutterer and its effect upon meaning. Dis. Abstr. 28:4745B.

Freund, H. 1966. Psychopathology and the Problem of Stuttering. Charles C Thomas, Publisher, Springfield, Illinois.

Giolas, T., and Williams, D. 1958. Children's reactions to nonfluencies in adult speech. J. Speech Hear. Res. 1:86–93.

Griffith, F. 1969. Uses of the Sheehan Sentence Completion Test in speech therapy for stuttering. J. Speech Hear. Disord. 34:342–349.

Hansen, R. 1964. A study of self-concepts of stutterers as measured by the semantic differential test. Unpublished thesis, Michigan State University.

Haynes, W. 1976. Disfluency changes as a function of systematic modification of linguistic complexity in children. Unpublished doctoral dissertation. Bowling Green State University, Bowling Green, Ohio.

Haynes, W., and Hood, S. 1977. An investigation of linguistic and fluency variables in nonstuttering children from discrete chronological age groups. J. Fluency Disord. In Press.

Hood, S. 1970. Projective testing in speech pathology. Ohio J. Speech Hear. 5:145–151.

Hood, S. 1969. Investigation of the effect of communicative stress on the audible, inaudible and avoidance-escape components of stuttering. Doctoral dissertation. University of Wisconsin, Madison.

Hood, S. 1974a. Clinical assessment of the moment of stuttering. J. Fluency Disord. 1:22–34.

Hood, S. 1974b. Effect of communicative stress on the frequency and form-type of disfluent behavior in adult stutterers. J. Fluency Disord. 1:38–51.

Hood, S., and Stigora, J. 1972. Perceptions of stuttering severity based on auditory, visual and auditory-visual cues. Presented at the American Speech and Hearing Association National Convention.

Jakobovits, L. 1966. Utilization of semantic satiation in stuttering: A theoretical analysis. J. Speech Hear. Disord. 31:105–114.

Johnson, W., and associates. 1959. The Onset of Stuttering. University of Minnesota Press, Minneapolis.

Johnson, W. 1961a. Measurements of oral reading and speaking rate and disfluency of adult male and female stutterers and nonstutterers. J. Speech Hear. Disord. Monogr. Suppl. 7:1–20.

Johnson, W. 1961b. Stuttering and What You Can Do About It. The Interstate Printers & Publishers, Inc., Danville, Illinois.

Johnson, W. 1963. Iowa Scale for Rating Severity of Stuttering. In: W. Johnson, F. Darley, and D. Spriestersbach, Diagnostic Methods in Speech Pathology. Harper & Row, Publishers, New York.

Johnson, W., Darley, F., and Spriestersbach, D. 1963. Diagnostic Methods in Speech Pathology. Harper & Row, Publishers, New York.

Kroll, R. and Hood, S. 1974. Differences in stuttering adaptation in oral reading and spontaneous speech. J. Commun. Disord. 7:227-237.

Kroll, R., and Hood, S. 1976. The influence of task presentation and information load on the adaption effect in stutterers and normal speakers. J. Commun. Disord. 9:95-110.

Lanyon, R. 1967. The measurement of stuttering severity. J. Speech Hear. Res. 10:836-843.

Lee, L. 1974. Developmental Sentence Analysis. Northwestern University Press, Evanston, Illinois.

Longhurst, T., and Grubb, S. 1974. A comparison of language samples collected in four situations. Lang. Speech Hear. Serv. Schools, 5:71-78.

Luper, H. 1959. Relative severity of stuttering rating from visual and auditory presentation of the same speech samples. South. Speech J. 25:107-114.

Luper, H., and Mulder, R. 1964. Stuttering Therapy for Children. Prentice-Hall Inc., Englewood Cliffs, New Jersey.

Machover, K. 1951. Drawing of the human figure: a method of personality investigation. In: H. Anderson and G. Anderson (eds.), An introduction to Projective Techniques.

McCarthy, D. 1929. A comparison of children's language in different situations and its relations to personality traits. J. Genet. Psychol. 36:583-591.

Minifie, F., Darley, F. and Sherman, D. 1963. Temporal reliability of seven language measures. J. Speech Hear. Res. 6:139-149.

Mintun, S. 1968. A preliminary investigation of certain procedures for eliciting varbalizations in EmH children. Unpublished thesis, Eastern Illinois University.

Mowrer, D. 1975. Stuttering: An Overview. Audio-Tape Lecture Series. Ideas, Tempe, Arizona.

Muma, J. 1971. Syntax of preschool fluent and disfluent speech: a transformational analysis. J. Speech Hear. Res. 14:428-441.

Murphy, A., and FitzSimons, R. 1960. Stuttering and Personality Dynamics. The Ronald Press Company, New York.

Osgood, C., Succi, J., and Tannenbaum, P. 1957. The Measurement of Meaning. University of Illinois Press, Urbana, Illinois.

Perry, C. 1975. The effect of difficulty of reading material on the disfluencies in the oral reading of nonstuttering children. Unpublished thesis. Bowling Green State University, Bowling Green, Ohio.

Prins, D. 1968. Pretherapy adaptation of stuttering and its relation to speech measures of therapy progress, J. Speech Hear. Res. 11:740-746.

Prins, D., and Lohr, F. 1968. A study of the behavioral components of stuttered speech. United States Department of Health, Education and Welfare. Office of Education, Bureau of Research. Final Report, Project No 6-2382, Grant No. OEG-3-6-062382-1882.

Riley, G. 1972. A stuttering severity instrument for children and adults. J. Speech Hear. Disord. 37:314-320.

Ryan, B. 1974. Programmed Therapy for Stuttering in Children and Adults. Charles C Thomas, Publisher, Springfield, Illinois.

Sander, E. 1965. Comments on investigating listener responses to speech disfluency. J. Speech Hear. Disord. 30:159–165.

Schlesinger, I., Forte, M. Fried, B., and Melkman, R. 1965. Stuttering, information load, and response strength. J. Speech Hear. Dis. 30:32–36.

Shames, G., and Egolf, D. 1975. Operant Conditioning and the Management of Stuttering. Prentice-Hall Inc., Englewood Cliffs, New Jersey.

Shearer, W., and Williams, J. 1965. Self-recovery from stuttering. J. Speech Hear Disord. 30:288–290.

Sheehan, J. 1968. Stuttering as a self-role conflict. In: H. Gregory (ed.), Learning Theory and Stuttering Therapy, pp. 72–83. Northwestern University Press, Evanston, Illinois.

Sheehan, J. 1970. Stuttering: Research and Therapy. Harper & Row, Publisher, New York.

Sheehan, J., Cortese, P. and Hadley, R. 1962. Guilt, shame and tension in the graphic projections of stuttering. J. Speech Hear. Disord. 27:129–139.

Sheehan, J., and Martyn, M. 1966. Spontaneous recovery from stuttering. J. Speech Hear. Res. 9:121–135.

Sheehan, J., and Martyn, M. 1970. Stuttering and its disappearance. J. Speech Hear. Res. 13:279–289.

Shumak, I. 1955. A speech situation rating sheet for stutterers. In: W. Johnson (ed.), Stuttering in Children and Adults. pp. 341–347. University of Minnesota Press, Minneapolis.

Silverman, E.-M. 1971a. Situational variability of preschooler's disfluency: A preliminary study. Percept. Motor Skills, 33:1021–1022.

Silverman, E.-M. 1971b. Situational variability of preschooler's disfluency: A preliminary study. Percept. Motor Skills, 33:1021–1022.

Silverman, E.-M. 1972. Generality of disfluency data collected from preschoolers. J. Speech Hear. Res. 15:84–92.

Silverman, E.-M. 1973. The influence of preschoolers' speech usage on their disfluency frequency. J. Speech Hear. Res. 16:474–481.

Silverman, E.-M. 1974a. Word position and grammatical function in relation to preschoolers' speech disfluency. Percept. Motor Skills, 39:267–272.

Silverman, F. 1974b. Disfluency behavior of elementary-school stutterers and nonstutterers. Lang. Speech Hear. Serv. Schools. 5:32–37.

St. Onge, K. 1963 The stuttering syndrome. J. Speech Hear. Res. 6:195–197.

Stephenson, W. 1953. The Study of Behavior. University of Chicago Press, Chicago.

Taylor, I. 1966. The properties of stuttered words. J. Verb. Learn. Verb. Behav. 5:112–118.

Tracy, K. 1974. An investigation of responses from speech clinicians and the lay public to the concept "Typical Adult Stutterer." Unpublished thesis. Bowling Green State University, Bowling Green, Ohio.

Van Riper, C. 1954. Speech Correction: Principles and Methods. 3rd Ed. Prentice-Hall Inc., Englewood Cliffs, New Jersey.

Van Riper, C. 1963. Speech Correction: Principles and Methods. 4th Ed. Prentice-Hall Inc., Englewood Cliffs, New Jersey.

Van Riper, C. 1971. The Nature of Stuttering. Prentice-Hall Inc., Englewood Cliffs, New Jersey.

Van Riper, C. 1972. Speech Correction: Principles and Methods. 5th Ed. Prentice-Hall Inc., Englewood Cliffs, New Jersey.

Van Riper, C. 1973. The Treatment of Stuttering. Prentice-Hall Inc., Englewood Cliffs, New Jersey.

Webster, L. 1965. An audio-visual exploration of the stuttering moment. Unpublished thesis. Southern Illinois University, Carbondale.

Williams, D. 1957. A point of view about stuttering! J. Speech Hear. Disord. 22:390–397.

Williams, D. 1968. Stuttering therapy: An overview. In: H. Gregory (ed.), Learning Theory and Stuttering Therapy, pp. 52–66. Northwestern University Press, Evanston, Illinois.

Williams, D. 1971. Stuttering therapy for children. In: L. Travis (ed.), Handbook of Speech Pathology and Audiology, pp. 1073–1093. Appleton-Century-Crofts, New York.

Williams, D. 1972. Some suggestions for adults who want to talk easily. In: S. Hood (ed.), To The Stutterer, pp. 99–103. Speech Foundation of America, Memphis, Tennessee.

Williams, D., and Kent, L. 1958. Listener evaluations of speech interruptions. J. Speech Hear. Res. 1:124–131.

Williams, D., Wark, M., and Minifie, F. 1963. Rating of stuttering by audio, visual and audiovisual cues. J. Speech Hear. Res. 6:91–100.

Wingate, M. 1962a. Evaluation and stuttering, Part I: Speech characteristics of young children. J. Speech Hear. Disord. 27:106–115.

Wingate, M. 1962b. Evaluation and stuttering, II: Environmental stress and critical appraisal of speech. J. Speech Hear. Dis. 27:244–257.

Wingate, M. 1962c. Evaluation and stuttering, III: Identification of stuttering and the use of a label. J. Speech Hear. Disord. 27:368–377.

Wingate, M. 1964. Recovery from stuttering. J. Speech Hear. Dis. 29:312–321.

Wolpe, J. 1969. The Practice of Behavior Therapy. Pergamon Press, New York.

Woolf, G. 1967. The assessment of stuttering as struggle, avoidance and expectancy. Br. J. Dis. Commun. 2:158–171.

Woods, C., and Williams, D. 1971. Speech clinicians' conceptions of boys and men who stutter. J. Speech Hear. Disord. 36:225–234.

Woods, C., and Williams, D. 1976. Traits attributed to stuttering and normally fluent males. J. Speech Hear. Res. 19:267–278.

Yairi, E., and Williams, D. 1970. Speech clinicians stereotypes of elementary-school boys who stutter. J. Commun. Disord. 3:161–170.

Zenner, A. 1971. A molecular analysis of stuttering and associated behaviors during massed oral readings of the same material: The adaptation and consistency of behaviors. Unpublished doctoral dissertation. Syracuse University, Syracuse, New York.

APPENDIX A

Speech and Hearing Clinic
Bowling Green State University
Stuttering Information: (Children)

IDENTIFICATION:
Name: Birthdate: Age:
Address: Telephone no:
Name of person answering questionnaire:
Relationship to client:
Father's name: Age:
Occupation:
Level of education:
Mother's name: Age:
Occupation:
Level of education:
Other children in family:
        Name   Age   Sex   Any speech problem

List other adults in the home:

STATEMENT OF PROBLEM:
Describe in your own words your child's way of talking:

When was his stuttering first noticed? By whom?

When is his stuttering most noticeable?

To what do you attribute his stuttering?

What do you do when he stutters?

Does his stuttering seem to bother him?

Has his speech gotten worse or better lately?

Does he repeat phrases and sentences?_____ words?_____
    syllables? _____ sounds? _____

Does he prolong sounds?

Does he stutter silently? _____ out loud? _____ or both? _____

If you were to indicate what factors may be related to your child's stuttering, which ones would you include? Circle as many as you think are possible:

Emotional	Neglect by father
Sibling rivalry	Neglect by mother
Overprotection by father	Overprotection
Overprotection by mother	Behavior problems
Environmental problems	Lack of playmates
Feeling of insecurity	Inconsistency of parental handling
Strong fears	Strong hates
Nervousness	Marital problems
Insecurity	Other (list)

What is the nature of your child's stuttering when he is (check the category that applies):

		Better than average	Average	Worse than average
a.	Very happy or pleased			
b.	Angry			
c.	Tired			
d.	Excited			
e.	Talking to teachers			
f.	Talking to pets			
g.	Talking before a group			
h.	Talking to good friends			
i.	Talking to parents			
j.	Asking permission			
k.	Talking on the telephone			
l.	Talking to strangers			

EDUCATIONAL INFORMATION:

School: Grade:

Address: Teacher's name:

Principal's name:

Has he ever failed a grade?   Which grades?

Does he excel in any subjects?

Does he have any serious difficulty in any?

How does the child feel about school and his teachers?

Has he ever had any psychological tests?   When?

    Where?   By whom?

Were the results interpreted to you?

If so, what were they?

DAILY BEHAVIOR

Does he sleep well?

Does he eat well?

Does your child have any difficulty in concentrating?

What are your child's favorite play activities?

How does your child amuse himself when alone?

Plays alone or with other children?

Age of playmates?

How does he get along with other children?

How does he get along with adults?

Is it difficult to discipline the child?

Would you describe your child as basically happy or unhappy?

GENERAL DEVELOPMENT: Indicate ages at which child accomplished the following:

Sat alone	Crawled
Stood alone	Walked alone
Bowel trained: waking,	sleeping
Bladder trained: waking,	sleeping
Dressed self satisfactorily	

Was child's rate of growth seemingly normal?

Was normal development interrupted by anything?

MEDICAL HISTORY:

	Age	Severity		Age	Severity
Tonsilitis			Influenza		
Pneumonia			Measles		
Pleurisy			Mumps		
Chicken pox			Head injury		
Earaches			Frequent colds		
High fevers			Allergies		
Tonsillectomy			Headaches		
Ear surgery			Adenoidectomy		

Has he ever experienced a severe shock or injury?   When?
Explain:

Is general health good?

Name of child's physician_____Address _____

_____

SPEECH AND HEARING HISTORY:

Did infant babble and coo during first 6 months?

When did he speak his first word?

When did he begin to use two-word sentences?

When did he first use words meaningfully?

Does he use speech frequently?   occassionally?   never?

Does he prefer to use speech or gestures? (Give examples.)

Which does the child prefer to use: Complete sentences?
    Phrases?   One or two words?

How well can child be understood by parents?   his brothers
    and sisters?   friends or playmates?
    strangers?

What other information can you supply that will enable us to better
    know and understand your child?

APPENDIX B

Speech and Hearing Clinic
Bowling Green State University
Descriptions of Stuttering

Child's name: Date of birth
Form completed by: Today's date

Which of the following have you observed in your child's speech in the past month? Please answer by placing an "X" in the appropriate column.

	Never	Once or twice	Some-times	Quite often	Most of the time
1. When he is experiencing difficulty with his speech, does he:					
a. Hold his breath?					
b. Blink his eyes?					
c. Close his eyes completely?					
d. Hold his eyes wide open?					
e. Stick out his tongue?					
f. Press his lips tightly together?					
g. Hold his mouth wide open?					
h. Jerk his head?					

		Never	Once or twice	Some- times	Quite often	Most of the time
i.	Make other types of facial grimaces?					
j.	Clench his fists?					
k.	Stamp his feet?					
l.	Make other types of bodily dis- tortions?					
m.	Keep repeating the sound or word on which he is stuck?					
n.	Hold onto the sound and pro- long it until he can force it out?					
o.	Repeat whole words?					
p.	Repeat parts of words?					
q.	Have a quiver in his voice?					
r.	Add extra words at the beginning of a sentence (such as *and* or *uh*)?					

	Never	Once or twice	Some-times	Quite often	Most of the time
s. Have this trouble on the small parts of speech, such as *and, in, the*?					
t. Have this trouble on the major parts of speech (nouns, verbs)?					
u. Seem to know ahead of time that he is going to have difficulty on a certain word?					
v. Continue with the stuttering block until it is completed?					
w. Give up on what he was trying to say and stop talking?					
x. Give up on what he was trying to say and substitute another word?					
y. Give up on what he was trying to say and change the subject?					

	Never	Once or twice	Some-times	Quite often	Most of the time
2. Does the child show frustration regarding his speech?					
3. After a stuttering block does he look frightened?					
4. After a stuttering block does he become bewildered?					
5. Does he become embarrassed by his speech?					
6. Does he seem to be worried or anxious about it?					
7. Does he get angry with himself after a block?					
8. Does he show any reaction after a block?					
9. Does he refuse to play with other children because of his speech?					
10. Does he avoid speaking?					

11.   Does he stutter during every sentence?   Yes   No

12.   Does he have periods when he stutters and periods when he does not?

Yes   No

If so, how long are the periods of stuttering?

If so, how long are the periods without stuttering?

13.   Are there some situations in which he stutters more than in others?

Yes   No

Describe

14.   Does he have trouble with the first word of a sentence?

Yes   No

15.   Does he have trouble with words that occur in the middle of a sentence?

Yes   No

16.   Does he have trouble with words that occur at the end of a sentence?

Yes   No

17.   Does he typically have trouble with the same words?

Yes   No

18.   Does he ask why he has trouble talking?   Yes   No

19.   Is he aware of his speech difficulty?   Yes   No

Additional Comments:

APPENDIX C

Speech and Hearing Clinic
Bowling Green State University
Stuttering Information (Adults)

Name   Birthdate   Sex

Address

Name of school   Year in school

Father's name   Address

Mother's name

Name and age

Brothers

Sisters

Your rank in family (1st, 2nd, 3rd, etc.)
1. Have there been any changes in the family (for example, accident, moving, separation, divorce, birth, etc.)?
2. Are there any other members of your family who stuttered (parents, brothers or sisters, near or distant relatives)? Specifically state their relationship to you.
3. Are you right or left handed? Did you ever show a preference for the other hand?
4. At what age did you begin to stutter? If you do not recall yourself, at what age do you recall being told you began?
5. What do you think caused you to stutter?
6. What is your stuttering like: Do you repeat sounds, words, or phrases? Do you have long pauses (silent "blocks")? Do you drag out sounds? Are some sounds particularly hard? If so, are they always the same sounds? If you feel that you will stutter, do you change a word, sentence, or the entire idea?
7. What things do you do to help you talk better or to avoid stuttering?
8. If your stuttering has changed in form, what was it like before?
9. Please describe your stuttering as it is now, in your own words.
10. What are your feelings and attitudes toward your stuttering?
11. Do you think your stuttering is severe, moderate, or mild?

12. Is your stuttering much worse at some times than at others? At what times or in what situations is your stuttering particularly severe?
At what times or in what situations do you stutter relatively little? Are there any situations in which you do not stutter at all? Describe:

13. What is the nature of your stuttering when you are:

   a). Very happy or pleased
   b). Angry
   c). Tired
   d). Excited
   e). Talking to teachers
   f). Talking to pets or animals
   g). Talking before a group
   h). Talking to good friends
   i). Talking to parents

14. Did any other people let you know they were aware you stuttered?

15. Did you receive any special help for your speech (that is, from parents, a speech therapist, psychologist, teacher, physician, etc.)?

16. At what age(s) did you receive help? How frequently and for how long did you receive this help?

17. Of all the things you have tried, what helped you the most? What things were least helpful?

18. What bothers you the most about your stuttering: the way stuttering looks? The way stuttering sounds? The way you feel when you stutter? The way others react to your speech?

19. Is there anything else that you feel is important about yourself and would help us to know in working with you?

APPENDIX D

Speech Situations Check List For Adults
Gene J. Brutten, Ph.D.
Donald J. Shoemaker, Ph.D.
Southern Illinois University

Name:
Address:
Birthdate:
Date:

Instructions

The items in this check list refer to speech situations; situations where you are involved in talking. Talking in these situations may or may not currently cause you some negative emotion (e.g. fear, tension, anxiety or other unpleasant feelings). In the emotional reaction column put the number that best describes how much each of these speech situations disturbs you nowadays.

1. not at all
2. a little
3. a fair amount
4. much
5. very much

Talking in these situations may currently disrupt your speech. You may hesitate or be unable to say a word. You may repeat and prolong part of words. In the column marked speech disruption put one of the five numbers that best describes how much, if at all, each of these situations disturbs your speech nowadays.

---

1. not at all   2. a little   3. a fair amount   4. much   5. very much

---

	Emotional Reaction	Speech Disruption
1. talking on the telephone		
2. talking to a stranger		

1. not at all   2. a little   3. a fair amount   4. much   5. very much

	Emotional Reaction	Speech Disruption
3. giving your name		
4. talking with a young child		
5. saying a sound or word that has in the past been troublesome		
6. placing on order in a restaurant		
7. talking to an animal		
8. placing a person to person call		
9. talking with a close friend		
10. arguing with parents		
11. talking with a sales clerk		
12. talking in a rap or bull session		
13. being criticized		
14. meeting someone for the first time		
15. talking after being teased about your speech		
16. saying hello		
17. reading an unchangeable passage aloud		
18. being misunderstood		

1. not at all   2. a little   3. a fair amount   4. much   5. very much

	Emotional Reaction	Speech Disruption
19. answering a specific question		
20. asking for information		
21. being interviewed for a job		
22. trying to get across your own point of view		
23. introducing yourself		
24. giving directions		
25. talking when "high"		
26. talking to barber or beautician		
27. talking when trying to make a good impression		
28. talking when generally unhappy		
29. talking with teachers		
30. making an appointment with a secretary		
31. asking questions about your speech		
32. asking the teacher a question		
33. being asked to repeat your answer		
34. being asked to give your name		

1. not at all   2. a little   3. a fair amount   4. much   5. very much

	Emotional Reaction	Speech Disruption
35. making introductions		
36. being asked to give personal information		
37. asking if someone is at home		
38. buying a plane, bus, or train ticket to a specific place		
39. telling taxicab driver where to take you		
40. asking a gas-station attendant for a specific amount of gas		
41. speaking before a group		
42. making an appointment		
43. giving a prepared speech		
44. being rushed when speaking		
45. apologizing		
46. being with a member of the opposite sex		
47. refuting a criticism		
48. giving a telephone number		
49. giving an ad-lib report		

1. not at all 2. a little 3. a fair amount 4. much 5. very much		
	Emotional Reaction	Speech Disruption
50. returning a call		
51. selling a product		

APPENDIX E

Southern Illinois University

Speech Situations Check List For Children

Name
Birthdate
Age
Grade

Instructions

How is your speech when you talk? Is talking hard for you? Are there times when the same sound or word comes out over and over again, or you can't get the sound or word out at all? Is talking easy for you? You don't have trouble speaking. The sounds or words are easy for you to say and you talk without any stops. For example, how is your speech when you are talking at a picnic? If talking at a picnic gives you a little trouble, you would circle, a little trouble.

a. Talking at a picnic   No trouble   (A little   More than a   Much   Very much
                           at all   trouble)   little trouble   trouble   trouble

If talking at a picnic gives you very much trouble, you would circle, very much trouble.

b. Talking at a picnic   No trouble   A little   More than a   Much   (Very much
                           at all   trouble   little trouble   trouble   trouble)

Read everything on the list and circle how much trouble you have when you talk.

	No trouble at all	A little trouble	More than a little trouble	Much trouble	Very much trouble
1. Talking to a new kid in school	No trouble at all	A little trouble	More than a little trouble	Much trouble	Very much trouble
2. Talking at the dinner table	No trouble at all	A little trouble	More than a little trouble	Much trouble	Very much trouble
3. Talking when excited	No trouble at all	A little trouble	More than a little trouble	Much trouble	Very much trouble
4. Talking with an older person	No trouble at all	A little trouble	More than a little trouble	Much trouble	Very much trouble
5. Asking for money	No trouble at all	A little trouble	More than a little trouble	Much trouble	Very much trouble
6. Talking to the doctor	No trouble at all	A little trouble	More than a little trouble	Much trouble	Very much trouble
7. Having to answer a question in class when you don't really know the answer	No trouble at all	A little trouble	More than a little trouble	Much trouble	Very much trouble
8. Talking after having a fight with a friend	No trouble at all	A little trouble	More than a little trouble	Much trouble	Very much trouble

	No trouble at all	A little trouble	More than a little trouble	Much trouble	Very much trouble
9. Talking to yourself	No trouble at all	A little trouble	More than a little trouble	Much trouble	Very much trouble
10. Talking to your dad while he's reading the newspaper	No trouble at all	A little trouble	More than a little trouble	Much trouble	Very much trouble
11. Asking for help with your homework	No trouble at all	A little trouble	More than a little trouble	Much trouble	Very much trouble
12. Reciting in class	No trouble at all	A little trouble	More than a little trouble	Much trouble	Very much trouble
13. Asking for a certain kind of candy at a store	No trouble at all	A little trouble	More than a little trouble	Much trouble	Very much trouble
14. Telling a story	No trouble at all	A little trouble	More than a little trouble	Much trouble	Very much trouble
15. Spelling words in a spelling bee	No trouble at all	A little trouble	More than a little trouble	Much trouble	Very much trouble
16. Talking to a kid you don't know	No trouble at all	A little trouble	More than a little trouble	Much trouble	Very much trouble

	No trouble at all	A little trouble	More than a little trouble	Much trouble	Very much trouble
17. Talking at a party	No trouble at all	A little trouble	More than a little trouble	Much trouble	Very much trouble
18. Raising your hand to talk in class	No trouble at all	A little trouble	More than a little trouble	Much trouble	Very much trouble
19. Talking to a baby	No trouble at all	A little trouble	More than a little trouble	Much trouble	Very much trouble
20. Telling a lie	No trouble at all	A little trouble	More than a little trouble	Much trouble	Very much trouble
21. Talking about something you don't like	No trouble at all	A little trouble	More than a little trouble	Much trouble	Very much trouble
22. Talking when embarrassed	No trouble at all	A little trouble	More than a little trouble	Much trouble	Very much trouble
23. Talking on the telephone	No trouble at all	A little trouble	More than a little trouble	Much trouble	Very much trouble
24. Talking with a stranger	No trouble at all	A little trouble	More than a little trouble	Much trouble	Very much trouble

	No trouble at all	A little trouble	More than a little trouble	Much trouble	Very much trouble
25. Saying certain sounds or words	No trouble at all	A little trouble	More than a little trouble	Much trouble	Very much trouble
26. Talking after someone has hurt your feelings	No trouble at all	A little trouble	More than a little trouble	Much trouble	Very much trouble
27. Talking to an animal	No trouble at all	A little trouble	More than a little trouble	Much trouble	Very much trouble
28. Talking to your parents	No trouble at all	A little trouble	More than a little trouble	Much trouble	Very much trouble
29. Talking with a best friend	No trouble at all	A little trouble	More than a little trouble	Much trouble	Very much trouble
30. Talking after being yelled at	No trouble at all	A little trouble	More than a little trouble	Much trouble	Very much trouble
31. Reading aloud from a book	No trouble at all	A little trouble	More than a little trouble	Much trouble	Very much trouble
32. Talking with an adult	No trouble at all	A little trouble	More than a little trouble	Much trouble	Very much trouble

	No trouble at all	A little trouble	More than a little trouble	Much trouble	Very much trouble
33. Talking after being misunderstood	No trouble at all	A little trouble	More than a little trouble	Much trouble	Very much trouble
34. Answering a question	No trouble at all	A little trouble	More than a little trouble	Much trouble	Very much trouble
35. Talking after you have given the wrong answer	No trouble at all	A little trouble	More than a little trouble	Much trouble	Very much trouble
36. Telling people what you think	No trouble at all	A little trouble	More than a little trouble	Much trouble	Very much trouble
37. Telling someone your name	No trouble at all	A little trouble	More than a little trouble	Much trouble	Very much trouble
38. Talking when trying to make people think you are nice	No trouble at all	A little trouble	More than a little trouble	Much trouble	Very much trouble
39. Talking when unhappy	No trouble at all	A little trouble	More than a little trouble	Much trouble	Very much trouble
40. Telling someone where something is	No trouble at all	A little trouble	More than a little trouble	Much trouble	Very much trouble

	No trouble at all	A little trouble	More than a little trouble	Much trouble	Very much trouble
41. Talking to boys your own age	No trouble at all	A little trouble	More than a little trouble	Much trouble	Very much trouble
42. Asking your teacher a question	No trouble at all	A little trouble	More than a little trouble	Much trouble	Very much trouble
43. Talking after being asked to repeat your answer	No trouble at all	A little trouble	More than a little trouble	Much trouble	Very much trouble
44. Telling someone about yourself	No trouble at all	A little trouble	More than a little trouble	Much trouble	Very much trouble
45. Asking if your friend is home	No trouble at all	A little trouble	More than a little trouble	Much trouble	Very much trouble
46. Talking on the playground	No trouble at all	A little trouble	More than a little trouble	Much trouble	Very much trouble
47. Talking in front of class	No trouble at all	A little trouble	More than a little trouble	Much trouble	Very much trouble
48. Giving a speech	No trouble at all	A little trouble	More than a little trouble	Much trouble	Very much trouble

	No trouble at all	A little trouble	More than a little trouble	Much trouble	Very much trouble
49. Talking to girls your own age	No trouble at all	A little trouble	More than a little trouble	Much trouble	Very much trouble
50. Talking when you are in a hurry	No trouble at all	A little trouble	More than a little trouble	Much trouble	Very much trouble
51. Telling someone your phone number	No trouble at all	A little trouble	More than a little trouble	Much trouble	Very much trouble
52. Talking to your teacher when you know she is angry with you	No trouble at all	A little trouble	More than a little trouble	Much trouble	Very much trouble
53. Telling someone your address	No trouble at all	A little trouble	More than a little trouble	Much trouble	Very much trouble
54. Asking a saleslady to show you something	No trouble at all	A little trouble	More than a little trouble	Much trouble	Very much trouble
55. Telling someone you are sorry	No trouble at all	A little trouble	More than a little trouble	Much trouble	Very much trouble

APPENDIX F

Behavior Check List
Gene J. Brutten, Ph.D.
Donald J. Shoemaker, Ph.D.

Name:
Address:
Birthdate:
Date:

Instructions

Many different behaviors are contained in this check list. Some of them may occur nowadays when you get ready to speak or are speaking. The others listed do not describe the way you behave at the present time.

Carefully think about each of the listed behaviors. For each one that occurs nowadays when you speak put a check in the first column. Do not check those behaviors if they do not describe the way you behave currently.

Some of the behaviors that you have identified by putting a check in column 1 may be used by you either to avoid or get out of speaking difficulties. Indicate which, if any, of the behaviors you have checked in column one are those that you use to help yourself speak with less trouble by putting a check in column 2. Remember, put a check in column 2 only if they were previously checked in column 1 and only if you use those behaviors as speech aids nowadays.

	Current Behaviors	Speech Aids
Touching hair		
Wrinkling of the forehead		
Closing of the eyes		
Eye-blinking		

	Current Behaviors	Speech Aids
Increased opening of eyes		
Raising eyebrow		
Quivering of eyelid		
Looking up		
Looking down		
Looking to the side		
Avoiding eye contact		
Wrinkling of nose		
Opening or moving the nostril		
Pressing lips together		
Pursing the lips		
Movement of the lip to the side		
Smacking lips		
Lip quivering		
Tongue clicking		
Pressing tongue to teeth		
Pressing tongue to roof of mouth		
Protuding of tongue		
Dropping jaw (Opening mouth)		

	Current Behaviors	Speech Aids
Moving jaw to either side		
Silent repetition of a phrase		
Prolongation of a sound (nnnnnnobody)		
Addition of a sound		
Addition of a syllable (I went to uh-uh-uh-uh see him last week)		
Addition of a word		
Addition of a phrase		
Omission of a sound		
Omission of a syllable		
Omission of a word		
Omission of a sentence		
Omission of a phrase		
Substitution of one sound for another		
Subsitution of one syllable for another		
Subsitution of one phrase for another		
Failure to complete word		
Failure to complete phrase		
Failure to complete sentence		

	Current Behaviors	Speech Aids
Pausing before attempting to speak a word		
Pausing (breaking) in the middle of a word (I am g—oing home)		
Movement of body to side		
Forward movement of body		
Backward movement of body		
Tightening of muscles in forehead		
Tightening of facial muscles		
Tightening of muscles in chin		
Tightening of leg muscles		
Tightening of abdominal muscles		
Tightening of neck muscles		
Leg movement to side		
Leg movement up		
Leg movement down		
Leg kick		
General movements of the body		
Foot tap		
Curling toes		

	Current Behaviors	Speech Aids
Repetition of a sound (s—s—s—s—say)		
Repetition of a syllable (bas-bas-basket-ball)		
Repetition of whole word (I always-always-always go home this way)		
Repetition of a phrase (How are you, how are you this morning)		
Silent repetition of a sound		
Silent repetition of a syllable		
Silent repetition of a word		
Pitching head at an angle		
Turning head to the side (left or right)		
Moving head up		
Moving head down		
Sudden inhalation		
Extended inhalation		
Extended exhalation		
Irregular exhalation		
Holding breath		
Gasping		

	Current Behaviors	Speech Aids
Speaking on inhalation		
Speaking after exhalation		
Raising shoulder or shoulders		
Turning of shoulder or shoulders		
Arm-swinging		
Other movements of the arm		
Hand-swinging		
Other movements of the hand		
Snapping of fingers		
Tapping of finger or fingers		
Swinging the finger		
Other movements of the finger		
Pausing in the middle of a phrase		
Slowing down rate of speaking		
Speeding up rate of speaking		
Rythmic speech (sing song pattern)		
Gesturing in place of speech		
Answering with gestures		
Evasion through speech (I don't know)		

	Current Behaviors	Speech Aids
Decreasing intensity of speech		
Increasing intensity of speech		

OTHER BEHAVIORS

APPENDIX G

Southern Illinois University
Modification of Fear Survey
Schedule Inventory

Name:
Address:
Birthdate:
Date:

The items in this questionnaire refer to things and experiences that may cause fear or other unpleasant feelings. Write the number of each item in the column that describes how much you are disturbed by it nowadays.

	Not at all	A little	A fair amount	Much	Very much
1. Sharp objects					
2. Being a passenger in a car					
3. Dead bodies					
4. Suffocating					
5. Failing a test					
6. Looking foolish					
7. Being a passenger in an airplane					
8. Worms					
9. Arguing with parents					
10. Rats and mice					
11. Life after death					
12. Hypodermic needles					
13. Being criticized					
14. Meeting someone for the first time					
15. Roller coasters					
16. Being alone					
17. Making mistakes					

	Not at all	A little	A fair amount	Much	Very much
18. Being misunderstood					
19. Death					
20. Being in a fight					
21. Crowded places					
22. Blood					
23. Heights					
24. Swimming alone					
25. Being a leader					
26. Illness					
27. Being with drunks					
28. Illness or injury to loved ones					
29. Being self-conscious					
30. Driving a car					
31. Meeting authority					
32. Mental illness					
33. Closed places					
34. Boating					
35. Spiders					
36. Thunderstorms					
37. Not being a success					
38. God					
39. Snakes					
40. Cemeteries					
41. Speaking before a group					
42. Seeing a fight					
43. Death of a loved one					
44. Dark places					
45. Strange dogs					
46. Deep water					
47. Being with a member of the opposite sex					
48. Stinging insects					
49. Untimely or early death					
50. Losing a job					
51. Auto accidents					

APPENDIX H

Fear Survey Schedule Inventory For Children

Below is a list of things and experiences that may currently cause you to be afraid or have unpleasant feelings. Look at each one and circle the word which describes how much you think you are disturbed by it nowadays. Circle "None" if it does not bother you at all.

1.	Giving an oral report	None	A little	Some	Much	Very Much
2.	Riding in the car or on the bus	None	A little	Some	Much	Very Much
3.	Getting punished by my mother	None	A little	Some	Much	Very Much
4.	Lizards	None	A little	Some	Much	Very Much
5.	Looking foolish	None	A little	Some	Much	Very Much
6.	Ghosts or spook things	None	A little	Some	Much	Very Much
7.	Sharp objects	None	A little	Some	Much	Very Much
8.	Having to go to the hospital	None	A little	Some	Much	Very Much
9.	Death or dead people	None	A little	Some	Much	Very Much
10.	Getting lost in a strange place	None	A little	Some	Much	Very Much
11.	Snakes	None	A little	Some	Much	Very Much
12.	Talking on the phone	None	A little	Some	Much	Very Much
13.	Roller coasters or carnival rides	None	A little	Some	Much	Very Much
14.	Getting sick at school	None	A little	Some	Much	Very Much
15.	Being sent to the principal	None	A little	Some	Much	Very Much
16.	Riding on the train	None	A little	Some	Much	Very Much
17.	Being left at home with a sitter	None	A little	Some	Much	Very Much
18.	Bears or wolves	None	A little	Some	Much	Very Much
19.	Meeting someone for the first time	None	A little	Some	Much	Very Much
20.	Bombing attacks— being invaded	None	A little	Some	Much	Very Much

21.	Getting a shot from the nurse or doctor	None	A little	Some	Much	Very Much
22.	Going to the dentist	None	A little	Some	Much	Very Much
23.	High places like on mountains	None	A little	Some	Much	Very Much
24.	Being teased	None	A little	Some	Much	Very Much
25.	Spiders	None	A little	Some	Much	Very Much
26.	A burglar breaking into our house	None	A little	Some	Much	Very Much
27.	Flying a plane	None	A little	Some	Much	Very Much
28.	Being called in unexpectantly by the teacher	None None	A little A little	Some Some	Much Much	Very Much Very Much
29.	Getting poor grades	None	A little	Some	Much	Very Much
30.	Bats or birds	None	A little	Some	Much	Very Much
31.	My mother criticizing me	None	A little	Some	Much	Very Much
32.	Guns	None	A little	Some	Much	Very Much
33.	Being in a fight	None	A little	Some	Much	Very Much
34.	Fire—getting burned	None	A little	Some	Much	Very Much
35.	Getting a cut or injury	None	A little	Some	Much	Very Much
36.	Being in a crowd	None	A little	Some	Much	Very Much
37.	Thunderstorms	None	A little	Some	Much	Very Much
38.	Having to eat some food I don't like	None	A little	Some	Much	Very Much
39.	Cats	None	A little	Some	Much	Very Much
40.	Failing a test	None	A little	Some	Much	Very Much
41.	Being hit by a car or truck	None	A little	Some	Much	Very Much
42.	Having to go to school	None	A little	Some	Much	Very Much
43.	Playing rough games during physical education	None	A little	Some	Much	Very Much
44.	Having my parents argue	None	A little	Some	Much	Very Much
45.	Dark rooms or closets	None	A little	Some	Much	Very Much
46.	Having to perform or play at a recital	None	A little	Some	Much	Very Much
47.	Ants or beetles	None	A little	Some	Much	Very Much
48.	Being criticized by others	None	A little	Some	Much	Very Much

49.	Strange-looking people	None	A little	Some	Much	Very Much
50.	The sight of blood	None	A little	Some	Much	Very Much
51.	Going to the doctor	None	A little	Some	Much	Very Much
52.	Strange or mean dogs	None	A little	Some	Much	Very Much
53.	Cemeteries	None	A little	Some	Much	Very Much
54.	Getting a report card	None	A little	Some	Much	Very Much
55.	Getting a hair cut	None	A little	Some	Much	Very Much
56.	Deep water or the ocean	None	A little	Some	Much	Very Much
57.	Nightmares	None	A little	Some	Much	Very Much
58.	Falling from high places	None	A little	Some	Much	Very Much
59.	Getting shock from electricity	None	A little	Some	Much	Very Much
60.	Going to bed in the dark	None	A little	Some	Much	Very Much
61.	Getting car sick	None	A little	Some	Much	Very Much
62.	Being alone	None	A little	Some	Much	Very Much
63.	Having to wear clothes different from others	None	A little	Some	Much	Very Much
64.	Getting punished by my father	None	A little	Some	Much	Very Much
65.	Having to stay after school	None	A little	Some	Much	Very Much
66.	Making mistakes	None	A little	Some	Much	Very Much
67.	Mystery movies	None	A little	Some	Much	Very Much
68.	Loud sirens	None	A little	Some	Much	Very Much
69.	Doing something new	None	A little	Some	Much	Very Much
70.	Germs or getting a serious illness	None	A little	Some	Much	Very Much
71.	Closed places	None	A little	Some	Much	Very Much
72.	Earthquakes	None	A little	Some	Much	Very Much
73.	Russia	None	A little	Some	Much	Very Much
74.	Elevators	None	A little	Some	Much	Very Much
75.	Dark places	None	A little	Some	Much	Very Much
76.	Not being able to breathe	None	A little	Some	Much	Very Much
77.	Gettin a bee sting	None	A little	Some	Much	Very Much
78.	Worms or snails	None	A little	Some	Much	Very Much
79.	Rats or mice	None	A little	Some	Much	Very Much
80.	Taking a test	None	A little	Some	Much	Very Much

APPENDIX I

Sheehan's Sentence Completion Test

Name _____ Age _____ Date _____

Education_____Circle: male   female

Directions: Complete these sentences as honestly as you can. Work
rapidly, and write down the first thing you think of.

1. I admire people who . . .
2. I feel happiest when . . .
3. I feel closest to people who . . .
4. My hardest situation . . .
5. When I talk most people . . .
6. I boil up when . . .
7. People in authority . . .
8. Words that give me most trouble are . . .
9. A brother . . .
10. When I get down in the dumps . . .
11. I like children who are . . .
12. I used to daydream about . . .
13. When I'm treated unfairly . . .
14. The work I like best . . .
15. It is wrong to make people . . .
16. I hate to talk because . . .
17. When I think about marriage . . .
18. If I tried harder . . .
19. I often fool people about . . .
20. He failed because . . .
21. Girls who cannot talk right . . .
22. If I were president . . .
23. Most mothers . . .
24. I can achieve . . .
25. I get blocked when I talk to . . .
26. I secretly regret . . .
27. A lot of people think I'm . . .
28. If I could get over my problem, I would . . .
29. I hate people who . . .
30. My greatest desire . . .
31. Most females act as though . . .
32. Most of all I want . . .

33. People who are domineering toward others . . .
34. I often wished . . .
35. A sister . . .
36. Rather than have my problem I would . . .
37. Most men . . .
38. I like to get out of . . .
39. On a date . . .
40. One good thing about being myself . . .
41. If I were the boss . . .
42. I am . . .
43. My father . . .
44. I might fail if . . .
45. Most people I talk to . . .
46. My chief assets . . .
47. The person who most wanted me to work on my problem . . .
48. If I only . . .
49. When she refused me . . .
50. When I am successful . . .
51. My mother . . .
52. Whenever I am especially fluent . . .
53. Most males act as though . . .
54. My proudest accomplishment . . .
55. Most strangers . . .
56. In the future I'll be . . .
57. Fathers are likely to . . .
58. My greatest fault . . .
59. Most women . . .
60. If my problem suddenly disappeared, things would be different because . . .
61. My happiest childhood experience . . .
62. I feel sad about . . .
63. Quarreling . . .
64. Someday . . .
65. When he made love to her . . .
66. What annoys me most . . .
67. When I am alone I . . .
68. I feel guilty when . . .
69. Whenever . . .
70. I felt ashamed when . . .
71. Affection . . .

72. I could kill someone who . . .
73. My home . . .
74. My greatest fear . . .
75. I sometimes wonder . . .
76. I get blocked when I talk about . . .
77. Faith . . .
78. When I am nervous . . .
79. Sex and love . . .
80. When I get angry . . .

Scoring Key (Sheehan)
  I. Levels of conflict:

    1. Word—8 only
    2. Situation—4 only
    3. Feelings—Even numbers from 62–80
    4. Relationships—1, 3, 5, 7, and all odd numbers to 59 inclusive
    5. Defenses—All even numbers from 12–60 inclusive

 II. Unstructed—Odd numbers from 61–79 inclusive.

III. Suggestions for interpretation:

    1. Assume most material autobiographical, unless contrary evidence.
    2. Assemble response clusters for unstructured and for each conflict dimension.
    3. For each response in each area ask: 1) What sort of a person would he have to be to make such a response? 2) What does he bring in unnecessarily? 3) What is conspicuously omitted? A shorthand form of these questions is: 1) What gives? 2) Who asked him? 3) Where's Charley?
    4. Try to develop as many hypotheses as you can about the person without necessarily treating them as fact.
    5. Particularly on feelings and relationships, it is sometimes quite revealing to examine at some stage in interpretation only the cluster of responses, independent of the formal stimulus. Preoccupations and consistent personality traits often show through very well this way.

Caution: The test is now in preliminary form and is offered primarily as a research tool to throw light on conflict areas in stuttering. Although it has been designed to give some indication of prognostic potential, no person not otherwise qualified in the interpretation of projective techniques should attempt to base important clinical decisions on findings at this stage of test development.

For a different approach to scoring see Griffith (1969).

APPENDIX J

(From Woolf, 1967; reprinted by permission.)

Perceptions of Stuttering Inventory (PSI)

The symbols S, A, and E after each item denote struggle (S), avoidance (A), and expectancy (E). In practice, these symbols are not included in the Inventory, but are listed on a separate scoring key.

<u>S   A   E</u>

Name_____Age_____#_____
Examiner_____Date_____%_____

Directions

Here are sixty statements about stuttering. Some of these may be characteristic of *your* stuttering. Read each item carefully and respond as in the examples below.

Characteristic of me

_____ Repeating sounds

Put a check mark (✔) under "*characteristic of me*" if "repeating sounds" is part of *your* stuttering; if it is *not characteristic*, leave the space blank.

"*Characteristic of me*" refers only to what you do *now*, not to what was true of your stuttering in the past and which you no longer do; and not what you think you should or should not be doing. Even if the behavior described occurs only occasionally or only in some speaking situations, if you regard it as characteristic of your stuttering, check the space under "*characteristic of me*."

Characteristic
  of me

_____   1.   Avoiding talking to people in authority (e.g., a teacher, employer, or clergyman). (A).

*Characteristic
of me*

_____   2. Feeling that interruptions in your speech (e.g., pauses, hesitations, or repetitions) will lead to stuttering. (E).

_____   3. Making the pitch of your voice higher or lower when you expect to get "stuck" on words. (E).

_____   4. Having extra and unnecessary facial movements (e.g., flaring your nostrils during speech attempts). (S).

_____   5. Using gestures as a substitute for speaking (e.g., nodding your head instead of saying "yes" or smiling to acknowledge a greeting). (A).

_____   6. Avoiding asking for information (e.g., asking for directions or inquiring about a train schedule). (A).

_____   7. Whispering words to yourself before saying them or practising what you are planning to say long before you speak. (E).

_____   8. Choosing a job or a hobby because little speaking would be required. (A).

_____   9. Adding an extra and unnecessary sound, word, or phrase to your speech (e.g., "uh", "well", or "let me see") to help yourself get started. (E).

_____   10. Replying briefly using the fewest words possible. (A).

_____   11. Making sudden, jerky, or forceful movements with your head, arms, or body during speech attempts (e.g., clenching your fist, jerking your head to one side). (S).

_____   12. Repeating a sound or word with effort. (S).

_____   13. Acting in a manner intended to keep you out of a conversation or discussion (e.g., being a good listener, pretending not to hear what was said, acting bored, or pretending to be in deep thought). (A).

_____   14. Avoiding making a purchase (e.g., going into a store or buying stamps in the post office). (A).

_____   15. Breathing noisily or with great effort while trying to speak. (S).

Characteristic
of me

_____ 16. Making your voice louder or softer when stuttering is expected. (E).

_____ 17. Prolonging a sound or word (e.g., m-m-m-m-my) while trying to push it out. (S).

_____ 18. Helping yourself to get started talking by laughing, coughing, clearing your throat, gesturing, or some other body activity or movement. (E).

_____ 19. Having general body tension during speech attempts (e.g., shaking, trembling, or feeling "knotted up" inside). (S).

_____ 20. Paying particular attention to *what* you are going to say (e.g., the length of a word, or the position of a word in a sentence). (E).

_____ 21. Feeling your face getting warm and red (as if you are blushing) as you are struggling to speak. (S).

_____ 22. Saying words or phrases with force or effort. (S).

_____ 23. Repeating a word or phrase preceding the word on which stuttering is expected. (E).

_____ 24. Speaking so that no word or sound stands out (e.g., speaking in a singsong voice or in a monotone). (E).

_____ 25. Avoiding making new acquaintances (e.g., not visiting with friends, not dating, or not joining social, civic, or church groups). (A).

_____ 26. Making unusual noises with your teeth during speech attempts (e.g., grinding or clicking your teeth). (S).

_____ 27. Avoiding introducing yourself, giving your name, or making introductions. (A).

_____ 28. Expecting that certain sounds, letters, or words are going to be particularly "hard" to say (e.g., words beginning with the letter "s"). (E).

_____ 29. Giving excuses to avoid talking (e.g., pretending to be tired or pretending lack of interest in a topic). (A).

_____ 30. "Running out of breath" while speaking. (S).

_____ 31. Forcing out sounds. (S).

*Characteristic
of me*

_____	32.	Feeling that your fluent periods are unusual, that they cannot last, and that sooner or later you will stutter. (E).
_____	33.	Concentrating on relaxing or not being tense before speaking. (E).
_____	34.	Substituting a different word or phrase for the one you had intended to say. (A).
_____	35.	Prolonging or emphasizing the sound preceding the one on which stuttering is expected. (E).
_____	36.	Avoiding speaking before an audience. (A).
_____	37.	Straining to talk without being able to make a sound. (S).
_____	38.	Co-ordinating or timing your speech with a rhythmic movement (e.g., tapping your foot or swinging your arm). (E).
_____	39.	Rearranging what you had planned to say to avoid a "hard" sound or word. (A).
_____	40.	"Putting on an act" when speaking (e.g., adopting an attitude of confidence or pretending to be angry). (E).
_____	41.	Avoiding the use of the telephone. (A).
_____	42.	Making forceful and strained movements with your lips, tongue, jaw, or throat (e.g., moving your jaw in an unco-ordinated manner). (S).
_____	43.	Omitting a word, part of a word, or a phrase which you had planned to say (e.g., words with certain sounds or letters). (A).
_____	44.	Making "uncontrollable" sounds while struggling to say a word. (S).
_____	45.	Adopting a foreign accent, assuming a regional dialect, or imitating another person's speech. (E).
_____	46.	Perspiring much more than usual while speaking (e.g., feeling the palms of your hands getting clammy). (S).
_____	47.	Postponing speaking for a short time until certain you can be fluent (e.g., pausing before "hard" words). (E).

*Characteristic
    of me*

_____ 48. Having extra and unnecessary eye movements while speaking (e.g., blinking your eyes or shutting your eyes tightly). (S).

_____ 49. Breathing forcefully while struggling to speak. (S).

_____ 50. Avoiding talking to others of your own age group (your own or the opposite sex). (A).

_____ 51. Giving up the speech attempt completely after getting "stuck" or if stuttering is anticipated. (A).

_____ 52. Straining the muscles of your chest or abdomen during speech attempts. (S).

_____ 53. Wondering whether you will stutter or how you will speak if you do stutter. (E).

_____ 54. Holding your lips, tongue, or jaw in a rigid position before speaking or when getting "stuck" on a word. (S).

_____ 55. Avoiding talking to one or both of your parents. (A).

_____ 56. Having another person speak for you in a difficult situation (e.g., having someone make a telephone call for you or order for you in a restaurant). (A).

_____ 57. Holding your breath before speaking. (S).

_____ 58. Saying words slowly or rapidly preceding the word on which stuttering is expected. (E).

_____ 59. Concentrating on *how* you are going to speak (e.g., thinking about where to put your tongue or how to breathe). (E).

_____ 60. Using your stuttering as the reason to avoid a speaking activity. (A).

FORM 14. SCALE FOR RATING SEVERITY OF STUTTERING

From *Diagnostic Methods in Speech Pathology*, by Wendell Johnson, Frederic L. Darley, and D. C. Spriestersbach, New York: Harper and Row, 1963.

Speaker _____ Age _____ Sex _____ Date _____

Rater _____ Identification _____

INSTRUCTIONS:

Indicate your identification by some such term as "speaker's clinician," "clinical observer," "clinical student," or "friend," "mother," "father," "classmate," etc.
Rate the severity of the speaker's stuttering on a scale from 0 to 7, as follows:

0   No stuttering

1   Very mild—stuttering on less than 1 percent of words; very little relevant tension; disfluencies generally less than one second in duration; patterns of disfluency simple; no apparent associated movements of body, arms, legs, or head.

2   Mild—stuttering on 1 to 2 percent of words; tension scarcely perceptible; very few, if any, disfluencies last as long as a full second; patterns of disfluency simple; no conspicuous associated movements of body, arms, legs, or head.

3   Mild to moderate—stuttering on about 2 to 5 percent of words; tension noticeable but not very distracting; most disfluencies do not last longer than a full second; patterns of disfluency mostly simple; no distracting associated movements.

4   Moderate—stuttering on about 5 to 8 percent of words; tension occasionally distracting; disfluencies average about one second in duration; disfluency patterns characterized by an occasional complicating sound or facial grimace; an occasional distracting associated movement.

5   Moderate to severe—stuttering on about 8 to 12 percent of words; consistently noticeable tension; disfluencies average about 2 seconds in duration; a few distracting sounds and facial grimaces; a few distracting associated movements.

6   Severe—stuttering on about 12 to 25 percent of words; conspicuous tension; disfluencies average 3 to 4 seconds in duration; conspicuous distracting sounds and facial grimaces; conspicuous distracting associated movements.

7   Very severe—stuttering on more than 25 percent of words; very conspicuous tension; disfluencies average more than 4 seconds in duration; very conspicuous distracting sounds and facial grimaces; very conspicuous distracting associated movements.

If this rating was based on a single sample of speech, describe the speech sample and the situation in which you made the rating. If the rating was based on two or more specific samples of speech, describe the various speech samples and the situations in which you made the ratings:

If this rating was not based on one or more specific speech samples in one or more specific situations, but covers instead many observations made in a variety of situations over a period of time, indicate the period covered and the main general types of speech samples and situations observed.

Dates: from _____ to _____. Main types of samples and situations:

Additional copies of this form may be obtained from the Interstate Printers and Publishers, 19-27 North Jackson Street, Danville, Illinois, Reorder No. 773.

© Harper and Row. The royalties from the sale of this Form are assigned to the American Speech and Hearing Foundation, 1001 Connecticut Avenue, N.W., Washington 6, D. C.

FORM 15. IOWA SCALE OF ATTITUDE TOWARD STUTTERING

From *Diagnostic Methods in Speech Pathology*, by Wendell Johnson, Frederic L. Darley, and D. C. Spriestersbach, New York: Harper and Row, 1963.

Name _____Age _____ Sex _____

Examiner _____ Score _____Date _____

Purpose of Scale: This is not a test or quiz. It is a scale of attitude toward stuttering. In order to help stutterers, we must know their attitudes and the attitudes of other people in connection with stuttering. Please mark this questionnaire as carefully as you can. We went to know your attitude. Don't hesitate to put down what you believe.

First please fill out the following blanks. Disregard any items which do not apply to you.

Extent of education (circle one):   elementary school   high school
                                              college   graduate college

Fields of university major and minor (specify):

Have you ever taken courses in speech correction?   Yes_____   No_____

What relatives of yours have stuttered?

How severe was the stuttering of each?

With how many stutterers other than relatives have you been acquainted?
How severe was the stuttering of each?

Have you ever noticeably stuttered?   Yes   No   If yes, rate yourself on the following scale as to the severity of your stuttering. Indicate your rating of your stuttering severity by circling one of the division bars:

| | | | | |
| mild | | moderate | | severe |

How many brothers have you?   List ages:
How many sisters have you?   List ages:

Procedure: Now you are ready to begin marking the scale, which begins at the top of the next page: In responding to each item, you are to circle the response which best reflects your own attitude. Work accurately and as rapidly as possible. Don't spend a great deal of time analyzing wording. Mark all statements. If you

are not sure what your attitude is, mark the best guess you can and go on.
Remember: In responding to each item, circle the answer which best reflects your own attitude.

1. If a person at the family dinner table is about to stutter on a word, he should substitute another word for it and go on.
   Strongly agree   Moderately agree   Undecided   Moderately disagree   Strongly disagree

2. When giving a talk before a group of friends, a person should talk more slowly and prolong sounds in order to put off saying words he thinks he is going to stutter on.
   Strongly agree   Moderately agree   Undecided   Moderately disagree   Strongly disagree

3. A stutterer should not try out for the debating team.
   Strongly agree   Moderately agree   Undecided   Moderately disagree   Strongly disagree

4. A fellow should prefer to sit in silence rather than stutter to a girl he is with at a party.
   Strongly agree   Moderately agree   Undecided   Moderately disagree   Strongly disagree

5. A husband who stutters should try to have his wife answer the doorbell or telephone.
   Strongly agree   Moderately agree   Undecided   Moderately disagree   Strongly disagree

6. If while introducing two friends a person believes he will stutter, he should prolong the final sound of the preceding word or say "a-a-a" until he believes he can get the word out.
   Strongly agree   Moderately agree   Undecided   Moderately disagree   Strongly disagree

7. If he feels he will stutter while doing so, a father should avoid talking to his son about sex and marriage.
   Strongly agree   Moderately agree   Undecided   Moderately disagree   Strongly disagree

8. If a girl goes for an auto ride with a young man she likes and believes she will stutter, she should speak as little as possible.
   Strongly agree   Moderately agree   Undecided   Moderately disagree   Strongly disagree

9. If she stutters, a girl should not apply for a position as salesgirl in a department store.
   Strongly agree   Moderately agree   Undecided   Moderately disagree   Strongly disagree

10. When at a party you should talk as little as possible if you are a stutterer.
    Strongly agree   Moderately agree   Undecided   Moderately disagree   Strongly disagree

11. A person should not be a Boy or Girl Scout leader if he stutters.
    Strongly agree   Moderately agree   Undecided   Moderately disagree   Strongly disagree

12. If you stutter, you should not prepare yourself to be a salesman.
    Strongly agree   Moderately agree   Undecided   Moderately disagree   Strongly disagree

13. A person should be embarrassed if he stutters while telling a casual, chance acquaintance about a book he has read.
    Strongly agree   Moderately agree   Undecided   Moderately disagree   Strongly disagree

14. A stutterer should not volunteer to be class secretary.
Strongly agree   Moderately agree   Undecided   Moderately disagree   Strongly disagree

15. You should be embarrassed if you stutter while talking before a school assembly.
Strongly agree   Moderately agree   Undecided   Moderately disagree   Strongly disagree

16. A boy who stutters should not run for class or school president.
Strongly agree   Moderately agree   Undecided   Moderately disagree   Strongly disagree

17. If you feel you are going to stutter when answering the phone, you should try to boost up your courage by telling yourself you won't stutter.
Strongly agree   Moderately agree   Undecided   Moderately disagree   Strongly disagree

18. If one is telling a story at a party and thinks he is going to stutter on a word he should try to find an easier word to take its place.
Strongly agree   Moderately agree   Undecided   Moderately disagree   Strongly disagree

19. If a person believes he will stutter when applying at a certain time for a job as a janitor, he should wait until later to apply, when he believes his speech will cause him less embarrassment.
Strongly agree   Moderately agree   Undecided   Moderately disagree   Strongly disagree

20. When visiting a friend's house for the evening and asked what he would like to do or play, a stutterer should choose a game where he would have little talking to do.
Strongly agree   Moderately agree   Undecided   Moderately disagree   Strongly disagree

21. If a person stutters while talking in class, he should talk more loudly and act more confidently.
Strongly agree   Moderately agree   Undecided   Moderately disagree   Strongly disagree

22. A street car or bus conductor should be embarrassed if he stutters on the name of a street he is calling out.
Strongly agree   Moderately agree   Undecided   Moderately disagree   Strongly disagree

23. A stuttering woman should avoid going into a store to buy a hat if she believes the saleslady will feel sorry for her or secretly laugh at her because of her stuttering.
Strongly agree   Moderately agree   Undecided   Moderately disagree   Strongly disagree

24. If a person stutters while answering a question in class, he should just stop and start over again.
Strongly agree   Moderately agree   Undecided   Moderately disagree   Strongly disagree

25. A person should not try to tell jokes to a person of the opposite sex if he is likely to stutter while doing so.
Strongly agree   Moderately agree   Undecided   Moderately disagree   Strongly disagree

26. A girl should feel embarrassed if she stutters saying her escort's name when introducing him to some of her friends.
Strongly agree   Moderately agree   Undecided   Moderately disagree   Strongly disagree

27. A stutterer should try to be hired for jobs requiring little speaking—for example, janitor or wrapping clerk.
Strongly agree   Moderately agree   Undecided   Moderately disagree   Strongly disagree

28. A salesgirl should be embarrassed if she stutters while trying to sell an article.
Strongly agree   Moderately agree   Undecided   Moderately disagree   Strongly disagree

29. A person should try to avoid leading a prayer at church or Sunday school if he believes he will stutter.
Strongly agree   Moderately agree   Undecided   Moderately disagree   Strongly disagree

30. A stutterer should stay at home and listen to the radio or watch TV rather than go to a discussion group where he would stutter if called on to speak.
Strongly agree   Moderately agree   Undecided   Moderately disagree   Strongly disagree

31. If he feels he will stutter while asking a girl to go with him to a party, a fellow should put off asking, hoping that later on his speech will be more fluent.
Strongly agree   Moderately agree   Undecided   Moderately disagree   Strongly disagree

32. If he believes he will stutter, a husband should avoid embarrassing his wife by talking while at a dinner given by one of her close friends.
Strongly agree   Moderately agree   Undecided   Moderately disagree   Strongly disagree

33. At church, if a person believes he will stutter while introducing friends, he should wait until some time later when he feels less likely to stutter.
Strongly agree   Moderately agree   Undecided   Moderately disagree   Strongly disagree

34. A salesgirl should be embarrassed if she stutters while trying to sell a book to a man.
Strongly agree   Moderately agree   Undecided   Moderately disagree   Strongly disagree

35. A teacher who stutters should conceal this by substituting easy words for the hard ones he feels he will stutter on.
Strongly agree   Moderately agree   Undecided   Moderately disagree   Strongly disagree

36. A stutterer should not plan to be a lawyer.
Strongly agree   Moderately agree   Undecided   Moderately disagree   Strongly disagree

37. A wife who stutters should try to keep it from her husband's notice by speaking slowly or prolonging sounds until she thinks she can say her words better.
Strongly agree   Moderately agree   Undecided   Moderately disagree   Strongly disagree

38. If he stutters, a young man should not prepare himself to be a salesman.
Strongly agree   Moderately agree   Undecided   Moderately disagree   Strongly disagree

39. A teacher generally should not call upon a stutterer in his class for oral recitation.
Strongly agree   Moderately agree   Undecided   Moderately disagree   Strongly disagree

40. A stutterer should not be a bus driver.
Strongly agree   Moderately agree   Undecided   Moderately disagree   Strongly disagree

41. If a person stutters in one of your classes, you should feel sorry for him.
Strongly agree   Moderately agree   Undecided   Moderately disagree   Strongly disagree

42. If acquaintances come to visit the family, a stutterer should leave the talking to them up to non-stuttering members of the family.

Strongly agree   Moderately agree   Undecided   Moderately disagree   Strongly disagree

43. When asked at a party to choose between a game where he will have to talk a good deal and one where he could keep still, the stutterer should choose the one where he could keep still.

Strongly agree   Moderately agree   Undecided   Moderately disagree   Strongly disagree

44. A woman who stutters should avoid meeting and talking with her husband's influential friends.

Strongly agree   Moderately agree   Undecided   Moderately disagree   Strongly disagree

45. A barber who stutters should not stutter while giving haircuts.

Strongly agree   Moderately agree   Undecided   Moderately disagree   Strongly disagree

Scoring:

Number "Strongly Agree"   _____ × 4 = _____
Number "Moderately Agree"   _____ × 3 = _____
Number "Moderately Disagree"   _____ × 2 = _____
Number "Strongly Disagree"   _____ × 1 = _____

A. Total   _____
B. Total number of items answered
   "Strongly" or "Moderately" agree
   or disagree   _____

Score = A divided by B   _____

Additional copies of this form may be obtained from the Interstate Printers and Publishers, 19-27 North Jackson Street, Danville, Illinois, reorder number 774.

FORM 16. STUTTERER'S SELF-RATINGS OF REACTIONS TO SPEECH SITUATIONS

From *Diagnostic Methods in Speech Pathology*, by Wendell Johnson, Frederic L. Darley, and D. C. Spriestersbach, New York: Harper and Row, 1963.

Name _____ Age _____ Sex _____

Examiner _____ Date _____

After each item put a number from 1 to 5 in each of the four columns.

Start with right-hand column headed Frequency. Study the five possible answers to be made in responding to each item, and write the number of the answer that best fits the situation for you in each case. Thus, if you habitually take your meals at home and seldom eat in a restaurant, certainly not as often as once a week, write the number 5 in the Frequency column opposite item No. 1, "Ordering in a a restaurant." In like manner respond to each of the other 39 items by writing the most appropriate number in the Frequency column. When you have finished with this column fold it under so you cannot see the numbers you have written. This is done to keep you from being influenced unduly by the numbers you have written in the Frequency column when you write your responses to the 40 situations in the Stuttering column.

Now, write the number of the response that best indicates how much you stutter in each situation. For example, if in ordering meals in a restaurant you stutter mildly (for you), write the number 2 in the Stuttering column after item No. 1. In like manner respond to the other 39 items. Then fold under the Stuttering column so you will not be able to see the numbers you have written in it when you make your responses in the Reaction column.

Following the same procedure, write your responses in the Reaction column, fold it under, and, finally, write your responses in the Avoidance column.

Numbers, for each of the columns, are to be interpreted as follows:

A. Avoidance:
1. I never try to avoid this situation and have no desire to avoid it.
2. I don't try to avoid this situation, but sometimes I would like to.
3. More often than not I do not try to avoid this situation, but sometimes I do try to avoid it.
4. More often than not I do try to avoid this situation.
5. I avoid this situation every time I possibly can.

B. Reaction:
1. I definitely enjoy speaking in this situation.
2. I would rather speak in this situation than not.
3. It's hard to say whether I'd rather speak in this situation or not.
4. I would rather not speak in this situation.
5. I very much dislike speaking in this situation.

C. Stuttering:
1. I don't stutter at all (or only very rarely) in this situation.
2. I stutter mildly (for me) in this situation.
3. I stutter with average severity (for me) in this situation.
4. I stutter more than average (for me) in this situation.
5. I stutter severely (for me) in this situation.

D. Frequency:
1. This is a situation I meet very often, two or three times a day, or even more, on the average.
2. I meet this situation at least once a day with rare exceptions (except Sunday, perhaps).
3. I meet this situation from three to five times a week on the average.
4. I meet this situation once a week, with few exceptions, and occasionally meet it twice a week.
5. I rarely meet this situation—certainly not as often as once a week.

	Avoidance	Reaction	Stuttering	Frequency
1. Ordering in a restaurant				
2. Introducing myself (face to face)				
3. Telephoning to ask price, train fare, etc.				
4. Buying plane, train, or bus ticket				
5. Short class recitation (10 words or less)				
6. Telephoning for taxi				
7. Introducing one person to another				
8. Buying something from store clerk				
9. Conversation with good friend				
10. Talking with an instructor after class or in his office				
11. Long distance telephone call to someone I know				
12. Conversation with father				
13. Asking girl for date (or talking to man who asks me for a date)				
14. Making short speech (1 or 2 minutes) in familiar class				
15. Giving my name over telephone				
16. Conversation with my mother				
17. Asking a secretary if I can see her employer				
18. Going to house and asking for someone				
19. Making a speech to unfamiliar audience				
20. Participating in committee meeting				
21. Asking instructor question in class				

	Avoidance	Reaction	Stuttering	Frequency
22. Saying hello to a friend going by	_____	_____	_____	_____
23. Asking for a job	_____	_____	_____	_____
24. Telling a person a message from some-one else	_____	_____	_____	_____
25. Telling funny story with one stranger in a crowd	_____	_____	_____	_____
26. Parlor games requiring speech	_____	_____	_____	_____
27. Reading aloud to friends	_____	_____	_____	_____
28. Participating in a bull session	_____	_____	_____	_____
29. Dinner conversation with strangers	_____	_____	_____	_____
30. Talking with my barber (or beauty operator)	_____	_____	_____	_____
31. Telephoning to make appointment, or arrange meeting place with someone	_____	_____	_____	_____
32. Answering roll call in class	_____	_____	_____	_____
33. Asking at a desk for book, or card to be filled out, etc.	_____	_____	_____	_____
34. Talking with someone I don't know well while waiting for bus or class, etc.	_____	_____	_____	_____
35. Talking with other players during a playground game	_____	_____	_____	_____
36. Taking leave of a hostess	_____	_____	_____	_____
37. Conversation with friend while walking along the street	_____	_____	_____	_____
38. Buying stamps at post office	_____	_____	_____	_____
39. Giving directions or information to strangers	_____	_____	_____	_____
40. Taking leave of a girl (boy) after a date	_____	_____	_____	_____
Total	_____	_____	_____	_____
Average	_____	_____	_____	_____
No. of 1's	_____	_____	_____	_____
" " 2's	_____	_____	_____	_____
" " 3's	_____	_____	_____	_____
" " 4's	_____	_____	_____	_____
" " 5's	_____	_____	_____	_____

Additional copies of this form may be obtained from the Interstate Printers and Publishers, 19-27 North Jackson Street, Danville, Illinois, reorder number 775.

Index